PHYSIOLOGY AND PATHOPHYSIOLOGY OF THE ISLETS OF LANGERHANS

ADVANCES IN EXPERIMENTAL MEDICINE AND BIOLOGY

Recent Volumes in this Series

Volume 417
DENDRITIC CELLS IN FUNDAMENTAL AND CLINICAL IMMUNOLOGY, Volume 3
Edited by Paola Ricciardi-Castagnoli

Volume 418
STREPTOCOCCI AND THE HOST
Edited by Thea Horaud, Anne Bouvet, Roland Leclerq, Henri de Montclos, and Michel Sicard

Volume 419
ADP-RIBOSYLATION IN ANIMAL TISSUES: Structure, Function, and Biology of Mono (ADP-ribosyl) Transferases and Related Enzymes
Edited by Friedrich Haag and Friedrich Koch-Nolte

Volume 420
ADVANCES IN CIRRHOSIS, HYPERAMMONEMIA, AND HEPATIC ENCEPHALOPATHY
Edited by Vicente Felipo

Volume 421
CELLULAR PEPTIDASES IN IMMUNE FUNCTIONS AND DISEASES
Edited by Siegfried Ansorge and Jürgen Langner

Volume 422
DIETARY FAT AND CANCER: Genetic and Molecular Interactions
Edited under the auspices of the American Institute for Cancer Research

Volume 423
IN VITRO–IN VIVO CORRELATIONS
Edited by David Young, John G. Devane, and Jackie Butler

Volume 424
THE FATE OF THE MALE GERM CELL
Edited by Richard Ivell and Adolf-Friedrich Holstein

Volume 425
CHEMISTRY AND BIOLOGY OF SERPINS
Edited by Frank C. Church, Dennis D. Cunningham, David Ginsburg, Maureane Hoffman, Stuart R. Stone, and Douglas M. Tollefsen

Volume 426
PHYSIOLOGY AND PATHOPHYSIOLOGY OF THE ISLETS OF LANGERHANS
Edited by Bernat Soria

A Continuation Order Plan is available for this series. A continuation order will bring delivery of each new volume immediately upon publication. Volumes are billed only upon actual shipment. For further information please contact the publisher.

PHYSIOLOGY AND PATHOPHYSIOLOGY OF THE ISLETS OF LANGERHANS

Edited by

Bernat Soria

Miguel Hernandez University
Alicante, Spain

PLENUM PRESS • NEW YORK AND LONDON

Library of Congress Cataloging-in-Publication Data

Physiology and pathophysiology of the islets of Langerhans / edited by
Bernat Soria.
p. cm. -- (Advances in experimental medicine and biology ; v.
426)
"Proceedings of the First International Meeting of the Pancreatic
Islet Study Group, held November 25-28, 1994, in Alicante, Spain"-
-T.p. verso.
Includes bibliographical references and index.
ISBN 0-306-45702-4
1. Islands of Langerhans--Physiology--Congresses. 2. Islands of
Langerhans--Pathophysiology--Congresses. 3. Diabetes-
-Pathophysiology--Congresses. I. Soria, Bernat. II. International
Meeting of the Pancreatic Islet Study Group (1st : 1994 : Alicante,
Spain) III. Series.
[DNLM: 1. Islets of Langerhans--physiology--congresses. 2. Islets
of Langerhans--physiopathology--congresses. 3. Islets of Langerhans
Transplantation--congresses. W1 AD559 v.426 1997 / WK 800 P578
1997]
QP188.P26P47 1997
612.3'4--dc21
DNLM/DLC
for Library of Congress 97-27991
CIP

Proceedings of the First International Meeting of the Pancreatic Islet Study Group,
held November 25 – 28, 1994, in Alicante, Spain

ISBN 0-306-45702-4

A Division of Plenum Publishing Corporation
233 Spring Street, New York, N. Y. 10013

http://www.plenum.com

10 9 8 7 6 5 4 3 2 1

Printed in the United States of America

CONTENTS

I. PREFACE

II. STIMULUS SECRETION COUPLING: ARE $K_{(ATP)}$ CHANNELS ENOUGH?

A. Glucose Recognition

B. The Role for $K_{(ATP)}$ Channels

VII. PATHOPHYSIOLOGY OF THE NIDDM

VIII. ISLET GROWTH, REGENERATION, AND TRANSPLANTATION

Part I. PREFACE

1

WHY ARE ISLETS SO IMPORTANT?

Bernat Soria*

Center for Bioengineering
Department of Physiology
Miguel Hernandez University
Alicante, Spain

Why should a book such as a book on the *Physiology and Pathophysiology of the Islets of Langerhans* be published, bought, and even read?

Since their discovery by Paul Langerhans more than a century ago [1], pancreatic islets have attracted the attention of pathologists, histologists, physiologists, etc. It has become well established over the years that many of the clues indicating diabetic syndromes originate at the islets of Langerhans [2,3,4]. This book, which contains plenty of data supporting this point of view aims to present most of up to date thinking on the mechanisms of insulin release, islet pathophysiology and potential treatments for diabetes.

Although chapters may be read as separate contributions, they are grouped in sections devoted to a more broad topic. Chapters 9, 14 or 24, provide an introduction to each section,whilst others review an specific item. All chapters contain abundant experimental facts and observations which will be of help to those interested in the physiology and pathophysiology of the islet of Langerhans. The authors have presented their material in a broad and comprehensible manner in order to reach the widest possible audience.

For example, diabetologists will find Chapters 40 through 59 helpful reading. The integrated approach presented by Okamoto in Chapter 40 suggests some therapeutical approaches to stop β-cell damage and to promote their regeneration. Identifyng the final common pathway for agents that promote β-cell injury (DNA damage, polyADP-rybose synthetase activation and NAD^+ depletion) makes counteractive treatment possible. Furthermore, the detailed description of the prominent role ot the Reg gene in β-cell regeneration and the recent experimental results showing that the Reg protein can ameliorate diabetes in partially pancreatectomized rats strongly point to the use the subsequent protein as a new treatment for human diabetes. Valverde et al. (Chapter 32) discuss the current belief that in non-insulin dependent diabetes mellitus, the pancreatic B-cell suffers from a kind of blindness to D-glucose. Since the secretory response to hexose seems to be more affected than that evoked by other nutrient or non-nutrient secretagogues, methyl esters of succinic acid and glutamic acid have been proposed for the treatment of type II diabetes.

* E-mail: bernat.soria@umh.es

Physiology and Pathophysiology of the Islets of Langerhans, edited by Soria.
Plenum Press, New York, 1997.

Those interested in basic mechanisms will find of value Chapters 34 through 39 addressed to answering the question: how to build an homogeneous response from an heterogeneous population of cells? And more specifically, (i) Why do β-cells organize themselves in islets?, (ii) Why is there cell-to-cell coupling?, (iii) What is the role of non-β cells in the islet?, etc. To my knowledge this Section represents the only collection of single papers in which heterogeneity is analyzed from the biophysical, biochemical and cell biology points of view. The islet response, modelled by Sherman (Chapter 38) and reconstructed be Meda and Bosco (Chapter 39) represents a synthesis of the other chapters. It could be anticipated that this approach will be used by cell biologists and neurobiologists to model the behaviour of functionally coupled groups cells [5].

The first group of chapters is devoted to Stimulus-Secretion Coupling and grouped under the general title "*Glucose-induced insulin release: are ATP-regulated K^+ channels enough?*" Previous work by Dr. Henquin's group showed that glucose regulates insulin release at least at two sites. In addition to glucose-induced cell depolarization and Ca^{2+} entry [6,7], glucose also increases the β-cell secretory response by amplifyng the effectiveness of Ca^{2+} on the secretory process [8]. Dr. G. W. G. Sharp (Ithaca, USA), presents evidence that the role of K_{ATP} channels in fetal β-cells is not as crucial as in adults. In early stages of development, K_{ATP} channels are present, but apparently not used in glucose-stimulated insulin release. Drs. A. Niki and H. Niki (Nagoya, Japan) approached hexose recognition in a different way. Taking adavantage of the similarity between the pancreatic B-cell and gustatory cell, they explored the basic mechanisms which underly sugar recognition. Other chapters, including those of Drs. Santos et al. (Coimbra, Portugal) and Taguchi et al. (Matsumoto, Japan) analyze the contribution of sulphonylurea-sensitive K^+ channels in the generation of β-cell electrical activity and glucose-induced priming. It is broadly accepted that K_{ATP} channels are inhibited by ATP and activated by ADP acting by the intracellular side. Although the existence and first description of these channel properties began with two independent observations, an open discussion held in Alicante more than10 years ago established the identity of the channel. In 1984, two independent contributions showed that: (i) a K^+ channel with inward rectifier properties was blocked by increasing ATP in the cytosolic side [9] and (ii) increasing glucose concentration blocks a K^+ channel recorded in the cell-attached mode [10], then termed it the G channel. Some months later it was agreed in Alicante that the G-channels [10] were those K^+ channels blocked by increasing ATP on the cytosolic side [9], the tidy up marriage between these two concepts was witnessed by the scientists working in the field gathered together in Alicante in a Workshop on the *Biophysics of the Pancreatic β-cell*; Illani Atwater, Eduardo Rojas and myself acted as bestmen [11]. It was extremely exciting to find out that sulphonylureas also blocked this channel [12]. It was later demonstrated that both sulphonylureas and glucose produced an increase in the cytosolic Ca^{2+} which in turn induced exocytosis.

Independently of additional mechanisms existing in nutrient-induced insulin release, the central role played by the K_{ATP} channel is broadly accepted and therefore, cloning and sequencing of the channel became a worthwhile goal. Niki et al. (Chapter 8) have characterized the phosphorilation properties of the pancreatic β-cell sulphonylurea receptor, but we still cannot conclude from this if the receptor is the channel or an associated protein. Two recent studies by Aguilar-Bryan et al. [13] and Inagaki et al [14] have established that K_{ATP} channels are composed of at least two subunits. One subunit, K_{IR} 6.2, also termed BIR ("B-cell inward rectifier"), is a member of the inward rectifier pore protein family. The other is a larger protein belonging to the ATP-binding cassette (ABC) proteins which contain two nucelotide binding folds and the high affinity receptor for sulphonylureas (SUR1).

K_{IR} 6.2 and SUR1 need to be coexpressed to generate ion currents similar to the native channel. The genes which encode SUR1 and K_{IR} 6.2 are located in human chromosome 11. Defects in the SUR1 gene are believed to be associated with loss of functional K_{ATP} channels responsible of the persistent hyperinsulinaemic hypoglycaemia of infancy (PHHI) [15]. The central role of K_{ATP} conductance in β-cell stimulus-secretion coupling is highlighted by this observation which suggests that β-cells in PHHI children have no regulatory systems to counteract this absence.

Downstream from the Ca^{2+} signal: To be effective, Ca^{2+} changes should modify the activity or the location of "target" proteins. In Chapter 11 Dr. I. Niki and his colleagues show that the Ca^{2+}-binding protein calcyclin is present in the islet and that it might be involved in the control of insulin release in response to an increase in $[Ca^{2+}]_i$. Molecular cloning of the cDNA encoding β-cell Ca^{2+}-calmodulin-dependent proteinkinase II is described by Drs. V. Urquidi and S. J. H. Ashcroft (Oxford, UK) in Chapter 12. A large group of candidates including syntaxin, synaptotagmin, SNAP-25, etc. are supposed to constitute the exocytotic machinery. Most of their components have been identified in the pancreatic β-cell and their physiological roles established [16,17,18]. Cloning of these proteins and establishing the mechanism by which this engine leads to exocytotic release of insulin will open new approaches not only from the molecular point of view, but also to those interested in vesicle docking, recycling and release in this unique cell.

In addition to nutrients, β-cells are modulated by neurotransmitters and hormones. *Section 2* is devoted to the *Modulation of Islet Release*. Following a short overview by T. Yada (Kagoshima, Japan), the molecular properties of physiological and pharmacological modulators are described in chapters 14 to 23. Dr. G. M. Grodsky (San Francisco, USA) presents a study of sympathetic regulation in transgenic mice which exhibit islet hypersensitivity resulting from overexpression of nerve growth factor in β-cells. Dr. J. J. Gagliardino (Buenos Aires, Argentina) shows that the islet may release ACTH-like peptides and suggests a regulatory role for this relative newcomer. Pituitary adenylatecyclase activating polypeptide is shown to be localized within the pancreas and capable of potentiating insulin release by Dr. T. Yada and colleagues (Kagoshima and Tokyo, Japan), etc.

"*β-cell metabolism and calcium oscillations*" are discussed in *Section 3*. The unique capability of the β-cell to act as an integrator of metabolic and electrical properties is clearly introduced by Prof. Malaisse with a description of the reciprocal links between metabolism and ionic events in islet cells. Dr. L. Best suggests that glyceraldehyde, used to stimulate insulin release in tumoral β-cell lines which fail to respond to glucose, is poorly metabolized in these cells and, unlike glucose, it stimulates the β-cell by a mechanism which does not involve glycolytic metabolism. Nutrient-induced Ca^{2+} oscillations [19,20,21,22] and Ca^{2+} waves [20,23] are analyzed in Chapters 26 and 27. Dr. F. Martin (Alicante, Spain) demonstrates that α-ketoisocaproate, the first derivative of the amino acid leucine, causes slow $[Ca^{2+}]_i$ oscillations in pancreatic islets of Langerhans. Under these conditions, simultaneous insulin release which parallels $[Ca^{2+}]_i$ oscillations could be resolved, thus reinforcing the view that Ca^{2+} acts as a moment-to-moment regulator of insulin release. Other mechanisms contributing to build the Ca^{2+} signal are analyzed in Chapters 28 through 32. Finally, Nadal et al. (Chapter 33) postulate that glucose controls cytosolic Ca^{2+} at three different sites.

Chapters 34 through 39 (*Section 4*) bring together the most complete collection of work dedicated to "*β-cell heterogeneity: building an homogeneous response from an heterogeneous population.*" There are many facts supporting the view that isolated β-cells display heterogeneity: (i) β-cells segregated by fluorescence-activated sorting as a function of their metabolic responsiveness to glucose, differ in terms of insulin release, insulin biosynthesis, glucose utilization, glucose oxidation and the activities of glucokinase and hexokinase (F. Schuit, Chapter 36). Hence β-cell heterogeneity may result in part from differences in glucose metabolism; (ii) P. Meda (Chapter 39) reports that β-cells insensitive to glucose are recruited into secretion after contacting glucose-responsive β-cells. (iii) Responses to glucose as observed by plaque assay, by blockade of K_{ATP} or in terms of $[Ca^{2+}]_i$ changes are also heterogeneous but somehow correlated. For example, F. M. Ashcroft and colleagues (Chapters 34 and 35) show that cells in which K_{ATP} responses are mininal also form small size plaques, thereby explaining how β-cells, despite being endowed with the same set of ionic channels, are heterogeneous in terms of insulin release [24]; (iv) Individual β-cells display rather variable patterns of secretagogue induced $[Ca^{2+}]_i$ oscillations. By contrast, β-cells in contact exhibit $[Ca^{2+}]_i$ oscillations that are synchronized throughout the monolayer clusters and do not consistently originate from a same cell. Previous reports that the glucose-induced electrical activity of islet cells coincided with $[Ca^{2+}]_i$ oscillations of 10–60 sec intervals, suggests that all islet cells oscillate synchronously [20] and that $[Ca^{2+}]_i$ oscillates in the same way in different regions of the islet, with no region being consistently ahead of the others [20,22,23]. Computer simulation shows that heterogenous β-cells may burst in synchrony, provided that they are coupled (Chapter 38). Again, no evidence for a cell consistently leading the others has been found. There is a general acceptance of the following concepts: heterogeneity of insulin biosynthesis and secretion exists in β-cell populations and must be taken into account. The collective response to glucose of an islet cell population results from both a graded, increasing response of individual cells, as well as the recruitment of new secreting cells. Glucose stimulation results in the recruitment of at least some individual β-cells. A further recruitment is dependent on cell-to-cell interactions, as a result of cell communication presumably mediated by gap junctions or the extracellular diffusion of messengers. There is some debate as to whether β-cells may form distinct subpopulations (Chapter 37), or are distributed in a graded continuum of differing threshold levels for activation. It should be noted that the number of subpopulations which may be identified is strongly influenced by the experimental strategy chosen. However, in spite of the intrinsic heterogeneity of individual cells, islet cell populations show a synchronized activity, as evidenced by the synchronous oscillations of membrane potential and $[Ca^{2+}]_i$. A subpopulation of pacemaker β-cells able to consistently generate these oscillations to drive nearby cells has not been identified. Synchronization permits groups of cells to exhibit amplification, even if they are all-or-none responders when isolated. There is a broad consensus that gap junctional coupling is the most likely mechanism for synchronization [20,24,25].

"*IDDM: What went wrong? Mechanisms of β-cell destruction and defence*" is covered by *Section 5*. Most studies dealing with the pathogenesis of IDDM have emphasized the immune assault against β-cells, however, β-cell destruction of IDDM represents the net balance between β-cell damage and repair. In this Section β-cell damage is described in detail (Chapters 41, 43, 44, 45 and 47), whereas Chapters 40 (H. Okamoto) and 42 (A. Bone) are dealt with β-cell repair mechanisms. The role of cytokines (IL-1β) and nitric oxide (NO) in the selective destruction of pancreatic β-cells is reviewed by Dr. M. L. McDaniel (St. Louis, USA). He shows that IL-1β induces the expression of iNOS (inhibitor of nitric oxyde synthase) in β-cells purified by fluorescence activated cell sorting and that this results in the severe inhibition of glucose-stimulated insulin release. He reports on studies carried out on the induction of islet cyclooxygenase by IL-1β, and additionally, that NMMA, an inhibitor of NOS, inhibits production of PGE2, providing evidence for a direct effect by NO on islet cyclooxygenase. The NO releasing agent SIN-1 also potentiates the activity of both cCOX and iCOX, resulting in the overproduction of PGE2. McDaniel proposes that IL-1β-induced coexpression of INOS and ICOX in islets, together with the ability of NO to mediate β-cell disfunction and to activate ICOX activity, may contribute to autoimmune diabetes. Okamoto (Chapter 40) presents recent studies on the islet regenerating gene (reg). Although direct evidence for its role in growth stimulation of pancreatic β-cells has not yet been obtained, the effects of reg protein on pancreatic β-cell replication have been examined. To this end, 90% depancreatized rats and isolated islets were used. In depancreatized rats, reg protein significantly increases thymidine incorporation, suggesting that reg protein may act as a growth factor for β-cells. Okamoto also discuss recent data on the role played by cyclic ADPribose (cADPR) in Ca^{2+} release by islet microsomes and in insulin release by digitonin-permeabilized rat islets. It is proposed that cACPR rather that IP_3 mobilizes Ca^{2+} in islet microsomes, and that cACPR may play the role of messenger in glucose-induced Ca^{2+} mobilization from cellular stores. More specifically, Dr A. Bone and colleagues (Chapter 42) discuss the involvement of the islet regenerating gene (Reg) and its products in the repair and renewal response of islets in spontanneously diabetic BB/S rat. There is a significant increase in Reg mRNA levels in pancreatic biopsies taken at and around onset of disease in diabetes prone BB/S rats. In islets isolated from normal rats and exposed to glucose, amino acids and non-nutrient growth factors in culture increased DNA synthesis rates accompanied by increased Reg mRNA levels. In separate experiments, Reg protein was found to stimulate islet DNA synthesis in a dose-dependent manner. This evidence suggests that Reg gene and/or its products influence islet repair and regeneration in BB rats. The mechanisms by which macrophages, NO and oxidants damage β-cell function is discussed in Chapters 43 to 47.

Chapters 48 through 52 are devoted to the *Pathophysiology of NIDDM*. Results from a Spanish multicentre programme on islet cell transplantation are reported by Dr. R. Gomis and Dr. A. Novials from the Departament of Endocrinology and Diabetes at the Hospital Clinic of Barcelona (Spain). A surprising finding was the dissociation of the insulin and islet amyloid polypeptide (IAPP) secretory responses of human islets after seven days of culture, and a high glucose-induced increase in islet IAPP content. It was already known that islets prepared from four Type 2 human diabetic donors showed significant reduction in the activity of mitochondrial glycerol phosphate dehydrogenase [26]. It is not yet clear whether this is a primary or secondary defect, although it has been suggested that not all conditions associated with hyperglycaemia also exhibit a reduction in the activity of this enzyme. The enzyme has not yet been cloned and sequenced. The animal model of human Type 2 diabetes provided by the "sand rat" (*Psammomys obesus*) has been studied in detail by Drs. N. Kaiser, E. Cerasi, and colleagues at the Hadassah Medical Center (Jerusalem, Israel). Some animals develop diabetes on exposure to standard laboratory chow. The genetic basis for this has been established by isolating phenotipically stable lines differing in their susceptibility to diet-induced diabetes. Reversed-phase HPLC is used to study the relative amounts of insulin and proinsulin-like peptides in the plasma of diabetic animals. Marked increases in the concentrations of proinsulin and proinsulin conversion intermediates are observed. Fed diabetic animals exhibit a low pancreatic insulin content with a higher relative proportion of proinsulin and proinsulin conversion intermediates. Fasting diabetic animals partially corrected these abnormalities. It is concluded that these changes were related to the inability of β-cells to compensate for an increased insulin demand secondary to insulin resistance. Insulin-secreting cells, cultured under hyperglycaemic conditions show an altered secretory response (Chapter 50). β-cell hyperresponse in prediabetes and pregnacy is analyzed by Sato et al. (Chapter 51) and Koiter et al. (Chapter 52).

The last Section is dedicated to *Islet Growth, Regeneration, and Transplantation*. Needless to say, transplantation may constitute the definitive cure for Type I diabetes. Chapters 53 to 59 also illustrate that islet pathophysiology can be learned from transplantation. Chapter 54 by H. J. Hahn (Karlburg, Germany) reports on the use of syngeneic islet transplantation for conducting in vivo studies of the function, viability and vulnerability of pancreatic islets. This model has also been used to investigate grafted islets as a possible target for the autoimmune reactions characteristic of BB-rats and NOD mice. It is nicely demonstrated that there is a biphasic release of insulin in response to an acute glucose challenge when perfusing livers containing intraportally implanted islets in non-diabetic recipients. This response is already documented in 2 weeks post transplantation and, moreover, electrical stimulation of nerves in the hepatic artery and portal vein influenced the insulin secretory rates. These latter findings together with immunocytochemical and electron microscopical studies demonstrate reinnervation of the intraportally grafted islets. When syngeneic islets are grafted into spontaneoulsy diabetic BB rats or NOD mice, the grafted recipients relapse into hyperglycemia. The graft is characterized by a marked insulitis with a predominance of T–, IL–2R+ and CD4+ cells. Temporary immunosuppresion prevented β-cell destructionand the invasion of CD4+-cells into the islets. All in all these data suggest that syngeneic islet transplantation experiments may be very suitable for studying of the natural course of β-cell destruction in insulin-dependent diabetes. Montaña (Barcelona, Spain), Chapter 55, shows that an increase in the transplanted β-cell mass prevented the development of hyperglycaemia in rats pancreatectomized 14 days after islet transplantation. Likewise, the β-cell mass was increased in islet grafts transplanted into pancreatectomized rats. Such grafts also restored normoglycemia in most recipients. The increase in β-cell mass was associated with increased rates of β-cell replication and also to an increase in the size of individual β-cells. It was concluded that the transplanted β-cell mass can adapt to meet an increased metabolic demand in diabetic transplant recipients. Davies et al. (Chapter 57) introduce a new method for immunomagnetic purification of pancreatic islets. Finally, Madureira (Chapter 56) and Tormo et al. (Chapter 58) explore the behaviour of transplanted islets in dog's spleen and NIDDM rats.

Chapter 15 is most probably the last scientific contribution of Cris Boyd, who last visited Alicante in 1984 [27]. Sufffering from a fatal disease he told me by phone of his decision not to visit Alicante this time. It was our last opportunity to chat and joke on the phone as he passed away some months later. For those of us who had an opportunity to know and work with Cris it is a great honour to have this chapter from a great scientist and friend.

This book is the result of the First Meeting of the Pancreatic Islet Study Group of the European Association for the Study of Diabetes. Despite being held during Thanks Giving (I was the one responsible for this mistake) it was attended by 16 scientists from the USA. Our Japanese colleagues also deciced to travel more that 20 h. to be present. Since Alicante is a resort city, scientists from Europe were easily convinced to come. Thus, Swedish, British, Belgian, Danish and German were present. It was also a nice opportunity for Spanish diabetologists to create the Spanish Islet Group. The meeting organizers and attendees are indebted to the Fundación CAM, the Generalitat Valenciana, the Alicante City Council and the University of Alicante for their generous support. This book results from the effort of a wide group of people, including the authors who reviewed a particular aspect or included original data not previoulsy published. Both types of contribution will be appreciated by the readership. I am particularly indebted to my wife Verónica who "enjoyed" vacations and week-ends taking care of our little daughters, Aitana and Barbara, while her father was editing this book.

REFERENCES

1. Langerhans, P (1869) Beiträge zur mikroskopischen. Anatomie der Beauchspercheldrüse (Thesis). Friedrich-Wilhelms-Universität, Berlin.
2. Froguel P, Zouali H, Vionnet N, Velho G, Vaxillaire M, Sun F, Lesague S, Stoffel M, Takeda J, Passa P, Permutt A, Beckamn J, Bell GI, Cohen D (1993) Familial hyperglycaemia due to mutations in glucokinase. *N. Eng. J. Med. 328*: 697–702.
3. Porte Jr, D (1991) β-cells in type II diabetes mellitus. *Diabetes 40*: 166–180.
4. Soria B, Andreu E, Pertusa JG, Martin F, Ripoll C, Sanchez-André JV (1996) Target molecules as candidates to be defective in stimulus-secretion coupling in type II diabetes. *Endocrinologia 43(9)*: 321–328.
5. Andreu E, Soria B, Sanchez-Andrés JV (1997) Oscillations of the gap junction electrical coupling in the mouse pancreatic islet of Langerhans. *J.Physiol. (Lond) 498(3)*: 753–761.
6. Ashcroft FM, Rorsman P (1991) Electrophysiology of the pancreatic β-cell. *Progress in Biophysics and Molecular Biology 54*: 87–147.
7. Valdeolmillos M, Nadal A, Contreras D, Soria B (1992) The relationship between glucose-induced K(ATP) channel closure and the rise in $[Ca^{2+}]_i$ in single mouse pancreatic B-cells. *J. Physiol. (Lond) 455*: 173–186.
8. Gembal M, Detimary P, Gilon P, Gao ZY, Henquin JC (1993) Mechanisms by which glucose can control insulin release independently from its action on adenosine triphosphate-sensitive K^+ channels in mouse B cells. *J. Clin. Invest. 91*: 871–880.
9. Cook DL, Hales CN (1984) Intracellular ATP directly blocks K^+ channels in pancreatic β-cells. *Nature 311*: 271–273.
10. Ashcroft FM, Harrison DE, Ashcroft SJH (1984) Glucose induces closure of single potassium channels in isolated rat pancreatic β-cells. *Nature 312*: 446–448.
11. Atwater I, Rojas E, Soria B (1986) *Biophysics of the Pancreatic β-cell*. Plenum Press, New York.
12. Ashford MLJ, Sturgess NC, Cook DL, Hales CN (1986) K-channels in an Insulin-secreting Cell Line. In: *Biophysics of the Pancreatic β-cell* (Atwater, Rojas, and Soria, eds) Plenum Press, New York pp. 69–76.
13. Aguilar-Bryan L, Nichols CG, Wechsler SW, Clement JP, Boyd III AE, Gonzalez G, Herrera-Sosa H, Nguyk K, Bryan J, Nelson DA (1995) Cloning of the beta-cell high-affinity sulphonylurea receptor: a regulator of insulin secretion. *Science 268*: 372–373.
14. Inagaki N, Gonoi T, Clement JP, Namba N, Inazawa J, Gonzalez G, Aguilar-Bryan L, Seino S, Bryan J (1995) Reconstitution of KATP: an inward rectifier subunit plus the sulphonylurea receptor. *Science 270*: 1166–1170.
15. Kane C, Shepperd RM, Squires PE, Johnson PRV, James RFL, Milla PJ, Aynsley-Green A, Lindley KJ, Dunne MJ (1996) Loss of functional KATP channels in pancreatic β-cells causes persistent hyperinsulinaemic hypoglyccemia of infancy. *Nature Medicine 2(12)*: 1344–1347.
16. Jacobson G, Bean AJ, Scheller RH, Juntti-Berggren L, Deeney JT, Berggren P-O (1994) Identification of synaptic proteins and their isoform mRNAs in compartiments of pancreatic endocrine cells. *Proc. Natl. Acad. Sci. USA 91*: 12487–12491.
17. Martin F, Moya F, Gutierrez LM, Reig JA, Soria B (1995) Role of syntaxin in mouse pancreatic β-cell. *Diabetologia 38*: 860–863.
18. Martin F, Salinas E, Vazquez J, Soria B, Reig JA (1996) Inhibition of insulin release by synthetic peptides shows that the H3 region at the C-terminal domain of syntaxin-1 is crucial for calcium but not for GTP-S-induced secretion. *Biochem. J. 320*: 201–205.
19. Valdeolmillos M, Santos R, Contreras D, Soria B, Rosario LM (1989) Glucose-induced oscillations of intracellular Ca^{2+} concentration resembling bursting electrical activity in single mouse islets of Langerhans. *FEBS Letters 259*: 19–23.
20. Santos RM, Rosario LM, Nadal A, García-Sancho J, Soria B, Valdeolmillos M (1991) Widespread synchronous $[Ca^{2+}]_i$ oscillations due to bursting electrical activity in single pancreatic islets. *Pflügers Archiv 418*: 417–422.
21. Martin F, Sanchez-Andrés JV, Soria B (1995) Slow [Ca2+] oscillations induced by ketoisocaproate in mouse pancreatic islets. *Diabetes 44*: 300–305.

22. Martin F, Soria B (1995) Amino acid induced [Ca2+]i oscillations in single mouse pacreatic islets. *J. Physiol. (Lond) 486*: 361–371.
23. Valdeolmillos M, Nadal A, Soria B, García-Sancho J (1993) Fluorescence digital image analysis of glucose-induced [Ca^{2+}]i oscillations in mouse pancreatic islet of Langerhans. *Diabetes 42*: 1210–1214.
24. Soria B, Chanson M, Giordano E, Bosco D, Meda P (1991) Ionic channels in glucose responsive and unresponsive B-cells. *Diabetes 40*: 1069–1078.
25. Soria B (1994) First Meeting of the Pancreatic Islet Study Group. *Diabetologia 7*: 27–30.
26. Malaisse WJ (1995) Non-insulin dependent diabetes mellitus and islet B-cell mitochondrial glycerophosphate dehydrogenase deficiency. *Diabetes Med. 12*: 479–481.
27. Boyd III AE, Hill RS, Nelson TY, Oberwetter JM, Berg M (1986) In: *Biophysics of the Pancreatic β-cell* (I. Atwater, E. Rojas and B. Soria, eds). Plenum Press, New York, pp. 479–481.

Part II. STIMULUS SECRETION COUPLING: ARE $K_{(ATP)}$ CHANNELS ENOUGH?

Part II.A. Glucose Recognition

HEXOSE RECOGNITION BY THE PANCREATIC β-CELL AND THE GUSTATORY CELL

A. Niki and H. Niki

Department of Internal Medicine
Aichigakuin University School of Dentistry
Suemori, Chikusa, Nagoya, 464, Japan

INTRODUCTION

It is widely accepted that the signal for insulin release by D-glucose is generated by the metabolism of the sugar in the pancreatic β-cell, while the gustatory cell has a receptor for sugars.[1] However, these two cells phenomenally share the common properties in their stimulus-secretion coupling, as far as the stimulant is D-glucose.[2,3]

Well known is the ability of these cells to discriminate the α and β anomers of the sugars. The α anomer of D-glucose or D-mannose is more potent than the β anomer in inducing both insulin release[2,4] and sweet taste response.[5] Treatment with alloxan of the pancreatic β-cell and the gustatory cell inhibits their responses to D-glucose, although the responses to other stimuli are preserved.[6,7] Both of the cells are protected from alloxan toxicity by the co-existence of D-glucose; the α anomer is more potent than the β anomer in protecting the pancreatic β-cell[8], though the protective effects of the two anomers in the gustatory cell have not yet been studied.

A line of evidence to support the receptor hypothesis in the gustatory cell was obtained using inhibitors of sweet taste response.[5] We have studied the effects of the α and β anomers of the specific competitive inhibitors on glucose-induced insulin release and the interaction of alloxan and the inhibitors, using batch incubated islets isolated from rat pancreata.

MATERIALS AND METHODS

The specific competitive inhibitors used were *p*-nitrophenyl derivatives of hexoses; *p*-nitrophenyl-D-glucopyranoside (PNP-Glu), *p*-nitrophenyl-D-mannopyranoside (PNP-Man) and *p*-nitrophenyl-D-galactopyranoside (PNP-Gal). The α and β anomers of these compounds and alloxan were purchased from Sigma (St. Louis, MO).

Islets of Langerhans were isolated from the pancreata of fed male Wistar rats weighing 300–350g by the collagenase digestion method. All incubations were performed at

Physiology and Pathophysiology of the Islets of Langerhans, edited by Soria.
Plenum Press, New York, 1997.

37°C in gassed (95% O_2 and 5% CO_2) Krebs-Ringer bicarbonate solution (pH 7.4) containing 5 mg/ml bovine serum albumin (fraction V: Armour Kankakee, IL) as a basal medium. Islets were preliminary incubated for 60 min in the basal medium supplemented with 3 mmol/l D-glucose.

Alloxan treatments were made by incubating groups of islets for 5 min with media containing alloxan alone or alloxan with the compounds indicated, as described elsewhere in detail.[8] After washing, the islets were used to study glucose-induced insulin release.

Insulin release: Batches of 5 islets of comparable size were incubated for 60 min in 1 ml of the basal media containing the additions indicated. Insulin content of the media at the end of the incubation period was measured by solid phase radioimmunoassay.[9]

Glucose oxidation: Batches of 15 islets were incubated for 60 min in 0.2 ml of the media containing 10 mmol/l D-[U-^{14}C]glucose (New England Nuclear, Boston, MA) (0.25 mCi/mmol) with or without the compound indicated and the $^{14}CO_2$ formed was estimated as described previously.[10]

All results were expressed as mean ± SEM, and statistical analysis was performed by the unpaired Student's *t*-test.

RESULTS

Fig. 1 shows the effects of the α anomers of *p*-nitrophenyl-hexopyranosides on glucose-induced insulin release.[9] The α anomers of PNP-Glu and PNP-Man dose-dependently inhibited insulin release induced by 10 mmol/l D-glucose, while the α anomer of PNP-Gal did not. None of the β anomers of these compounds modified glucose-induced insulin release.[9] Phenyl-α-D-glucopyranoside, known to have no effect on sugar taste response, had no effect on glucose-induced insulin release.[9] *p*-Nitrophenol without hexose moiety completely inhibited the release.[9]

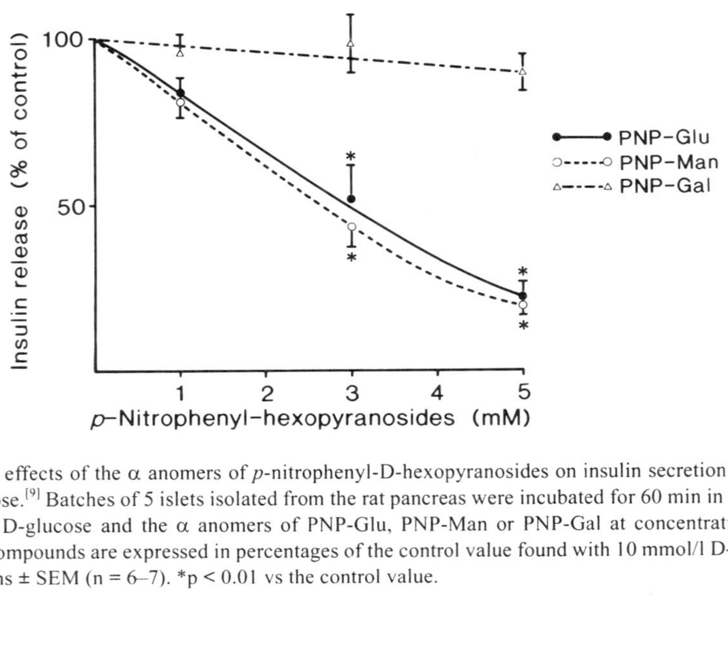

Figure 1. The effects of the α anomers of *p*-nitrophenyl-D-hexopyranosides on insulin secretion induced by 10 mmol/l D-glucose.[9] Batches of 5 islets isolated from the rat pancreas were incubated for 60 min in media containing 10 mmol/l D-glucose and the α anomers of PNP-Glu, PNP-Man or PNP-Gal at concentrations indicated. Effects of the compounds are expressed in percentages of the control value found with 10 mmol/l D-glucose alone. Values are means ± SEM (n = 6–7). *$p < 0.01$ vs the control value.

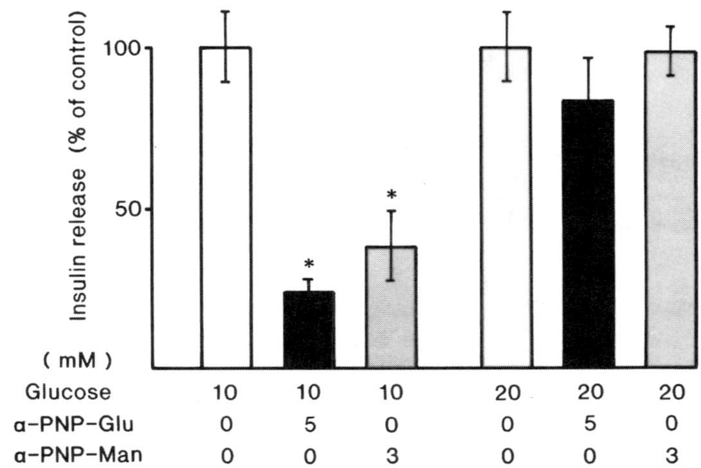

Figure 2. The effects of the α anomers of PNP-Glu and PNP-Man on insulin secretion induced by different concentrations of D-glucose. Batches of 5 islets isolated from the rat pancreas were incubated for 60 min in media containing indicated concentrations of D-glucose and the α anomers of PNP-Glu (5 mmol/l) or PNP-Man (3 mmol/l). Values are means ± SEM (n = 7–9). *p < 0.01 vs the control value with D-glucose alone.

As shown in Fig. 2, the inhibitory effects of the α anomers of PNP-Glu (5 mmol/l) and PNP-Man (3 mmol/l) on insulin release induced by 10 mmol/l D-glucose were eliminated when the glucose concentration was raised to 20 mmol/l. The inhibitory effects of these compounds were easily eliminated by washing the islets with the medium containing 3 mmol/l D-glucose.[11]

To examine whether these inhibitors exert the effects via inhibiting glucose metabolism in the pancreatic β-cell, we studied the effects of the compounds, which inhibited glucose-induced insulin release, on glucose oxidation in the islets. The α anomers of PNP-Glu and PNP-Man did not inhibit glucose oxidation, while *p*-nitrophenol completely inhibited the oxidation.[9]

Fig. 3 shows the protective effect of the α and β anomers of PNP-Glu against alloxan toxicity in islets. Pretreatment of islets with alloxan alone markedly diminished subsequent glucose-induced insulin release. When the islets were pretreated with alloxan together with the α anomer of PNP-Glu, subsequent glucose-induced insulin release was partially preserved; the protective effect was comparable to that observed with the same concentration of D-glucose. A less potent protection was observed with the β anomer than with the α anomer of PNP-Glu.

As shown in Fig. 4, D-mannoheptulose was itself a weak protector against alloxan, but attenuated the protective effect of the α anomer of PNP-Glu on subsequent glucose-induced insulin release.

DISCUSSION

In the gustatory cell, the findings obtained with inhibitors of sweet taste response are considered to support the receptor hypothesis on the mechanism of sugar recognition.[5] These inhibitors have been divided into three categories from a mechanistical point of

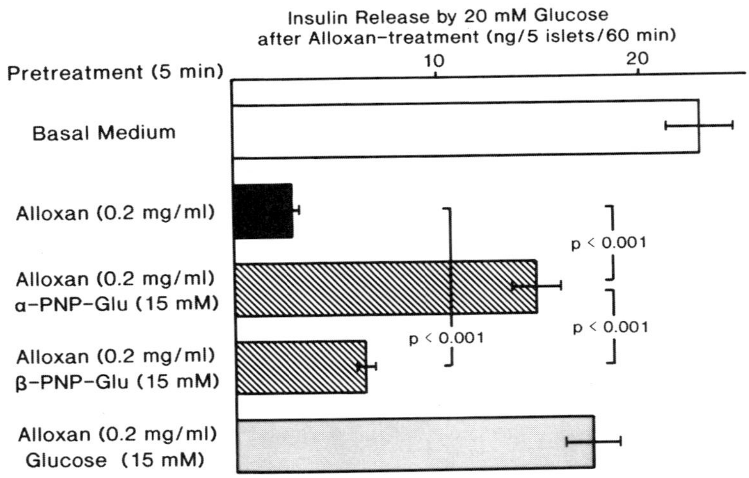

Figure 3. Effects of alloxan and interaction of alloxan with the α or β anomer of PNP-Glu on glucose-induced insulin secretion. Islets isolated from the rat pancreas were pretreated by incubating for 5 min in media containing alloxan (0.2 mg/ml) alone or alloxan with the compounds indicated. Islets incubated in the basal medium for 5 min were used as control. After washing, batches of 5 islets were incubated with 20 mmol/l D-glucose for 60 min. Values are means ± SEM (n=8).

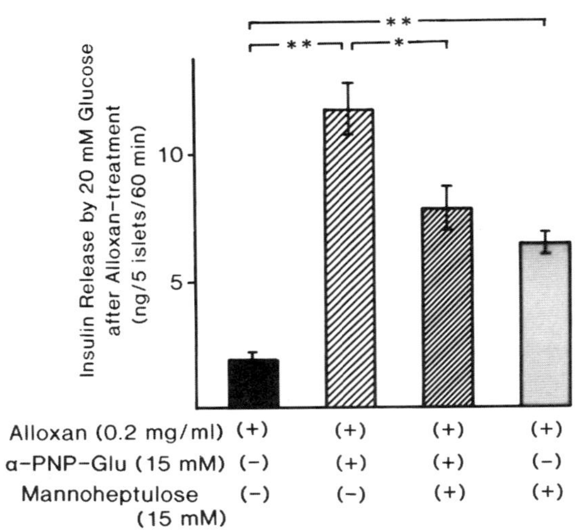

Figure 4. Effect of D-mannoheptulose on α-PNP-Glu protection against alloxan toxicity. Islets isolated from the rat pancreas were pretreated by incubating for 5 min in media containing alloxan (0.2 mg/ml) alone or alloxan with the compounds indicated. After washing, batches of 5 islets were incubated with 20 mmol/l D-glucose for 60 min. Values are means ± SEM (n=8). $^*p < 0.01$, $^{**}p < 0.001$.

view; namely non-specific, specific non-competitive and specific competitive inhibitors.[5] *p*-Nitrophenyl-hexopyranosides, PNP-Glu, PNP-Man and PNP-Gal, were reported to behave as specific competitive inhibitors of sugar taste response;[12] these compounds had no effect by themselves, but when added to sucrose solutions they did suppress sucrose taste responses. Evidence to support the concept of specific competitive inhibition includes the observations that high concentrations of sucrose surmounted the inhibitory effects of the compounds, that the α anomers of these compounds were more potent than the β anomers, and that the compounds did not affect other taste qualities.[12]

In the present studies, the α anomers of PNP-Glu and PNP-Man inhibited glucose-induced insulin release without affecting glucose oxidation in the pancreatic islets, while the β anomers of these compounds had no effect on insulin release. However, as distinct from sweet taste sensation, either anomer of PNP-Gal did not affect glucose-induced insulin release. The inhibitory action of the α anomer of PNP-Glu or PNP-Man was eliminated by raising the concentration of D-glucose, suggesting a competitive manner of the inhibition. The inhibition by these compounds also seems to be specific for glucose-induced insulin release, since insulin release induced by non-glucose secretagogues, such as arginine and tolbutamide, was not inhibited by PNP-Glu.[11]

D-Glucose and D-mannose are sweet substances and insulin secretagogues, the α anomers being more potent than the β anomers, while D-galactose is sweet, having the same anomeric preference, but has no physiological effect on the pancreatic β-cell.[2] Thus, the inhibitory effects of these compounds in the two cell types are intimately related to the physiological activities of the hexose moieties in these cells. *p*-Nitrophenol without hexose moiety completely inhibited both glucose-induced insulin release and glucose oxidation in islets. It is assumed, therefore, that the hexose moieties direct the compounds to a hexose recognition site in the pancreatic β–cell, and the *p*-nitrophenyl moiety exerts its inhibitory effect at the site. Though the exact nature of the site remains to be studied, the site may exist outside the major pathway of glucose metabolism in the pancreatic β-cell. It may be argued that the inhibitors act as a mitchondrial uncoupler and inhibit the production of ATP. This is not the case, since Tanigawa et al[13] recently observed in cell- attached patch clamp studies that α-PNP-Glu did not affect the K_{ATP} channel activity of the pancreatic β-cell in the presence of 10 mmol/l D-glucose.

Treatment of the gustatory cell and the pancreatic β-cell with alloxan, itself a sweet substance, results in unresponsiveness of these cells to D-glucose.[7,8] Certain hexoses, including D-glucose, are known to protect both types of cells against alloxan toxicity.[2] Mechanisms of the inhibitory actions of alloxan is still a matter of debate,[14] although in the gustatory cell it is considered to be a specific non-competitive inhibitor of sweet taste response.[5] D-Mannoheptulose, a seven carbon sugar, is widely used as an inhibitor of hexokinases. However, it was reported that D-mannoheptulose inhibited glucose-induced activation of phospholipase C in digitonin-permeabilized islets, in which glucose phosphorylating activity was not demonstrable.[15] Besides, D-mannoheptulose is a sweet sugar that may bind to a sweet taste receptor of the gustatory cell, and is known to exist almost exclusively in the α-pyranose form.[16]

In the present study, PNP-Glu protected islets against alloxan toxicity, the α anomer being more potent than the β anomer. The protective effect of α-PNP-Glu was attenuated by D-mannoheptulose. These observations suggest that D-mannoheptulose could compete for the site with the α anomer of PNP-Glu, bearing a higher affinity and a lower protective effect.

Our present findings suggest the possibility that, in the pancreatic β-cell, there is a glucose-recognizing mechanism that is independent of glucose metabolism and is similar to the mechanism of sugar recognition by the sweet taste receptor cell.

ACKNOWLEDGMENTS

This work was supported in part by a grant-in-aid for Scientific Research (02807229) from the Ministry of Education, Science and Culture of Japan. We thank Mrs. F. Furuta, Aichigakuin University, for her technical and secretarial assistance.

REFERENCES

1. Niki, A., and Niki, H., 1993, Hexose anomers and insulin release in nondiabetic and diabetic rats, with special reference to glucose recognition, in: *Lessons from animal diabetes IV. Biennial review volume 1992*, Shafrir, E., ed., Smith-Gordon, London, p. 27–37.
2. Niki, A., and Niki, H., 1980, Hexose anomers, insulin release, and diabetes mellitus, *Biomed. Res.* 1:189–205.
3. Niki, A., Niki, H., and Hashioka, T., 1989, Receptors of paraneurons, with special reference to glucoreceptors, *Arch. Histol. Cytol.* 52(Suppl.): 33–38.
4. Meglasson, M.D., and Matschinsky, F.M., 1986, Pancreatic islet glucose metabolism and regulation of insulin secretion, *Diabetes/Metab Rev* 2: 163–214.
5. Jakinovich, W., Jr., and Sugarman, D., 1988, Sugar taste reception in mammals, *Chemical Senses* 13:13–31.
6. Tomita, T., Lacy, P.E., Matschinsky, F.M., and McDaniel, M.L., 1974, Effect of alloxan on insulin secretion in isolated rat islets perifused *in vitro*, *Diabetes* 23: 517–524.
7. Zawalich, W.S., 1973, Depression of gustatory sweet response by alloxan, *Comp. Biochem. Physiol. A* 44: 903–909.
8. Niki, A., Niki, H., Miwa, I., and Lin, B.J., 1976, Interaction of alloxan and anomers of D-glucose on glucose-induced insulin secretion and biosynthesis in vitro, *Diabetes* 25: 574–579.
9. Niki, A., Niki, H., and Hashioka, T., 1993, Effects of specific competitive inhibitors of sweet taste response on glucose-induced insulin release, *Biomed. Res.* 14: 13–18.
10. Niki, A., Niki, H., and Hidaka, H., 1981, Effects of a new calmodulin inhibitor (W-7) on glucose-induced insulin release, *Biomed. Res.* 2: 413–417.
11. Niki, A., Niki, H., and Hashioka, T., 1989, An inhibitor of sweet taste response inhibits glucose-induced insulin release, *Biomed. Res.* 10: 169–172.
12. Vlahopoulos, V., and Jakinovich, W.J., 1986, Antagonism of the gerbil's sucrose taste response by p-nitrophenyl alpha-D-glucopyranoside and chloramphenicol, *J. Neurosci.* 6: 2611–2615.
13. Tanigawa, K., Furui, M., Hara, N., Sawada, M., and Kato, Y., 1992, An inhibitor of sweet taste response modulates glucose-induced phosphoinositide breakdown in rat pancreatic islets, *Endocrinol. Japan.* 39: 439–444.
14. Lenzen, S., and Panten, U., 1988, Alloxan: history and mechanism of action, *Diabetologia* 31: 337–342.
15. Wolf, B.A., Florholmen, J., Turk, J., and McDaniel, M.L., 1988, Studies of the Ca^{2+} requirements for glucose- and carbachol-induced augmentation of inositol trisphosphate and inositol tetrakisphosphate accumulation in digitonin-permeabilized islets. Evidence for a glucose recognition site in insulin secretion, *J. Biol. Chem.* 263: 3565–3575.
16. Pigman, W., and Isbell, H.S., 1968, Mutarotation of sugars in solutions: Part I History, basic kinetics, and composition of sugar solutions, in: *Advances in carbohydrate chemistry, Vol 23*, Wolfrom, M.L., and Tipson, R.S., eds., Academic Press, New York and London, p. 11–57.

3

GLUCOSE-INDUCED TIME-DEPENDENT POTENTIATION AND "RUN DOWN" OF INSULIN SECRETION IN ISLETS OF YOUNG RATS

Cheryl R. Bliss and Geoffrey W. G. Sharp

Department of Pharmacology
College of Veterinary Medicine
Cornell University
Ithaca, New York, 14853

SUMMARY

A "run down" phenomenon in isolated islets from young rats has been detected, in which the amount of insulin released in response to glucose decreases with time. This has been studied in conjunction with glucose-induced time-dependent potentiation (TDP) to see if the two are related. Islets, isolated from 7-day-old rats, exposed to 16.7 mM glucose for the first time after 30, 75 and 120 minutes of perifusion in Krebs-Ringer bicarbonate buffer (KRB) and 2.8 mM glucose, showed a progressive loss of responsiveness, and less insulin was released at the later times. This run down of the responses was prevented by successive challenges with 16.7 mM glucose and marked TDP was observed. The earlier the islets were exposed to glucose the more effectively was the run down prevented. Also, and perhaps causally related to the prevention of run down, the earlier the exposure to glucose the greater the TDP of a subsequent response. The results could possibly be explained in terms of a shift in metabolism in the isolated 7-day islets, with resultant diminution of the signals for the stimulation of insulin release and TDP. Early, and repeated exposure to high glucose would appear to minimize and delay the metabolic shift.

INTRODUCTION

Many reports have documented that insulin release in response to glucose by islets from young rats is small when compared with islets from adult rats[1-4]. To date, no satisfactory explanations are available to explain the reduced responses. Components of mature signal transduction mechanisms for glucose stimulated insulin secretion, the K_{ATP} channel, the L-type Ca channel, and adenylyl cyclase are present and functional in islets of 3-day-old rats[2,5], but their combined operation fails to evoke the magnitude of secretory response seen in the adult state. Recently, we reported on the possibility that the reduced response of islets from young rats could be due to the lack of "time-dependent potentiation" (TDP) in these animals[6]. Under experimental conditions in which glucose-induced TDP was easily detectable in islets from 21-day and 3-month-old rats, we were unable to demonstrate TDP in islets from 7- and 14-day-old rats. More importantly, for the purpose of the current work, it was found that the response to glucose in the 7-day islets deteriorated with time when the islets were incubated in a Krebs-Ringer bicarbonate (KRB) buffer. The "deterioration" appeared to result from a switch in metabolism which could be prevented by the inhibitor of fatty acid oxidation 2-bromostearate[6]. In fact, not only did 2-bromostearate prevent the "run down" of the glucose response, it also allowed glucose to induce TDP. It is clear, therefore, that islets from rats as young as 7 days do indeed have the capacity for TDP, and that failure to demonstrate the phenomenon previously could have been due to the run down under *in vitro* conditions. As this changed metabolism appeared to be time-dependent, we have reexamined TDP in islets from 7-day old rats and carried out the experiments in as short a time as possible, to minimize the run down. We found that under these conditions the islets were capable of TDP (unpublished data). Subsequently, the effects of time and repetitive glucose challenge on the presence and persistence of TDP were studied.

MATERIALS AND METHODS

Pregnant Wistar rats were maintained under controlled temperature conditions at 20–25°C, 50–70% humidity, and light (6:00 A.M. to 6:00 P.M.)/dark cycle both before and after giving birth to their litters. They had free access to regular laboratory chow at all times. At seven days of age, the rat pups were killed and the pancreases removed. Islets were isolated by the collagenase method[7] and placed into 70 μl perifusion chambers as previously described[6]. All procedures were carried out as quickly as possible in order to study the islet responses as soon as possible after the death of the animal. For each individual experiment, isolated islets from a common pool were perifused in four groups of twenty with Krebs-Ringer-bicarbonate (KRB) buffer containing (in mM) 119 NaCl, 25 $NaHCO_3$, 5 KCl, 1.2 KH_2PO_4, 1.2 $MgSO_4$, 2.5 $CaCl_2$, 10 N-2-hydroxyethylpiperizine-N′-2-ethanesulfonic acid, pH 7.4, and 0.25% bovine serum albumin with 2.8 mM glucose for different periods of time. Each experiment used batches of islets isolated from seven-day old rats from separate litters. The islets were exposed to KRB containing 16.7 mM glucose for twenty minute periods as follows; one group (n=10) was exposed at 30 minutes. Of these ten, five were exposed again at 75 minutes and the remaining five at 120 minutes. A second group (n=5) was exposed at 75 minutes and again at 120 minutes. A third group (n=5) was challenged only at 120 minutes. The fourth group (n=5) was challenged at 30, 75 and 120 minutes. After the twenty minute exposure periods, i.e. at 50 and 95 minutes, the islets were returned to KRB with 2.8 mM glucose. At 140 minutes the experiments were terminated. Perifusion flow rates were 1 ml/min throughout. Perifusion samples were collected every minute during exposure to KRB with 16.7 mM glucose. During exposure to KRB with 2.8 mM glucose the samples were collected every minute for the period 25–30 minutes and every 5 minutes thereafter. Samples were stored frozen at −20°C until radioimmunoassay[8]. Rats were purchased from and bred by Charles River (Kingston, NY).

Rat Chow was from Ralston Purina (Richmond, IN). Chemicals used were all reagent grade. Collagenase was from Accurate Chemical (Westbury, NY) and ^{125}I labeled insulin was obtained from Du-Pont New England Nuclear (Wilmington, DE).

RESULTS

The results shown in Figure 1 are from islets that were isolated from 7-day-old rats as rapidly as possible after they were killed, and then studied immediately under perifusion conditions. Prior to the first high glucose challenge, the equilibration period of perifusion with KRB and 2.8 mM glucose was reduced from the usual 45 minutes[6,9] to 30 minutes. In the presence of KRB and 2.8 mM glucose, insulin secretion from the islets was constant at around 16 to 17 pg/islet/minute from the start of sample collection at 25 minutes until 120 minutes. In Figure 1 (upper panel) are shown the effects of 16.7 mM glucose on insulin secretion when the islets were exposed to 16.7 mM glucose for the first time, 30, 75, and 120 minutes after the start of the perifusion (these data are all shown with open circles). It can be seen that the responses to the first exposures to glucose diminish with time with respect to both phases of release. The response to glucose at the 30 minute point (the "earliest" response to glucose) was characterized by a typically biphasic response. The first phase of release peaked after two to three minutes. A nadir after 5 to 6 minutes separated the first and second phases. The second phase showed continually increasing rates of insulin release from the nadir until the perifusion with 16.7 mM glucose was changed to 2.8 mM glucose at the 50th minute, i.e. after the islets had been exposed to the high glucose for 20 minutes. At this time, the rate of insulin release rapidly returned to basal values. The response to high glucose at 75 minutes was only slightly less than that of the first response. However, at 120 minutes the response has run down so far that the first phase of insulin release is barely detectable. In addition to documenting the run down, these experiments were designed to study TDP. Therefore, also shown in the upper panel of Figure 1, are the effects of a second exposure to glucose. One second response was measured at 75 minutes, i.e. 25 minutes after the first exposure, and the other second response to glucose was at 120 minutes, i.e. 70 minutes after the first exposure (both of these second exposures are illustrated by filled circles). At 75 minutes both test and control islets were exposed to 16.7 mM glucose. The control islets (open circles), seeing high glucose for the first time, gave a biphasic response which was similar to, but smaller than the response given by the paired test islets when exposed to high glucose 45 minutes earlier, as already mentioned. The test islets (closed circles) responded to their second exposure to high glucose with a prompt and vigorous release of insulin and exhibited strong TDP. First-phase release again peaked after 2 to 3 minutes and at a rate some three-fold higher than that of the control islets. The nadir exhibited a secretion rate that was double that seen in the controls and was followed by a rapid increase up to a second phase plateau which was again higher than the control values. In fact, the TDP was so strong in these test islets that the overall secretory response was even greater than the first response to glucose some 45 minutes earlier. Thus, under these conditions, with minimum delay after killing the 7-day-old rats and isolating the islets, marked TDP was evident. The memory for this effect was at least 70 minutes as can be seen by the second response to high glucose shown at 120 minutes (again illustrated by closed circles). Here, the first phase response to 16.7 mM glucose was some two and a half fold greater than the control response, although run down at this point and the decay of TDP had affected both the control and the potentiated responses.

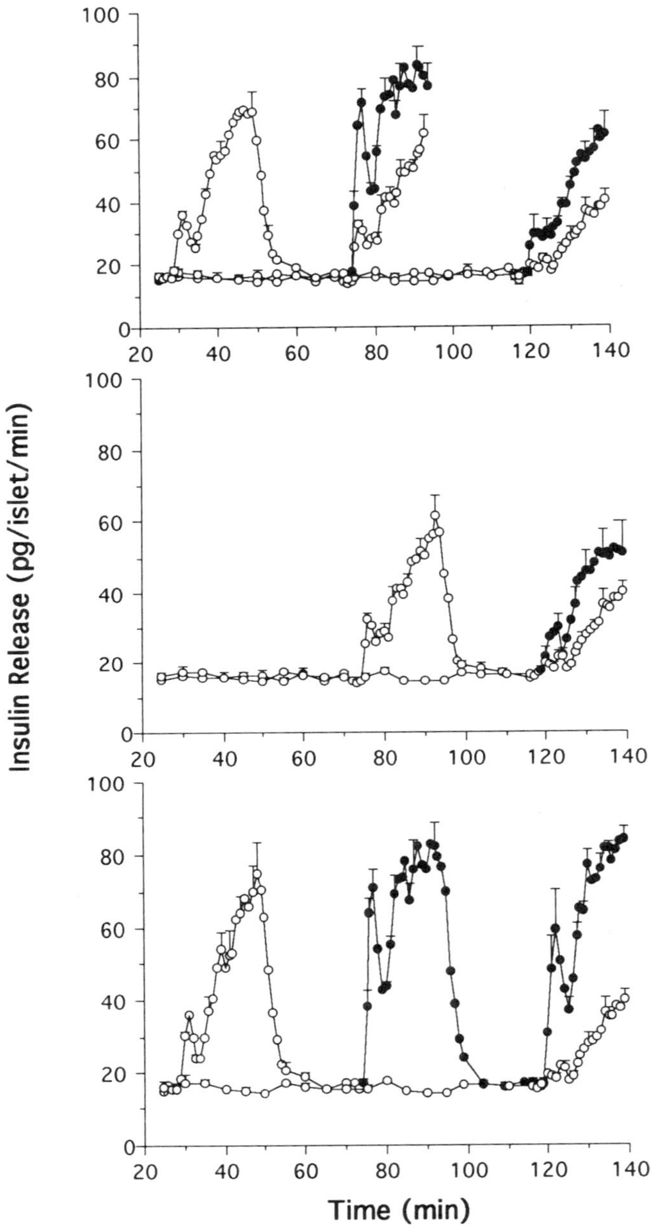

Figure 1. (**Upper**) Insulin release responses to 16.7 mM glucose given for the first time (open circles) at 30 (n=10), 75 (n=5) and 120 minutes (n=5). Two groups of paired islets exposed to 16.7 mM glucose at 30 minutes (each n=5) were subsequently exposed again either at 75 minutes or 120 minutes (closed circles). (**Middle**) Insulin release in response to 16.7 mM glucose given for the first time (open circles) at 75 minutes and 120 minutes (as seen in the upper panel). Islets exposed at 75 minutes were subsequently exposed again at 120 minutes (closed circles). n=5 in all cases. (**Lower**) Insulin release in response to 16.7 mM glucose given for the first time (open circles) at 30 minutes and 120 minutes (as seen in the upper panel). Islets exposed at 30 minutes were subsequently exposed at 75 minutes and then again at 120 minutes (closed circles). n=5 in all cases.

In the middle panel of Figure 1, data are shown which are derived from experiments in which the first exposure to glucose occurred at 75 minutes (these data are shown as open circles and are the same data as in the upper panel for this time point) and shows the effect of this on a subsequent response to glucose administered at 120 minutes (closed circles). Again TDP was detected. In this case, the potentiated response was comparable to that at the same time point in the upper panel, although not so well marked. Therefore, even though the time elapsed between the two glucose challenges was the same, the ability of glucose to induce TDP had diminished because of the additional time spent in low glucose before the first exposure. This illustrates the run down of both the response to glucose with time and the ability to generate TDP. Finally, in the lower panel of Figure 1 are shown the effects of two successive exposures to 16.7 mM glucose given at 30 (open circles) and 75 minutes (closed circles) on the insulin release response to a third exposure to glucose at 120 minutes (closed circles). The third glucose response was larger than any of the other responses at this time point whether they were responding to a first challenge with high glucose, or to a second challenge after an earlier exposure at 30 or 75 minutes. Thus repeated exposure to high glucose prevents "run down" and reinforces, or renews, the signal for TDP built up by the first exposure to glucose in these islets. There was a small time-dependent decrease in the magnitude of the first phase peak, from the highest value recorded during the 75 minute response to that occurring during the 120 minute response in these experiments. However there was no diminution of the second phase release rates.

DISCUSSION

The data presented in this paper show that islets from 7-day-old rats exhibit TDP in response to high glucose. In a previous report we had noticed that the response of these young (7-day) islets decreased (ran down) with time and that this was minimized by the presence of 2-bromostearate[6]. Furthermore, TDP in response to glucose was only observed in the presence of 2-bromostearate. It was considered possible that the young islets in simple KRB buffers were changing their metabolism and increasing the oxidation of fatty acids. The run down in glucose responsiveness, together with the restorative effect of 2-bromostearate, leads to the possibility that glucose metabolism in the young islet was failing to inhibit fatty acid oxidation as it does in the adult islet. Consequently, glucose was failing to give adequate signals to fully stimulate insulin secretion and generate TDP. Because of this, we tested the possibility that if we performed experiments on the 7-day islets in the shortest possible time after the rats were killed, then run down would be minimal, insulin release in response to glucose would be improved and TDP might be induced by high glucose alone. It is clear from the data presented that this was the case. It is also clear from these results that the young islet is difficult to study *in vitro*, because of its changing and diminishing responsiveness with time. Thus, experiments performed over prolonged time periods *in vitro* are unlikely to reflect accurately the performance or characteristics of the young islets as they exist in the animal. Further studies will be necessary to detail the time-dependent metabolic events and changes which occur in these islets.

ACKNOWLEDGMENTS

This work was supported by the National Institute of Diabetes and Digestive and Kidney Diseases Grants RO1 DK-34305 and R01 DK-42063. The authors are grateful for the skilled technical assistance of Ms. Shelley Nichols.

REFERENCES

1. Blazquez, E. L., Lipshaw, A., Blazquez, M., and Foa, P. P., 1975, The synthesis and release of insulin in fetal, nursing and young adult rats: studies in vivo and in vitro, *Pediat Res* 9: 17–25.
2. Grill, V., Asplund, K., Hellerstrom, C., and Cerasi, E., 1975, Decreased cyclic AMP and insulin response to glucose in isolated islets of neonatal rats, *Diabetes* 24: 746–752.
3. Grill, V., Lake, W., and Freinkel, N., 1981, Generalized diminution in the response to nutrients as insulin-releasing agents during the early neonatal period in the rat, *Diabetes* 30: 56–63.
4. Heinze, E., and Steinke, J., 1971, Glucose metabolism of isolated pancreatic islets; difference between fetal, newborn and adult rats, *Endocrinology* 88: 1259–1263.
5. Hole, R. L., Pian-Smith, M. C. M., and Sharp, G. W. G., 1988, Development of the biphasic response to glucose in fetal and neonatal rat pancreas, *Am J Physiol* 254: E167–E174.
6. Bliss, C. R., and Sharp, G. W. G., 1992, Glucose-stimulated insulin release in islets of young rats: time-dependent potentiation and effects of 2-bromostearate, *Am J Physiol* 263: E890–896.
7. Lacy, P., and Kostianovsky, M., 1967, Method for the isolation of intact islets of Langerhans from the rat pancreas, *Diabetes* 16: 35–39.
8. Herbert, V., Lau, K-S., Gottlieb, C. W., and Bleicher, S. J., 1965, Coated charcoal immunoassay of insulin, *J Clin Endocrinol* 25: 1375–1384.
9. Chalmers, J. A., and Sharp, G. W. G., 1989, The importance of Ca^{2+} for glucose-induced priming in pancreatic islets, *Biochim Biophys Acta* 1011: 46–51.

Part II.B. The Role for $K_{(ATP)}$ Channels

4

ATP-SENSITIVE K^+ CHANNEL CLOSURE IS NOT AN OBLIGATORY STEP FOR GLUCOSE-INDUCED PRIMING OF PANCREATIC B-CELL

N. Taguchi, T. Aizawa, and K. Hashizume

Shinshu University School of Medicine
3-1-1 Asahi, Matsumoto, Japan

INTRODUCTION

Exposure of the B-cell to high glucose has a priming effect so that insulin release in response to subsequent stimuli is enhanced[1]: the phenomenon is called "Time-Dependent Potentiation (TDP)". For glucose-induced insulin release, closure of the ATP-sensitive K^+ (K^+ATP) channel is an obligatory step because *all* of the response is eliminated by the presence of diazoxide, an opener of the channel. However, we[2] and others[3] found that there is a K^+ATP channel-independent branch of glucose-induced signaling in the B-cell, which is dependent on elevation of cytosolic Ca^{2+}. Here, we show that "glucose-induced priming of the B-cell" and "glucose-induced insulin release by the B-cell" are mechanistically distinct from each other: closure of K^+ATP channel is a pre-requisite for the latter but not for the former. Differential effects of lowering ambient Ca^{2+} concentration on glucose-induced TDP[4,5] and glucose-induced insulin release were also evaluated.

MATERIALS AND METHODS

Pancreatic islets were obtained from male Wistar rats by collagenase dispersion and insulin release was measured in incubation experiments: incubation was carried out using 5 islets/tube at 37°C in Krebs-Ringer bicarbonate buffer (KRBB) as reported.[2] KRBB contained 1.9 mM Ca^{2+}, 4.7 mM K^+ and 3 mM glucose unless otherwise stated.[2] The islets were first incubated in 1 ml KRBB containing 3 or 16.7 mM glucose for 45 min (priming). In some experiments, 150 mM diazoxide, 25 mM K^+ and 10 mM glyburide were included during the priming period. Ca^{2+}-omitted KRBB, Ca^{2+}-omitted KRBB containing EGTA (500 mM), and EGTA (500 mM)-containing KRBB with increased Ca^{2+} (2.4 mM) were also used during the priming period: Ca^{2+} concentration of the Ca^{2+}-omitted KRBB was 58

Physiology and Pathophysiology of the Islets of Langerhans, edited by Soria.
Plenum Press, New York, 1997.

Table 1. Effects of various additions to, and changes of, the media during the initial incubation on subsequent response to 25 mM K^+

Group	Additions to/Changes of KRBB during the initial incubation	Insulin release during the final incubation (pg/islet/20 min)
1.	None	335.4 ± 97.6
2.	16.7 mM glucose	868.9 ± 336.5[a]
3.	150 mM diazoxide + 16.7 mM glucose	519.3 ± 265.0[b]
4.	150 mM diazoxide + 25 mM K^+ + 16.7 mM glucose	520.6 ± 243.7[b]
5.	16.7 mM glucose in Ca^{2+}-omitted KRBB	915.0 ± 778.6[b]
6.	16.7 mM glucose in EGTA-containing, Ca^{2+}-omitted KRBB	142.3 ± 68.1
7.	16.7 mM glucose in EGTA-containing, Ca^{2+}-added KRBB	888.3 ± 248.3[a]
8.	10 mM glyburide	104.3 ± 74.4

During the final incubation, the islets were exposed to 25 mM K^+ in the presence of 3 mM glucose. [a] and [b], $P < 0.01$ and 0.05, respectively, compared to the value of Group 1. Number of determinations are 5–8 in each group.

mM (measured by atomic absorption). Upon removal of the initial incubation media, 4 ml regular KRBB was introduced and incubated for 15 min (wash-out). Then, the buffer was aspirated and 0.5 ml KRBB containing 25 mM K^+ was introduced and incubated for 20 min for the measurement of insulin release. Four ml of wash-out buffer was used to minimize "carry-over" of the buffer to the subsequent incubation. The "carry-over" was calculated to be less than 30 ml. Insulin was measured by radioimmunoassay using rat insulin as a standard.

RESULTS AND DISCUSSION

With the protocol employed, glucose unequivocally causes TDP (Table 1). As reported previously, glucose-induced insulin release (during the priming period) is eliminated by 150 mM diazoxide due to inhibition of K^+ATP channel closure (Table 2). However, TDP is clearly present in the islets primed with high glucose in the presence of diazoxide (Table 1). Glucose-induced potentiation is one third in the diazoxide-exposed,

Table 2. Effects of various additions to and changes of the regular KRBB on insulin release during the initial incubation

Group	Additions to/Changes of KRBB during the initial incubation	Insulin release during the initial incubation (pg/islet/20 min)
1.	None	927.4 ± 457.2
2.	16.7 mM glucose	2837.5 ± 604.3
3.	150 mM diazoxide + 16.7 mM glucose	941.5 ± 533.8[a]
4.	150 mM diazoxide + 25 mM K^+ + 16.7 mM glucose	1510.5 ± 212.0[b]
5.	16.7 mM glucose in Ca^{2+}-omitted KRBB	875.6 ± 477.3
6.	16.7 mM glucose in EGTA-containing, Ca^{2+}-omitted KRBB	930.3 ± 635.1
7.	16.7 mM glucose in EGTA-containing, Ca^{2+}-added KRBB	2364.5 ± 660.8[c]
8.	10 mM glyburide	1143.8 ± 442.5

Regular KRBB contained 4.7 mM K^+ and 3 mM glucose. [a], [b] and [c], $P < 0.01$, $P < 0.05$ and not significantly different, respectively, compared to the value of Group 2. Number of determinations are 5–8 in each group.

compared to non-diazoxide-exposed, B-cell, however. When the initial glucose priming is carried out in the presence of diazoxide plus depolarizing concentration of K^+, inhibition of TDP by diazoxide is not significantly eliminated (Table 1), indicating high K^+-induced depolarization/Ca^{2+} influx cannot be a substitute for glucose-induced K^+ATP channel closure. Alternatively, high concentration of diazoxide might possess suppressive action on the B-cell at a site other than K^+ATP channel.

Use of Ca^{2+}-omitted KRBB completely abolishes glucose-induced insulin release during the priming period (Table 2), however, it does not at all attenuate glucose-induced priming of the B-cell (Table 1). Complete removal of free Ca^{2+} by addition of 500 mM EGTA to the Ca^{2+}-omitted buffer eliminates both glucose-induced insulin release (Table 1) and glucose-induced priming of the B-cell (Table 2). This is not due to non-specific toxic effect of EGTA because normalization of Ca^{2+} concentration (1.9 mM) by adding 2.4 mM Ca^{2+} to the EGTA (500 mM)-containing buffer restores both glucose-induced TDP and insulin release (Table 1 and 2). Thus, very low extracellular Ca^{2+} (58 mM in the present study), but not zero Ca^{2+}, is able to support glucose-induced priming of the B-cell. When glyburide is used to close K^+ATP channel (with 3 mM glucose) during the initial incubation, potentiation of the B-cell does not occur, which implies that closure of K^+ATP channel alone cannot activate the mechanism of B-cell potentiation. The finding is compatible with the fact that closure of the channel is not obligatory step for glucose-induced TDP.

CONCLUSIONS

K^+ATP channel closure is not an obligatory step for glucose-induced TDP of the B-cell and extremely low extracellular Ca^{2+} (58 mM) is enough to support the TDP. Mechanism of glucose-induced initiation of insulin release and priming of the B-cell are thus distinct from each other.

ACKNOWLEDGMENT

This work was supported by a Grant-in-Aid for Scientific Research from the Ministry of Education, Science and Culture, Japan.

REFERENCES

1. Cerasi, E.,1975, Potentiation of insulin release by glucose in man. Quantitative analysis of the enhancement of glucose-induced insulin secretion by pretreatment with glucose in normal subjects, *Acta Endocrinol.* 79: 483–501.
2. Sato, Y., Aizawa, T., Komatsu, M., Okada, N., and Yamada, T., 1992, Dual functional role of membrane depolarization/Ca^{2+} influx in rat pancreatic B-cell, *Diabetes* 41: 438–443.
3. Gembal, M., Gilon, P., and Henquin, J.-C., 1992, Evidence that glucose can control insulin release independently from its action on ATP-sensitive K^+ channels in mouse B cells, *J. Clin. Invest.* 89: 1288–1295.
4. Grill, V., Adamson, U., and Cerasi, E., 1978 Immediate and time dependent effects of glucose on insulin release from rat pancreatic tissue, *J. Clin. Invest.* 61: 1034–1043.
5. Malaisse, W. J., and Sener, A., 1987 Interaction between D-glucose and Ca^{2+} in the priming of the pancreatic B-cell, *Diabet. Res.* 4: 5–8.

5

BURSTING ELECTRICAL ACTIVITY GENERATED IN THE PRESENCE OF K_{ATP} CHANNEL BLOCKERS

Pharmacology, Sensitivity to Intracellular pH and Modulation by Glucose Metabolism

Rosa M. Santos,[1,2] Rui M. Barbosa,[1,3] Célia M. Antunes,[1] Amélia M. Silva,[1] António P. Salgado,[1] Antero J. Abrunhosa,[1] Frederico C. Pereira,[1] Raquel M. Seiça,[1,4] and Luís M. Rosário[1,2]

[1]Center for Neurosciences of Coimbra
University of Coimbra, P-3049 Coimbra, Portugal
[2]Department of Biochemistry, Faculty of Sciences and Technology
University of Coimbra, P. O. Box 3126, P-3049 Coimbra, Portugal
[3]Laboratory of Instrumentation and Analysis, Faculty of Pharmacy
University of Coimbra, P-3049 Coimbra, Portugal
[4]Institute of Physiology, Faculty of Medicine
University of Coimbra, P-3049 Coimbra, Portugal

INTRODUCTION

The use of the patch-clamp technique has made possible the characterization of the glucose sensitivity of a number of cation channels present in the β-cell membrane. One of these channels, the ATP-dependent K^+ (K_{ATP}) channel, is specifically blocked by intracellular ATP and appears to play an essential role in the coupling of glucose metabolism to membrane depolarization and, hence, to Ca^{2+} influx and to the initiation of insulin release[1]. The available data indicate that the activity of the K_{ATP} channel is almost fully suppressed at 6 mM glucose, ie. a concentration which brings the membrane potential to a level just below the threshold for the appearance of electrical activity. At glucose concentrations above 7 mM the β-cell displays a pattern of bursting electrical activity which is remarkably sensitive to the hexose concentration, with the silent unexcited period ("silent phase") being progressively reduced and the depolarized active phase ("active phase") becoming progressively elongated as the size of the glucose stimulus increases[2]. We conclude that, while the glucose-mediated reduction in the activity of the K_{ATP} channels is indeed essential for the glucose-evoked initial depolarization of the β-cell, the modulation of bursting electrical

Physiology and Pathophysiology of the Islets of Langerhans, edited by Soria.
Plenum Press, New York, 1997.

activity by the hexose in the range 7–20 mM is apparently accounted for, at least in part, by a channel distinct from the K_{ATP} channel. The present account aims at providing evidence to support this hypothesis.

Previous reports from our laboratory have provided an experimental model of bursting whereby the β-cell is induced into a phasic pattern of electrical activity in the presence of sulphonylurea blockers of the K_{ATP} channel, thus ruling out an essential role for this channel in the bursting mechanism[3–5] (for review see Santos et al., 1994[6]). Although several agents (e.g. the L-type voltage-sensitive Ca^{2+} channel agonist Bay K 8644 and the delayed rectifier K^+ channel blocker tetraethylammonium) have the capability to change the β-cell tonic firing pattern, observed in the presence of tolbutamide, into a phasic pattern, the most effective and predictable experimental maneuver is simply to raise extracellular Ca^{2+} concentration to high levels (e.g. 13 mM) in the presence of the sulphonylurea[3,4]. This maneuver appears to act by promoting the interaction of Ca^{2+} influx with the putative intracellular Ca^{2+} concentration ($[Ca^{2+}]_i$)-sensitive conductance underlying the burst[4,6]. The specific aim of this report is to explore the intrinsic sensitivity of the β-cell bursting mechanism to intracellular processes which also interfere with the K_{ATP} channel (e.g. glucose metabolism, intracellular pH and drugs), thus uncovering actions normally obscured by the free operation of the latter channel.

MATERIALS AND METHODS

The membrane potential was recorded from microdissected mouse islets using high-resistance glass microelectrodes essentially as reported[4]. The $[Ca^{2+}]_i$ and the intracellular pH (pH_i) were recorded from single collagenase-isolated mouse islets or from single β-cells using the fluorescent indicators fura-2 and BCECF, respectively, essentially as reported[7,5].

RESULTS AND DISCUSSION

Effect of Reducing Extracellular Ca^{2+} Concentration on Bursting Electrical Activity

The physiological significance of bursting electrical activity for β-cell function and insulin release has been occasionally undervalued by the claim that this bursting pattern is lost when the Ca^{2+} concentration in the solution is reduced from the typical 2.56 mM, used in the electrical activity studies, to the levels normally found in the plasma, ie. approximately 1–2 mM[8]. This claim is totally unwarranted, as demonstrated by previous studies[9] and by recent experiments from our laboratory (C.M. Antunes, R.M. Barbosa, L.M. Rosário, R.M. Santos and P. Bergsten, manuscript in preparation), both demonstrating that the mechanisms that normally operate at 2.56 mM Ca^{2+} are also operative at 1.28 mM Ca^{2+}. Fig. 1 shows the typical effect of halving the external Ca^{2+} concentration on the electrical activity recorded from a cell exposed to 11 mM glucose. Although the cell is paradoxically activated by reducing extracellular Ca^{2+}, it is apparent that the cell does undergo prominent bursting. An interesting feature of the effect of lowering external Ca^{2+} is the pronounced hyperpolarization of the burst active phase, which entirely accounts for the dramatic reduction of the amplitude of the underlying slow wave (Fig. 1).

Previous studies have shown that bursting electrical activity is on the basis of the fast $[Ca^{2+}]_i$ oscillations and the pulsatile insulin release measured from single islets[10–12].

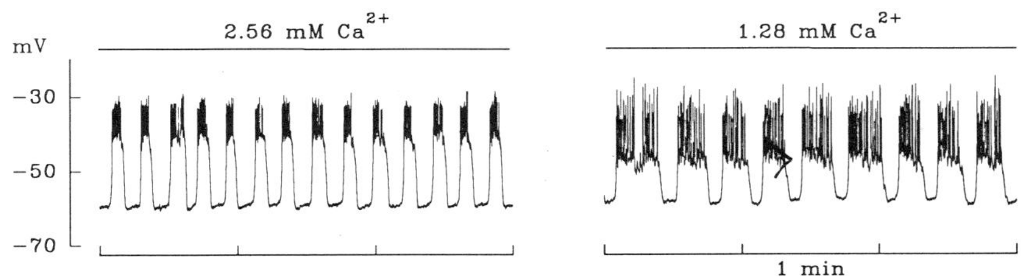

Figure 1. Effect of reducing extracellular Ca^{2+} concentration from 2.56 to 1.28 mM on bursting electrical activity. Glucose concentration was 11 mM.

Thus, the experiment depicted in Fig. 1 suggests that the oscillatory electrical activity has the potential to serve as an effective regulator of *in vivo* Ca^{2+} influx and insulin secretion.

Intrinsic Sensitivity of the Bursting Mechanism to Glucose Metabolism

We have assessed whether glucose may enhance bursting electrical activity in the absence of functional K_{ATP} channels, as is the case when the activity of these channels is left free to change according to the metabolic energy status of the cells. To this end, we have investigated the modulation by glucose of bursting electrical activity generated in the presence of tolbutamide and high Ca^{2+} (R.M. Barbosa, R.M. Santos and L.M. Rosário, manuscript in preparation). In these experiments the glucose concentration was increased stepwise from 3 to 11 mM in the continued presence of tolbutamide and 13 mM Ca^{2+}. Fig. 2 shows that glucose increased the burst active phase duration and concomitantly decreased the silent phase duration, thus increasing the fraction of time that the β-cells spend in the active phase of the bursts.

In a series of parallel experiments, we have observed that α-ketoisocaproic acid (KIC), a metabolic substrate that bypasses glycolysis and feeds directly the mitochondrial Krebs' cycle, enhances bursting electrical activity recorded in the presence of tolbutamide and high Ca^{2+} in a glucose-like manner. Fig. 3 shows that the glycolytic inhibitor iodoacetic acid (IAA), administered to islets otherwise exposed to 11 mM glucose, tolbutamide and high Ca^{2+}, suppressed bursting electrical activity after a lag time of several minutes. Interestingly, the IAA-mediated suppression of the electrical activity was accompanied by an hyperpolarization of the β-cell membrane of approximately 10 mV. Subsequently exposing the islets to 11 mM KIC, in the continued presence of all the above agents, evoked a triphasic electrical response consisting of an initial burst of spikes, an after-burst hyperpolarization lasting 2–3 min and a phase of complete resumption of bursting electrical activity (Fig. 3). The transient hyperpolarization and cessation of electrical activity that follows the initial surge of spikes is reminescent of the initial effect of raising glucose concentration on bursting electrical activity, recorded in the presence of tolbutamide and high Ca^{2+} (not apparent in Fig. 2).

The fact that IAA, but not long term exposures to glucose-free solutions (R.M. Barbosa, R.M. Santos and L.M. Rosário, unpublished observations), suppresses the electrical activity recorded in the presence of tolbutamide and high Ca^{2+}, indicates that the β-cell can utilize energy reserves other than exogenous carbohydrates and that this endogenous pool (e.g. fatty acids, glycogen) is effectively used when the external carbohydrate pool is depleted. Thus, the fact that the mitochondrial substrate KIC can support bursting electri-

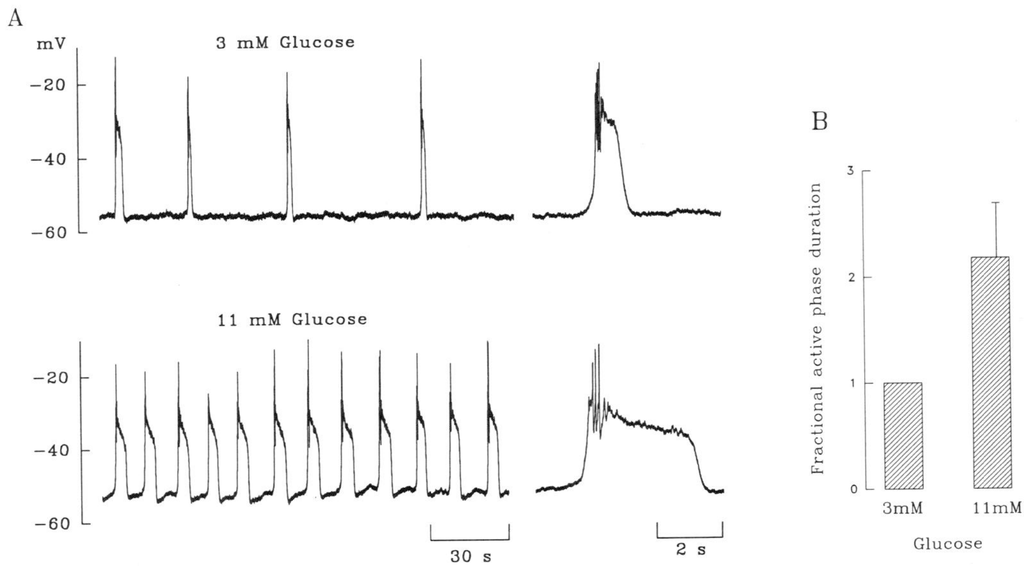

Figure 2. Effect of raising glucose concentration on bursting electrical activity recorded in the presence of tolbutamide and high Ca^{2+}. **A:** The islet was sequentially exposed to 3 and 11 mM glucose for 15 min periods in the continued presence of 100 μM tolbutamide and 12.8 mM external Ca^{2+}. The traces depicted are representative of the last 2 min of the steady-state electrical activity recorded at each glucose concentration. Representative bursts on an expanded time scale are shown to the right of each trace. Identical results were obtained using 500 μM tolbutamide. **B:** The fraction of time spent at the burst active phase was normalized to the activity recorded in 3 mM glucose. The data are plotted ± S.E.M. from 5 experiments similar to that depicted in panel A.

cal activity as effectively as glucose, under conditions where glycolysis has been interrupted, together with the fact that it has glucose-like effects on bursting electrical activity recorded in the presence of tolbutamide and high Ca^{2+}, attributes to the mitochondria the origin of the glucose effect depicted in Fig. 2. Several possible mechanisms may account for the latter effect, including enhanced phosphorylation of a critical component of the bursting mechanism (e.g. the voltage-dependent Ca^{2+} channel) and/or stimulation of intracellular Ca^{2+} buffering mechanisms. Preliminary experiments indicate that the enhancement of the electrical activity observed in the absence of functional K_{ATP} channels is not caused by phosphorylation reactions mediated by protein kinases acting on serine/threonine aminoacid residues (C.M. Antunes, L.M. Rosário and R.M. Santos, manuscript in preparation). Although we suspect that a rise in cytosolic ATP may mediate the glucose enhancement of the electrical activity, the available data are not contradictory with the possibility that alternative metabolites and/or second messengers might be involved.

Intrinsic Sensitivity of the Bursting Mechanism to Intracellular pH Changes

Since the K_{ATP} channels are activated by raising the pH at the cytoplasmic face of the channel[13], knowledge of the modulation of the mechanism underlying the burst by pH_i changes has been hampered by the effect of pH_i on the background activity of these channels. Using the K_{ATP} channel-free bursting model described above, we have recently found that an alkalinizing pH_i shift (exposure to 20 mM NH_4Cl) enhances the time spent at the

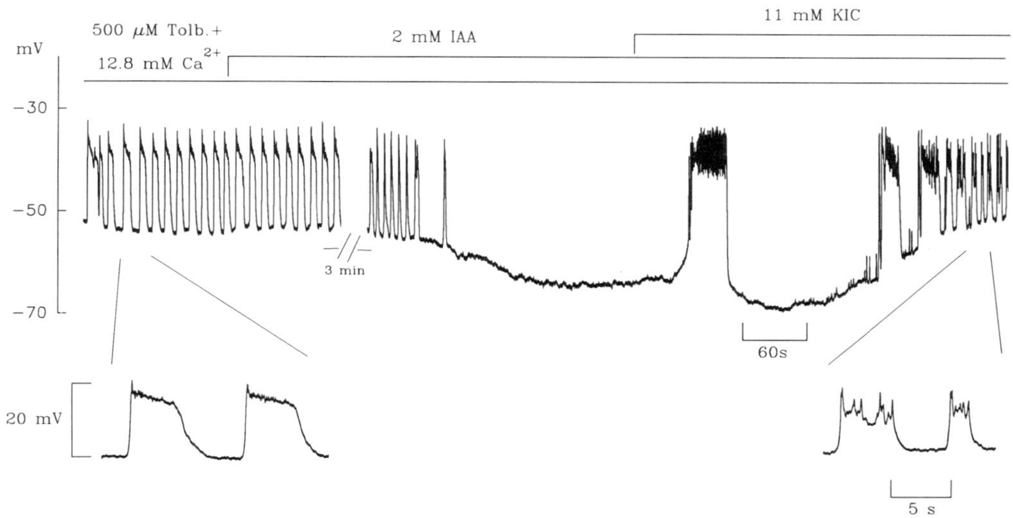

Figure 3. Glucose-like effects of α-ketoisocaproic acid on bursting electrical activity recorded in the presence of tolbutamide and high Ca^{2+}. Exposure to the glycolytic inhibitor iodoacetic acid (IAA) in the continued presence of 11 mM glucose, 500 μM tolbutamide and 12.8 mM Ca^{2+} hyperpolarized the β-cell membrane and suppressed bursting electrical activity. This activity resumed following administration of the mitochondrial substrate α-ketoisocaproic acid (KIC), in the continued presence of all the above agents. The data are representative of three similar experiments.

burst active phase and that, conversely, an acidifying shift (NH_4Cl withdrawal) hyperpolarizes the cell and suppresses bursting electrical activity[5] (Fig. 4A). This stands in sharp contrast to the effects of alkalinizing and acidifying pH_i shifts on the bursting electrical activity recorded under control conditions (i.e. 2.56 mM Ca^{2+} and 11 mM glucose)[14], which are likely to be mediated by the K_{ATP} channel[5]. We conclude that the bursting mechanism is intrinsically sensitive to pH_i, with an alkalinizing shift promoting a net depolarization to the burst active phase. Moreover, the experiment depicted in Fig. 4A emphasizes the potential of the K_{ATP} channel-free model described in this paper for investigations concerning the specific role of the bursting mechanism in processes triggered by drugs, metabolites and other agents.

We have plotted the fractional active phase duration, observed in response to 20 mM NH_4Cl from experiments similar to that depicted in Fig. 4A, against the respective pH_i values, measured from separate islets using the fluorescent pH indicator BCECF as depicted in Fig. 4B. The result is a "titration curve" with two inflexion points, one around 6.65–6.8 and another around 7.4–7.45 (Fig. 4C). This analysis suggests that the bursting mechanism is controlled by a pH-sensitive channel with two pKs in the range 6.65–7.45. This channel is unlikely to be a Ca^{2+}-dependent K^+ channel, since a pH_i rise would be expected to enhance the affinity of its gate to Ca^{2+}, thereby activating the channel and hyperpolarizing the membrane.

Possible Involvement of Non-selective Cation Channels in the Bursting Mechanism

A feed-back regulatory mechanism involving calcium-activated, non-specific cation (CAN) channels and $[Ca^{2+}]_i$ changes appears to underlye bursting electrical activity in

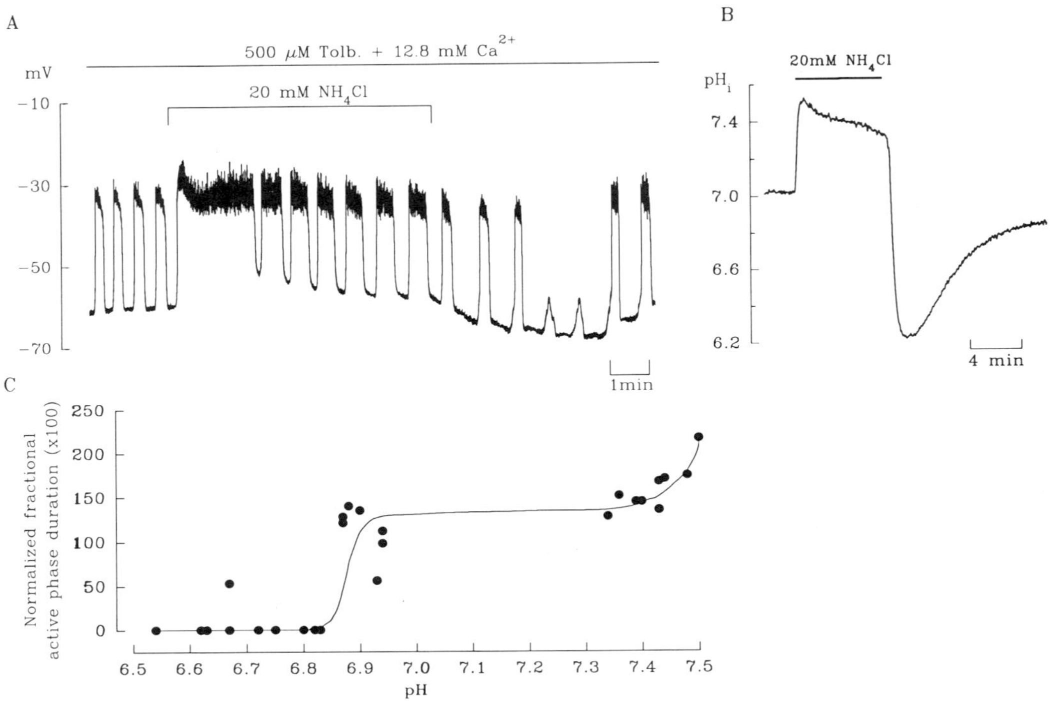

Figure 4. Modulation of bursting electrical recorded in the presence of tolbutamide and high Ca^{2+} by pH_i changes. **A:** Ammonium chloride was added to and withdrawn from the perifusion solution in the continued presence of 11 mM glucose, 500 μM tolbutamide and 12.8 mM Ca^{2+}, as indicated by the square bracket. **B:** Effect of an ammonium pulse on the intracellular pH, recorded from a single collagenase-isolated islet loaded with BCECF. **C:** Plot of the fraction of time spent at the burst active phase, normalized to the electrical activity recorded immediately prior to ammonium delivery, against the pH_i. The pH_i values used for the plot were taken from the average single islet responses to 20 mM NH_4Cl (3 experiments similar to that depicted in B).

Helix burster neurones[15]. CAN channels with an altered sensitivity to Ca^{2+} arising from patch excision have been described in human and rat insulinoma cells[16,17]. Importantly, a channel of similar conductance and kinetics has been detected in cell-attached patches on β-cells[1]. Thus, the CAN channel has the potential to be a "burster" channel in the β-cell.

By recording the $[Ca^{2+}]_i$ responses of whole islets to stepwise increases in external Ca^{2+}, we have recently found that β-cells are very leaky to Ca^{2+} under conditions where the voltage-sensitive Ca^{2+} channel is blocked[7]. The high Ca^{2+}-evoked $[Ca^{2+}]_i$ rises recorded from single whole islets are relatively insensitive to glucose metabolism, are not dependent on Ins 1,4,5-P_3-linked internal Ca^{2+} stores and can be suppressed by Ni^{2+} and diphenylamine-2-carboxylate (DPC)[7]. Since the latter drug is an effective blocker of non-selective cation channels[18,19], it can be used to probe the involvement of these channels in physiological processes provided that the fact that it also behaves as a potent Cl^- channel blocker[20] is taken into consideration.

Fig. 5A depicts the sensitivity of high Ca^{2+}-evoked $[Ca^{2+}]_i$ rises, recorded from single mouse β-cells, to DPC. The cell was superfused with DPC during continued exposure to the high Ca^{2+} solution, resulting in a slow but pronounced $[Ca^{2+}]_i$ fall. The effect of DPC was reversible, as assessed by the prompt $[Ca^{2+}]_i$ return to higher levels following

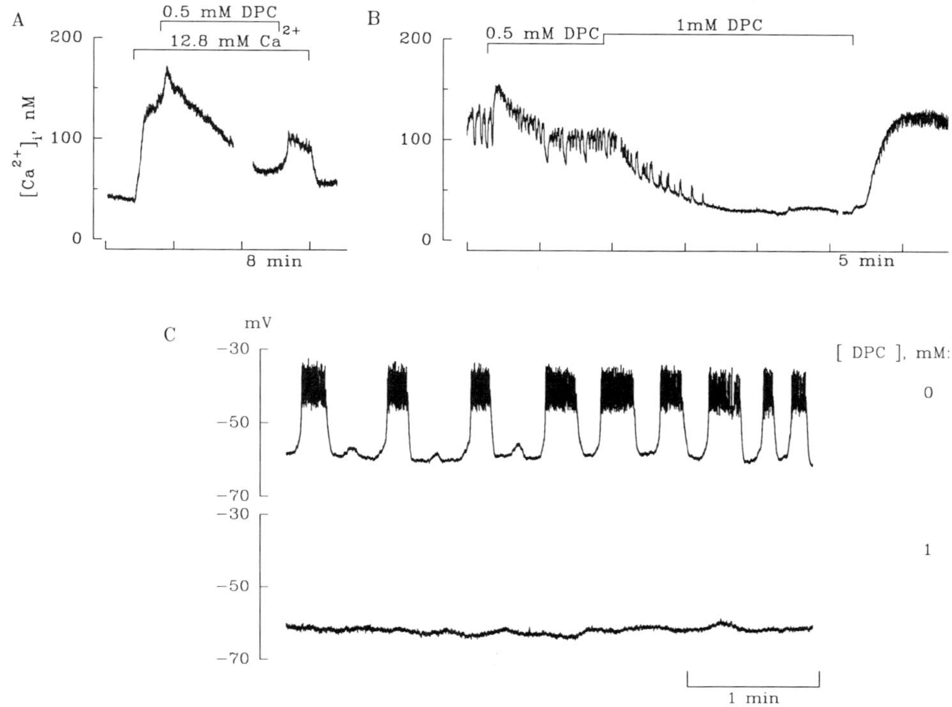

Figure 5. Effects of the non-selective cation channel blocker diphenylamine-2-carboxylate on fast $[Ca^{2+}]_i$ transients and on the underlying bursts of electrical activity. **A:** $[Ca^{2+}]_i$ recording from a single β-cell. The external Ca^{2+} concentration was raised from 0.2 to 12.8 mM and 0.5 mM diphenylamine-2-carboxylate (DPC) was temporarily applied during high Ca^{2+} perifusion, as denoted by the square bracket. Glucose concentration was 3 mM throughout. **B:** $[Ca^{2+}]_i$ recording from a single collagenase-isolated islet. The islet was exposed to 0.5 and 1 mM DPC in the continued presence of 11 mM glucose. **C:** Membrane potential recording from a microdissected islet. Perifusion with a solution containing 1 mM DPC (lower trace) suppressed the bursting electrical activity invoked by 11 mM glucose (upper trace).

DPC withdrawal from the solution. The experiment depicted in Fig. 5A is critical for the interpretation of the data gathered from whole islets, since it rules out the possibility that the DPC-sensitive Ca^{2+} influx mechanism might originate from neurotransmitter release processes within the islets, as previously hypothesized[7].

We have investigated the effects of DPC on the $[Ca^{2+}]_i$ oscillatory activity (Fig. 5B) and bursting electrical activity (Fig. 5C) recorded from single collagenase-isolated islets and from microdissected islets exposed to 11 mM glucose, respectively. DPC was indeed effective in suppressing both types of oscillatory activity, although the concentration required to suppress the oscillations (c. 1 mM) was significantly higher than the concentration necessary to block the high Ca^{2+}-evoked $[Ca^{2+}]_i$ transients recorded from single islets (c. 0.3 mM, ie. approximately twice the respective IC_{50}[7]).

The slight membrane hyperpolarization and the concomitant suppression of bursting electrical activity caused by 1 mM DPC are highly unlikely to originate from blockade of Cl^- channels, since the respective reversal potential is probably close to the K^+ equilibrium potential and, thus, blockade of the channels would be expected to depolarize the cells. The possible blockade by DPC of voltage-dependent Ca^{2+} channels is dismissed by control experiments showing that the drug does not affect high K^+-evoked $[Ca^{2+}]_i$ transients (A.M. Silva, L.M. Rosário and R.M. Santos, manuscript in preparation). We conclude that the DPC effect on bursting is mediated by a non-selective cation channel, but whether this channel is essential to the bursting mechanism or, alternatively, plays a permissive role for the development of the underlying slow wave cannot be assessed at present.

CONCLUSIONS

We have shown that the bursting mechanism is intrinsically sensitive to glucose metabolism. Thus, the graded β-cell electrical response observed in the intermediate-high glucose concentration range may, at least in part, originate from the fact that the channels underlying the burst are sensitive to metabolically derived signals. We have also determined that the latter channels are intrinsically sensitive to pH_i, with an alkalinizing shift promoting a net depolarization to the burst active phase. The nature of the channel responsible for the slow wave remains elusive. We now know that the K_{ATP} channel and the large conductance, charybdotoxin-sensitive Ca^{2+}-dependent K^+ channel are not essential for the bursting mechanism, but whether a recently discovered DPC-sensitive non-selective cation channel simply plays a permissive role in the bursting mechanism by providing the β-cells with a sustained depolarizing drive or, alternatively, might be essential for the operation of the bursting cycle is currently under investigation.

ACKNOWLEDGMENTS

This work was partially financed by JNICT (PMCT/C/CEN/394/90), Calouste Gulbenkian Foundation (Lisbon) and the EC SCIENCE Program (SC1-CT92-0833).

REFERENCES

1. Ashcroft, F.M., and Rorsman, P. , 1989, Electrophysiology of the pancreatic β-cell, Prog. Biophys. mol. biol. 54: 87–143
2. Atwater, I., Carroll, P., and Li, M.X., 1989, Electrophysiology of the pancreatic β-cell, in: "Insulin secretion", Alan R. Liss, Inc., pp. 49–68
3. Santos, R.M., Barbosa, R.M., Silva, A.M., Antunes, C.M., and Rosario, L.M., 1992, High external Ca^{2+} levels trigger membrane potential oscillations in mouse pancreatic β-cells during blockade of K(ATP) channels, Biochem. Biophys. Res. Commun. 187: 872–879
4. Rosário, L.M., Barbosa, R.M., Antunes, C.M., Silva, A.M., Abrunhosa, A.J., and Santos, R.M., 1993, Bursting electrical activity in pancreatic β-cells: evidence that the channel underlying the burst is sensitive to Ca^{2+} influx through L-type Ca^{2+} channels, Pflugers Arch. 424: 439–447
5. Barbosa, R.M., Salgado, A.P., Santos, R.M., and Rosário, L.M., 1993, Differential modulation of pancreatic β-cell bursting by intracellular pH in the presence and absence of a K-ATP channel blocker, FEBS Lett. 332: 9–13
6. Santos, R.M., Barbosa, R.M., Silva, A.M., Antunes, C.M., and Rosario, L.M., 1994, $[Ca^{2+}]_i$-sensitive conductance in the regulation of pancreatic B-cell bursting, in: "Insulin secretion and pancreatic B-cell research", P.R. Flatt and S. Lenzen, eds., Smith-Gordon, USA, pp. 181–186
7. Silva, A.M., Rosário, L.M., and Santos, R.M., 1994, Background Ca^{2+} influx mediated by a dihydropyridine- and voltage-insensitive channel in pancreatic β-cells: modulation by Ni^{2+}, diphenylamine-2-carboxylate, and glucose metabolism, J. Biol. Chem. 269: 17095–17103
8. Harkness, J.E., and Wagner, J.E., 1989, "The Biology and Medicine of Rabbits and Rodents", Lea & Febiger, Philadelphia and London
9. Atwater, I., Frankel, B.J., Rojas, E., and Grodsky, G.M., 1983, β-cell membrane potential and insulin release: role of calcium and calcium:magnesium ratio, Quart. J. Exp. Physiol. 68: 233–245

10. Valdeolmillos, M., Santos, R.M., Contreras, D., Soria, B., and Rosario, L.M., 1989, Glucose-induced oscillations of intracellular Ca^{2+} concentration resembling bursting electrical activity in single mouse islets of Langerhans, FEBS Lett. 259: 19–23
11. Santos, R.M., Rosario, L.M., Nadal, A., Garcia-Sancho, J., Soria, B., and Valdeolmillos, M., 1991, Widespread synchronous $[Ca^{2+}]_i$ oscillations due to bursting electrical activity in single pancreatic islets, Pflugers Arch. 418: 417–422
12. Rosario, L.M., Atwater, I., and Scott, A.M., 1986, Pulsatile insulin release and electrical activity from single ob/ob mouse islets of Langerhans, in: "Biophysics of the pancreatic B-cell", I. Atwater, E. Rojas and B. Soria, eds., Plenum Publishing Corporation, pp. 203–215
13. Misler, S., Gillis, K., and Tabcharani, J., 1989, Modulation of gating of a metabolically regulated, ATP-dependent K^+ channel by intracellular pH in B cells of the pancreatic islet, J. Membrane Biol. 109: 135–143
14. Rosario, L.M., and Rojas, E., 1986, Modulation of K^+ conductance by intracellular pH in pancreatic β-cells, FEBS Lett. 200: 203–209
15. Partridge, L.D., and Swandulla, D., 1988, Calcium-activated non-specific cation channels, TINS 11: 69–720
16. Sturgess, N.C., Hales, C.N., and Ashford, M.L.J., 1987, Calcium and ATP regulate the activity of a non-selective cation channel in a rat insulinoma cell line, Pflugers Arch. 409: 607–615
17. Sturgess, N.C., Carrington, C.A., Hales, C.N., and Ashford, M.L.J., 1987, Nucleotide-sensitive ion channels in human insulin producing tumour cells, Pflugers Arch. 410: 169–172
18. Gogelein, H., and Pfannmuller, B., 1989, The nonselective cation channel in the basolateral membrane of rat exocrine pancreas, Pflugers Arch. 413: 287–298
19. Cook, D.I., Poronnik, P., and Young, J.A., 1990, Characterization of a 25-pS nonselective cation channel in a cultured secretory epithelial cell line, J. Membrane Biol. 114: 37–52
20. Di Stefano, A., Wittner, M., Schlatter, E., Lang, H.J., Englert, H., and Greger, R., 1985, Diphenylamine-2-carboxylate, a blocker of the Cl^--conductive pathway in Cl^--transporting epithelia, Pflugers Arch. 405 (Suppl.1): S95–S100

6

MODULATION OF THREE TYPES OF POTASSIUM SELECTIVE CHANNELS BY NAD AND OTHER PYRIDINE NUCLEOTIDES IN HUMAN PANCREATIC β-CELLS

NAD and K^+ Channels in Human β-Cells

E. A. Harding,[1] C. Kane,[1] R. F. L. James,[2] N. J. M. London,[2] and M. J. Dunne[1]

[1]Department of Biomedical Science
The University of Sheffield
Western Bank
Sheffield, S10 2TN, United Kingdom
[2]The University of Leicester Department of Surgery
School of Medicine
Clinical Sciences Building, Leicester Royal Infirmary
Leicester, LE2 7LX, United Kingdom

INTRODUCTION

ATP-regulated potassium (K^+ATP) channels play a major role in control of the cell membrane potential in pancreatic β-cells, and therefore, nutrient-induced insulin secretion (for recent reviews see 1–4). It has been well documented that glucose-induced closure of these channels is involved in the initial depolarisation of the membrane[(5)], and widely accepted that this may occur through an increase in the intracellular ATP:ADP ratio which is responsible for coupling metabolic events to ionic events at the plasma membrane[(1,2,4)]. However, other intracellular modulators of K^+ATP channels could also be involved in the regulation of the complex cycles of electrical activity exhibited by the cells in response to glucose stimulation. Changes in the redox potential of the nicotine adenine dinucleotides NAD(P)/NAD(P)H have for many years been thought to be important intracellular signals that could mediate the effects of nutrient secretagogues on insulin secretion[(6–9)]. In more recent studies it has been demonstrated using rodent β-cells stimulated with glucose that increases in the concentration of NAD(P)H occur prior to an increase in $[Ca^{2+}]_i$[(10,11)], and also that all four of the pyridine nucleotides will modulate the gating of ATP-sensitive K^+ channels in the RINm5F insulin-secreting cell line[(12)]. Using patch clamp techniques we have now examined the effects of NAD and other pyridine nucleotides on the gating of three types of K^+ channel in human pancreatic β-cells; the K^+ATP channel, the Ca^{2+} and voltage gated channel, and a novel NAD-activated K^+ channel.

MATERIAL AND METHODS

All experiments were performed on transplantable human pancreatic β-cells isolated (with permission) from non-diabetic, heart beating cadaver organ donors. Islets of Langerhans were isolated using a collagenase digestion technique under aseptic conditions following similar procedures to those described previously[13,14]. In brief, the pancreatic duct was cannulated and the pancreas distended with 2 ml/g of collagenase solution (concentration 3 mg/ml Serva, Heidelberg, Germany). The pancreas was then placed into a stainless steel chamber and gradually warmed to 39°C whilst the chamber was gently agitated. The fluid from the chamber was sampled on a regular basis and when islets were seen and confirmed by dithizone staining, the digest was collected. Islets were purified from the digest using continuous gradients of BSA (bovine serum albumin) on a COBE 2991 cell processor and then placed into standard tissue culture conditions for short-term maintenance[13,14]. Before use, islets were hand-picked, and gentle trituration employed to dissociate them into isolated cells, and small clusters of cells. Whole islets and isolated cells were maintained for up to 16 days in RPMI 1640 tissue culture media, supplemented with 10% foetal calf serum, and 100 IU/ml penicillin and 100 μg/ml streptomycin in a humidified atmosphere of 95% O_2 and 5% CO_2 at a temperature of 37°C.

For electrophysiology studies patch clamp micropipettes were filled with a Na^+ rich solution of the following composition (mM): 140 NaCl, 4.7 KCl, 1.13 $MgCl_2$, 2.5 glucose, 10 N-[2-hydroxylethyl] piperazine-N′-[2 ethanesulphonic acid] (HEPES) and 2.5 $CaCl_2$; pH 7.4 with NaOH. Prior to experiments, the cells were repeatedly washed to remove excess tissue culture media, and upon isolation of the patch, the internal face of the membrane bathed in a K^+ rich solution containing (mM): 140 KCl, 10 NaCl, 1.13 MgCl, 2.5 glucose, 10 HEPES, and 1 EGTA; pH 7.2 with KOH. EGTA was removed from this solution and 1 μM $CaCl_2$ added when studies of NAD on the Ca^{2+}-induced activation of the K^+_{Ca} channel were investigated. The osmolality of all solutions was 290 ± 5 mosm/Kg^{-1}. All chemicals were obtained from Sigma Chemical Co. (Poole, Dorset, UK) in the $^+$ form.

RESULTS

Modulation of K^+ Channels by NAD, NADH, NADP, and NADPH

Human islets of Langerhans were isolated from two separate pancreata, as described. As in all other studies of K^+_{ATP} channels[15,16], upon forming excised patches these channels undergo spontaneous run-down or inactivation. This is demonstrated in Figure 1, a continuous current record that begins 10 seconds after forming the inside-out patch. In this particular record intracellular addition of ATP (1mM) causes channel closure and 10M concentrations of NAD, NADH, NADP and NADPH all activate K^+_{ATP} channels, partially reversing the rate of channel inactivation. Generally we found the process of K^+_{ATP} channel run-down in human β-cells to be rapid and in this typical experiment whilst we observed openings from a large number of channels upon forming the patch, 50% of the current—corresponding to probably 20 channels, was lost over the first 4 minutes of the experiment. Higher concentrations of the pyridine nucleotides had predominantly the same effect: 1mM

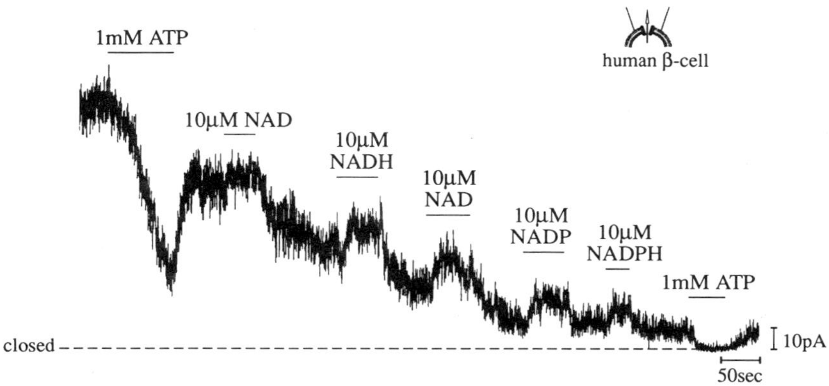

Figure 1. Activation of K^+_{ATP} channels in a human pancreatic β-cell membrane following the addition of 10M NAD, NADH, NADP and NADPH to the intracellular face of an excised inside-out patch (see cartoon). The record begins approximately 10 seconds after the patch was formed. Note how rapidly K^+_{ATP} channels run-down in human β-cells and how each of the pyridine nucleotides can reverse the effects of channel inactivation.

NAD, NADH and NADP causing channel activation, whilst 1mM NADPH evoked channel closure. Average values for their actions on K^+_{ATP} channels are shown in Figure 2A. These data indicate that only NADPH resulted in a concentration-related block (at 1mM) and activation (at 10μM) of channels. For comparison, we have also included some of our previous data for the effects of 10μM and 1mM of the pyridine nucleotides on K^+_{ATP} channels in RINm5F cells; the only other study to address the actions of these nucleotides on ion channels in insulin-secreting cells[(12)].

Pyridine-Nucleotide Dependent Gating of the Large Ca^{2+}- and Voltage-Gated K^+ Channel (K_{Ca})

Under normal testing conditions K_{Ca} channels are not operational in pancreatic β-cells. In order to record openings from these channels in excised patches, the membrane must either be depolarised or the intracellular Ca^{2+} concentration elevated. In our experiments when 1 μM Ca^{2+} was added to the inside face of the cell membrane, we found NAD was able to inhibit K_{Ca} channels in a concentration-dependent manner (1 μM–500 μM), Fig. 3A. However, if the membrane was depolarised in the presence of nominal $[Ca^{2+}]_i$, NAD had the opposite effect by promoting K^+_{Ca} channel activation, Fig. 3B. The mechanisms that underlie these effects are currently under investigation in the laboratory.

Interactions between NAD and ATP

Figures 4 and 5 summarise interactions between ATP (1mM) and NAD (1mM) on K^+ channels in human β-cells. In the record shown in Figure 4A, the data suggest that NAD can reverse the inhibitory effects of ATP on K^+_{ATP} channels by causing channel activation in the presence of 1 mM ATP. Figure 4B shows that the NAD-evoked activation of K^+_{ATP} channels can be reversed by ATP. Note how 1mM ATP will only inhibit the maximal K^+_{ATP} current to approximately 50% of the pre-control value in the presence of NAD, and how the actions of NAD are probably under-estimated because of the inherent problems of channel run-down

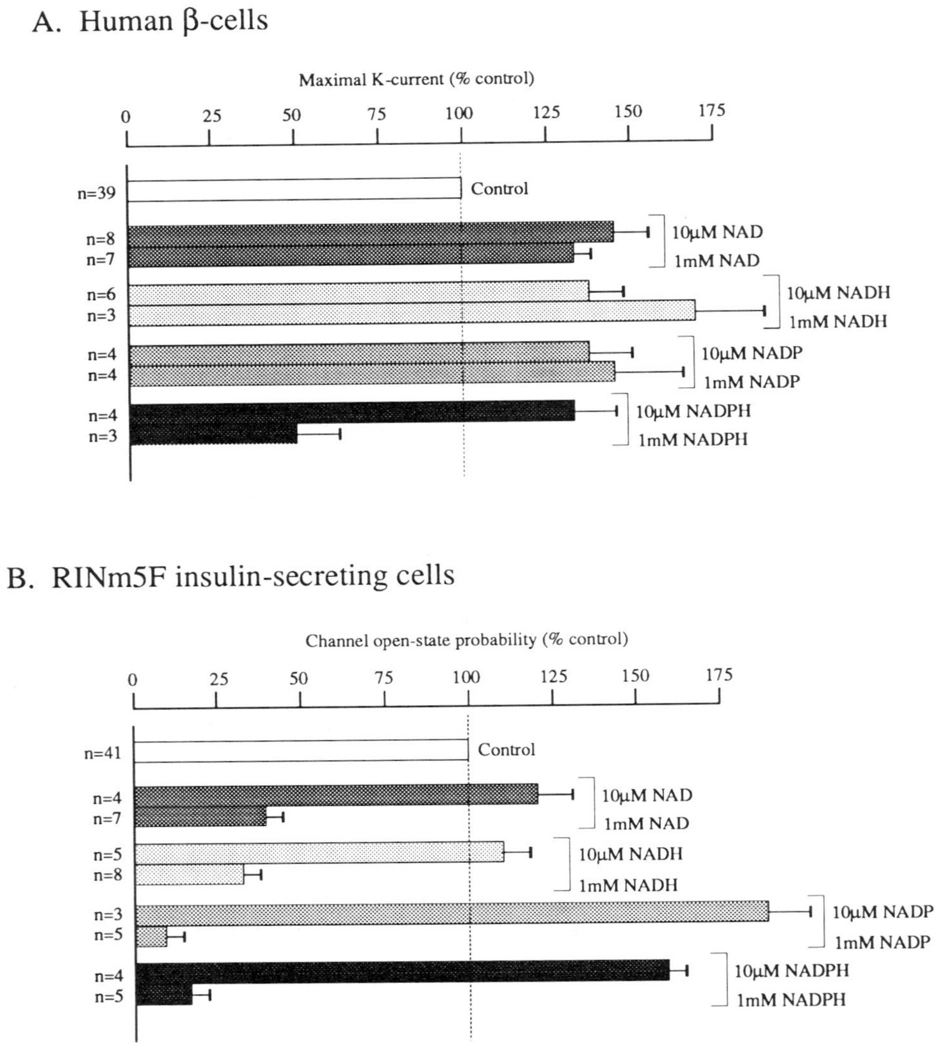

Figure 2. Average effects of 1mM and 10μM concentration of the pyridine nucleotides on K^+_{ATP} channels in human β-cells (Panel A) and RINm5F insulinoma cells (Panel B). RINm5F cell data has been re-plotted from (12) for comparative purposes.

in human β-cells, Fig 4B. In the presence of both ATP and NAD we also observed regular openings from a second type of K^+ channel (Fig. 5). This channel appeared to be activated by NAD, and exhibited different gating properties to the K^+_{ATP} channel — opening for longer periods of time, and with a much reduced conductance. Figure 5A is a extract of current data taken from the same experiment as that shown in Fig. 4A. It is evident from this trace that in the combined presence of intracellular ATP and NAD openings from several small K^+ channels (designated k_1–k_4) are recorded simultaneously with that of the K^+_{ATP} channel. (The same channel was also seen in the absence of NAD (panels 1 and 3 of Fig. 4A) but with a much reduced frequency of opening.) We can conclude that the NAD-acti-

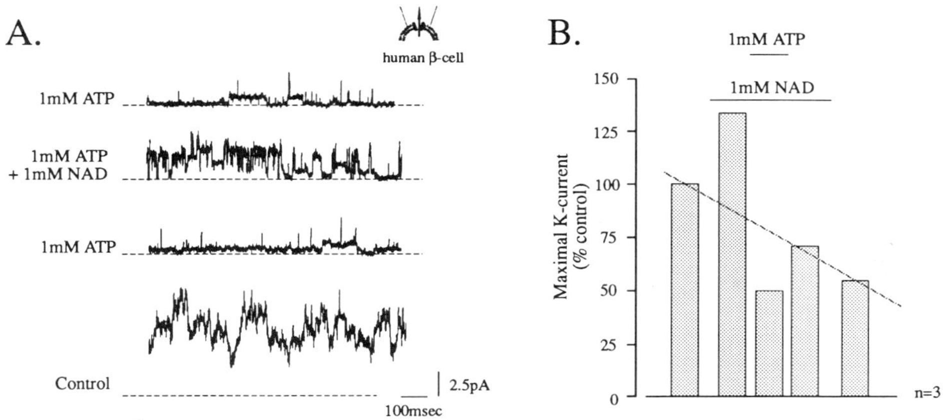

Figure 3. Modulation of K_{Ca} channels by NAD produced inhibition of channels in the presence of 1 μM $[Ca^{2+}]_i$, and activation when the membrane is depolarised in the presence of high intracellular Ca^{2+}.

vated channel is K^+ selective since under our experimental conditions only K^+ could give rise to an outward current (see 'Methods & Materials'). For comparison with the K^+_{ATP} channel the unitary current amplitude for this channel in the presence of 1mM ATP at OmV voltage-clamp was found to be approximately 0.7pA, Fig. 5B.

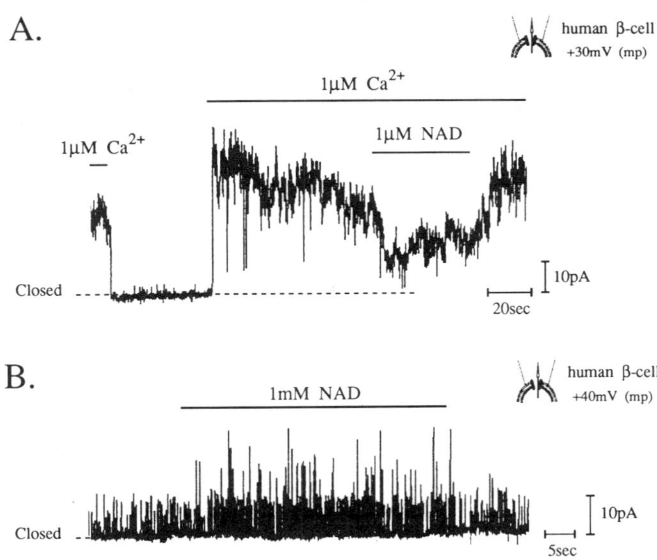

Figure 4. **Panel A:** Effects of NAD (1mM) on ATP (1mM) — inhibited K^+_{ATP} channels. All current traces are taken from the same patch over approximately 4 minutes. OP values: 0.98×10^{-3} ATP; 10.8×10^{-3} ATP + NAD. Note the appearance of a smaller K^+ selective channel in the presence of ATP and NAD. **Panel B:** Average effects of ATP on NAD-activated K^+ channels. Data were obtained from 3 separate patches. Overall the interactions between ATP and NAD are clearly represented, but because of the marked degree of channel run down in human β-cell patches, these effects are probably under-represented. A dashed line has been added to indicate the level of channel inactivation between the average maximal K-current in the initial and final control solutions.

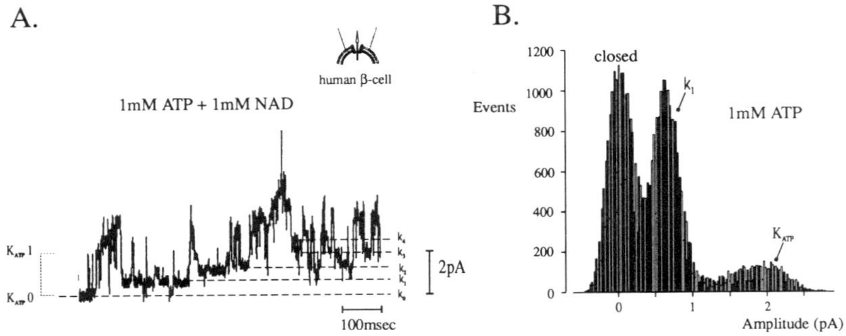

Figure 5. NAD-induced activation of a novel K^+ channel. **Panel A:** In the presence of ATP and NAD we show open events from the K^+_{ATP} channel, and several lower-conductance K^+ channels. Openings from the smaller channel are more sustained than the K^+_{ATP} channel. In this patch, taken from the same experiment shown in Fig 4A, we can identify at least four levels of coincidence from the smaller K^+ channel — designated, k_1, k_2, k_3 and k_4. **Panel B:** shows comparative amplitude histogram profiles (single-channel current amplitude vs. number of events) for the small K^+ channel (k_1) and the K^+_{ATP} channel (K^+_{ATP}). Data were obtained from an excised inside-out patch continually exposed to 1mM ATP.

DISCUSSION

This study has demonstrated for the first time the effects of pyridine nucleotides on three types of potassium selective channels in transplantable human pancreatic β-cells. Despite an extensive literature of electrophysiological events in rodent and clonal insulin-secreting cells, we know relatively little of the regulation of ion channels in human tissue[3,17–23]. One of the more important aspects of this paper, is that our data indicate differences in the nucleotide-dependent gating of K^+_{ATP} channels in human β-cells when compared to the RINm5F insulin-secreting cell line. In a previous study using the RINm5F cells, we demonstrated that low concentrations (< 100μM) of all four nucleotides caused K^+_{ATP} channel activation, whilst concentrations > 100μM promoted inhibition (summarised in Fig. 2B). Interactions between ATP and NAD were also examined in RINm5F cells, and we showed that in the presence of 1mM ATP, 1mM NAD promoted further channel inhibition[12]. Therefore in human β-cells, pyridine nucleotide-dependent gating of K^+_{ATP} channels is different in several ways: (1) NAD, NADH and NADP all activate K^+_{ATP} channels at concentrations up to 1mM, and only high concentrations of NADPH tended to close channels; (2) stimulation of K^+_{ATP} channels by NAD, NADH, and NADP was not concentration-related; (3) in the presence of ATP, 1mM NAD caused activation of channels, and not further inhibition: (4) in human β-cells we also found that NAD had complex effects on the K_{Ca} channel and (5) in the presence of ATP, NAD caused the activation of a novel K^+ channel that was not previously described in clonal cells. Despite the fact that access to human material is extremely limited and patches contained large numbers of K^+_{ATP} channels, we were able to show that the NAD-activated channel was smaller in conductance under our experimental conditions than the K^+_{ATP} channel and that it also exhibited a different pattern of channel opening and closure; in general remaining open for much longer periods than the ATP-regulated K^+ channel (Fig. 5). The NAD-activated channel is somewhat similar in conductance and gating properties to the non-selective cation channel, which has been identified in human β-cells[18] and the clonal insulin-secreting cell line CR1-G1[24].

In unstimulated rodent insulin-secreting cells the concentration of the pyridine nucleotides have been estimated to be approximately: 200–350μM for NAD, 20–70μM NADH, 30–100μM NADPH and 30–70μM NADPH (see 12 for references). If these were to be translated to the intracellular nucleotide concentrations in human β-cells, our data suggests that the pyridine nucleotides would tend to promote activation of K^+_{ATP} channels in the intact cell. In the presence of intracellular ATP the nucleotides would also cause channel activation, and this may partly explain why K^+_{ATP} channels with an apparent high sensitivity to ATP in excised patches (Ki = approximately 70μM; reviewed by 1, 2), can readily open in the intact cell where the intracellular ATP concentration far exceeds this value. Therefore the significance of our data is that we can suggest that the pyridine nucleotides, along with intracellular ADP may be responsible for reducing the sensitivity of K^+_{ATP} channels to ATP, and thereby possibly contribute to K^+_{ATP} channel-gating under basal conditions. Whether these nucleotides are involved with coupling metabolic changes in the nutrient status of the cell to electrophysiological events, is somewhat speculative at this stage. We do have evidence from this study that in the human β-cells NADPH can elicit concentration-related changes in channel activity (Fig. 2). With this data and the results of other studies carried out using rodent β-cells suggesting that glucose can induce an increase in NAD(P)H concentration, and that this precedes a rise in cytosolic Ca^{2+},[(10,11)] it is possible that the pyridine nucleotides could play an important modulatory role in the regulation of β-cell electrical activity.

ACKNOWLEDGMENTS

Human β-cell studies have been supported by the British Diabetic Association (M.J.D., R.F.L.J., N.M.J.L.), the Wellcome Trust (M.J.D.) and the University of Sheffield.

REFERENCES

1. Ashcroft, F.M., and Rorsman, P., 1989, Electrophysiology of the pancreatic β-cell, *Prog. Biophys. Mol. Biol.* 54: 87–143.
2. Dunne, M.J., and Petersen, O.H., 1991, Potassium selective ion channels in insulin secreting cells: physiology, pharmacology and their role in stimulus-secretion coupling, *Biochem. Biophys. Acta* 1071: 67–82.
3. Misler, S., Barnett, D.W., Gillis, K.D., and Pressel, D.M., 1992 , Electrophysiology of stimulus-secretion coupling in human beta-cells *Diabetes* 41: 1221–1228.
4. Dunne, M.J., Harding, E.A., Jaggar, J.H., and Squires, P.E., 1994, Ion channels and the molecular control of insulin secretion, *Biochem. Soc. Trans.* 22: 6–12.
5. Ashcroft, F.M., Harrison, D.E., and Ashcroft, S.J.H., 1984, Glucose induces closure of single potassium channels in isolated rat pancreatic beta-cells, *Nature* 312: 446–448.
6. Panten, U., Christians, J., Kriegstein, E. von, Poser, W., and Hasselblatt, A., 1973, Effects of carbohydrates upon fluorescence of reduced pyridine nucleotides from perifused isolated pancreatic islets, *Diabetologia* 9: 477–482.
7. Ashcroft, S.J.H., and Christie, M.R., 1979, Effects of glucose on the cytosolic ratio of reduced/oxidised nicotinamine-adenine di-nucleotide phosphate in rat islets of Langerhans, *Biochem J* 184: 697–700.
8. Malaisse, W.J., Hutton, J.C., Kawazu, S., Herchuelz, A., Valverde, I., and Sener, A. 1979, The stimulus secretion coupling of glucose-induced insulin release: XXXV. The links between metabolic and cationic events, *Diabetologia* 16: 331–341.
9. Matschinsky, F.M., Gosh, A.K., Meglasson, M.D., Prentki, M., June, V., and Allman, D. von, 1986, Metabolic concomitants in pure, pancreatic beta cells during glucose-stimulated insulin secretion, *J. Biol. Chem.* 261: 14057–14061.
10. Pralong, W.F., Bartley, C., and Wollheim, C.B., 1990, Single islet beta-cell stimulation by nutrients: relationship between pyridine nucleotides, cytosolic calcium and secretion, *EMBO J.* 9: 53–60.

11. Gilon, P., and Henquin, J.C., 1992, Influence of membrane potential changes on cytoplasmic calcium concentration in an electrically excitable cell, the insulin-secreting pancreatic β-cell, *J. Biol. Chem.* 267: 20713–20720.
12. Dunne, M.J., Findlay, I., and Petersen, O.H., 1988, The effects of pyridine nucleotides on the gating of ATP-sensitive K^+ channels in insulin-secreting cells, *J. Membr. Biol.* 102: 205–216.
13. London, N.J.M., James, R.F.L., and Bell, P.R.F., 1992, Islet purification. In: Pancreatic islet cell transplantation. Ed C. Ricordi, pp 113–123. RG Landes Press, UK.
14. Squires, P.E., James, R.F.L., London, N.J.M., and Dunne, M.J. 1994, ATP-induced intracellular Ca^{2+} signals in isolated human insulin-secreting cells, *Pflugers Arch.,* 427: 181–183.
15. Findlay, I., and Dunne, M.J., 1986 ATP maintains ATP-inhibited K^+ channels in an operational state, *Pflugers Arch.* 407: 238–240.
16. Misler, S., Falke, L.C., Gillis, K.D., and McDaniel, M.L., 1986, A metabolite regulated potassium channel in rat pancreatic β-cells, *Proc Natl Acad Sci USA* 83: 7119–7123.
17. Ashcroft, F.M., Kakei, M., Gibson, J.S., Gray, D.W., Sutton, R., 1989, The ATP- and tolbutamide sensitivity of the ATP-sensitive potassium channel from human pancreatic beta cells, *Diabetologia* 32: 591–598.
18. Misler, S., Gee, W.M., Gillis, K.D., Scharp, D.W., Falke, L.C., 1989, Metabolite-regulated ATP-sensitive potassium channel in human pancreatic islet cells, *Diabetes* 38: 422–427.
19. Pressel, D.M., and Misler, S., 1990, Sodium channels contribute to action potential generation in canine and human pancreatic islet B cells, *J. Membr. Biol.* 116: 273–280.
20. Kelly, R.P., Sutton, R., and Ashcroft, F.M., 1991, Voltage-activated calcium and potassium currents in human pancreatic beta-cells, *J. Physiol.* 443: 175–192.
21. Misler, S., Barnett, D.W., and Falke, L.C., 1992, Effects of metabolic inhibition by sodium azide on stimulus-secretion coupling in β-cells of human islets of Langerhans, *Pflugers Arch.* 421: 289–291.
22. Misler, S., Barnett, D.W., Pressel, D.M., Gillis, K.D., Scharp, D.W., Falke, L.C., 1992, Stimulus-secretion coupling in beta-cells of transplantable human islets of Langerhans: Evidence for a critical role for calcium entry, *Diabetes* 41: 662–670.
23. Williams, B.A., Smith, P.A., Leow, K., Shimizu, S., Gray, D.W., and Ashcroft, F.M. 1993, Two types of potassium channel regulated by ATP in pancreatic β-cells isolated from a type-2 diabetic human, *Pflugers Arch.* 423: 265–273.
24. Sturgess, N.C., Hales, C.N., and Ashford, M.L.J., 1986, Inhibition of a calcium-activated non-selective cation channel in a rat insulinoma cell line, by adenine derivatives, *FEBS Letts* 208: 397–400.

7

NOVEL ACTIONS OF THE POTASSIUM CHANNEL MODULATOR SDZ PCO 400 ON ATP-REGULATED POTASSIUM CHANNELS IN INSULIN SECRETING CELLS

SDZ PCO 400 and β-Cells

E. A. Harding and M. J. Dunne

Cell Biology Research Group
Department of Biomedical Science
The University
Sheffield, S10 2TN, United Kingdom

INTRODUCTION

Potassium channel openers are a novel group of compounds that have potent effects upon a number of tissues. In general, their actions are most pronounced in smooth muscle cells, where they may prove to be an important group of agents effective against a number of pathophysiological disorders such as angina, hypertension, genitourinary dysfunction, asthma, etc. (for reviews see references 1 and 2). Despite the fact that diazoxide was the first synthetic compound shown to be directly capable of opening potassium ion channels[(3,4)], prominent interest in the K^+ channel modulators was only stimulated when the physiological and pharmacological effects of cromakalim (BRL 34915) were first described[(5,6)]. Since then, cromakalim, and its active enantiomer levcromakalim, have become widely accepted as the 'prototypical molecule,' although there are several other structures capable of modulating K^+ channels e.g. pinacidil, nicorandil, RP 49356, BPDZ44, etc.[(1,2,7)], see Table 1. Through the activation of K^+ channels, these compounds elicit a marked hyperpolarisation of the cell membrane potential, leading to the inhibition of voltage-gated calcium channels and a subsequent lowering of the free intracellular calcium ion concentration ($[Ca^{2+}_i]$). The principal site of action of the K^+ channel activators is the ATP-gated potassium (K^+ATP) channel. As has been well documented, this group of K^+ channels play an important role in the regulation of insulin secretion from the β-cells of the pancreatic islets of Langerhans (for reviews see 8–11). Glucose-induced closure of K^+_{ATP} channels initiates a depolarisation of the membrane, and the opening of voltage-gated Ca^{2+} channels[(12)]. Diazoxide and several other K^+ channels modulators therefore

Physiology and Pathophysiology of the Islets of Langerhans, edited by Soria.
Plenum Press, New York, 1997.

Table 1. Typical synthetic potassium channel openers

Chemical class	Member	Source
Benzothiadiazine	Diazoxide	Schering
Benzopyran	Cromakalim	SmithKline Beecham
	SR 44866	Sanofi
	SDZ PCO-400	Sandoz
Nicotinamide	Nicorandil	Chugai
Cyanoguanidine	Pinacidil	Leo
Thioformamide	RP 49356	Rhone Poulenc
Pyridothiadiazine	BPDZ 44	see Pirotte et al., 1993

inhibit secretion by promoting a hyperpolarisation of the membrane[13]. In β-cells even though the precise nature of the interaction with the K^{+}_{ATP} channel is unknown, the actions of diazoxide, cromakalim and other K^{+} channel modulators have been described[4,14–20]. In a recent series of experiments we have been studying the action of compounds analogous in structure to the more established K^{+} channel openers. Using human and rodent β-cells, we have described how the pyridothiadizine BPDZ44 — a compound structurally analogous to diazoxide[21] will act as a potent activator of K^{+}_{ATP} channels[22] and in this paper we describe effects of a levcromakalim analogue — SDZ PCO 400, on insulin-secreting cells. Both SDZ PCO 400 and levcromakalim are benzopyran derivatives, but differ in structure at the fourth substituted carbon on the pyran ring (Figure 1)[7,23]. Like levcromakalim, SDZ PCO 400 has marked effects on airways and vascular smooth muscle cells tone[24,25], however, unlike levcromakalim we find that in insulin-secreting cells, SDZ PCO 400 is an inhibitor of ATP-regulated K^{+} channels.

METHODS AND MATERIALS

Experiments were performed either upon the clonal insulin-secreting cell line RINm5F, or upon primary cultured rat pancreatic β-cells. Islets of Langerhans were isolated from fed male Wistar rats (180–220 g body weight) following described procedures[26] and cultured overnight in RPMI 1640 tissue culture media supplemented with 10% (v/v) heat-inactivated foetal calf serum, 100 U penicillin/ml and 100 μg streptomycin/ml. The patch clamp technique was used to examine the effects of SDZ PCO 400 upon; (i) individual ion channel currents using excised inside-out patches and open-cells, and (ii) changes in the cell

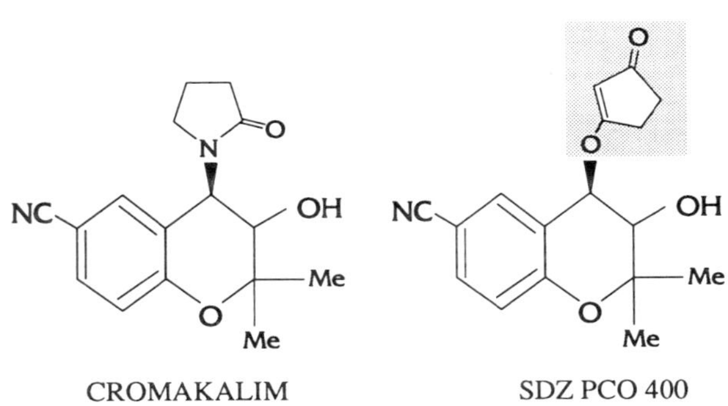

Figure 1. Schematic diagram of the benzopyrans cromakalim (levcromakalim) and SDZ PCO 400.

membrane potential using the whole-cell current-clamp recording configuration. The extracellular Na^+ rich solution used throughout these experiments contained (mM): 140 NaCl, 4.7 KCl, 1.13 $MgCl_2$, 2.5 $CaCl_2$ and 10 HEPES. The pH was adjusted to 7.2 with NaOH. This solution was used to fill the patch-clamp pipette during single-channel current experiments and was added to the bath for whole-cell studies. The standard K^+-rich solution contained (mM): 140 KCl, 10 NaCl, 1.13 $MgCl_2$, 10 HEPES and 1 EGTA. No $CaCl_2$ was added and the pH was adjusted to 7.2 using KOH. This solution was used in the bath for inside-out and open-cell experiments, and was added to the pipette solution along with 1 mM ATP for whole-cell studies. All experiments were carried out at ambient temperature. Stock solutions of SDZ PCO 400 (a gift from Sandoz Pharmaceuticals, Basel, Switzerland), diazoxide and tolbutamide were made up in dimethylsulphoxide (DMSO).

Insulin secretion was assessed by radioimmunoassay. Prior to experimentation the islets of Langerhans were removed from tissue culture and placed into isolation media for 1 hour. Insulin secretion in response to 2 mM or 20 mM glucose containing 50 μM or 100 μM SDZ PCO 400, or 100 μM diazoxide was determined using static incubations (3 islets/ 0.6 ml media for 60 minutes). After this period, 200 μl of the incubation media was diluted to 1ml with borate buffer (containing (mM); 133 boric acid, 68 NaOH, 15 Na azide, 10 EDTA, and 1 g/lt. BSA at pH 8.0), and stored at −70°C. The insulin content of the islets was determined by sonication (1 min, 120 Watts) of 10–20 cultured islets in 200μl acidified ethanol (absolute ethanol:H_2O:concentrated HCl 52:17:1 (v/v)), followed by 20–40 hours extraction at 4°C. The extract was then centrifuged for 5 minutes at 11,500 rpm and finally diluted 1:100, 1:200, 1:400, 1:800 with borate buffer. Insulin release and total cellular insulin were determined using a standard radioimmunoassay protocol. Iodinated insulin (70 TBq-mMol), insulin antibodies and insulin standard were supplied as a gift by Dr. Peter Jones of the Dept Biomedical Sciences, King's College, London. A standard curve was set up for each radioimmunoassay (10–0.08 ng/ml of rat insulin standard, approximately 10,000 cpm/tube, and 100 μl insulin antibody). Unknowns were sampled in duplicate, with reference tubes for non-specific binding, maximum binding and total radioactivity being performed in triplicate. All tubes were mixed and incubated for 60–72 hours at 4°C to reach equilibrium. The reaction was terminated by addition of 1 ml of fresh precipitating buffer to each tube, except the totals. The precipitating solution consisted of phosphosaline buffer (containing (mM); 19 NaCl, 7.8 NaH_2PO_4, 0.7 KH_2PO_4), and an equal volume of 30% aqueous polyethylene glycol, 1 mg/ml gamma globulins, and 0.05% Tween. The antibody/antigen complex was obtained by centrifugation in an MSE Coolspin at 2,100 rpm, 4°C for 30 minutes, followed by removal of the supernatant using a vacuum pump. The pellet radioactivity was then measured using a Rackgamma counter and the results expressed as a log-logit plot (log bound antigen/antibody divided by maximum bound value, versus insulin concentration ng/ml).

RESULTS

Standard patch-clamp whole-cell recordings of individual RINm5F cells were used to examine the actions of 50–100 μM SDZ PCO 400, phentolamine (5 μM) and tolbutamide (50 μM) on the cell electrical activity. The resting transmembrane potential was found to be approximately −65/−70 mV (−66 ± 5 mV, n = 12). In the record shown in Figure 2, membrane potential data begins 5 minutes after forming the nystatin-perforated patch. At the points indicated 5 μM phentolamine and 50 μM SDZ PCO 400 were added to the bath solution, and the cell underwent a sharp, sustained depolarisation which was

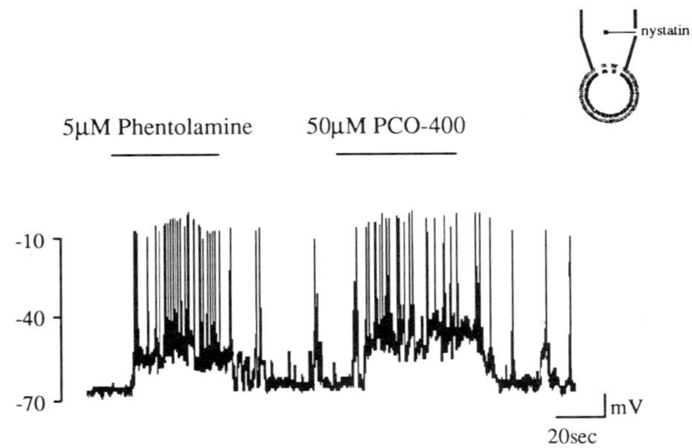

Figure 2. Effects of phentolamine (5 μM) and SDZ PCO 400 (50 μM) on the cell electrical activity of an individual RINm5F cell. Data was obtained using the perforated patch-clamp technique with the cell bathed in a 140 mM NaCl-rich solution containing 2.5 mM glucose. Both phentolamine and SDZ PCO 400 elicit a sharp depolarisation of the membrane and the generation of action potential-like spikes.

associated with the rapid generation of Ca^{2+} action potentials. This finding is in marked contrast to the action of diazoxide and other K^+ channel openers in these cells which have been previously shown to abolish glucose-induced changes in the cell electrical activity and elevation of $[Ca^{2+}]_i$[27]. The magnitude of the SDZ PCO 400-induced depolarisation — on average 28 ± 3 mV (mean ± S.E.M.) (n = 8) was similar to that evoked by either phentolamine (5 μM) 29 ± 5 mV (n = 6) or tolbutamide (50 μM) 25 ± 3 mV (n = 5).

As the overall effects of tolbutamide and phentolamine on insulin-secreting cells have previously been shown to be mediate through closure of ATP-regulated K^+ channels[28,29], inside-out patches and open-cells were used to examine the effects of SDZ PCO 400 on individual K^+_{ATP} channel current events. From these experiments we found that SDZ PCO 400 inhibited K^+_{ATP} channels, Figure 3. In other studies we have also shown that

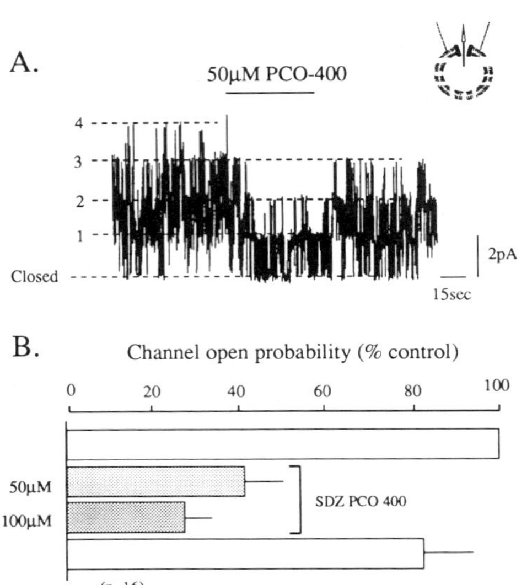

Figure 3. A–B. Inhibition of ATP-regulated K^+ channels by SDZ PCO 400. Single-channel current data in panel A commences approximately 35 minutes after the recording configuration was established. The maximum number of coincident channel openings in the patch was 14. As the record begins, at least 4 channels were operational. Channel open-state probability was significantly, and reversibly reduced by the addition of SDZ PCO 400 to the inside face of the membrane: control = 0.08, SDZ PCO 400 = 0.03, control = 0.06. Data in panel B shows average effects of SDZ PCO 400 (50–100 μM) on K^+_{ATP} channels. Data were obtained from 16 separate patches exposed to both 50 and 100 μM SDZ PCO 400. Values for changes in open-state probability (mean ± S.E.M.) have been expressed a fraction of the pre-control value (100%).

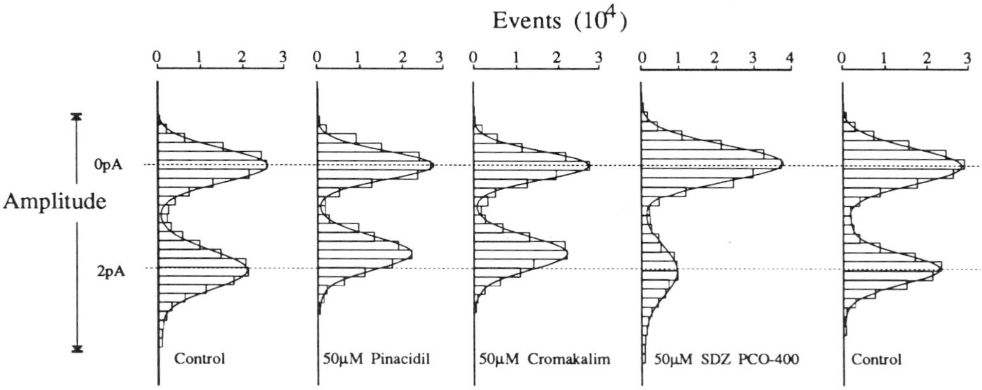

Figure 4. Effects of 50 μM SDZ PC0 400, cromakalim and pinacidil on single-channel current amplitude. All plots come from the same inside-out patch of membrane. A maximum of 3 coincident channel events were seen as the patch was formed, but for the sake of clarity, our analysis was restricted to that part of the experiment when only a single channel was operational. Each plot was composed from a minimum of 40 seconds of continuous data.

under certain experimental conditions, both diazoxide[(4)] and K^+ channel openers[(16)] will block ATP-sensitive K^+ channels. These effects only occur if the compounds are added to the internal face of the membrane in the absence of cytosolic ATP, and are associated with a decrease in the amplitude of the single-channel current events [there is no change in channel open-state probability under these conditions[(4,16)]]. As SDZ PCO 400 inhibits K^+_{ATP} channels in the absence and the presence of internal ATP (n = 4), we therefore examined in more detail the mechanism of channel inhibition. Figure 4 shows data from an inside-out patch and summarises the actions of 50 μM concentrations of SDZ PCO 400, cromakalim and pinacidil on the amplitude of K^+_{ATP} single channel current events. In this experiment a maximum of 3 coincident K^+_{ATP} channels openings were seen within seconds of forming the recording configuration, but our analysis was only performed when 1 channel was operational. From the plot of current amplitude vs. frequency of events, it is clear that in both the control situation and in the presence of SDZ PCO 400, open events occur at approximately 2 pA [with SDZ PCO 400 more events are recorded at zero pA consistent with a decrease in channel open-state probability]. However, in the presence of both pinacidil and cromakalim openings occur with a reduced amplitude — on average 1.6 ± 0.03 pA (n = 6) (mean ± S.E.M.), indicating that both compounds are able to induce block of K^+_{ATP} channels. Finally, insulin radioimmunoassay studies were carried out in order to examine the effects of SDZ PCO 400 on secretion from isolated rat islets of Langerhans. The results of these experiments are summarised in Figure 5. Over the concentration range 50 and 100 μM we found that despite its action of ion channels and the cell membrane potential in RINm5F cells, SDZ PCO 400 had no significant influence upon either basal (2 mM) or 20 mM-glucose stimulated insulin secretion, whereas 100 μM diazoxide markedly inhibited glucose-induced secretion under the same conditions.

DISCUSSION

The physiological and pharmacological effects of K^+ channel openers and their mechanisms of action have been widely studied and extensively reviewed. What is unique

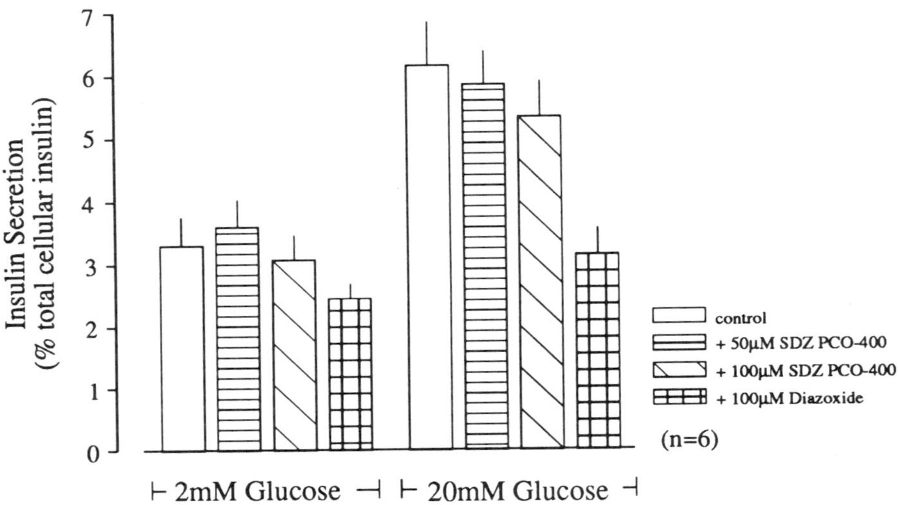

Figure 5. Effects of SDZ PC0 400 and diazoxide on basal and glucose-stimulated insulin secretion from isolated rat islets of Langerhans. Values have been expressed as a fraction of total cellular insulin content for 50 and 100 μM SDZ PCO 400 and 100 μM diazoxide on unstimulated, and 20 mM glucose-stimulated islets of Langerhans. Data points, expressed as mean ± S.E.M., were obtained from 6 separate animals (n = 6) with multiple assays per animal.

about these type of compounds, is their ability to hyperpolarise the cell membrane, and thereby prevent the voltage-gated entry of Ca^{2+} into the cell, whilst also preventing mobilization of $[Ca^{2+}]_i$[30]. Many K^+ channel modulators are effective at activating K^+_{ATP} channels in pancreatic β-cells; diazoxide, cromakalim, nicorandil, pinacidil, RP49356, etc[14,16,27]. As we have recently found that the diazoxide analogue BPDZ44 is more potent at activating these channels than diazoxide[22] it was therefore somewhat surprising to find that the benzopyran SDZ PCO 400 — a molecule very similar in structure to cromakalim (Fig. 1), was in fact able to inhibit and not activate K^+_{ATP} channels in these cells. These actions explain the pronounced depolarisation of the cell membrane potential shown in Fig. 2. It is important to point out that the action of SDZ PCO 400 on K^+_{ATP} channels in insulin-secreting cells occurs at 10–50 fold higher concentrations than those used to relax airways smooth muscle[24,25] and there were no effects of SDZ PCO 400 on K^+ channels below 50 μM, with or without ATP present. Nevertheless the actions of SDZ PCO 400 were consistent, reproducible and certainly intriguing. We have previously shown for diazoxide and other K^+ channel openers, that under certain experimental conditions these compounds will also inhibit K^+_{ATP} channels. This occurs through a mechanism associated with a reduction in the single-channel current amplitude and may be evidence that these compounds bind to, or interact with a site on the channel closely associated with the pore of the ion channel[20]. In this study, we have therefore closely compared the effects of SDZ PCO 400, cromakalim and pinacidil in a number of patches, and whilst these experiments re-affirmed the blocking action of pinacidil and cromakalim, they also demonstrated that SDZ PCO 400 mediates its effects by different mechanism(s); not through changes in the amplitude of single channel currents, but by reducing channel open-state probability (Fig 4). Our data also indicate that although SDZ PCO 400 is a novel modulator of K^+_{ATP} channels in the β-cell, it has relatively little influence upon the secretory responses of the rat pancreatic islets of Langerhans (Figure 5).

We can suggest that even though there were effects of SDZ PCO 400 on changes in the cell electrical activity in individual cells, these actions are not potent enough to elicit secretion from the intact islet of Langerhans at similar concentrations. This is in agreement with in vivo studies which indicate that at concentrations used to promote vasodilation there is no effect upon blood glucose levels[31].

In summary, SDZ PCO 400 is a novel regulator of K^+_{ATP} channels, effective as a vasodilator in smooth muscle tissues, but having an inhibitory effect on K^+_{ATP} channels in the β-cell. One of the major implications of these data is that it extends the suggestion[32] that K^+_{ATP} channels have discrete pharmacology in different tissues. This was based upon the observations that, diazoxide, one of the most effective β-cell channel modulators, is in fact an inhibitor of myocardial K^+_{ATP} channels.

ACKNOWLEDGMENTS

We are very grateful to Drs Peter Jones and Shanta Persaud, MRC Research Fellows at Department of Biomedical Science, Kings College (Kensington), The University of London, for their help in establishing radioimmunoassay techniques in our laboratory. Experiments were supported by project grants to MJD from the Wellcome Trust, The British Diabetic Association, The Yorkshire Cancer Research Campaign and the University of Sheffield. EAH is a BDA-funded research fellow.

REFERENCES

1. Cook, N.S., 1988, The pharmacology of potassium channels and their therapeutic potential. *Trends Pharmacol. Sci.* 9: 21–28.
2. Quast, U., and Cook, NS, 1989, Moving together, K^+ channel openers and ATP-sensitive K^+ channels, *Trends in Pharmacol. Sci.* 10: 431–435.
3. Trube, g., Rorsman, p., and Ohno-Shosaku, T., 1986, Opposite effects of tolbutamide and diazoxide on the ATP-dependent K^+ channel in mouse pancreatic β-cells, *Pflugers Arch.* 407: 493–499.
4. Dunne, M.J., Ilott, M.C., and Petersen, O.H., 1987, Interactions of diazoxide, tolbutamide and ATP^{4-} on nucleotide-dependent K^+ channels in an insulin-secreting cell line, *J. Membr. Biol.* 99: 215–224.
5. Hamilton, T.C., Weir, S.W., and Weston, A.H., 1986, Comparison of the effects of BRL 34915 and verapamil on electrical and mechanical activity in rat portal vein, *Br. J. Pharmacol.* 88: 103–111.
6. Weir, S.W., and Weston, A.H., 1986, The effects of BRL34915 and nicorandil on electrical and mechanical activity and on $^{86}Rb^+$ efflux in rat blood vessels, *Br. J. Pharmacol.* 88: 113–120.
7. Edwards, G., and Weston, A.H., 1990, Structure-activity relationships of K^+ channel openers, Trends Pharmacol. Sci. 11: 417–423.
8. Petersen, O.H., and Findlay, I., 1987, Electrophysiology of the pancreas, *Physiol. Rev.* 67: 1054–1116.
9. Ashcroft F.M., and Rorsman P., 1989, Electrophysiology of the pancreatic β-cell, *Prog. Biophys. Mol. Biol.* 54: 87–143.
10. Dunne, M.J., and Petersen, O.H., 1991, Potassium selective ion channels in insulin-secreting cells, physiology, pharmacology and their role in stimulus-secretion coupling, *Biochim. Biophys. Acta* 1071: 67–82.
11. Lebrun, P., Antoine M.-H., and Herchuelz, A., 1992, Mini review: K^+ channel openers and insulin release, *Life Sciences* 51: 795.
12. Ashcroft, F.M., Harrison, D.E., and Ashcroft, S.J.H., 1984, Glucose induces closure of single potassium channels in isolated rat pancreatic β-cells, *Nature* 312: 446–448.
13. Henquin, J.C., and Meissner, H.P., 1982, Opposite effects of tolbutamide and diazoxide on ^{86}Rb fluxes and membrane potential in mouse pancreatic B-cells, *Biochemical Pharmacology* 31: 1407–1413.
14. Dunne, M.J., Aspinall, R.J., and Petersen, O.H., 1990a, Cromakalim (BRL 34915) opens ATP-sensitive potassium channels in insulin-secreting cells, *Br. J. Pharmacol.* 99: 169–175.
15. Dunne, M.J., 1989, Protein phosphorylation is required for diazoxide to open ATP-sensitive potassium channels in insulin (RINm5F) secreting cells, *FEBS Lett.* 250: 262–266.

16. Dunne, M.J., 1990, Effects of pinacidil, RP 49356 and nicorandil on ATP-sensitive potassium channels in insulin-secreting cells, *Br. J. Pharmacol.* 99: 487–492.
17. Kozlowski, R.Z., Hales, C.N., and Ashford, M.L.J., 1989, Dual effects of diazoxide on ATP-K^+ currents recorded from an insulin-secreting cell line. *Br. J. Pharmacol.* 97: 1039–1050.
18. Kozlowski, R.Z., and Ashford, M.L.J., 1992, Nucleotide-dependent activation of K^+_{ATP} channels by diazoxide in CRI-GI insulin-secreting cells. *Br. J. Pharmacol.* 107: 34–43.
19. Harding, E.A., Jaggar, J.H., Ayton, B.J., and Dunne, M.J. 1993, Properties of diazoxide and cromakalim-induced activation of potassium channels in insulin-secreting cells; Effects of GTP, *Exp. Physiol.* 78: 25–34.
20. Jaggar, J.H., Harding, E.A., Ayton, B.J., and Dunne, M.J., 1993, Interaction of diazoxide and cromakalim with ATP-regulated potassium channels in insulin-secreting cells, *J. Mol. Endocrinol* 10: 59–70.
21. Pirotte, B., De Tullio, P., Lebrun, P., Antoine, M.-H., Masereel, B., Schynts, M., Dupont, L., Herchuelz, A., and Delarge, J., 1993, 3-Alkylamino-4H-pyrido[4,3-e][1,2,4]thiadiazine 1,1-dioxides as powerful inhibitors of insulin release from pancreatic B cells, *J. Med. Chem.* 36: 3211.
22. Kane, C., Harding, E.A., Antoine, M.-H., Lebrun, P., Pirotte, B., James, R.F.L., Johnson, P.R.V., Lindley, K.J., and Dunne, M.J., 1995, Activation of potassium channels in human and rodent β-cells by BPDZ-44 and BPDZ-62 — mechanisms of action and effect in human neonatal nesidioblastosis, *Diabetologia* 38: A24.
23. Evans, J.M., Hadley, M.S., and Stemp, G., 1992, Potassium channel activators, Structure-activity relationships. In: Potassium Channel Modulators, by A.H. Weston and T.C. Hamilton, pp 341–368. Blackwell, UK.
24. Chapman, I.D., Kristersson, A., Meathelin, G., Schaemblin, E., Mazzoni, L., Boubekeur, K., Murphy, N., and Morley, J., 1992, Effects of a potassium channel activator (SDZ PCO 400) on guinea pig and human pulmonary airways, *Br. J. Pharmacol.* 106: 423–429.
25. Small, R.C., Berry, J.L., Foster, R.W., Blarer, S., and Quast, U., 1992, Analysis of the relaxant action of SDZ PCO 400 in airway smooth muscle from ox and guinea pig, *Eur. J. Pharmacol.* 219: 81–88.
26. Sutton, R., Peters, M., McShane, P., Gray, D.W.R., and Morris, P.J., 1986, Isolation of pancreatic islets by ductal injection of collaginase, *Transplantation* 42: 689–691.
27. Dunne, M.J., Yule, D.I., Gallacher, D.V., and Petersen, O.H., 1990b, A comparative study of the effects of cromakalim BRL 34915., and diazoxide on membrane potential, $[Ca^{2+}]_i$ and ATP-sensitive potassium currents in insulin-secreting cells, *J. Membr. Biol.*, 114: 54–61.
28. Sturgess, N., Ashford, M.L.J., Cook, D.L., and Hales, C.N., 1985, The sulphonylurea receptor may be an ATP-sensitive potassium channel, *Lancet* 8453: 474–475.
29. Dunne, M.J. 1991, Block of ATP-regulated potassium channels by phentolamine and other α-adrenoceptor antagonists, *Br. J. Pharmacol.* 103: 1847–1850.
30. Quast, U., 1993, Do the K^+ channel openers relax smooth muscle by opening K^+ channels? *Trends in Pharmacol. Sci.*, 14: 332–337.
31. Fozard, J.R., Menninger, K., Cook, N.S., Blarer, S., and Quast, U., 1990, The cardiovascular effects of SDZ PCO-400 in vivo, *Br. J. Pharmacol.* 99: 77P.
32. Faivre, J.-J., and Findlay, I., 1989, Effects of tolbutamide, glibenclamide and diazoxide upon action potentials recorded from rat ventricular muscle, *Biochim. Biophys. Acta* 984: 1–5.

8

EFFECTS OF PROTEIN PHOSPHORYLATION ON THE SULPHONYLUREA RECEPTOR OF THE PANCREATIC β-CELL

Ichiro Niki,* Barbara Coles, Frances M. Ashcroft and Stephen J. H. Ashcroft

Nuffield Department of Clinical Biochemistry
John Radcliffe Hospital Headington
Oxford OX3 9DU, United Kingdom
University Laboratory of Physiology
Parks Road, Oxford OX3 1PT, United Kingdom

INTRODUCTION

There is evidence that protein phosphorylation may modulate the action of diazoxide on the β-cell K-ATP channel [1] and the sulphonylurea receptor [2–3]. In this paper, we have further investigated the role of phosphorylation in the action of diazoxide on the β-cell sulphonylurea receptor by carrying out time-course studies on inhibition of [^{3}H]-glibenclamide binding by MgATP and diazoxide, and by examining effects of phosphatase inhibitors on binding. We also investigated the presence of protein kinase and protein phosphatase activities in β-cell membrane fractions.

METHODS

HIT T15 β-cells (passage numbers 80–95) were cultured [4] and membranes were prepared[5] as previously described. For measurement of [^{3}H]-glibenclamide binding to isolated membranes, aliquots of HIT cell membranes (150–200 μg protein/ml) were incubated for 5–120 min at 37°C with [^{3}H]-glibenclamide in 0.24 ml (final volume) of 0.1 mM $CaCl_2$/50 mM-MOPS (pH 7.4 with NaOH) in the presence or absence of test substances. In some experiments, okadaic acid, microcystin or NaF were added at 15 min after the start of the incubation. EDTA when added was at a final concentration of 0.25 mM. Bound radioactivity was separated from free by rapid filtration on Whatman GF/F filters which were then washed four times with 5 ml of distilled water at 4°C. Non-specific binding was

* Dr. Niki's present address: Dept. of Pharmacology, Nagoya University School of Medicine, Japan.

taken as the residual binding in the presence of 1 μM unlabelled glibenclamide. HIT cell membranes were solubilised by incubation for 1 hr at 4°C in 50 mM-Tris (pH 8)/ 10% (vol/vol) glycerol containing 2% CHAPS plus the protease inhibitors 0.2 mM-phenyl-methyl-sulphonylfluoride, 1 mM-EDTA, 1 mM-benzamidine, 10 μM-leupeptin and 1 mM-iodoacetamide. The membranes were spun at 100,000 g for 40 min and the supernatant was retained for binding studies [5].

Solubilized HIT cell membranes (approximately 0.5 mg protein/ml final concentration) were incubated in 0.5 ml (final volume) of the same buffer containing 0.8% CHAPS for 60 min at 4°C with 3–4 nM [^{3}H]-glibenclamide in the presence or absence of test substances. [^{3}H]- Glibenclamide binding of solubilized fractions was assayed by rapid gel filtration [5].

For assay of ATPase activity [6], HIT cell membranes (200 μg protein/ml) were incubated for up to 2 h at 37°C in 0.1 mM-$CaCl_2$/50 mM-MOPS (pH 7.4 with NaOH) containing 0.1–1 mM MgATP and [γ-^{32}P]-ATP (6.6 dpm/pmol). At the end of the incubation, 100 μl of the assay mixture were added to 1 ml of 5 mg/ml charcoal suspended in 1 N-HCl. Samples were vortexed and spun down at 10,000 g for 2 min. Radioactivity in the supernatant was counted.

For phosphorylation studies, 100 μl of membranes (400 μg protein) were incubated at 25°C with 125 μl of incubation buffer (pH 7.4) containing 40 mM MOPS/0.25 mM EGTA/5 mM $MgCl_2$. Inhibitors and distilled water were added as appropriate to give a final volume of 250 μl. In some experiments $MgCl_2$ was omitted from the incubation buffer, or 2 mM-EDTA was added. Phosphorylation was started by the addition of 3 μl of 5 mM [γ-^{32}P]-ATP (1 μCi), giving a final ATP concentration of 60 μM. Aliquots were removed at intervals and added to a sample buffer to give a final concentration of 62.5 mM-Tris-HCl (pH 6.8)/2% SDS/10% glycerol/5% mercaptoethanol/0.002% bromophenol blue, and boiled for 2–3 min. Samples were analysed using 8% acrylamide gels with a 4% stacking gel and stained with Coomasie Brilliant Blue R-250. Phosphoproteins were detected by autoradiography using Kodak X-Omat AR-5 film. In some experiments membranes were incubated with 5 mM [α-^{32}P]-ATP instead of [γ-^{32}P]-ATP.

To study the effects of phosphatases on dephosphorylation, membranes were first phosphorylated by incubation in incubation buffer with 3 μl of 5 mM [γ-^{32}P]-ATP for 5 min at 25°C. An aliquot was then removed and processed as above. A phosphatase inhibitor (or distilled water) was added to the remainder of the sample, which was incubated for a further 30 mins. Aliquots were then removed and processed as above.

All gels shown are representative of two to four similar experiments.

RESULTS

ATPase Activity of HIT Cell Membranes

[^{32}P]-phosphate release from [γ-^{32}P]-ATP was measured during a 120 min incubation. In the presence of 100 μM, 300 μM and 1 mM ATP, HIT cell membranes hydrolysed ATP completely by the end of 15, 30 and 120 min incubations, respectively (Fig 1).

[^{3}H]-Glibenclamide Binding to HIT Cell Membranes

Fig 2 shows the time-course of binding of [3H]-glibenclamide to HIT cell membranes over a period of 5–120 min in the absence or presence of different concentrations of MgATP. The same batch of the membranes as that used for the measurement of ATPase

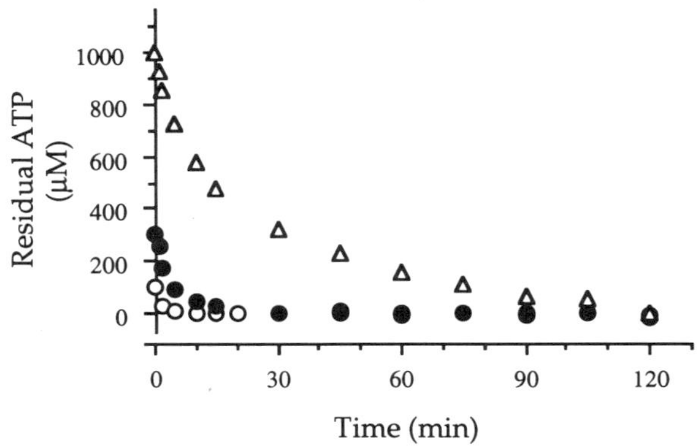

Figure 1. Time-course of ATP hydrolysis by HIT cell membranes. HIT cell membranes (200 μg/ml) were incubated for 1–120 min at 37°C in the presence of 100 μM (○), 300 μM (●), or 1 mM (△) ATP. [^{32}P]-phosphate released from [γ-^{32}P]-ATP was assayed using charcoal separation. Each symbol is the mean of duplicate determinations.

activity was used in these studies. When membranes were incubated at 37°C in the absence of MgATP, binding was maximal at 30–60 min and a slow decrease was observed after 1 hr. This decline was not obvious when membranes were incubated at room temperature (data not shown). MgATP caused a dose- and time-dependent inhibition of binding. Inhibition of binding by 100 or 300 μM MgATP disappeared at 30 min or 90 min after the start of the incubation, respectively, whereas 1 mM-MgATP caused persistent inhibition of binding throughout a 2 hr incubation. At all these concentrations of MgATP, further inhibition of binding was observed in the simultaneous presence of 300 μM-diazoxide. Inhibition by diazoxide was no longer evident after 60 min with 100 μM-MgATP but was still apparent after 2 h for the two higher ATP concentrations.

When similar experiments were carried out using ATP-γS instead of ATP (Fig. 3), a small inhibition of [^{3}H]-glibenclamide binding (which reached significance at 30 min) was observed with 1 mM-MgATP-γS, but 300 μM-MgATP-γS was ineffective. However, at both concentrations this ATP analogue was able to reveal inhibition of binding by 300 μM-diazoxide. In the presence of MgATP-γS, inhibition by diazoxide persisted for 120 min.

Studies to assess whether MgATP must be present throughout the incubation for diazoxide to be effective, as would be expected if the drug worked by activation of a protein kinase, are shown in Table 1. The maximum binding measured in control samples after a 15 min incubation was reduced by 100 μM-MgATP and further inhibited by the additional presence of 300 μM-diazoxide.

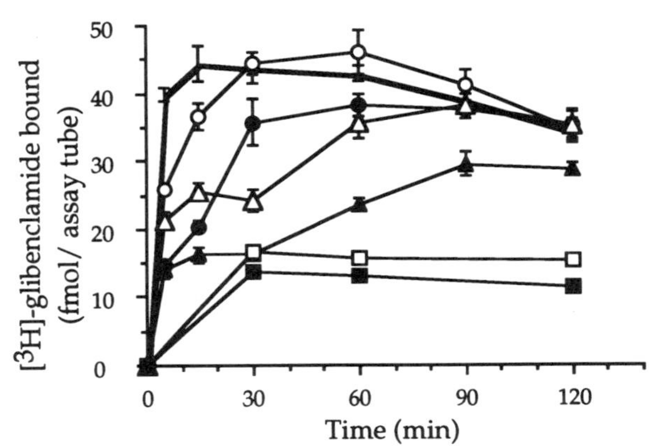

Figure 2. Effects of MgATP and diazoxide on the time-course of [^{3}H]-glibenclamide binding to HIT cell membranes. HIT cell membranes (200 μg/ml) were incubated for 5–120 min with 3 nM [^{3}H]-glibenclamide and 1 mM-$MgSO_4$ in the presence of 100 μM (○, ●), 300 μM (△, ▲) or 1 mM ATP (○, ■) in the absence (○, △, □) or presence (●, ▲, ■) of 300 μM-diazoxide. Control data (without ATP or diazoxide) are indicated by the bold line (no symbols). Bound ligand was separated from free using filtration through a glassfibre GF/F filter. Data are expressed as mean ± SEM for 6 observations.

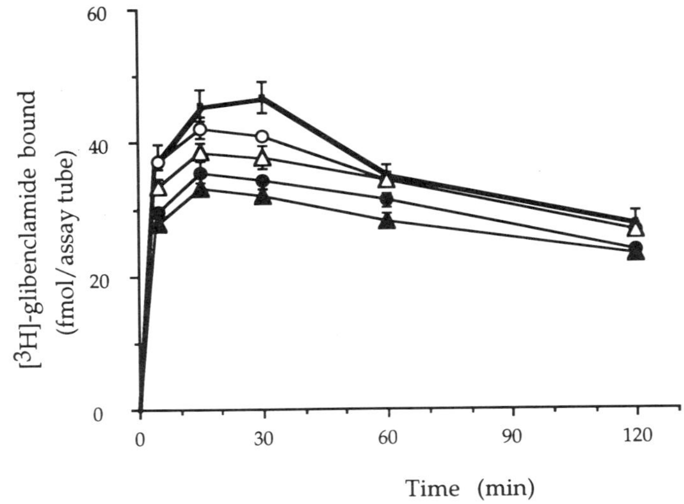

Figure 3. Effects of MgATP-γS and diazoxide on the time-course of [^{3}H]-glibenclamide binding to HIT cell membranes. HIT cell membranes (200 μg/ml) were incubated for 5–120 min with 3 nM [^{3}H]-glibenclamide and 1 mM-$MgSO_4$ in the presence of 300 μM (○, ●) or 1 mM ATP-γS (△, ▲) with (●, ▲) or without (○, △) 300 μM-diazoxide. Control data are indicated by the bold line (no symbols). Data are expressed as mean ± SEM for 5 observations.

When diazoxide was added 15 min after the start of the incubation, by which time ATP may be expected to be completely hydrolysed, the drug reduced glibenclamide binding to the same extent as that found when diazoxide was present from the start of the incubation.

The effects of phosphatase inhibitors were tested on membranes incubated for up to 90 min with [^{3}H]-glibenclamide. As shown in Table 2, 50 mM-NaF was able to increase or prolong the inhibition by MgATP and diazoxide. However neither okadaic acid (4 μM) nor microcystin (4 μM) had any effects on binding (results not shown).

Effects of MgATP and Diazoxide on Solubilized HIT Cell Membranes

In the presence of 1 mM-$MgSO_4$, 3 mM-ATP inhibited [^{3}H-]glibenclamide binding to solubilized HIT cell membranes to a similar extent to that shown in Table 2 for particulate fractions (75.7 ± 2.1% of control, n=8: $p<0.001$). The inhibitory effect of ATP required the presence of Mg^{2+} since it was abolished by substitution of 1 mM EDTA for $MgSO_4$ (108.6 ± 4.5% of control, n=4). However, in contrast to particulate fractions, in soluble membranes

Table 1. Inhibition of [^{3}H]-glibenclamide binding to HIT cell membranes by diazoxide

[^{3}H]-glibenclamide bound (% of maximum value)		
15 min incubation	30 min incubation	Addition control
100.0 ± 1.5 (11)	89.8 ± 3.0 (9)	100 μM MgATP
83.2 ± 1.2 (11)[a]	86.1 ± 1.8 (8)	100 μM MgATP + 300 μM diazoxide at 0 min
52.6 ± 1.6 (11)[a]	56.5 ± 3.2 (6)[a]	100 μM MgATP + 300 μM diazoxide at 15 min – 59.5 ± 2.3 (7)[a]

[a]$P < 0.001$ vs. control value at the same time-point.

Table 2. Effect of NaF on inhibition of [^{3}H]-glibenclamide binding to HIT cell membranes by ATP and diazoxide

Time	Incubation additions		[^{3}H]glibenclamide bound
(min)	no NaF	50 mM-NaF	(% of maximum value)
15	None	100.0 ± 2.1 (6)	
	100 μM-MgATP	76.5 ± 3.3 (6)	
	100 μM-MgATP + 300 μM-diazoxide	47.8 ± 1.5 (6)	
30	None	87.2 ± 3.5 (12)	
	100 μM-MgATP	77.5 ± 2.5 (10)	74.6 ± 4.8 (6)
	100 μM-MgATP + 300 μM-diazoxide	55.0 ± 2.6 (6)	46.1 ± 2.6 (6)[a]
90	None	80.0 ± 3.1 (8)	
	100 μM-MgATP	84.5 ± 4.0 (6)	73.0 ± 4.1 (6)[a]
	100 μM-MgATP + 300 μM-diazoxide	69.5 ± 2.6 (5)	50.6 ± 1.3 (6)[a]

[a]P.001 vs value under the same conditions in the absence of NaF.

no further inhibition of binding in the presence of MgATP was elicited by 300 μM-diazoxide (76.5 ± 2.1% of control, n=8: not significantly different from MgATP alone).

Protein Kinase and Phosphatase Activities in HIT Cell Membranes

Fig. 4 shows that there was substantial incorporation of ^{32}P from [γ-^{32}P]-ATP into HIT cell membrane proteins (second two lanes). In the absence of Mg (first two lanes), most of this radioactivity was not evident, suggesting that it results from protein phosphorylation. In support of this idea, no labelling was found when the experiment was repeated with [α-^{32}P]-ATP. Since exogenous kinases were not added to the incubation buffer, these data suggest the presence of endogenous kinases in HIT cell membranes. It appears that the kinase(s) involved are not strongly Ca^{2+}-dependent as phosphorylation occurred in the presence of 0.25 mM EGTA.

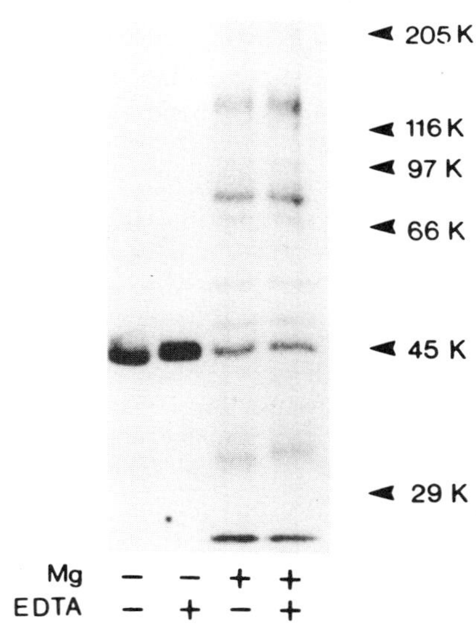

Figure 4. Phosphorylation of HIT cell membrane proteins. HIT cell membranes (400 μg/ml) were incubated with 60 μM [γ-^{32}P]-ATP for 30 min in the presence or absence of 5 mM-$MgCl_2$ and 2 mM-EDTA as indicated.

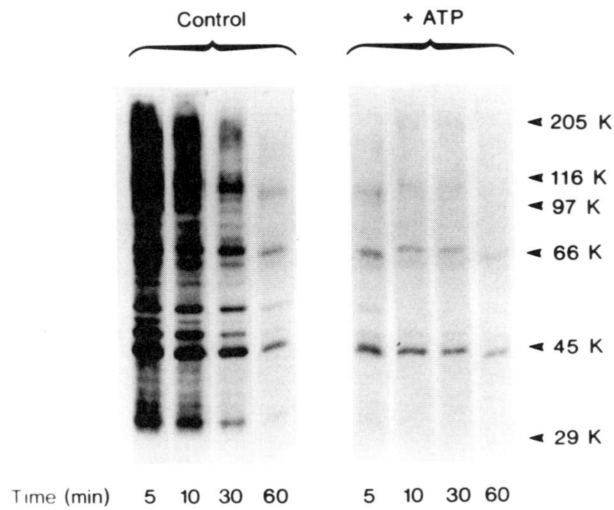

Figure 5. Time course of phosphorylation of HIT cell membrane proteins. HIT cell membranes (400 μg/ml) were incubated with 60 μM [γ-^{32}P]-ATP and 5 mM-$MgCl_2$ for the times indicated (lanes labelled "Control"). Unlabelled ATP (5 mM) was then added to samples incubated for 60 min and incubation continued for up to 60 min as indicated (lanes labelled "+ATP").

The time course of incorporation of [γ-^{32}P] into HIT cell membrane proteins is shown in Fig. 5. Phosphorylation was maximal after 5 min and declined thereafter. This decline in phosphorylation is indicative of endogenous phosphatase activity; after 5 min, the [γ-^{32}P]-ATP in the incubation mixture (60 μM) would have been completely hydrolysed (see above) and rephosphorylation should therefore not occur. Consistent with this idea, radioactivity continued to decline but there was no change in the rate of dephosphorylation, following addition of non-radioactive ATP to a final concentration of 5 mM at 60 min. Since dephosphorylation occurs in the absence of Ca^{2+}, the phosphatases involved do not have a high Ca^{2+} requirement.

The effects of protein kinase inhibitors on the incorporation of [γ-^{32}P] into HIT cell membranes are shown in Fig. 6. Protein kinase A inhibitor peptide (10 μM) slightly reduced labelling of a 100 kDa band but was without effect on most labelled species. PKC-inhibitor peptide (10 μM) was without effect. Tyrphostin, an inhibitor of tyrosine kinases, at 100 μM, almost completely abolished phosphorylation of an 80 kDa band and decreased labelling of bands at 115 kDa and 68 kDa. These results suggest that PKA and tyrosine kinase activity are present in HIT cell membranes but that substrate proteins are few. An unidentified kinase is responsible for most phosphorylation.

We next examined the effects on dephosphorylation of HIT cell membranes of a number of agents known to inhibitor activate protein phosphatases (Figs 7–8). In these experiments membranes were first phosphorylated for 5 min. A sample was then removed (lanes a, b, c, ...) and the membranes incubated for a further 30 min in the presence or absence of various inhibitors or activators (lanes a1, b1, c1, ...). Fig. 7 shows the effect of two non-specific phosphatase inhibitors NaF and Na_3VO_4 on dephosphorylation of HIT cell membrane proteins. Considerable decrease in radioactivity is seen in the control samples (compare lane c with c1 and lane d with d1). 40 mM-NaF caused marked preservation of label in several proteins, particular those of 45, 50, 54 and 57 kDa (lanes e1 and f1).

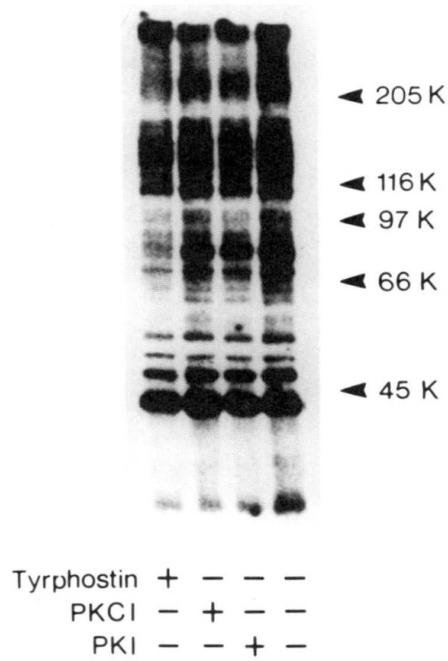

Figure 6. Effects of protein kinase inhibitors on phosphorylation of HIT cell membrane proteins. HIT cell membranes (400 μg/ml) were incubated with 60 μM [γ-^{32}P]-ATP and 5 mM-$MgCl_2$ for 5 min in the absence of inhibitors (right hand lane) or in the presence of 100 μM-tyrphostin, 10 μM protein kinase C inhibitor peptide (PKCI) or 10 μM protein kinase A inhibitor peptide (PKI) as indicated.

Na_3VO_4 also strongly decreased dephosphorylation, both at 1 mM (lanes a1 and b1) and at 100 μM (data not shown). In addition to the proteins affected by NaF, phosphorylation of a 115 kDa protein was completely preserved.

Fig. 8 shows the effect of the phosphatase inhibitor microcystin at two concentrations, 0.4 μM (lanes a1 and b1) and 4 μM (lanes e1 and f1). Microcystin produced a dose-

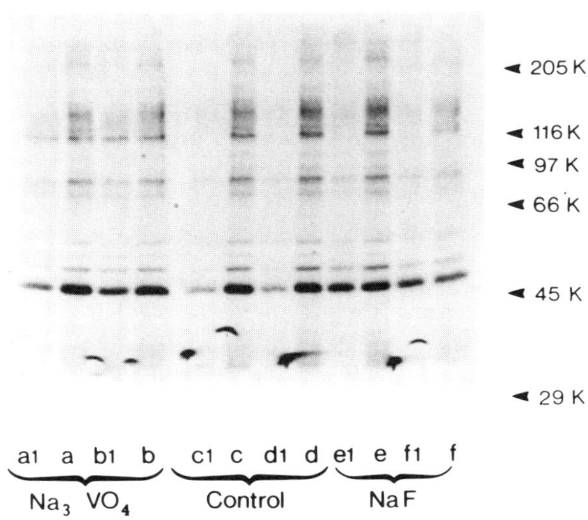

Figure 7. Effects of Na-fluoride and Na-vanadate on dephosphorylation of HIT cell membrane proteins. HIT cell membranes (400 μg/ml) were incubated with 60 μM [γ-^{32}P]-ATP and 5 mM-$MgCl_2$ for 5 min. Aliquots were then taken from each of 5 tubes and processed (lanes a,b,c,d,e and f). The remaining samples were incubated for a further 30 min in the absence of phosphatase inhibitor (lane c1 and d1) or in the presence of 40 mM-NaF (lanes e1 and f1) or 1 mM-Na_3VO_4 (lanes a1 and b1). A second aliquot was then removed from the same tube.

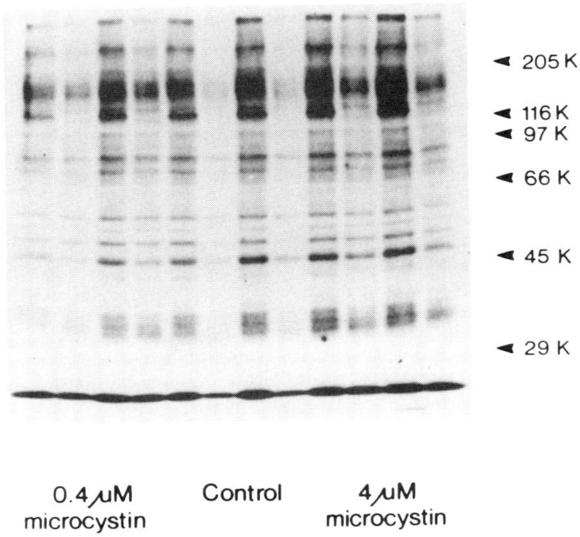

Figure 8. Effects of microcystin on dephosphorylation of HIT cell membrane proteins. HIT cell membranes (400 μg/ml) were incubated with 60 μM [γ-^{32}P]-ATP and 5 mM-$MgCl_2$ for 5 min. Aliquots were then taken from each of 5 tubes and processed (lanes a, b, c, d, e and f). The remaining samples were then incubated for a further 30 min in the absence of phosphatase inhibitor (lane c1 and d1) or in the presence of 4 μM (lanes e1 and f1) or 0.4 μM microcystin (lanes a1 and b1). A second aliquot was then removed from the same tubes.

dependent inhibition of dephosphorylation of 45, 50, 54, 60, 68 and 135 kDa bands; the 115 kDa protein was unaffected.

Addition of 5 mM $CaCl_2$, which might be expected to activate Ca-dependent phosphatases, markedly potentiated dephosphorylation of a 45 kDa protein but did not significantly alter dephosphorylation of most bands (Fig 9, lane b1).

We finally tested the possibility that diazoxide influences endogenous kinase and phosphatase activity in HIT cell membranes. At a concentration of 300 μM, diazoxide was without effect on the incorporation of radioactivity into HIT cell proteins, or on dephosphorylation of HIT cell membranes (Figure 10).

DISCUSSION

The binding studies described here provide further evidence in support of the idea that protein phosphorylation enables diazoxide to displace [^{3}H]-glibenclamide binding from HIT cell membranes [2–3]. Several possible sites of phosphorylation could be involved. First, the sulphonylurea receptor itself may be subject to phosphorylation. Secondly, a separate diazoxide receptor may be the target of phosphorylation, since it is currently unclear if K-channel openers bind to the same site as sulphonylureas or to a different protein. Thirdly, phosphorylation of an unrelated protein may influence the interaction between the diazoxide receptor and the sulphonylurea receptor.

We exclude the possibility that diazoxide either activates a kinase or inhibits a phosphatase which modulates the sulphonylurea receptor, since the K-channel opener had no effect on either phosphorylation or dephosphorylation of HIT cell membranes. Furthermore, the time course studies show that the inhibitory effect of diazoxide on [^{3}H]-gliben-

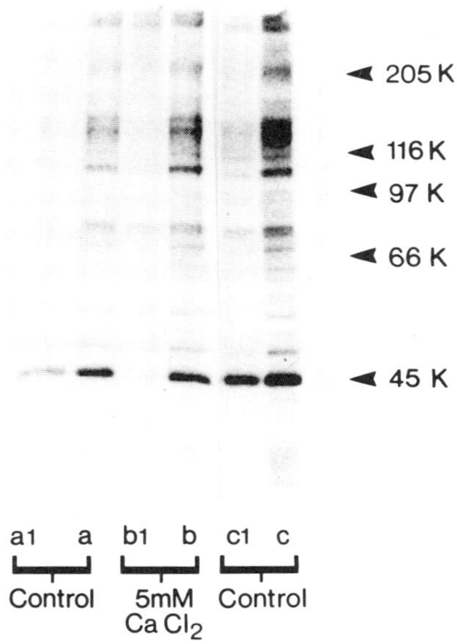

Figure 9. Effects of calcium on dephosphorylation of HIT cell membrane proteins. HIT cell membranes (400 μg/ml) were incubated with 60 μM [γ-^{32}P]-ATP and 5 mM-$MgCl_2$ for 5 min. Aliquots were then taken from each of 3 tubes and processed (lanes a,b,c). The remaining samples were then incubated for a further 30 min in the absence (lanes a1, c1) or presence of 5 mM-$CaCl_2$ (lane b1) and a second aliquot was then removed.

clamide binding persists for some time after all exogenous ATP was hydrolysed, supporting the idea that diazoxide does not activate a kinase; and inhibition of phosphatase action (with NaF) did not alter the inhibitory effect of diazoxide on [^{3}H]-glibenclamide binding arguing against the possibility that the drug inhibits a phosphatase.

[^{3}H]-Glibenclamide binding to the solubilized receptor inhibited by the presence of MgATP was not further decreased by diazoxide. This would be consistent with the dissociation of the sulphonylurea receptor from the diazoxide receptor on solubilization and suggests they may be separate proteins.

The growing evidence that the ability of MgATP both to displace [^{3}H]-glibenclamide binding and to permit diazoxide to reduce [^{3}H]-glibenclamide binding involves protein phosphorylation argues that HIT-cell membranes contain endogenous kinase and phos-

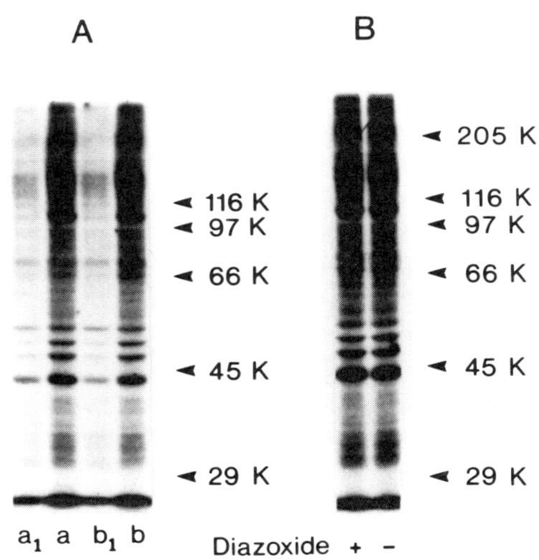

Figure 10. Effects of diazoxide on (A) dephosphorylation and (B) phosphorylation of HIT cell membrane proteins. **A:** HIT cell membranes (400 μg/ml) were incubated with 60 μM [γ-^{32}P]-ATP and 5 mM-$MgCl_2$ for 5 min. Aliquots were then taken from each of 2 tubes and processed (lanes a,b). The remaining samples were then incubated for a further 30 min in the absence (b1) or presence (a1) of 300 μM-diazoxide. **B:** HIT cell membranes (400 μg/ml) were incubated with 60 μM [γ-^{32}P]-ATP and 5 mM-MgCl2 for 5 min in the absence or presence of 300 μM-diazoxide as indicated. (Data of Ashcroft et al., 1994.)

phatase activity. The present paper demonstrates that this is indeed the case. Phosphorylation of endogenous membrane proteins occurred in the absence of cyclic AMP or Ca^{2+} and most of the kinase activity was unaffected by inhibitors of PKA and PKC, indicating that these kinases are not responsible. The phosphorylation of several bands was decreased by tyrphostin, suggesting the presence of tyrosine kinase activity. However, the large amount of phosphorylation resistant to all kinase inhibitors tested, and to the absence of Ca^{2+}, suggests the presence of additional kinase(s) which remain to be identified.

Microcystin reduced dephosphorylation of many proteins, suggesting the presence of membrane-bound protein phosphatases 1 and/or 2A. Substantial preservation of label was found in some of these proteins, and in additional bands, in the presence of the non-specific phosphatase inhibitors NaF and Na_3VO_4. This suggests the presence of other protein phosphatases, distinct from those inhibited by microcystin. Calcium enhanced dephosphorylation of a 45 kDa protein suggesting the additional presence of an endogenous Ca^{2+}-dependent phosphatase. It is of interest that phosphorylation of a 115 kDa species whose phosphorylation was reduced by tyrphostin was markedly and specifically enhanced by 1 mM Na_3VO_4, which at this concentration inhibits phosphotyrosine phosphatases. This provides further evidence that the 115 kDa substrate protein is phosphorylated on tyrosine residues.

Proteins of 140–175 kDa [7–8], 65 kDa [2, 9], and 38 kDa [10] have all been postulated to constitute the sulphonylurea receptor(s). Proteins of similar Mr were subject to phosphorylation and dephosphorylation in our studies. However, our experiments do not directly address the issue of whether phosphorylation of the sulphonylurea receptor itself modulates its binding activity; for this the purified protein must be used. The molecular weight of the diazoxide receptor and its relationship to the sulphonylurea receptor has not yet been determined.

ACKNOWLEDGMENTS

The technical assistance of Ling Weng is highly appreciated. Glibenclamide and $[^3H]$-glibenclamide were generous gifts from Hoechst. Diazoxide was kindly provided by Glaxo Inc. These studies have been supported by grants from the Medical Research Council, the British Diabetic Association, the Wellcome Trust, the EP Abraham Fund and Glaxo Research Laboratories.

REFERENCES

1. Dunne M.J., 1989, Protein phosphorylation is required for diazoxide to open ATP-sensitive potassium channels in insulin (RIN m5F) secreting cells, FEBS Letts. 250: 262–266
2. Niki, I. and Ashcroft, S.J.H, 1992, Possible involvement of protein phosphorylation in the regulation of the sulphonylurea receptor of a pancreatic β cell line, HIT T15, Biochim. Biophys. Acta. 1133: 95–101
3. Schwanstecher, M., Löser, S., Rieze, I. and Panten, U., 1991,Phosphate and thiophosphate group donating adenine and guanine nucleotides inhibit glibenclamide binding to membranes from pancreatic islets, Naunyn-Schmiedeberg's Arch. Pharmacol. 343: 83–89
4. Ashcroft, S.J.H., Hammonds, P. and Harrison, D.E., 1986, Insulin secretory responses of a clonal cell line of simian virus 40-transformed B cells, Diabetologia 29: 727–733
5. Niki, I., Welsh, M., Berggren, P.-O., Hubbard, P., and Ashcroft, S.J.H., 1991, Characterization of the solubilized glibenclamide receptor in a hamster pancreatic β-cell line, HIT T15, Biochem. J. 277: 619–624
6. Cooper, R.H., Randle, P.J. and Denton, R.M., 1974, Regulation of heart muscle pyruvate dehydrogenase kinase, Biochem. J. 143: 625–641

7. Aguilar-Bryan, L., Nelson, D.A., Vu, Q.A., Humphrey, M.B. and Boyd, A.E., III, 1990, Photoaffinity labeling and partial purification of the beta cell sulfonylurea receptor using a novel, biologically active glyburide analog, J. Biol. Chem. 265: 8218–8224
8. Skeer, J.M., Dégano, P., Coles, B., Potier, M., Ashcroft, F.M. and Ashcroft, S.J.H., 1994, Determination of the molecular mass of the native beta-cell sulfonylurea receptor, FEBS Lett. 338: 98–102
9. Kramer, W., Müller, G., Girbig, F., Gutjahr, U., Kowalewski, S., Hartz, D. and Summ, H.-D., 1994, Differential interaction of glimepiride and glibenclamide with the beta-cell sulfonylurea receptor. II. Photoaffinity labeling of a 65 kDa protein by [^{3}H]glimepiride, Biochim. Biophys. Acta 1191: 278–290
10. Schwanstecher, M., Löser, S., Chudziak, F. and Panten, U., 1994, Identification of a 38-kDa high affinity sulfonylurea-binding peptide in insulin-secreting cells and cerebral cortex, J. Biol. Chem. 269: 17768–17771

Part II.C. Intracellular Messengers

9

INTRACELLULAR SECOND MESSENGERS

Stephen J. H. Ashcroft

Nuffield Department of Clinical Biochemistry
John Radcliffe Hospital
Headington, Oxford OX3 9DU, United Kingdom

INTRODUCTION

In the β-cell, the effects of extracellular signals are mediated by changes of concentration of intracellular second messengers. Complex interrelationships among the signalling pathways determine the rate of insulin release and also can modulate the rate of insulin biosynthesis. This short overview summarises some key properties of the known second messenger systems of the β-cell. References cited are, where possible, to reviews in order to keep the reference list to a reasonable size.

CALCIUM

Calcium plays the key role in the insulin secretory response both to the main physiological regulator, glucose, and to the pharmacologically important sulfonylureas. The increase in insulin release in response to elevation of blood glucose involves an increase in the rate of glucose metabolism within the β-cell — the key component of this metabolic response is the high K_m for the rate-limiting step for glucose utilisation which is phosphorylation of the sugar [1]. This step constitutes a substrate-cycle composed of glucokinase and glucose 6-phosphatase. Increased generation of ATP and increase in cytosolic [ATP]/[ADP] ratio leads to closure of ATP-sensitive K-channels (K_{ATP} channels) in the β-cell plasma membrane [2]. The resultant depolarisation elicits opening of voltage-dependent Ca-channels and influx of calcium ions. Sulfonylureas bypass the metabolic steps and directly close K_{ATP} channels by interacting with a K_{ATP} channel regulatory protein containing high affinity sulfonylurea-binding sites [3]. Diazoxide causes β-cell hyperpolarisation and inhibits insulin secretion by opening K_{ATP} channels; however, it is not yet known whether diazoxide binds to the channel itself or to the sulfonylurea receptor. In addition to entry via L-type Ca-channels, the intracellular free Ca-concentration is determined by the balance between uptake into and release from intracellular storage sites in the endoplasmic reticulum (ER) and extrusion from the β-cell by the plasma membrane Ca-Mg-ATPase and Na-Ca-exchanger [4]. Release from the ER store can be elicited by IP_3 or by cyclic ADP- ribose

Physiology and Pathophysiology of the Islets of Langerhans, edited by Soria.
Plenum Press, New York, 1997.

(see below). In addition there is evidence for Ca-induced Ca-release (CICR), in which a relatively small influx of Ca across the plasma membrane leads directly to a greater release from the ER [5]. As a consequence of these multiple pathways for regulation of Ca-concentration within the β-cell, the response to stimulation displays complex kinetics; oscillations in intracellular Ca-concentration are observed when individual β-cells are examined [6]. In the islet, these oscillations appear to be synchronised such that an oscillating intracellular Ca response is seen throughout the islet which can be correlated with insulin release [7]. L-type Ca-channels have been cloned from the β-cell [8], but currently the other components of the Ca regulatory systems, the plasma membrane and ER Ca-pumps, the ER Ca-release system(s) and the Na–Ca- exchanger, have not been characterised at the molecular level in the β-cell.

The mechanism by which an increase in intracellular Ca triggers insulin release has not been defined. There is considerable evidence that one component is activation of a Ca/calmodulin-dependent protein kinase. The evidence for this is as follows. Firstly, Ca- and calmodulin-dependent protein phosphorylation can be demonstrated in extracts of islets or β-cells; the main phosphorylated species detected has an M_r of 53 kDa and appears to represent autophosphorylation of the kinase [9]. From studies of the substrate specificity and sensitivity to inhibitors it was concluded that the β-cell kinase may be similar or identical to calcium/calmodulin-dependent protein kinase II [10,11]. Evidence from both Northern hybridization and immunoblotting have supported this view [12,13]. Secondly, an increase in the extent of autophosphorylation of CaMK II, diagnostic of activation of the enzyme, within islets exposed to elevated glucose has been demonstrated [14]. Thirdly, an inhibitor of CaMK II, KN62, inhibits insulin release [15,16]. However, this effect is ambiguous since KN62 also inhibited L-type Ca-channels [16]. Fifthly, in patch clamp studies using the perforated patch technique and monitoring exocytosis by measurement of membrane capacitance, a peptide inhibitor of CaMK II was shown to decrease insulin release induced by Ca [17]. Sixthly, the loss of Ca-inducible insulin release from permeabilised islets was paralleled by a loss of autophosphorylation of Ca/calmodulin-dependent protein kinase [18].

Little is yet known of the way in which activation of CaMKII may increase insulin release.

Ca-binding proteins in addition to calmodulin could also be involved in the control of insulin release by Ca. Calcyclin, a member of the EF-hand family of Ca-binding proteins, has been demonstrated immunologically in rabbit islets of Langerhans; and in permeabilised rat islets calcyclin enhanced Ca-stimulated insulin release [19]. There is some evidence from studies of reporter gene expression in transfected β-cells that Ca may also be a trigger for insulin gene expression [20] . However another study using this approach found no evidence that Ca was involved in transcriptional control of the insulin gene [21].

CYCLIC AMP

The level of cAMP in the β-cell is controlled by the relative activities of plasma membrane adenylcyclase (AC) and one or more phosphodiesterases (PDE). AC is activated by extracellular signals interacting with receptors linked to AC via the activatory G-protein G_s22. AC in the β-cell may also be activated in response to an increase in glucose [23] but the mechanism of this effect has not been established (see Hughes and Ashcroft [24] for discussion). Activation of AC is involved in the potentiation of insulin secretion by glucagon, by GLP-1 and by GIP [22]. Inhibition of AC may also occur via receptors coupled to G_i. Such an inhibition may be exerted by adrenaline, somatostatin and galanin; however this is only one component, possibly not the major one, of the inhibitory effect of these agents [22].

The effects of cAMP on insulin release are mediated by activation of protein kinase A. Since the insulin gene contains a cAMP-responsive element [25], a consensus sequence for binding of the transcription factor CREB, protein kinase A may also be involved in regulation of insulin gene expression.

It is unknown how activation of protein kinase A modulates insulin release. However, the effect is potentiatory rather than initiatory since activation of protein kinase A in the absence of stimulation by glucose elicits little or no increase in insulin secretion [24]. Moreover protein kinase A activation is not involved in glucose-stimulated insulin release [26]. There is considerable evidence that this potentiation involves an increase in sensitivity of the secretory system to Ca ions [24]. Evidence for this has come from studies on intact islets and β-cells, in which the curve relating glucose-stimulated insulin release to extracellular Ca concentration (shown to be paralleled by intracellular Ca concentration) is shifted to the left by agents which increase β-cell cAMP [27,28]. A similar leftward shift for the dependence of secretion on Ca has been found in permeabilised islets [29]. Additionally, patch clamp studies have shown that the extent of secretion observed with a given Ca stimulus was markedly increased by addition of protein kinase A [30].

CYCLIC GMP

It is unclear whether cGMP is a physiological modulator of insulin release although RINm5F cells possess receptors for atrial natriuretic peptide (ANP) and a functioning cGMP system. The level of cGMP in cells is determined by the relative activities of guanyl cyclase (GC) and cGMP phosphodiesterase(s) [31]. In contrast to AC, GC has both soluble and membrane-bound forms. The latter have a dual role as both ligand receptor and enzyme. Soluble GC can be activated by nitric oxide (NO). There is currently considerable interest in the possible importance of NO in the effects of cytokines on β-cells [32]. Treatment of islets with interleukin-1 (IL-1) results in an inhibition of glucose-stimulated insulin release shown to be dependent on metabolism of L-arginine to NO and accompanied by an increase in cGMP [33,34], E.P.R. spectroscopy has been used to show that the formation of NO mediates destruct ion of iron-sulfur centres of iron-containing proteins which results in impairment of islet mitochondrial function [33]. Streptozotocin contains a nitroso moiety and there is evidence that similar deleterious effects to those exerted by IL-1 on the β-cell can be obtained as a consequence of liberation of NO from streptozotocin [35].

INOSITOL TRIPHOSPHATE

Receptors linked to phospholipase C-β (PLC) via G_q elicit hydrolysis of membrane-bound phosphatidylinositol bisphosphate to inositol triphosphate (IP_3) and diacylglycerol (DAG) [36]. In the β-cell such receptors include the muscarinic cholinergic receptors mediating the important physiological effects of acetylcholine on insulin release [22]. IP_3 binds to receptor sites on the Ca-release channels of the ER to cause mobilization of intracellular Ca. The operation of this signalling system in the β-cell is well documented [5,37,38]. Thus IP_3 was shown to elicit Ca-release from β-cell microsomes [39] or permeabilised β-cells [40]. An increase in IP_3 has been measured under conditions expected to activate PLC [41]. The nature and precise location of the Ca-stores sensitive to IP_3 are not established but a model incorporating compartmentalised uptake and release compartments has been suggested [22].

DIACYLGLYCEROL

The other branch of the phospholipase C signalling pathway involves generation of DAG and activation of protein kinase C. Measurements of DAG in β-cells have demonstrated that DAG is elevated in response to cholinergic agents; however glucose is ineffective in increasing DAG [42]. This is consistent with much data indicating that activation of protein kinase C is not involved in glucose-stimulated insulin release [43]. Nor does an increase in β-cell Ca elicited by high potassium or tolbutamide lead to an increase in DAG [42]. Current evidence favours the view that activation of protein kinase C is of most physiological importance in the potentiatory effect of acetylcholine on insulin release [43].

The consequences of activation of protein kinase C are complex. As for protein kinase A, the main effect is a potentiation of the secretory response to an initiator such as glucose [24,43]. Again the mechanism appears to involve an increase in the sensitivity of the secretory system to Ca. Evidence for this has come from studies on intact and permeabilised cells [27,28,44]. Particularly striking is the situation in HIT T15 β-cells, where activation of protein kinase C by the phorbol ester 12-O-tetradecanoyl-phorbol 13-acetate (TPA) lowered the level of intracellular Ca found in the presence of glucose and totally abolished the very marked rise in Ca normally elicited in these cells by vasopressin [45]. Despite these negative effects on Ca, the net effect on secretion was stimulatory. Patch clamp studies have also supported the idea of a sensitizing action of protein kinase C on the secretory system [46].

Activation of protein kinase C has been shown to be accompanied by translocation of the kinase from the β-cell cytosol to a membrane-bound location [43]. However, with the exception of MARCKS (myristoylated alanine-rich C-kinase substrate) [47], the identity of the endogenous β-cell substrates for protein kinase C and their role in secretion have not been defined. The modulation of insulin release induced by an activator (phorbol ester) and an inhibitor (clomiphene) of protein kinase C paralleled the phosphorylation of a 37 kDa islet membrane protein but the nature of this phosphoprotein is unknown [48]. A complication in assessing the role of protein kinase C in the β-cell is that the enzyme consists of a family of at least eight closely related subtypes which differ in their localization and activation properties [49]. The β-cell expresses several different isoforms including a novel form, PKCt [50]. The predominant form in adult β-cells is PKC-α [51].

Protein kinase C may also play a role in regulation of insulin gene expression. In HIT T15 β-cells, TPA increased the level of prepronsulin mRNA two-fold [52]. However species differences in the insulin gene transcriptional response to activators of proten kinase C have been observed; in human islets, TPA *decreased* preproinsulin mRNA level [53].

CYCLIC ADP RIBOSE

Cyclic ADP ribose (cADPR), a novel intracellular messenger formed from NAD, has been detected in various cell types [54]. A role in β-cell function has been proposed based on the findings that cADPR, but not IP_3, induced Ca-release from islet microsomes and in digitonin-permeabilised islets cADPR and Ca, but not IP3, elicited insulin release [55]. However these findings have been challenged in a study using electropermeabilised RINm5F cells and mouse pancreatic β-cells in which no effects of cADPR on Ca-release could be demonstrated [56].

ARACHIDONIC ACID

Amplification of glucose-induced insulin secretion by arachidonate and its metabolites via activation of phospholipase A2 (PLA2) has been suggested to be of importance for β-cell function [57,58]. Pharmacologic inhibition of arachidonate metabolism by both lipoxygenase and cyclooxygenase pathways suppressed glucose-induced insulin secretion from perifused human islets, and the selective cyclooxygenase inhibitor indomethacin enhanced insulin secretion [59]. These findings suggest that arachidonate metabolites may modulate glucose-induced insulin secretion in humans. Islets have been shown to possess Ca-independent PLA2 activity specific to the β-cells [60]. Inhibition of arachidonate release by secretagogue-stimulated pancreatic islets suppresses both insulin secretion and the rise in β-cell cytosolic calcium ion concentration [61]. Arachidonic acid was shown to increase phosphorylation of an 18 kDa protein in islets of Langerhans [62]. However arachidonate-induced insulin secretion was not mediated by protein phosphorylation [63].

Despite the considerable evidence that arachidonate or one of its numerous potential metabolites is involved in control of insulin secretion [38] depletion of RINm5F β-cells of arachidonate to levels undetectable by gas chromatography did not modify insulin synthesis, basal and potassium-induced insulin release, cell growth (cell number and protein), membrane depolarization and increases in cytosolic Ca^{2+} concentration [64].

PLA2-mediated hydrolysis of phospholipid produces a lysophospholipid in addition to a fatty acid. Lysophospholipids were shown to increase the free Ca^{2+} concentration in the incubation medium of permeabilized ob/ob mouse pancreatic islets [65]. Since activation of both PLC and PLA2 may occur in glucose-induced insulin secretion, the interaction of the PLC reaction product IP_3 with a lysophospholipid or an unsaturated fatty acid may affect the extent and/or duration of the glucose-induced rise in cytosolic Ca^{2+} concentration and hence insulin secretion.

REFERENCES

1. Ashcroft, S.J.H., and Ashcroft, F.M., 1992, In: "Insulin. Molecular Biology to Pathology", F.M. Ashcroft and S.J.H. Ashcroft, eds., IRL Press, pp 37–63.
2. Ashcroft, F.M., Williams, B., Smith, P.A. and Fewtrell, C.M.S., 1992, Ion channels involved in the regulation of nutrient-stimulated insulin secretion. In: Nutrient regulation of insulin secretion (P.R. Flatt, ed.) Portland Press: 193–212.
3. Ashcroft, S.J.H., and Ashcroft, F.M., 1992, The sulfonylurea receptor, Biochim. Biophys. Acta Mol. Cell Res 1175: 45–59.
4. Hellman, B., Gylfe, E., Grapengiesser, E., Lund, P.-E., and Marcström, A., 1992, Cytoplasmic calcium and insulin secretion. In: "Nutrient regulation of insulin secretion," P.R. Flatt, ed., Portland Press: 213–246.
5. Berggren, P.-O., Arkhammar, P., Islam, M.S., Juntti-Berggren, L., Khan, A., Kindmark, H., Köhler, M., Larsson, K., Larsson, O., Nilsson, T., Sjöholm, A., Szecowka, J., and Zhang, Q., 1993, Regulation of cytoplasmic free Ca^{2+} in insulin-secreting cells, Adv. Exp. Med. Biol 334: 25–45.
6. Hellman, B., Gylfe, E., Grapengiesser, E., Lund, P.-E., and Berts, A., 1992, Cytoplasmic Ca^{2+} oscillations in pancreatic beta-cells, Biochim. Biophys. Acta Rev. Biomembr. 1113: 295–305.
7. Valdeolmillos, M,, Santos, R.M., Contreras, D., Soria, B.,and Rosario, L.M., 1989, Glucose-induced oscillations of intracellular Ca^{2+} concentration resembling bursting electrical activity in single mouse islets of Langerhans, FEBS Lett 259: 19–23.

8. Yaney, G.C., Wheeler, M.B., Wei, X., Perez-Reyes, E., Birnbaumer, L., Boyd, A.E., III, and Moss, L.G., 1992, Cloning of a novel alpha1-subunit of the voltage-dependent calcium channel from the beta-cell, Mol. Endocrinol. 6: 2143–2152.
9. Harrison, D.E., Ashcroft, S.J.H., Christie, M.R., and Lord, J.M., 1984, Protein phosphorylation in the pancreatic β-cell, Experientia 40: 1057–1084.
10. Harrison, D.E., Poje, M., Rocic, B. & Ashcroft, S.J.H., 1986, Effects of dehydrouramil on protein phosphorylation and insulin secretion in rat islets of Langerhans, Biochem. J. 237: 191–196.
11. Hughes, S.J., Smith, H., and Ashcroft, S.J.H., 1993, Characterization of Ca^{2+}/calmodulin-dependent protein kinase in rat pancreatic islets, Biochem J 289: 795–800.
12. Niki, I., Okazaki, K., Saitoh, M., Niki, A., Niki, H., Tamagawa, T., Iguchi, A., and Hidaka, H., 1993, Presence and possible involvement of Ca/calmodulin-dependent protein kinases in insulin release from the rat pancreatic beta cell, Biochem. Biophys. Res. Commun 191: 255–261.
13. Urquidi, V., and Ashcroft, S.J.H., 1993, Ca^{2+}/calmodulin-dependent protein kinase (CaM kinase) of pancreatic β-cells exhibits homology with CaM kinase II: immunological and genetic evidence, Diabetologia 36 [Suppl 1]: A113.
14. Wenham, R.M., Landt, M., and Easom, R.A., 1994, Glucose activates the multifunctional Ca^{2+}/calmodulin-dependent protein kinase II in isolated rat pancreatic islets, J. Biol. Chem. 269: 4947–4952.
15. Wenham, R.M., Landt, M., Walters, S.M., Hidaka, H., and Easom, R.A., 1992, Inhibition of insulin secretion by KN-62, a specific inhibitor of the multifunctional Ca^{2+}/calmodulin-dependent protein kinase II, Biochem. Biophys. Res. Commun., 189: 128–133.
16. Li, G., Hidaka, H., and Wollheim, C.B., 1992, Inhibition of voltage-gated Ca^{2+} channels and insulin secretion in HIT cells by the Ca^{2+}/calmodulin-dependent protein kinase II inhibitor KN-62: Comparison with antagonists of calmodulin and L-type Ca^{2+} channels, Mol Pharmacol 42: 489–498.
17. Ämmälä, C., Eliasson, L., Bokvist, K., Larsson, O., Ashcroft, F.M., and Rorsman, P., 1993, Exocytosis elicited by action potentials and voltage-clamp calcium currents in individual mouse pancreatic B-cells, J. Physiol. (Lond.) 472: 665–688.
18. Jones, P.M., Persaud, S.J., and Howell, S.L., 1992, Ca^{2+}-induced insulin secretion from electrically permeabilized islets: Loss of the Ca^{2+}-induced secretory response is accompanied by loss of Ca^{2+}-induced protein phosphorylation, Biochem. J. 285: 973–978.
19. Okazaki, K., Niki, I., Iino, S., Kobayashi, S. & Hidaka, H. (1994) A role of calcyclin, a Ca^{2+}-binding protein, on the Ca^{2+}-dependent insulin release from the pancreatic beta cell. J. Biol. Chem. 269: 6149–6152.
20. German, M.S., Moss, L.G., and Rutter, W.J., 1990, Regulation of insulin gene expression by glucose and calcium in transfected primary islet cultures, J. Biol. Chem. 265: 22063–22066.
21. Goodison, S., Kenna, S., and Ashcroft, S.J.H., 1992, Control of insulin gene expression by glucose. Biochem. J. 285: 563–568.
22. Berggren, P.-O., Rorsman, P., Efendic, S., Östenson, G., Flatt, P.R., Nilsson, T., Arkhammar, P., and Juntti-Berggren , L., 1992, Mechanisms of action of entero-insular hormones, islet peptides and neural input on the insulin secretory process. In: "Nutrient regulation of insulin secretion," P.R. Flatt, ed., Portland Press: 289–318.
23. Capito, K., and Hedeskov, C.J., 1977, Effects of glucose, glucose metabolites and calcium ions on adenylate cyclase activity in homogenates of mouse pancreatic islets, Biochem. J. 162: 569–573.
24. Hughes, S.J., and Ashcroft, S.J.H., 1992, Cyclic AMP, protein phosphorylation and insulin release. In: "Nutrient Regulation of Insulin Secretion," P.R. Flatt, ed., Portland Press: 271–288.
25. Philippe, J., 1991, Structure and pancreatic expression of the insulin and glucagon genes, Endocr. Rev. 12: 252–271.
26. Persaud, S.J., Jones, P.M., and Howell, S.L., 1990, Glucose-stimulated insulin secretion is not dependent on activation of protein kinase A, Biochem. Biophys. Res. Commun. 173: 833–839.
27. Hughes, S.J., Christie, M.R., and Ashcroft, S.J.H., 1987, Potentiators of insulin secretion modulate Ca^{2+} sensitivity in rat pancreatic islets, Mol. Cell Endocrinol 50: 231–236.
28. Hughes, S.J., Chalk, J.G., and Ashcroft, S.J.H., 1989, Effects of secretagogues on cytosolic free Ca^{2+} and insulin release at different extracellular Ca^{2+} concentrations in the hamster clonal β-cell line HIT-T15, Mol. Cell Endocrinol. 65: 35–41.
29. Jones, P.M., Salmon, D.M.W., Howell, S.L., 1988, Protein phosphorylation in electrically permeabilised islets of langerhans. Effects of Ca^{2+}, cyclic AMP, a phorbol ester and noradrenaline, Biochem. J. 254: 397–403.
30. Ämmälä, C., Ashcroft, F.M., and Rorsman, P., 1993, Calcium-independent potentiation of insulin release by cyclic AMP in single beta-cells, Nature 363: 356–358.
31. Garbers, D.L., 1992, Guanylyl cyclase receptors and their endocrine, paracrine, and autocrine ligands, Cell 71: 1–4.

32. Purrello, F., and Buscema, M., 1993, Effects if interleukin-1β on insulin secretion by pancreatic beta-cells, Diab. Nutr. Metab. 6: 295–304.
33. Corbett, J.A., Wang, J.L., Hughes, J.H., Wolf, B.A., Sweetland, M.A., Lancaster, J.R., Jr., and McDaniel, M.L., 1992, Nitric oxide and cyclic GMP formation induced by interleukin 1beta in Islets of Langerhans. Evidence for an effector role of nitric oxide in islet dysfunction, Biochem. J. 287: 229–235.
34. Corbett, J.A., Sweetland, M.A., Wang, J.L., Lancaster, J.R., Jr., and McDaniel, M.L., 1993b, Nitric oxide mediates cytokine-induced inhibition of insulin secretion by human islets of Langerhans, Proc. Natl. Acad. Sci. USA 90: 1731–1735.
35. Turk, J., Corbett, J.A., Ramanadham, S., Bohrer, A., and McDaniel, M.L., 1993, Biochemical evidence for nitric oxide formation from streptozotocin in isolated pancreatic islets, Biochem. Biophys. Res. Commun. 197: 1458–1464.
36. Berridge, M.J., 1993, Inositol trisphosphate and calcium signalling, Nature 361: 315–325.
37. Prentki, M., and Matchinsky, F.M., 1987, Ca^{2+}, cAMP and phospholipid-derived messengers in coupling mechanisms of insulin secretion, Physiol Rev 67: 1185.
38. Morgan, N.G., and Montague, W., 1992, Phospholipids and insulin secretion. In: "Nutrient regulation of insulin secretion", P.R. Flatt, ed., Portland Press: 125–155.
39. Prentki, M. Biden, T.J., Janjic,D., Irvine, R.F., Berridge,M.J., and Wollheim C.B., 1984, Rapid mobilization of Ca^{2+} from rat insulinoma microsomes by inositol-1,4,5-triphosphate, Nature 309: 562–564.
40. Biden, T.J., Prentki, M., Irvine, R.F., Berridge, M.J., and Wollheim, C.B., 1984, Inositol 1,4,5-trisphosphate mobilizes intracellular Ca^{2+} from permeabilised insulin-secreting cells, Biochem. J. 223: 467–473.
41. Biden, T.J., Prugue, M.L., and Davison, A.G.M., 1992, Evidence for phosphatidylinositol hydrolysis in pancreatic islets stimulated with carbamoylcholine. Kinetic analysis of inositol polyphosphate metabolism, Biochem. J. 285: 541–549.
42. Weng, L., Davies, M., and Ashcroft, S.J.H., 1993, Effects of cholinergic agonists on diacylglycerol and intracellular calcium levels in pancreatic beta-cells, Cell. Signal. 5: 777–786.
43. Persaud, S.J., Jones, P.M., and Howell, S.J., 1992, The role of protein kinase C in insulin secretion. In: "Nutrient regulation of insulin secretion", P.R. Flatt, ed, Portland Press: 247–269.
44. Hughes, S.J., Chalk, J.G., and Ashcroft, S.J.H., 1990, The role of cytosolic free Ca^{2+} and protein kinase C in acetylcholine-induced insulin release in the clonal beta-cell line, HIT-T15, Biochem. J. 267: 227–232.
45. Hughes, S.J., Carpinelli, A., Niki, I., Nicks, J.L., and Ashcroft, S.J.H., 1992, Stimulation of insulin release by vasopressin in the clonal beta-cell line, HIT-T15: The role of protein kinase C, J. Mol. Endocrinol. 8: 145–153.
46. Ämmälä C., Eliasson, L., Bokvist, K., Berggren, P.-O, Honkanen, R.E., Sjöholm, A., and Rorsman, P., 1994, Activation of protein kinases and inhibition of protein phosphatases play a central role in the regulation of exocytosis in mouse pancreatic beta cells, Proc. Natl. Acad. Sci. USA 91: 4343–4347.
47. Calle, R., Ganesan, S., Smallwood, J.I. and Rasmussen, H., 1992, Glucose-induced phosphorylation of myristoylated alanine-rich C kinase substrate (MARCKS) in isolated rat pancreatic islets. J. Biol. Chem. 267: 18723–18727.
48. Hughes, S.J., and Ashcroft, S.J.H., 1988, Effects of a phorbol ester and clomiphene on protein phosphorylation and insulin secretion in rat pancreatic islets, Biochem. J. 249: 825–830.
49. Dekker, L.V., and Parker, P.J., 1994, Protein kinase C. A question of specificity, Trends Biochem. Sci. 19: 73–77.
50. Selbie, L.A., Schmitz-Peiffer, C., Sheng, Y., and Biden, T.J., 1993, Molecular cloning and characterization of PKCiota, an atypical isoform of protein kinase C derived from insulin-secreting cells, J. Biol. Chem. 268: 24296–24302.
51. Fletcher, D.J. and Ways, D.K., 1991, Age-dependent expression of protein kinase C isoforms in rat islets, Diabetes 40: 1496–1503.
52. Hammonds, P., Schofield, P.N., and Ashcroft, S.J.H., 1987, Glucose regulates preproinsulin messenger RNA levels in a clonal cell line of simian virus 50-transformed β-cells. FEBS Lett. 213: 149–154.
53. Hammonds, P., Schofield, P.N., Ashcroft, S.J.H., Sutton, R., and Gray, D.W.R., 1987, Regulation and specificity of glucose-stimulated insulin gene expression in human islets of Langerhans. FEBS Lett. 223: 131–137.
54. Galione, A., 1993, Cyclic ADP-ribose: A new way to control calcium, Science 259: 325–326.
55. Takasawa, S., Nata, K., Yonekura, H., and Okamoto, H., 1993, Cyclic ADP-ribose in insulin secretion from pancreatic beta cells, Science 259: 370–373.
56. Islam, M.S., Larsson, O, and Berggren, P.-O., 1993, Cyclic ADP-ribose in β cells, Science 262: 584–585.
57. Turk, J., Gross, R.W., and Ramanadham, S., 1993, Amplification of insulin secretion by lipid messengers, Diabetes 42: 367–374.
58. Jones, P.M., and Persaud, S.J., 1993, Arachidonic acid as a second messenger in glucose-induced insulin secretion from pancreatic beta-cells, J. Endocrinol. 137: 7–14.

59. Turk, J., Hughes, J.H., Easom, R.A., Wolf, B.A., Scharp, D.W., Lacy, P.E. and McDaniel, M.L., 1988, Arachidonic acid metabolism and insulin secretion by isolated human pancreatic islets, Diabetes 37: 992–996.
60. Gross, R.W., Ramanadham, S., Kruszka, K.K., Han, X., and Turk, J., 1993, Rat and human pancreatic islet cells contain a calcium ion independent phospholipase A2 activity selective for hydrolysis of arachidonate which is stimulated by adenosine triphosphate and is specifically localized to islet beta-cells, Biochemistry 32: 327–336.
61. Ramanadham, S., Gross, R.W., Han, X., and Turk, J., 1993, Inhibition of arachidonate release by secretagogue-stimulated pancreatic islets suppresses both insulin secretion and the rise in beta-cell cytosolic calcium ion concentration, Biochemistry 32: 337–346.
62. Basudev, H., Jones, P.M., Persaud, S.J., and Howell, S.L., 1992, Arachidonic acid induces phosphorylation of an 18 kDa protein in electrically permeabilised rat islets of Langerhans, FEBS Lett 296: 69–72.
63. Basudev, H., Jones, P.M., Persaud, S.J., and Howell, S.L., 1993, Arachidonic acid-induced insulin secretion from rat islets of Langerhans is not mediated by protein phosphorylation, Mol. Cell. Endocrinol. 91: 193–199.
64. Safayhi, H., Koopmann, I., and Ammon, H.P.T., 1993, Insulin secretion without the participation of arachidonic acid, Mol. Cell. Endocrinol. 91: 143–148.
65. Rustenbeck, I., and Lenzen, S., 1992, Effect of lysophospholipids, arachidonic acid and other fatty acids on regulation of Ca^{2+} transport in permeabilized pancreatic islets, Cell Calcium 13: 193–202.

10

IMMUNOLOGICAL ANALYSIS OF G-PROTEIN EXPRESSION IN THE ENDOCRINE PANCREAS

Nicholas S. Berrow, Rosemary J. Lacey, Ian J. White, and Noel G. Morgan

Cellular Pharmacology Group
Department of Biological Sciences
Keele University
Keele, Staffs ST5 5BG

INTRODUCTION

Inhibition of insulin secretion by agonists acting at cell surface receptors (e.g. α_2-agonists, somatostatin, galanin) is mediated by one or more guanine-nucleotide binding (G) proteins that serve as substrates for pertussis toxin[1]. Recent work has established that a family of such proteins exist and that at least 3 subtypes (G_{i2} and two forms of G_o) are present in rat islet cells[2,3].

Multiple pertussis toxin sensitive G-proteins are also expressed in cultured HIT-T15 and RINm5F cells[4–10] although it is not clear whether the complement of these proteins is similar in normal islet B-cells and the cell lines. Despite this, cultured insulin secreting cells are used widely to study receptor-mediated inhibition of insulin secretion. It remains an important objective, therefore, to establish whether coupling of cell surface receptors to G-proteins is similar in clonal pancreatic B-cells and normal islets.

In the present work we have used immunoblotting techniques to compare the expression of pertussis toxin sensitive G-protein subtypes in normal rat islets and in the clonal B-cell line, HIT-T15. The results suggest that these cells express similar forms of G_o but that there may be important differences in their expression of G_i isoforms.

MATERIALS AND METHODS

Preparation of Rat Islet, Brain, and HIT-T15 Cell Membranes

Freshly isolated rat islets (500–1000) or cultured HIT-T15 cells were homogenised in Tris/sucrose/phenylmethylsulphonylfluoride (TSP) buffer, pH 7.2. The homogenate was centrifuged at 32000g to generate cytosolic and total membrane fractions. Differential centrifugation was also used to prepare membranes from rat brain[11]. All samples were

Physiology and Pathophysiology of the Islets of Langerhans, edited by Soria.
Plenum Press, New York, 1997.

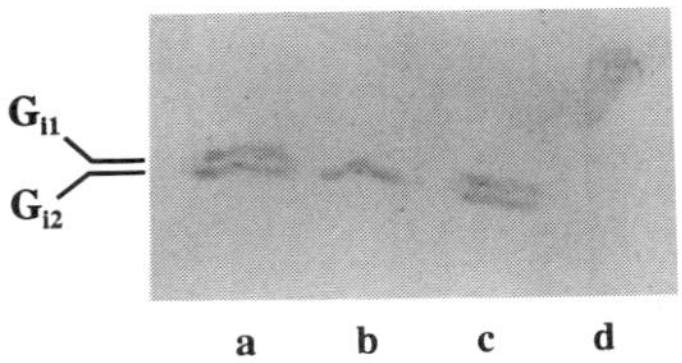

Figure 1. Detection of Gi subforms in rat brain and rat islets. Rat brain membrane proteins (20μg, lanes a and c) rat islet cell membrane proteins (50μg, lane b) and rat islet cytosolic proteins (50μg, lane d) were probed with antiserum SG1 (diluted 1:50). The location of G_{i1} and G_{i2} is indicated.

diluted with SDS-PAGE buffer, heated to 100°C for 5 min and loaded onto SDS-PAGE mini-gels (12% acrylamide) for electrophoresis. The proteins were then transferred to either nitrocellulose or charged nylon membranes by electroblotting.

Immunoblotting Protocols

Immobilised proteins were probed with antisera as described previously[2]. Visualisation of immunoreactive bands was achieved using either biotinylated second antibody/streptavidin-alkaline phosphatase or immunogold and silver staining.

RESULTS

Characterisation of G_i Subtypes Present in Rat Islets and HIT-T15 Cells

Probing of rat islet and rat brain membrane proteins with antiserum SG1 (which recognises both G_{i1} and G_{i2}) revealed the presence of two labelled bands in brain (Figure 1). These corresponded to proteins of 40 and 41kDa in molecular mass. In contrast only a single immunoreactive band was observed in islet membranes (Figure 1).

Use of antiserum I1C (G_{i1}-specific) to probe rat brain membranes revealed a single immunoreactive band (Figure 2). In HIT cell membranes this antiserum also labelled a corresponding band (Figure 2). In addition, a number of other immunoreactive proteins were also observed (Figure 2). From several experiments it was possible to identify at least 7 such bands corresponding to proteins with molecular masses ranging from 30 to 56kDa. None of these were present in either islet cell membranes or cytosol (Figure 2) consistent with the absence of G_{i1} in this tissue[2].

Presence of G_o in Rat Islets and HIT-T15 Cells

Using an antiserum (OC1) specific for α-subunits of members of the G_o family, immunoreactive bands corresponding to the presence of two forms of G_o were observed in rat brain and rat islet membranes, and also in membranes from HIT cells (Figure 3).

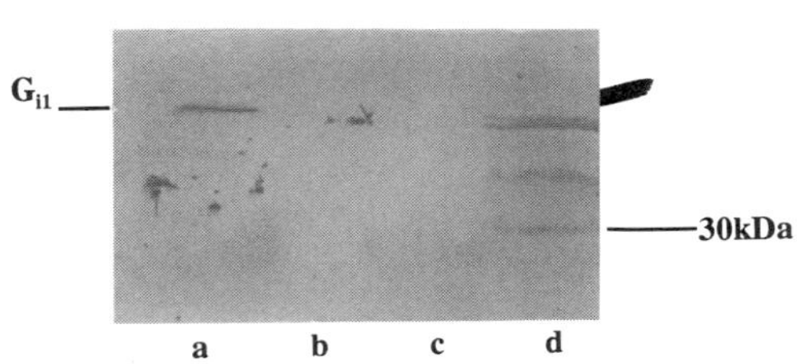

Figure 2. Detection of G_{i1} in rat brain, rat islets and HIT-T15 cells. Rat brain membrane proteins (20μg, lane a), rat islet cell membrane proteins (30μg, lane b) islet cytosolic proteins (30μg, lane c) and HIT-T15 cell membrane proteins (30μg, lane d) were probed with antiserum I1C. The position of G_{i1} is shown.

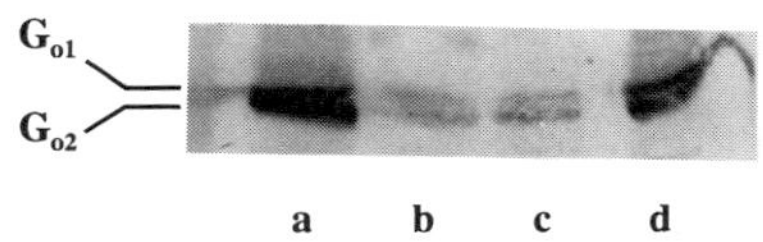

Figure 3. Detection of G_o isoforms in rat brain, rat islets and HIT cells. Rat brain membrane proteins (20µg, lanes a and d), islet cell membrane proteins (30µg, lane b) and HIT-T15 cell membrane proteins (30µg, lane c) were probed with antiserum OC1. The positions of G_{o1} and G_{o2} are indicated.

In order to ascertain which group(s) of G_o α-subunits are present in rat islets and HIT-T15 cells, an antiserum specific to the α-subunit of G_{o1} was used (O1A). This labelled only a single immunoreactive band in rat brain, rat islet membranes and HIT-T15 cell membranes (Figure 4). In some experiments the mobility of the band from islets and HIT cells was slightly different from that of rat brain (Figure 4) suggesting that the immunoreactive protein may exhibit slightly different characteristics in these tissues.

DISCUSSION

The data obtained during this investigation confirm that at least two G-proteins of the G_o subtype are present in rat islets of Langerhans[2] and demonstrate that similar proteins are also present in HIT-T15 cells. In both islets and HIT cells only one of the proteins was labelled by a G_{o1} specific antiserum, suggesting that both G_{o1} and G_{o2} are present in the cells. This is consistent with the results of Northern blot analysis which has revealed the expression of G_{o1} and G_{o2} mRNA in HIT cells[12]. It should be emphasised that we cannot draw the firm conclusion that the two forms of G_o are necessarily expressed in the same cell type within rat islets, although the results with HIT cells would support this.

HIT cells were found to express a protein recognised by a specific G_{i1} antiserum (I1C) which migrated in a similar position to G_{i1} from rat brain. This protein was not detected in rat islets. In support of this, antiserum SG1 labelled only a single band in rat islets (corresponding to brain G_{i2}) but recognised 2 proteins in brain (Figure 1) and HIT cells (not shown). Surprisingly, antiserum I1C also reacted with several other proteins in HIT cell membranes in addition to the band of 41kDa corresponding to brain G_{i1}. Additonal bands were not seen in either rat brain or rat islets, nor were they labelled by SG1 in HIT cells. The identity of these proteins remains to be established but it is possible that some of them may represent proteolytic products of G_{i1} produced during preparation of the membranes. This cannot, however, account for labelling of proteins that are apparently larger than native G_{i1} (>41kDa).

The observation that cultured HIT cells express G_{i1}, a G-protein that appears to be absent from the majority of rat islet cells, suggests that there could be important differences in the coupling of cell surface receptors to intracellular effectors in HIT cells and normal islets. Thus, when HIT cells are employed as a model system to study receptor-mediated inhibition of insulin secretion, it will be important to ensure that any responses measured also occur in intact islets. Similar considerations apply to RINm5F cells which have also been found to express G_{i1} by several groups[6,7] (I.J. White and N.G. Morgan, unpublished observations) although this finding has not been universal[8].

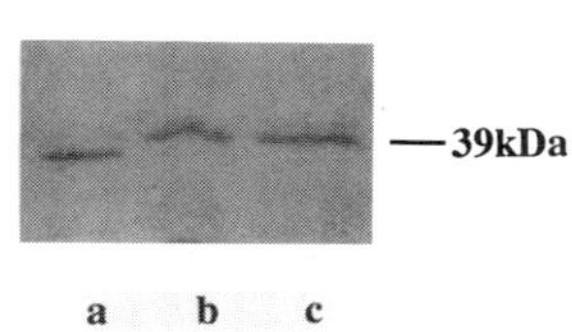

Figure 4. Detection of G_{o1} in rat brain, rat islets and HIT-T15 cells. Rat brain membrane proteins (20µg, lane a), islet cell membrane proteins (30µg, lane b) and HIT-T15 cell membrane proteins (30µg, lane c) were probed with antiserum O1A. The expected position of G_{o1} (39kDa) is shown.

ACKNOWLEDGMENTS

We are grateful to Dr. G. Milligan (University of Glasgow) for providing the anti-G-protein sera used in this study. Financial support from the British Diabetic Association, Wellcome Trust and MRC is also acknowledged with gratitude.

REFERENCES

1. A.M. McDermott and G.W.G. Sharp, Inhibition of insulin secretion: a fail- safe system, *Cell.Signalling* 5: 229 (1993).
2. N.S. Berrow, G. Milligan and N.G. Morgan, Immunological characterisation of the guanine-nucleotide binding proteins G_i and G_o in rat islets of Langerhans. *J.Mol.Endocrinol.* 8:103 (1992).
3. N.S. Berrow, R.D. Hurst, S.L.F. Chan and N.G. Morgan, Immunoprecipitation of a pertussis toxin substrate of the G_o family from rat islets of Langerhans, *Biosci.Rep.* 12:95 (1992).
4. R.P. Robertson, E.R. Seaquist and T.F. Walseth, G proteins and modulation of insulin secretion, *Diabetes* 40:1 (1991).
5. E.R. Seaquist, A. Robertson-Neal, K.D. Shoger, T.F. Walseth and R.P. Robertson, *Diabetes* 41:1390 (1992).
6. M. Cormont, Y. Le Marchand-Brustel, E. Van Obberghen, A.M. Spiegel and G.W.G. Sharp, Identification of G-protein α-subunits in RINm5F cells and their selective interaction with galanin receptors. *Diabetes* 40:1170 (1991).
7. A. Schmidt, J. Hescheler, S. Offermanns, K. Spicher, K-D. Hinsch, F-J. Klinz, J. Codina, L. Birnbaumer, H. Gausepoh, R. Frank, G. Schultz and W. Rosenthal, Involvement of pertussis toxin sensitive G-proteins in the hormonal inhibition of dihydropyridine sensitive Ca currents in an insulin secreting cell line (RINm5F), *J.Biol.Chem.* 266:18025 (1991).
8. A. Remaury and H. Paris, The insulin secreting cell line RINm5F expresses an alpha-2D adrenoceptor and nonadrenergic idazoxan binding sites. *J.Pharmacol.Exp.Ther.* 260:417 (1992).
9. S.L. Gillison and G.W.G. Sharp, ADP-ribosylation by cholera toxin identifies three G-proteins that are activated by the galanin receptor: studies with RINm5F cell membranes, *Diabetes* 43:24 (1994).
10. E.R. Seaquist, T.F. Walseth, J.B. Redmon and R.P. Robertson, G-protein regulation of insulin secretion, *J.Lab.Clin.Med.* 123:338 (1994).
11. P.C. Sternweis and J.D. Robishaw, Isolation of two proteins with high affinity for guanine nucleotides from membranes of bovine brain *J.Biol.Chem.* 259:13806 (1984).
12. P. Bertrand, J. Sanford, U. Rudolph, J. Codina and L. Birnbaumer, At least three alternatively spliced mRNAs encoding two alpha subunits of the G_o GTP-binding protein can be expressed in a single tissue, *J.Biol.Chem.* 265:18576 (1990).

11

CALCYCLIN, A CALCIUM-BINDING PROTEIN, WHICH REGULATES INSULIN SECRETION FROM THE PERMEABILIZED PANCREATIC β-CELL

Ichiro Niki, Katsuo Okazaki, Satoshi Iino, Sigeru Kobayashi, and Hiroyoshi Hidaka

Departments of Pharmacology and Anatomy
Nagoya University School of Medicine
65 Tsuruma-cho, Showa-ku, 466, Nagoya, Japan

INTRODUCTION

Although it is widely accepted that an increase in intracellular Ca^{2+} is a crucial event in the stimulus-secretion coupling in the pancreatic β-cell [1], we have limited knowledge on the later steps in the signal transduction pathway. Calcium binding proteins are considered to be involved in the control of Ca^{2+}-dependent cellular functions including hormone release [2]. Various types of calcium-binding proteins such as calmodulin, calbindin and S-100b protein are identified in the islet cells biochemically or immunohistochemically [3,4]. Calmodulin, the best characterized calcium binding protein, was demonstrated to exist in the pancreatic islet cells by Sugden et al [5]. The pancreatic β-cell possesses the kinase activity which is dependent on Ca^{2+}/calmodulin [6]. Involvement of calmodulin and calmodulin-dependent protein kinases in insulin release has been suggested mainly based on the inhibitory effect of calmodulin antagonists on the release [7,8,9], albeit there is the argument against this idea [10].

Calcyclin is a 10.5 kDa Ca-binding protein with two EF-hands. It was reported that expression of calcyclin is dependent on cell cycle [11]. There is a report that a calcyclin-like mouse decidual protein may be involved in the secretion of lactogen-II [12]. In this study, we aimed to elucidate the role of calcyclin in insulin release from the rat pancreatic islets.

METHODS AND MATERIALS

Immunoblot Analysis

The polyclonal antibodies against calcyclin were raised in a guinea pig by injecting rabbit lung calcyclin. For immunoblot analysis, pancreatic islets were isolated from

Physiology and Pathophysiology of the Islets of Langerhans, edited by Soria.
Plenum Press, New York, 1997.

female rabbits of the Japanese White strain using collagenase digestion. The islets were homogenated in 1mM EGTA and 20mM Tris-HCl (pH 7.5), and centrifuged at 100,000g. The supernatant was loaded onto SDS-PAGE and transferred to PVDF membranes. The procedure of Burnette [13] was then followed with minor modifications.

Light-Microscopic Immunohistochemistry

The sections of rabbit pancreas were incubated in 10% goat serum for 30min and then in anti-calcyclin or anti-insulin antibodies for 12hrs. After washing in phosphate-buffered saline (PBS) with 5mM Tris-HCl (pH 7.6), the sections were incubated in the biotinylated goat anti-guinea pig antibody for 30min. The tissue was washed in PBS, incubated in avidin horseradish-peroxidase for 30min and washed again in PBS. Finally, the bound antibody was visualized by peroxidase reaction.

Permeabilization of Pancreatic Islets with Streptolysin-O (STLO)

Pancreatic islets were isolated from male Wistar rats by collagenase digestion. The solution used during the isolation was Hepes-buffered Krebs-Ringer bicarbonate buffer containing 119mM NaCl, 4.75mM KCl, 5mM $NaHCO_3$, 2.54mM $CaCl_2$, 1.2mM $MgSO_4$, 1.2mM KH_2PO_4 and 20mM Hepes (pH 7.4 with NaOH) supplemented with 3mM glucose. Groups of size-matched 5 islets were preincubated at 37°C for 1hr in the same buffer with 5mg/ml bovine serum albumin gassed with 95% O_2/5% CO_2. The islets were then washed twice with 0.8ml of the glutamate buffer containing 100mM K-glutamate, 42mM Na-glutamate, 16mM Hepes, 5mg/ml bovine serum albumin, 1mM EGTA and 3mM Mg-ATP. The islets were permeabilized by incubation with 0.125 IU/ml STLO (Eiken, Tokyo, Japan) in the same glutamate buffer with various additions. After the 45min incubation, the amount of released insulin was measured by enzyme-linked immunoassay.

Others

Rabbit calcyclin was isolated from rabbit lungs as described previously [14]. For the secretion experiments, calcyclin was dialyzed against the glutamate buffer with 10^{-7} M Ca^{2+}. Calgizzarin was prepared from chicken gizzard as described elsewhere [15]. W-77 ((S)-P-(2-aminoethyloxy)-N-[2-(4-benzyloxy-carbonylpiperazinyl)-1-(P-methyoxy-benzoyl)ethyl]-N-methylbenzene-sulfonamide dihydrochloride) was synthesized by Hidaka et al. [16].

RESULTS AND DISCUSSION

Immunological Identification of Calcyclin in the Pancreatic Islet Cells

Fig. 1a demonstrates the presence of calcyclin-like immunoreactivity in the pancreatic islet cells. Immunohistochemical experiments revealed the presence of calcyclin-like immunoreactivity with some heterogenous distribution in the rabbit islet cells. The reactivity was partly co-localized with the insulin-like immunoreactivity, but not found in the pancreatic acinar cells. Fig. 1b shows immunoblot analysis of the rabbit islet homogenate using the anti-calcyclin antibody. It resulted in two immunopositive bands at 10.5 and 21kDa in the positive control (purified rabbit lung calcyclin; lane 1) and the islet homogenate (lane 2). The higher band at approx. 98kD, however, was observed only in purified

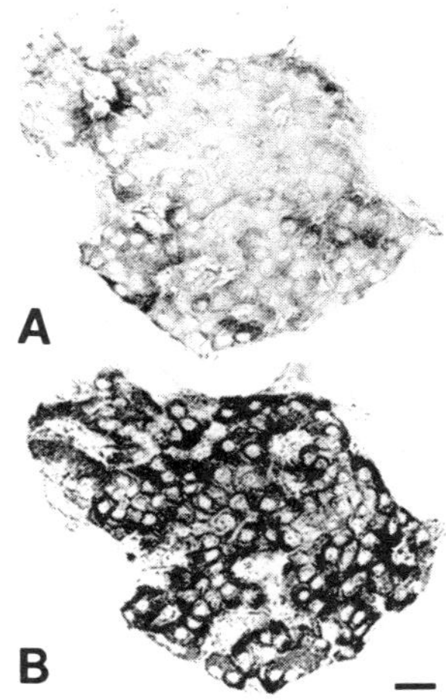

Figure 1. Presence of calcyclin in rabbit pancreatic islets. **a)** Sequential sections of the rabbit pancreas were stained by the anti-calcyclin (A) or anti-insulin (B) antibodies. **b)** Western blotting for the rabbit islet homogenate (lane 1) and purified calcyclin from rabbit lungs (lane 2) using the polyclonal anti-calcyclin antibody.

calcyclin. These findings indicate that calcyclin exists in the pancreatic islet cells including the β-cell. We consider that the 21kDa band is a dimer form of calcyclin.

Effects of Calcyclin and Calgizzarin on Ca^{2+}-Dependent Insulin Release from STLO-Treated Rat Pancreatic Islets

In the preliminary experiments, we found that increasing concentrations of Ca^{2+} (from 10^{-8} to 10^{-4} M) resulted in a dose-dependent increase in insulin release from rat pancreatic islets treated with 0.125 U/ml STLO (data not shown). The threshold of Ca^{2+} for the release was between 10^{-7} and 10^{-6} M, which agrees with the results from previous reports using different permeabilization methods [17,18].

Calcyclin at 100 nM and 1μM enhanced insulin release from the permeabilized islets stimulated by 10^{-5} M Ca^{2+}. Calcyclin did not increase insulin release from the permeabilized β-cell at 10^{-7} M Ca^{2+} (102±14 without calcyclin vs 79±6 with calcyclin pg/islet/45min, n=5). This Ca-binding protein in the presence of 10^{-5} M Ca^{2+} failed to change the release without treatment with STLO (47.2±10 without calcyclin vs 31.2±2 with calcyclin pg/islet/45min,

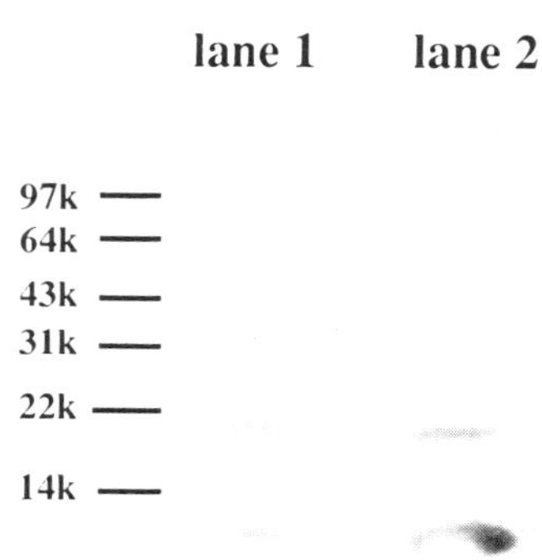

Figure 2. Dose-dependent increase by calcyclin in insulin release from the STLO-permeabilized islets. Five size-matched pancreatic islets were incubated in the co-presence of 10^{-5} M Ca^{2+}, 0.125 IU/ml STLO and various concentrations of calcyclin. Each value is the mean ± SEM for 4–5 observations.

n=5), which means that the action of calcyclin is intracellular. Calgizzarin, another Ca^{2+}-binding protein which has a partial homology with calcyclin, failed to increase the release in a parallel condition (576±78 without calgizzarin vs 600±80 with calgizzarin pg/islet/45min, n=4). These findings suggest that calcyclin may enhance Ca^{2+}-mediated insulin release in response to the increased intracellular Ca^{2+} concentration.

One interesting nature of calcyclin is that calcyclin binds to annexins [19,20] which are suggested to be involved in exocytosis [21]. It is, nevertheless, too early to say whether annexins are acting as target proteins of calcyclin in the pancreatic β-cell.

CONCLUSION

Calcyclin is present in the pancreatic islet cells and may be involved in the control of insulin release in response to an increase in the intracellular Ca^{2+}.

REFERENCES

1. M. Prentki and F.M. Matschinsky, Ca^{2+}, cAMP and phospholipid-derived messengers in coupling mechanisms of insulin secretion. Physiol.Rev. 67: 1185 (1987).
2. J.C. Hutton, Calcium-binding proteins and secretion. Cell Calcium, 7:339 (1986).
3. W.J. Malaisse F. Blachier, R. Pochet, B. Manuel-y-Keenoy, A. Sener, Calmodulin and calbindin in pancreatic islet cells. Adv.Exp.Med.Biol. 269:127 (1990).
4. T. Uchida and T. Endo, Identification of cell types containing S-100b protein-like immunoreactivity in the islets of Langerhans of the guinea pig pancreas with light and electron microscopy. Cell Tissue Res. 255:379 (1989).
5. M.C. Sugden,M.R. Christie and S.J.H. Ashcroft, Presence and possible role of calcium-dependent regulator (calmodulin) in rat islets of Langerhans. FEBS lett 105:95 (1979).
6. U.K. Schubart, J. Erlichman and N. Fleischer, The role of calmodulin in the regulation of protein phosphorylation and insulin release in hamster insulinoma cells. J.Biol.Chem. 255:4120 (1980).
7. H. Niki, A. Niki and H. Hidaka, Effects of a new calmodulin inhibitor (W-7) on insulin release and biosynthesis. Biomed.Res. 2:413 (1981).
8. Y. Krauz, C.B. Wollheim, E. Siegel and G.W.G. Sharp, Possible role for calmodulin in insulin release. J.Clin.Invest. 66:603 (1980).
9. I. Niki, K. Okazaki, M. Saitoh, A. Niki, H. Niki, T. Tamagawa, A. Iguchi and H. Hidaka, Presence and possible involvement of Ca/calmodulin-dependent protein kinases in insulin release from the rat pancreatic β-cell. Biochem.Biophys.Res.Commun. 191:255 (1993).
10. G.C. Yaney and G.W.G. Sharp, Calmodulin and insulin secretion: use of naphthalenesulphonamide compounds. Am.J.Physiol. 259:E856 (1990).
11. R.R. Hirschhorn, P. Aller, Z.-A. Yuan, C.W. Gibson and R. Baserga, Cell-cycle specific cDNAs from mammalian cells temperature sensitive for growth. Proc.Natl.Acad.Sci.USA 81:6004 (1984).
12. G. Thordarson, J.N. Southard and F. Talamantes, Purification and characterization of mouse decidual calcyclin: a novel stimulator of mouse placental lactogen-II secretion. Endocrinology 129:1257 (1991).
13. W.N. Burnette, “Western blotting” electrophoretic transfer of proteins from sodium dodecyl sulfate-polyacrylamide gels to unmodified nitrocellulose and radiographic detection with antibody and radioiodinated protein A. Anal.Biochem. 112:195 (1982).
14. H.Tokumitsu, R.Kobayashi and H.Hidaka, A Calcium-binding protein from rabbit lung cytosol identified as the product of growth-regulated gene and its binding proteins. Arch.Biochem. Biophys. 288:202 (1991).
15. H. Todoroki, R. Kobayashi, M. Watanabe, H. Minami and H. Hidaka, Purification, characterization and partial sequence analysis of a newly identified EF-hand type 13-kDa Ca^{2+}-binding protein from smooth muscle and non-smooth muscle tissues. J.Biol.Chem. 266:18668 (1992).
16. H. Hidaka, M. Inagaki, S. Kawamoto and Y. Sasaki, Isoquinolinesulpfnamides, novel and potent inhibitors of cyclic nucleotide dependent protein kinase and protein kinase C. Biochemistry 23:5036 (1984).
17. T. Tamagawa, A. Niki, H. Niki and I. Niki, Regulation of insulin release independent of changes of changes of cytosolic Ca^{2+} concentration. in: “Biophysics of the pancreatic B-cell.” (I. Atwater, E. Rojas and Soria B. eds.), Plenum Pub. Co. New York, pp293 (1987).

18. P.M. Jones, and S.L. Howell, Insulin secretion studied in islet permeabilized by high voltage discharge. in: Biophysics of the pancreatic B-cell (I. Atwater, E. Rojas and Soria, eds.) Plenum Pub. Co. New York. pp. 279 (1987).
19. H. Tokumitu, A. Mizutani, H. Minami, R. Kobayashi and H. Hidaka, A calcyclin-associated protein is a newly identified member of the Ca^{2+}/phospholipid-binding proteins, annexin family. J. Biol. Chem. 267: 8919 (1992).
20. Knoll S. and Savion N. Characterization of the cellular binding domain and the effects of monoclonal antibodies and thrombin inhibitors on the binding and internalization of the anti-thrombin complex by cultured cells. Eur. J. Biochem. 195:801 (1991).
21. Creutz, C.E. The annexins and exocytosis. Science 258:924 (1992).

12

MOLECULAR CLONING OF THE cDNA ENCODING β-CELL CALCIUM/CALMODULIN-DEPENDENT PROTEIN KINASE II

Virginia Urquidi and Stephen J. H. Ashcroft

University of Oxford
Nuffield Department of Clinical Biochemistry
John Radcliffe Hospital, Headington
Oxford OX3 9DU, United Kingdom

INTRODUCTION

Current hypotheses postulate that the metabolism of glucose within islets results in a transient increase in the ATP:ADP ratio, leading to depolarization and opening of voltage-dependent Ca^{2+} channels, promoting influx of Ca^{2+} into the β-cell. The increase in intracellular calcium may activate Ca^{2+}-dependent protein kinases, which in turn phosphorylate key components in the secretory machinery. The nature and identity of these components are at present unclear. In addition, the β-cell contains a high (15–50 μM) concentration of calmodulin (CaM) and it has been shown that inhibitors of CaM block insulin secretion. Possible candidates for Ca^{2+}/calmodulin-dependent protein kinases acting as regulatory enzymes in the exocytotic release process are phosphorylase kinase, myosin light chain kinase and CaM kinases.

Ca^{2+}/calmodulin-dependent protein kinase II (CaMkII) is a multifunctional kinase that has been implicated in the regulation of a variety of cellular processes, including contractility, gene expression and neurotransmitter release and synthesis.[1,2] It has been purified and characterized from mammalian brain and several nonneuronal tissues and from Drosophila. Molecular cloning indicates that at least four distinct genes encode CaMkII isoforms: α, β, γ and δ subunits and their variants originated by alternative splicing of the gene transcripts[3–6]. The α and β subunits are expressed primarily in brain and the γ and δ are the predominant forms in peripheral tissues[7]. The kinase is a multimer of 4–12 subunits, with subunit size ranging from 51–60 kDa on SDS-PAGE, depending on the isoform and tissue. CaMkII autophosphorylates in its autoinhibitory domain in the presence of Ca^{2+}, calmodulin and MgATP. Autophosphorylation at this site converts the kinase to a Ca^{2+}-independent or autonomous enzyme.

Physiology and Pathophysiology of the Islets of Langerhans, edited by Soria.
Plenum Press, New York, 1997.

Support for a role of a β-cell CaM kinase (CaMk) in the secretory process is provided by evidence that alloxan, a diabetogenic agent, and KN-62, a specific inhibitor of CaMkII inhibit both glucose-induced insulin secretion and CaMkII activity[8–10].

In order to identify the β-cell CaMk and its relationships to CaMkII, we have investigated: a) the expression of mRNA for CaMkII in the rat β-cell line RINm5F by Northern analysis; b) the aminoacid homology of the enzyme expressed in rat islets with brain CaMkII by immunoreactivity; c) the Ca^{2+}/calmodulin-dependent phosphorylation activity of islet extracts; d) the inhibition of β-cell CaMk by KN-62 and e) the expression of CaMkII in rat pancreatic islets by screening a cDNA library.

Since the characterization of β-cell CaMk will ultimately involve purification to homogeneity and comparison of kinetic and structural properties of this enzyme with those of CaMkII, we have used the baculovirus expression system to purify mg amounts of a subunit of brain CaMkII and have isolated a clone from a rat islet cDNA library to be expressed in the same way.

MATERIALS AND METHODS

Autophosphorylation Assay

Isolated rat islets were lysed by sonication in 50 mM HEPES pH 7.5–1% NP-40 and incubated for 3 min at room temperature with 0.5 pmol of [γ-^{32}P]-ATP (5000 Ci/mmol) in final concentrations of 10 mM $MgCl_2$; 25 mM HEPES pH 7.5; 10 mM $CaCl_2$ and 20 μM calmodulin (CaM), in a reaction volume of 100 μl. Parallel assays were conducted in the absence of Ca^{2+} and CaM, and with the addition of 1 mM EGTA; 1 mM trifluoperazine (TFP), and 30 μM KN62, individually or in combination. The reaction was terminated by the addition of 0.25 vol. of 5X dissociation buffer (250 mM Tris-Cl pH 6.8; 10% SDS; 5% β-mercaptoethanol; 50% glycerol and 0.5% bromophenol blue) and heating at 100°C for 3 min. The reaction products were resolved by SDS-PAGE, transferred to PVDF membranes for immunoanalysis and subsequently subjected to autoradiography.

Immunoblot Analysis

A synthetic peptide representing residues 281–309 of the α-subunit of brain CaMkII (which is identical in the α, β, γ and δ isozymes with the exception of 3 residues) was used to raise rabbit polyclonal antibodies. The specificity of the immune serum was tested by reaction with affinity purified mouse brain CaMkII α-subunit, expressed in a baculovirus system .

The products of the phosphorylation assay of rat islet proteins were resolved by SDS-PAGE and the proteins electroblotted onto PVDF membranes (Immobilon, Millipore). The membranes were soaked in blocking solution (5% nonfat dry milk; 0.02% Tween-20) for 1 hour and subsequently incubated for 12 hours at 4°C with the anti-CaMkII antibody in blocking solution. After washing steps in PBS-0.02% Tween-20 the membranes were incubated with alkaline phosphatase conjugated anti-rabbit IgG and immune complexes were detected by the addition of the chromogenic substrate NBT/BCIP.

Northern Hybridization Analysis

Total RNA extracted from RINm5F β-cells was resolved in a 1% methylmercury agarose gel, transferred and fixed to a nylon membrane (Hybond N, Amersham). A cDNA clone of mouse brain CaMkII α-subunit (kindly provided by A.R. Means, Baylor College of Medicine, Houston TX) was subcloned into pBluescript (Stratagene), which contains T3 and T7 RNA polymerase promoters. Antisense RNA probes were synthesized by in vitro transcription of the linearized plasmid in the presence of [α-^{32}P]-UTP and used in hybridization analysis with RINm5F RNA. After hybridization at 42°C for 16 hours, the filters were washed twice for 1 hour at 65°C with a solution consisting of 0.1 × SSC–0.1% SDS (20 × SSC is 3 M NaCl; 300 mM sodium citrate, pH 8.00) and subsequently subjected to autoradiography.

Cloning and Sequencing of a β-cell CaMk

A rat islet cDNA library in pCDM8, provided by B. Michelsen (Hagedon Research Laboratory, Denmark), was screened using a random-primer [^{32}P]-labelled cDNA probe corresponding to the α-subunit of CaMkII, by standard colony hybridization procedures. The DNA sequence of the positive clones was determined by the dideoxynucleotide-chain termination method and analyzed for homologous sequences in the GenBank and EMBL nucleic acid databases using the University of Wisconsin Genetic Computer Group software package.

Expression and Purification of Brain CaMkII

The coding region of a cDNA clone of the α-subunit of CaMkII was subcloned into pAcCL29 baculovirus transfer vector (kindly provided by I. Jones, NERC-IOVEM Oxford) downstream from the polyhedrin promoter and used in co-transfections with AcNPV (Autographa californica Nuclear Polyhedrosis virus) DNA into Spodoptera frugiperda (Sf) 9 cells. Recombinant baculovirus containing the CaMkII DNA were isolated by three rounds of plaque purification and grown to high titer. Recombinant clones expressed a polypeptide of approximate M_r of 50 kDa that was recognized by rabbit polyclonal antibodies in Western analysis. Purification of CaMkII by $[NH_4]_2SO_4$ precipitation and calmodulin affinity chromatography produced ca. 15 mg of protein per liter of Sf9-infected cells. The purity of the preparation was estimated to be 95% by silver staining of polyacrylamide gels. The activity of the purified enzyme was assessed by Ca^{2+}/calmodulin dependent autophosphorylation. (Data not shown).

RESULTS AND DISCUSSION

CaMkII Activity and Immunoreactivity in the β-Cell

In order to confirm that the autophosphorylation activity corresponded to CaMk in the β-cell, anti CaMkII antibodies were used with the phosphorylation products in Western analysis. Crude extracts of rat islets were subjected to a phosphorylation reaction in the presence or absence of Ca^{2+}, CaM, EGTA, TFP and KN62. The reaction products, resolved by SDS-PAGE were analyzed by immunoblotting and autoradiography (Fig. 1). The anti CaMkII antibody recognized a polypeptide of approximate M_r of 50 kDa (Fig. 1A) which was phosphorylated in a Ca^{2+}/calmodulin-dependent manner (Fig. 1B). The separate addition of EGTA, TFP and KN62 reduced the extent of phosphorylation (data not shown), and when they were jointly present in the reaction the phosphorylation of the 50 kDa protein was almost completely abolished.

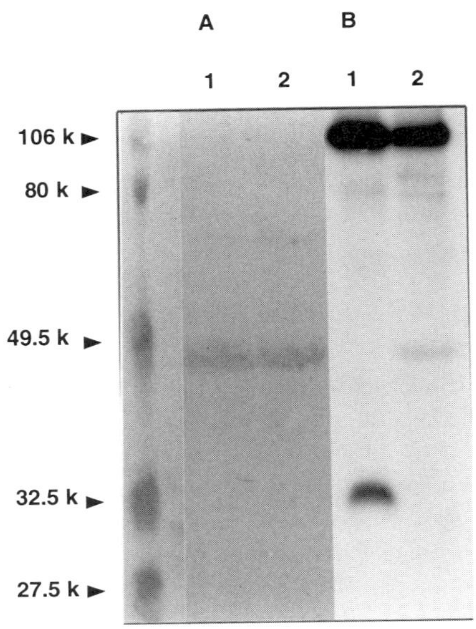

Figure 1. **A:** Immunoreactivity of anti CaMkII antibodies with rat islets proteins previously subjected to a phosphorylation reaction: Lane 1: in the presence of 1 mM EGTA; 1 mM TFP and 30 μM KN62. Lane 2: in the presence of 10 mM $CaCl_2$ and 20 μM calmodulin. **B:** Autoradiograph of the PVDF membrane in (A) showing the products of the phosphorylation reaction. Pre-stained molecular weight markers are shown on the left side panel.

Calcium/calmodulin-dependent phosphorylation of a protein of M_r 51–53 kDa has been previously reported in β–cells[11,9] The involvement of the β-cell CaMk in the secretory process has also been documented[10,12]. Our evidence for the presence of a protein with KN-62-inhibited Ca^{2+}/calmodulin-dependent phosphorylation activity that is recognized by anti-CaMkII antibodies strongly supports the view that the β-cell CaMk is closely related to CaMkII.

Northern Analysis of RINm5F β-Cells

Without previous data on the type of CaMk subunit/s expressed in the β-cell, and since all subunits exhibit high degree of homology in the catalytic (NH2-terminus) and the

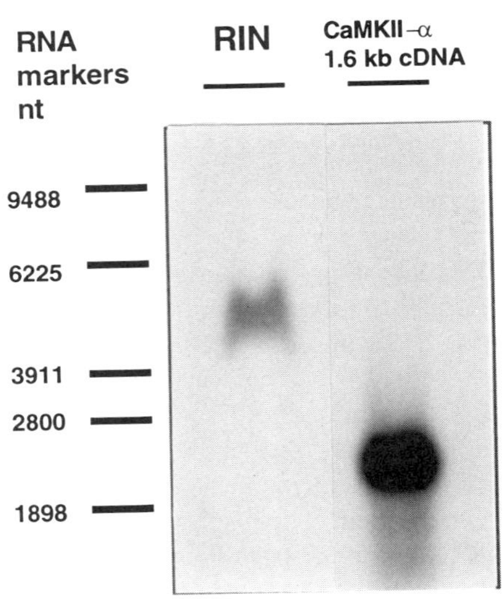

Figure 2. Northern analysis of RINm5F cells total RNA using a [^{32}P]-labelled riboprobe, transcribed from a brain CaMkII clone, included in the blot as a positive hybridization control. The position of ethidium bromide-stained molecular weight markers is indicated on the left side.

association (COOH-terminus) domains, the entire coding region of the α-subunit of the brain enzyme was arbitrarily chosen for the generation of the hybridization probe. An anti-sense riboprobe was preferred to DNA probes for the increased stability of RNA-RNA hybrids under equivalent stringency hybridization conditions.

The results of Northern analysis of total RNA extracted from RINm5F β-cells are shown in Fig. 2. The probe hybridized specifically with a single RNA band after high stringency washing steps. The length of the hybridizable fragment was estimated to be between 4500 and 5000 nucleotides, by comparison with ethidium bromide-stained RNA molecular weight markers.

Isolation of β-Cell CaMk Clones

The screening of a rat islet cDNA library with a brain CaMkII derived probe resulted in the isolation of several positive clones. The sequence of one of the clones, that encompassed the entire coding region, proved to be 88% homologous to the rat brain CaMkII β-subunit, exhibiting less degree of homology to all the other cloned subunits. Details of the cloned β-cell CaMk will be published elsewhere (manuscript in preparation).

The isolation of a rat islet cDNA clone homologous to the β-subunit of CaMkII constitutes conclusive evidence for the identity of at least one of the subunits of the β-cell CaMk. In addition to neuronal tissue, CaMkII activity has been reported in heart, liver, smooth muscle, and in cells of epithelial or sympathetic origin, but its functions have not been correlated with isoforms of the enzyme. Northern analyses of several rat tissues have revealed that the α (4.8 kb) and β (4.2 kb) mRNAs are primarily expressed in brain whereas γ (3.9 kb) and δ (4–4.2 kb) mRNAs are expressed in various other tissues[7]. The size of the CaMk-specific mRNA in RINm5F β-cells is compatible with that corresponding to the α or δ subunits, and the polypeptide identified in Western analysis appears to have a M_r closer to that of the α subunit or to one of the splice variants of the δ-subunit[6]. However, comparison of the predicted sizes of different cloned subunits with the apparent M_r indicates anomalous migration in SDS polyacrylamide gels[5]. These differences may be accounted for by post-translational modifications of the enzymes. We have observed two immunoreactive bands with CaMkII antibodies in several cultured β-cell lines (results not shown), indicating that more than one type of subunit is expressed. Our results demonstrating the expression of the β-subunit of CaMk in pancreatic islets do not provide information on the predominant form of the enzyme in the β-cell. Northern analysis with subunit-specific probes will provide a more conclusive answer to the identity of the expressed isozymes.

It has been shown that different isoforms of the enzyme are developmentally regulated and exhibit diverse cellular localization[7,13]. The variety and differential expression of the various subunits suggest that they have specialized functions in multiple tissues. There is evidence for the participation of CaMkII in neurotransmitter release[14,15] and the predominant isoforms in neuronal tissue appear to be the α and β-subunits. These data together with the implication of CaMk in insulin secretion[8–10,12] and the presence of the β isoform in rat islets suggest that this particular subunit is functionally related to the regulation of secretory processes.

CONCLUSIONS

We have identified the β-cell calcium/calmodulin-dependent protein kinase as CaMkII, by cloning from rat islets. Autophosphorylation of the β-cell CaMk occurs in a calcium/

calmodulin-dependent manner and is inhibited by KN62. The nucleotide sequence of one of the positive clones isolated from a cDNA library corresponds to that of the β isoform of the kinase. The expression of CaMkII was confirmed by Northern analysis of RINm5F β-cells RNA and by immunoreactivity of the pancreatic islet enzyme with CaMkII antibodies.

The cloning and determination of the nucleotide sequence of the β-cell CaMk provide the basis for studies on the regulation of the enzyme expression and its involvement in insulin secretion. Expression of the β isoform in the baculovirus system will allow further functional and structural characterization of the pancreatic CaMk.

ACKNOWLEDGMENTS

This study has been supported by grants from the Medical Research Council and the British Diabetic Association. We thank A. R. Means for CaMkII cDNA clones; B. Michelsen for the rat islet cDNA library and I. Jones for the baculovirus transfer-vector.

REFERENCES

1. Colbran, R.J. and Soderling, T.R. (1990). Curr. Topics Cell. Regul. 31: 181–221.
2. Hanson, P.I. and Schulman, H. (1992). Annu. Rev. Biochem. 61: 559–601.
3. Bulleit, R.F., Bennett, M.K., Molloy, S.S., Hurley, J.B., and Kennedy, M.B. (1988). Neuron 21: 63–72.
4. Nghiem, P., Saati, S.M., Martens, C.L., Gardner, P. and Schulman, H. (1993). J. Biol. Chem. 268: 5471–5479.
5. Schworer, C.M., Rothblum, L.I., Thekkumkara, T.J. and Singer, H.A. (1993). J. Biol. Chem. 268: 14443–14449.
6. Edman, C.F. and Schulman, H. (1994). Biochim Biophys. Acta 1221: 89–101.
7. Tobimatsu, T. and Fujisawa, H. (1989). J. Biol. Chem. 264: 17907–17912.
8. Colca J.R., Kotogal, N., Brooks, C.L., Lacy, P.E., Landt, M., and Mc Daniel, M.L. (1983). J. Biol. Chem. 258: 7260–7263.
9. Hughes, S., Smith, H. and Ashcroft, S.J.H. (1993). Biochem J. 289: 795–800.
10. Wenham, R.M., Landt, M. Walters, S.M., Hidaka, H. & Easom, R.A. (1992). Biochem. Biophys. Res. Com. 189: 128–133.
11. Cohn, J.A., Kinder, B., Jamieson, J.D., Delahunt, N.G. and Gorelick, F.S. (1987). Biochem. Biophys. Acta 928: 320–331.
12. Ämmälä, C., Eliasson, B., Wäppling-Raaholt, B., Bokvist, K., Larsson, O., Ashcroft, F.M. and Rorsman, P. (1993). Nature 363:356–358.
13. Takaishi, T., Saito, N. and Tanaka, C. (1992). J. Neurochem. 58: 1971–1974.
14. Llinas,R., Mc Guiness, T.L., Leonard, C.S., Sugimori, M. and Greengard, P. (1985). Proc. Natl. Acad. Sci. 82: 3035–3039.
15. Nichols, R.A., Sihra, T.S., Czernik, A.J., Nairn, A.C. and Greengard, P. (1990). Nature 343: 647–651.

13

TRANS-ACTING FACTOR(S) CONFER GLUCOSE-RESPONSIVE TRANSCRIPTIONAL REGULATION IN THE INSULIN GENE

Steve Goodison and Stephen J. H. Ashcroft

University of Oxford
Nuffield Dept. of Clinical Biochemistry
John Radcliffe Hospital
Headington, Oxford, United Kingdom

INTRODUCTION

In adult mammals the production of insulin is restricted to the β-cells of the islets of Langerhans. The β-cell specificity of insulin gene expression has been shown to be dependent on cis-acting sequences in the upstream non-coding region of the gene (1). Transfection studies have used mammalian insulin gene promoters to express reporter genes in a number of β-cell lines and have demonstrated that specific sequences exert positive or negative effects upon gene expression (2,3).

β-cell insulin biosynthesis is co-ordinated with the perception of metabolisable nutrient levels, the main physiological regulator molecule being glucose. Regulation of the synthesis of the insulin protein occurs at many levels and transcriptional regulation appears to be a key point of control. Glucose has been shown to stimulate increases in steady-state levels of preproinsulin mRNA in both islet preprartions and in β-cell lines (4,5) and more recently this nutrient controlled transcriptional regulation has been conferred upon reporter gene expression in β-cells when promoted by specific sequences of insulin gene 5′ sequences (6,7). The elements and sequences involved in the glucose response have been defined by 5′ deletion and subsequent transfection experiments (7,8), the putative "glucose-response element" lying between −193 to −227 bp of the insulin promoter within the region known as the FF-minienhancer (−196 to −247). Enhancer elements are thought to operate by influencing the binding of nuclear transcription factors to the gene promoter and these "glucose-sensitive" sequences have begun to be studied in order to identify the specific factors which may be involved in the glucose regulation of the insulin gene. The sequence −206 to −227 has been shown to bind up to three complexes in gel retardation experiments and furthermore the binding intensity of one of these complexes appears to be regulated by pre-incubation of rat islets with glucose (8).

Physiology and Pathophysiology of the Islets of Langerhans, edited by Soria.
Plenum Press, New York, 1997.

This study has attempted to detect glucose-responsive binding in a number of β-cell lines to correlate transcriptional activity of the insulin gene promoter and the binding profile of the "glucose-sensitive element."

METHODS

RNA analysis; Total RNA Northern blots were performed using MOPS denaturing gels with quantitation by autoradiography and densitometry.

Reporter gene studies; Calcium phosphate co-transfection of β-cell lines with β-galactosidase and rat insulin-1 promoted CAT expression plasmids. Enzyme activities were assayed 48 h post-transfection. Gel retardation assays; β-cell line nuclear extracts were bound to radio-labeled double-stranded GSE probe (–206 to –227) and visualised by high ionic strength polyacrylamide electrophoresis and autoradiography with densitometric quantitation.

RESULTS

Four different β-cell lines (HIT-T15, βTC3, RIN5mF and MIN-6) were tested for transcriptional responses to increased glucose concentrations. The steady-state level of pre-proinsulin RNA was monitored by RNA extraction and subsequent Northern blotting and quantitated by densitometry. All cell lines were incubated at 1 mM glucose overnight and then challenged with 11 mM glucose for a further 4 h. Both the HIT-T15 β-cell line and the MIN-6 β-cell line showed 2 to 3-fold increases in steady-state levels of preproinsulin mRNA (Fig. 1) whereas neither the RIN5mF or βTC3 cell lines showed any such increase in response to increased glucose.

This pattern of glucose responsiveness was repeated in the reporter gene transfection studies. An eukaryotic expression plasmid containing the reporter gene chloramphenicol acetyltransferase (CAT) under the transcriptional control of the rat insulin-1 sequences of –345 to +1 was co-transfected into the β-cell lines with a constitutively expressed β-galac-

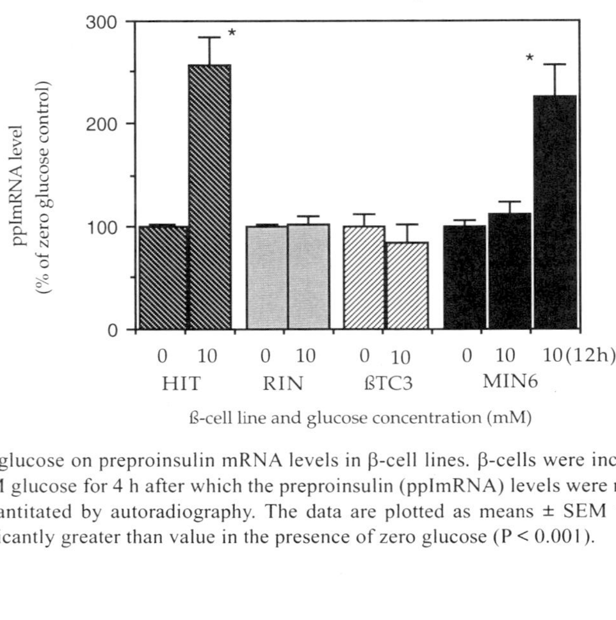

Figure 1. Effect of glucose on preproinsulin mRNA levels in β-cell lines. β-cells were incubated in the absence or presence of 10 mM glucose for 4 h after which the preproinsulin (pplmRNA) levels were measured by Northern blot analysis and quantitated by autoradiography. The data are plotted as means ± SEM for three independent observations. *Significantly greater than value in the presence of zero glucose ($P < 0.001$).

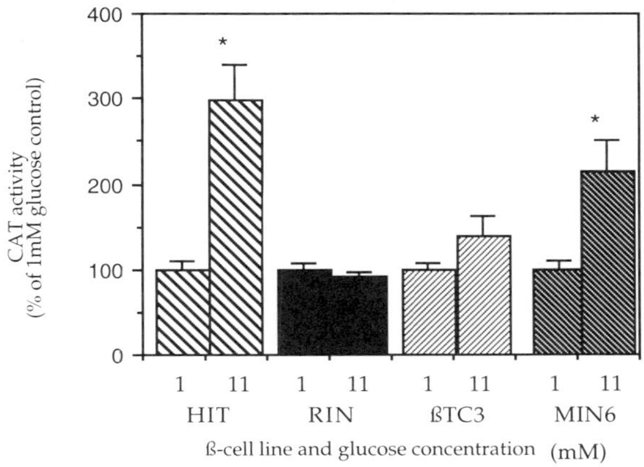

Figure 2. Effect of glucose on insulin promoter-driven CAT expression in transfected β-cell lines. β-cell lines were co-transfected with a RSV-promoted β-galactosidase expression plasmid and a rat insulin-1 promoted (–345 to +1) CAT reporter gene expression plasmid. 24 h after transfection the β-cells were incubated at 1 or 11 mM glucose for a further 24 h before extraction and assay of enzyme activities. The data are plotted as means ± SEM for three independent observations. *Significantly greater than value at 1mM glucose ($P < 0.001$).

tosidase plasmid for monitoring of insulin promoter regulated gene expression. The glucose challenge was as described for the mRNA experiments although the transfected cells needed 24 h recovery after the calcium phosphate mediated transfection before incubation in 1 mM glucose overnight. As in the RNA study neither the RIN5mF or the βTC3 cell lines responded to high glucose but both the HIT-T15 and the MIN-6 cells showed significantly increased reporter gene expression under high glucose conditions (Fig. 2).

Nuclear proteins were extracted from the various β-cell lines during the same passages and these extracts were used to analyse the binding profile of the putative "glucose-responsive element" by gel retardation experiments. The probe was synthesised to contain the sequences within the rat insulin-1 FF-minienhancer from –206 to –227 (GSE). The single-stranded probe was labelled with radioactive phosphate by T4 polynucleotide kinase and then annealed to the complementary strand to create the double-stranded DNA probe. Aliquots of nuclear protein were incubated with the labelled probe under the conditions described in the legend to Fig. 3. and then the DNA/protein complexes were separated on non-denaturing polyacrylamide gels. The specific complexes were visualised by autoradiography. A number of complexes were observed (P1-P4). Complexes P1–P3 were shown to bind specifically by competition with the unlabelled GSE probe and by using rat insulin-1 fragments containing block mutations. One complex, P2, was found to be consistently glucose-sensitive. β-cell cultures were incubated overnight (16 h) in 1 mM or 11 mM glucose media and nuclear extracts were isolated. Under these conditions the P2 complex was found to bind the labelled probe with an increased intensity of some 2-fold (Fig. 3).

However only extracts from those β-cell lines which retained glucose-responsive transcriptional regulation as measured by the mRNA and reporter gene studies showed such an increase in binding activity.

CONCLUSIONS

It therefore appears that there is a close correlation between the ability to regulate the binding of a specific protein to the rat insulin-I DNA sequences between base pair

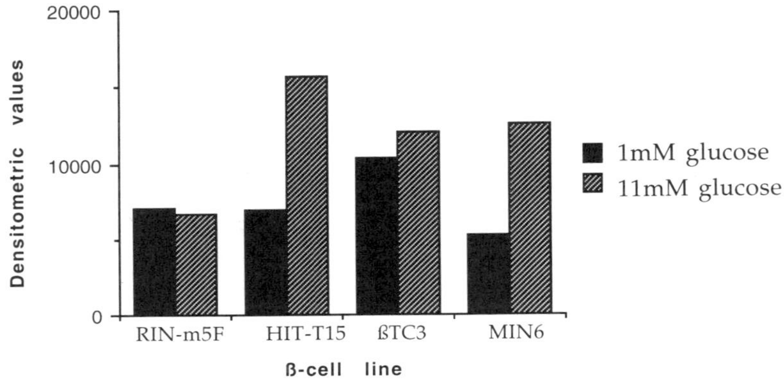

Figure 3. Binding activity of P2 complex. Nuclear extracts (2 μg) from β-cell lines incubated under 1 mM or 11 mM glucose conditions were assayed by binding to a labelled rat insulin-1 double stranded probe (−206 to −227). Gel retardation of equivalent protein concentrations was followed by densitometric quantificaton of P2 complex binding intensity.

positions −206 and −227 of the promoter and the ability to retain glucose-responsive transcriptional regulation. This particular protein may thus play a pivotal role at this level of nutrient regulation in the β-cell.

REFERENCES

1. Walker, M.D., Edlund, T., Boulet, A.M., Rutter, W.J. (1983). Nature 306, 557–61.
2. Boam, D.S.W., Clark, A.R., Docherty, K. (1990). J. Biol. Chem. 265, 8285–91.
3. Karlsson, O., Edlund, T., Barnet-Moss, J., Rutter, W.J., Walker, M.D. (1987). Proc. Natl. Acad. Sci. USA 84, 8819–23.
4. Welsh, M., Nielsen, D.A., MacKrell, A.J., Steiner, D.F. (1985). J. Biol. Chem. 260, 13590–94.
5. Permutt, M.A. (1974). J. Biol. Chem. 249, 2738–2742.
6. Goodison, S., Kenna, S., Ashcroft, S.J.H. (1992). Biochem. J. 285, 563–568.
7. German, M.S., Moss, L.G., Rutter, W.J. (1990). J. Biol. Chem. 265, 22063–66.
8. Melloul, D., Ben-Neriah, Y., Cerasi, E. (1993). Proc. Natl. Acad. Sci. USA 90, 3865–69.

Part III. MODULATION OF ISLET RELEASE

14

EXTRACELLULAR MESSAGES FOR PANCREATIC B-CELLS

Toshihiko Yada

Department of Physiology
Kagoshima University School of Medicine
8-35-1 Sakuragaoka
Kagoshima 890, Japan

Insulin secretion from pancreatic B-cells is subject to fine regulation by a variety of extracellular messages, which include nutrients of dietary origin, physiological messengers of neural and hormonal origins, and pharmacological agents. In this article, I will briefly review the major, classical messages of each type, and then focus on new studies on the substances that have recently been discovered or developed. Particular attention will be paid on their origin, action mechanisms in pancreatic B-cells, and potential physiological or pharmacological significance in the regulation of insulin release.

NUTRIENT MESSAGES

A unique and important aspect of insulin secretion from the islets of Langerhans is its regulation by nutrients as well as neuronal and hormonal factors.

Sugars

D-Glucose. Among nutrients, glucose is the most important stimulator of insulin release. Carbohydrates in the diet are digested in the gastrointestinal tract to finally yield monosaccharides: D-glucose, D-galactose and D-fructose. D-glucose represents more than 80 per cent of the final products of carbohydrate digestion. D-glucose, as well as D-galactose, is rapidly absorbed into the portal blood by the following mechanisms in the small intestine. Glucose is transported from the lumen to the interior of the cells by the Na^+-glucose co-transporter present in the luminal, brush-border membrane of the epithelial absorptive cells. By using the Na^+ gradient as a driving force, this Na^+-coupled transport mechanism is capable of moving glucose to the interior of the cells to a level higher than

Physiology and Pathophysiology of the Islets of Langerhans, edited by Soria.
Plenum Press, New York, 1997.

that in the lumen, thereby exhibiting the nature of the active transport. The accumulated glucose within the cells then diffuses into the blood by the passive, facilitative glucose transporter present in the basolateral membrane of the epithelial cells. A resultant rise in the blood glucose concentration, above the threshold level around 5 mM, initiates insulin release from pancreatic islets mainly by the following mechanisms. Glucose enters B-cells through a high K_m (around 15 mM) facilitative glucose transporter (GLUT-2) that is specific to B-cells and hepatocytes. It is now believed that glucose is metabolized by islet B-cells to raise intracellular ATP level, the key factor that inhibits the ATP-sensitive K^+ channel[1]. A resultant depolarization leads to an activation of the voltage-dependent L-type Ca^{2+} channel of the B-cell plasma membrane, and an increase in the cytosolic free Ca^{2+} concentration ($[Ca^{2+}]_i$)[2], a triggering signal for exocytosis of insulin[3,4]. Other signal transduction mechanisms are also provoked by glucose in B-cells[5], some of which appear to play an important role in the modulation of insulin release. Glucose is the primary stimulus or initiator, a concept given for the substance that stimulates insulin release in the absence of any other secretagogues. D-galactose is absorbed by the same route as glucose in the intestine, but it is neither metabolized by B-cells nor does it stimulate insulin release. D-mannose, another metabolized sugar in B-cells, can stimulate insulin release by similar mechanisms to those for glucose.

D-Fructose. D-fructose represents less than 10 percent of the final products of carbohydrate digestion. Fructose is absorbed into the portal blood by the facilitative transporters equipped in the intestinal epithelial cells. Fructose is metabolized by B-cells but at a much smaller rate than glucose, and therefore it can only potentiate the glucose-induced insulin release.

Amino Acids

Amino acids, like carbohydrates, are major components of food which control insulin secretion. Among ten essential amino acids, L-leucine, L-arginine and L-lysine stimulate insulin release. Leucine and arginine have been most thoroughly studied and are now recognized as insulin secretagogues of physiological relevance.

L-Leucine. L-leucine, an electrically neutral amino acid, qualifies as an initiator as well as potentiator, since it stimulates insulin release both at basal and elevated glucose concentrations[6]. Leucine is metabolized by pancreatic B-cells, thereby leading to a sequence of events similar to that evoked by glucose[7]. Leucine acts also through allosteric activation of glutamate dehydrogenase and resultant activation of the mitochondria TCA cycle in pancreatic B-cells[7].

L-Arginine. L-arginine is one of the cationic amino acids that possess positively charged side chains. Arginine is a strong potentiator of insulin release. The major mode of the arginine-induced insulin release is that a membrane depolarization produced by accumulation of the cationic arginine leads to a voltage-dependent activation of L-type Ca^{2+} channels, and a consequent increase in $[Ca^{2+}]_i$ triggers exocytosis[7]. Arginine is also metabolized by islet cells, yielding L-ornithine and urea, or, producing nitric oxide (NO). Although the available evidence suggests that the metabolism seems not to be directly linked to the stimulation of insulin release, the arginine-NO system might be involved in the late phase of insulin release, and also in the impaired insulin secretion and/or the destruction of B-cells in diabetes[7].

NEURONAL MESSAGES

Stimulators

Acetylcholine (ACh). ACh is an important neurotransmitter, which largely accounts for the vagal stimulation of insulin release[6]. Both *in vivo* and *in vitro*, ACh initiates insulin release at basal glucose concentrations, though modestly, and potently augments the glucose-induced insulin release[6]. ACh is thus considered to be a modest initiator as well as a strong potentiator of insulin secretion. ACh and its agonists, such as carbamylcholine (CCh), are thought to act on the muscarinic receptor of M_3 subtype in B-cells[8] that is linked to phospholipase C via a subtype of GTP-binding proteins (G_p). The muscarinic activation thus leads to a formation of IP_3 associated with Ca^{2+} release from intracellular stores and an activation of protein kinase C[5]. Muscarinic stimulation involves a depolarization of membrane potential, an increase in $[Ca^{2+}]_i$, and a rise in the membrane permeability for Na^+ in B-cells[9].

Vasoactive Intestinal Peptide (VIP). VIP-like immunoreactivity has been identified in the nerve fibres supplying pancreatic ganglia and blood vessels in humans, dogs, cats and rats[10]. It is suggested that preganglionic fibres entering the pancreas control the activity of the post-ganglionic, VIPergic nerve fibres that appear to be intrinsic to the pancreas[10]. VIP is released to the effluent of isolated, perfused pancreas following electrical stimulation of the vagal fibres[11]. VIP stimulates insulin release in rats, mice and dogs[10]. VIP is thus suggested to be a physiological neuropeptide. It is likely that VIP acts on B-cells via activating a stimulatory subtype of GTP-binding protein (G_s) that is coupled to adenylyl cyclase, thereby stimulating cAMP production. An increase in $[Ca^{2+}]_i$ has also recently been demonstrated in rat B-cells[12].

Gastrin-Releasing Peptide (GRP). Immunoreactivity for GRP and for a related peptide bombesin has been demonstrated in the pancreatic nerve fibres of several species[10]. GRP is released to the effluent of isolated, perfused pancreas following electrical stimulation of the vagal fibres[13]. GRP stimulates insulin secretion in dogs and calves. GRP is thus suggested to be a physiological neuropeptide.

Cholecystokinin (CCK). CCK, a well known insulinotropic peptide, is identified in nerve fibres in pancreas and probably acts as a neurotransmitter at peptidergic synapses in islets. The peptide stimulates insulin release from B-cells due to intracellular mechanisms similar to those evoked by ACh, except a rise in the Na^+ permeability which has not yet evidenced for CCK. Whether CCK is released to the effluent following neural stimulation remains to be demonstrated[10].

Pituitary Adenylate Cyclase Activating Polypeptide (PACAP). PACAP, a new member of the glucagon/VIP family of peptides[14], was originally isolated from bovine hypothalamus in 1989[15]. PACAP occurs as a 27- (PACAP27) or a 38-residue peptide (PACAP38), and is present in a variety of tissue, abundant in the central nervous system, posterior pituitary, adrenal, and testis[14]. PACAP-like immunoreactivity has been demonstrated in the nerve fibers of rat pancreas[12,16]. PACAP stimulates insulin release in a glucose-dependent manner[12]. PACAP is thus a putative neuromodulator of the glucose-induced insulin secretion.

Inhibitors

Noradrenalin. Noradrenalin (norepinephrine) is a well established neurotransmitter released from sympathetic nerve endings in the pancreas[6]. It has been believed that the adrenergic mechanism largely contributes to the sympathetic attenuation of insulin secretion. Noradrenalin, as well as adrenalin (epinephrine) that is released from the adrenal medulla, inhibits insulin release by activating α_2-adrenoceptors in B-cells[17]. The receptor is coupled to the adenylyl cyclase by an inhibitory subtype of GTP-binding proteins (G_i). Activation of the receptor causes a reduction of cAMP level in B-cells, an inhibitory signal for insulin release. It also involves opening of K^+ channels associated with membrane hyperpolarization, decreased Ca^{2+} influx through Ca^{2+} channels, and attenuation of the $[Ca^{2+}]_i$ activity in B-cells. It is suggested that catecholamines may also act directly on a subtype of GTP-binding proteins (G_e) that regulates exocytosis.

Galanin. Galanin-like immunoreactivity has been demonstrated in the pancreatic nerve fibres of several species[10]. Galanin is released from sympathetic nerve endings in the pancreas. This peptide potently inhibits insulin and somatostatin release as well as stimulating glucagon release. Consequently, it produces a marked hyperglycemia. The specific receptor for galanin has been demonstrated in B-cells. Activation of the receptor that is coupled to G_i leads to inhibition of adenylyl cyclase and other changes in signal transduction similar to those evoked by catecholamines[17].

Calcitonin Gene-Related Peptide (CGRP). CGRP containing fibers have been demonstrated in pancreas. This peptide inhibits insulin release[10].

Substance P. Substance P containing fibers have been identified in pancreas and this peptide inhibits insulin release. Substance P is suggested to be an inhibitory neuromodulator[10].

Opioids. Enkephalin containing fibers have been demonstrated in pancreas. Enkephalin inhibits insulin release and is suggested to be an inhibitory neuromodulator[10]. Opioids have also stimulatory effects on insulin release depending upon the species and concentration of the peptides used[17].

ENTERO-INSULAR AXIS

The insulin secretory response of pancreas is much larger after oral glucose than after intravenous infusion of glucose achieving identical plasma glucose levels. The functional connection from the intestine to the endocrine pancreas is called "entero–insular axis." The term "incretin" was introduced for a humoral factor which is released from the intestine upon food intake and potentiates the glucose-induced insulin secretion. Though the chemical structure of incretin has not thoroughly been determined, glucagon-like peptide-1 and gastric inhibitory polypeptide are currently considered to be physiological incretins[18–20].

Humoral Messages

Glucagon-Like Peptide-1 (GLP-1). GLP-1 is produced from proglucagon, a precursor of glucagon, by post-translational processing in the intestine, first as a form of GLP-1(1-37), which is further cleaved to yield GLP-1(7-37) and GLP-1(7-36)amide. GLP-1(7-37) and GLP-1(7-36)amide, the truncated GLP-1 (tGLP-1), are the active forms of the peptide. tGLP-1 is released from the distal small intestine to the circulation after oral ingestion of food. tGLP-1, in the physiological concentration range of 10^{-11} to 10^{-9} M, potently stimulates insulin release in a glucose-dependent manner in humans, rats, pigs and dogs. GLP-1 thus qualifies as a physiological incretin[18–20]. tGLP-1 also stimulates proinsulin expression and proinsulin biosynthesis, suggesting that this peptide is also a trophic hormone for insulin. Furthermore, tGLP-1 suppresses glucagon secretion and stimulates somatostatin secretion, thereby acting as a potent hypoglycemic hormone[19,20].

GLP-1 is a member of the glucagon/VIP family of peptides. A specific receptor for tGLP-1 has been cloned[21]. The GLP-1 receptor in B-cells appears to be coupled to adenylyl cyclase through G_s. An elevation of intracellular cAMP in response to tGLP-1 was demonstrated in rat, mouse and hamster insulinoma cell lines[19,22]. It has been demonstrated that tGLP-1 increases $[Ca^{2+}]_i$ by enhancing the activity of L-type Ca^{2+} channels in the plasma membrane in rat pancreatic B-cells[23] and HIT insulinoma cells[22], and that the $[Ca^{2+}]_i$ increase is produced by a cAMP-operative mechanism. The Ca^{2+} and cAMP messengers, thus activated by tGLP-1, could act synergistically to result in an eloquent insulin release, since a marked potentiation by cAMP of the Ca^{2+}-induced exocytosis has recently been demonstrated[24].

Gastric Inhibitory Polypeptide (GIP). GIP, a 30 amino acid residue peptide, is also a member of the glucagon/VIP family of peptides. GIP is produced and released from the upper small intestine to the circulation in response to oral ingestion of food[19]. GIP, in a nanomolar concentration range, increases insulin release in a glucose-dependent manner. Immunoneutralization with antisera against GIP abolished the incretin effect but only by 20–30%[18,20]. GIP, unlike tGLP-1, stimulates glucagon secretion. It appears that GIP stimulates insulin release from B-cells largely by similar mechanisms to those for tGLP-1 including increases in intracellular cAMP and $[Ca^{2+}]_i$ [22].

Nervous Messages

The possible role of the nervous system in the "entero-insular axis" is little understood. Electrophysiological studies indicated that glucoreceptors are present in the intestine and that glucose infusion in the intestinal tract leads to insulin release via vagal reflex[25]. An interesting idea that GLP-1, a humoral messenger for the "entero–insular axis," could additionally provoke a nervous mechanism has been proposed: intraportal administration of physiologic concentrations of tGLP-1, but not GLP-1(1-37), increased both the hepatic afferent and pancreatic efferent vagal activities within a few min[26].

INTRA-PANCREATIC MESSAGES

Stimulators

Glucagon. Glucagon is synthesized and released from islet A-cells. Glucagon potentiates the glucose-induced insulin secretion, and this effect is likely to be linked with increases in cAMP and $[Ca^{2+}]_i$ in B-cells[2]. It has long been thought that glucagon released from A-cells exerts a paracrine action on B-cells. However, in the light of the anatomy of islets that the local circulation is from the core of islets where B-cells are present to the mantle of islets where A-cells are present[17], the paracrine role of glucagon in the regulation of B-cell function needs to be reconsidered.

Activin. Activin, a 25K dalton protein composed of the dimer of b subunit of inhibin, was originally isolated in 1986 as a stimulatory factor for FSH release[27]. Activin was later shown to stimulate insulin release from rat islets in the presence of both basal and stimulatory concentrations of glucose[28]. Thus, activin is considered to be an initiator as well as an potentiator. Activin was also shown to increase $[Ca^{2+}]_i$, which was inhibited by nifedipine and diazoxide, indicating that activin stimulates Ca^{2+} influx through voltage-dependent Ca^{2+} channels in B-cells[29]. Immunocytochemical study in rat islets demonstrated that activin is localized both in glucagon and somatostatin granules[30]. It is therefore suggested that activin may be released together with glucagon from A-cells and with somatostatin from D-cells, and that it may modulate B-cell responsiveness to glucose by a paracrine influence. A stimulatory effect of activin was also observed on glucose output from the liver. However, a definitive physiological role of activin is yet to be ascertained.

ACTH-Like Peptide. ACTH-like immunoreactivity has recently been identified in pancreatic islets[31]. The ACTH-like peptide is released together with insulin from B-cells. In the presence of glucose, it stimulates insulin release, and this effect is due to an increase in $[Ca^{2+}]_i$ in B-cells.

Pacap. PACAP-like immunoreactivity has been demonstrated in rat pancreatic islets as well as in nerve fibers[12]. Both PACAP27 and PACAP38 as low as 10^{-14}–10^{-13} M stimulate insulin release in a glucose-dependent manner. A $[Ca^{2+}]_i$ measurement combined with immunocytochemical identification of islet cell species has revealed that PACAP at 10^{-13} M selectively and directly targets B-cells to increase $[Ca^{2+}]_i$ [12]. A subtype of PACAP receptors (PACAPR-3) is expressed in MIN6 insulinoma and islet cells[32]. The available evidence indicates that the $[Ca^{2+}]_i$ increase is due to a stimulated Ca^{2+} entry through L-type Ca^{2+} channels, and that the $[Ca^{2+}]_i$ increase triggers the insulin secretory response[33]. A striking feature is that PACAP appears to be at least 3 logs more potent than any of the insulinotropic peptides known to date. These findings suggest that PACAP could serve as a local hormonal regulator of the glucose-induced insulin secretion.

ATP. ATP amplifies insulin release, at least in certain species, by activating extracellular P_{2y}-purinergic receptors in B-cells[17]. It is known that ATP, a neurotransmitter, is also rich in the secretory granules. An interesting concept that ATP co-released with hormones from islet cells during exocytosis exerts a direct action on B-cells remains to be evidenced.

Inhibitors

Somatostatin. Somatostatin14 is synthesized and released from islet D-cells, whereas somatostatin28 is released by the gut. Somatostatin markedly inhibits insulin secretion stimulated by glucose and many other secretagogues. Several somatostatin receptor subtypes have been cloned[34]. It appears that somatostatin acts on one or a couple of the receptor subtypes in B-cells that are linked to G_i, and thereby leads to a sequence of inhibitory events including inhibition of adenylyl cyclase in a manner similar to catecholamines and galanin. It has long been thought that somatostatin released from D-cells exerts a paracrine action on B-cells. However, D-cells are located predominantly near A-cells but not B-cells, and somatostatin14, the form present in pancreatic islet D-cells, inhibits insulin release 3 log orders less potently than glucagon release[35]. Therefore, the role of somatostatin14 released from D-cells in the control of B-cell activity appears to be less important, if any, than previously thought, whereas its inhibitory action on glucagon release from A-cells is of physiological importance.

Pancreastatin. Pancreastatin, a peptide structurally similar to chromogranin A, modestly inhibits insulin release induced by glucose and other secretagogues[17].

Neuropeptide Y. It has recently been shown that neuropeptide Y is released from isolated perifused rat islets, and that immunoneutralization with neuropeptide Y antiserum increased insulin release[36]. It is thus suggested that islet neuropeptide Y could act as a paracrine hormone and constrain insulin release.

Islet Amyloid Polypeptide (IAPP). IAPP, a peptide structurally related to CGRP, is synthesized in B-cells and released with insulin[17]. IAPP, only in pharmacologically high concentrations, inhibits insulin secretion. It has been speculated that overproduction and excessive secretion of IAPP, observed in some NIDDM, may inhibit insulin release from B-cells by an autocrine mechanism[37]. However, whether and to what extent IAPP is involved in the impaired glucose tolerance in NIDDM are still disputed.

PHARMACOLOGICAL AGENTS

Insulin release is modulated by various pharmacological agents, which include inhibitors of metabolism, receptor agonists and antagonists, and activators and inhibitors of ion channels in the plasma membrane and ER membrane in B-cells. Here, however, the attention is focused only on the activators and inhibitors of ATP-sensitive K^+ channels and voltage-dependent Ca^{2+} channels of the B-cell plasma membrane.

ATP-Sensitive K^+ Channel Modulators

Sulfonylureas. Sulfonylureas, such as tolbutamide and glibenclamide, are currently used for treating patients with NIDDM. It is well established that the major action of sulfonylureas is to inhibit ATP-sensitive K^+ channels in B-cell plasma membrane[1]. This consequently depolarizes the membrane, activates voltage-dependent Ca^{2+} channels and increases $[Ca^{2+}]_i$, leading to insulin release.

Non-Sulfonylurea Moiety of Sulfonylureas. The activity to inhibit ATP-sensitive K^+ channels or Rb^+ efflux and to stimulate insulin release has been shown for derivatives of the second-generation sulfonylureas having only the non-sulfonylurea moiety of the mother compounds, which include HB699 derived from glibenclamide, UL-DF9 derived from gliquidone and AZ-DF-265[38].

Linogliride. The activity to inhibit ATP-sensitive K^+ channels and stimulate insulin release has been shown also for a non-sulfonylurea compound linogliride[38].

D-Phenylalanine Derivative A-4166. N-[(*trans*-4-isopropylcyclohexyl)-carbonyl]-D-phenylalanine (A-4166), a derivative of D-phenylalanine, is a new non-sulfonylurea oral hypoglycemic agent. It reduces blood glucose levels in nondiabetic and diabetic animals in a quicker and shorter-lasting manner than sulfonylureas due to a stimulated release of insulin. A-4166 increases $[Ca^{2+}]_i$ in B-cells presumably by an inhibition of ATP-sensitive K^+ channels[39].

Imidazoline RX821002. Imidazoline RX821002, an α_2-adrenoceptor antagonist, enhances insulin release due to a reduction of K^+ flux via ATP-sensitive K^+ channels[40]. An imidazoline binding site that could be responsible for regulation of ATP-sensitive K^+ channels has been identified in RIN cell plasma membrane.

Diazoxide. Diazoxide has been used to treat chronic hypoglycemia induced by hyperinsulinemia. Diazoxide opens ATP-sensitive K^+ channels and thereby repolarizes the membrane, closes voltage-dependent Ca^{2+} channels, reduces $[Ca^{2+}]_i$, and consequently attenuates insulin release[1].

Pyridothiadiazine Derivative, BPDZ. It has been shown that a newly synthesized pyridothiadiazine derivative, BPDZ 44 or BPDZ 62, inhibits insulin releasing process by activating ATP-sensitive K^+ channels[41]. The compounds could be useful pharmacological tools for characterizing the structural requirements for the ATP-sensitive K^+ channel activation and selectivity.

Ca^{2+} Channel Modulators

Dihydropyridine or Phenylalkylamine Inhibitor. Dihydropyridines, such as nitrendipine and nifedipine, or phenylalkylamines, such as verapamil and D-600, block the voltage-dependent L-type Ca^{2+} channel in B-cells, and thereby antagonize the action of a variety of depolarizing agents, including glucose, to increase $[Ca^{2+}]_i$ [1].

Dihydropyridine Activator. Dihydropyridine derivatives, Bay K 8644 and CGP-28392, increase the mean open time of the L-type Ca^{2+} current in B-cells[1]. They therefore potentiate the insulin release stimulated by depolarizing agents.

Non-Dihydropyridine Activator. A non-dihydropyridine Ca^{2+} channel activator, FPL 64176, has been found to produce an increase in $[Ca^{2+}]_i$ and a subsequent release of insulin from βTC3 cells[42]. This may be related to the background Ca^{2+} influx mediated by a dihydropyridine-insensitive Ca^{2+} channel recently reported in mouse pancreatic B-cells[43].

ACKNOWLEDGMENTS

Studies from my laboratory referred to in this article were supported in part by grants from the Ministry of Education, Science and Culture of Japan and from Japan Diabetes Foundation.

REFERENCES

1. Ashcroft, F.M., Rorsman, P. 1989, Electrophysiology of the pancreatic β-cells, *Prog. Biophys. Molec. Biol.* 54:87–143.
2. Hellman, B., Gylfe, E., Grapengiesser, E., Lund, P.-E., and Marcström, A. 1992, Cytoplasmic calcium and insulin secretion, In: "Nutrient regulation of insulin secretion," P.R. Flatt, ed., pp. 213–246, Portland Press Ltd., London.

3. Penner, R., and Neher, E. 1988, The role of calcium in stimulus secretion coupling in excitable and non-excitable cells, *J. Exp. Biol.* 139:329–345.
4. Ämmälä, C., Eliasson, L., Bokvist, K., Larsson, O., Ashcroft, F.M., and Rorsman, P. 1993b, Exocytosis elicited by action potentials and voltage-clamp calcium currents in individual mouse pancreatic B-cells, *J. Physiol.* 472:665–688.
5. Prentki, M., and Matschinsky, F.M., 1987, Ca^{2+}, cAMP, and phospholipid-derived messengers in coupling mechanisms of insulin secretion, *Physiol. Rev.* 67:1185–1248.
6. Wollheim, C.B., and Sharp, G.W.G., 1981, Regulation of insulin release by calcium, *Physiol. Rev.* 61:914–973.
7. Yada, T. 1994, Action mechanisms of amino acids in pancreatic B-cells, In: "Frontiers of Pancreatic B-cell Research," P.R. Flatt, ed., Smith Gordon and Co. Ltd., London, pp. 129–135.
8. Verspohl, E.J., Tacke, R., Mutschler, E., and Lambrecht, G., 1990, Muscarinic receptor subtypes in rat pancreatic islets: binding and functional studies, *Eur. J.Pharmacol.* 178:303–311.
9. Henquin, J.-C., Garcia, M.-C., Bozem, M., Hermans, M.P., and Nenquin, M., 1988, Muscarinic control of pancreatic B cell function involves sodium dependent depolarization and calcium influx, *Endocrinology* 122:2134–2142.
10. Ahren, B., Taborsky, G.J., and Porte, D., 1986, Neuropeptidergic versus cholinergic and adrenergic regulation of islet hormone secretion, *Diabetologia* 29:827–836.
11. Holst, J.J., Fahrenkrug, J., Knuhtsen, S., Jensen, S.L., Poulsen, S.S., and Nielsen, O.V., 1984, Vasoactive intestinal polypeptide (VIP) in the pig pancreas: role of VIPergic fibers in control of fluid and bicarbonate secretion, *Regul. Pept.* 8:245–249.
12. Yada, T., Sakurada, M., Ihida, K., Nakata, M., Murata, F., Arimura, A., and Kikuchi, M., 1994, Pituitary adenylate cyclase activating polypeptide is an extraordinarily potent intra-pancreatic regulator of insulin secretion from islet, β-cells, *J. Biol. Chem.* 269:1290–1293.
13. Knuhtsen, S., Holst, J.J., Jensen, S.L., and Nielsen, O.V., 1985, Gastrin-releasing peptide: effect on exocrine secretion and release from isolated perfused pig pancreas, *Am. J. Physiol.* 248:G281–G287.
14. Arimura, A., 1992, Pituitary adenylate cyclase activating polypeptide (PACAP): discovery and current status of research, *Regul. Pept.* 37:287–303.
15. Miyata, A., Arimura, A., Dahl, R.R., Minamino, N., Uehara, A., Jiang, L., Culler, M.D., and Coy, D.H., 1989, Isolation of a novel 38 residue-hypothalamic polypeptide which stimulates adenylate cyclase in pituitary cells, *Biochem. Biophys. Res. Commun.* 164:567–574.
16. Fridolf, T., Sundler, F., and Ahren, B., 1992, Pituitary adenylate cyclase-activating polypeptide (PACAP): occurrence in rodent pancreas and effects on insulin and glucagon secretion in the mouse, *Cell Tissue Res.* 269:275–279.
17. Henquin, J.-C., 1994, Cell biology of insulin secretion, In: "Joslin's Diabetes Mellitus," C.R. Kahn and G.C. Weir, eds., pp. 56–80, Lea & Febiger, Malvern.
18. Fehmann, H.-C., Göke, R., and Göke, B., 1992, Glucagon-like peptide-1(7-37)/(7-36)amide is a new incretin, *Mol. Cell. Endocrinol.* 85:C39–C44.
19. Orskov, C., 1992, Glucagon-like peptide-l, a new hormone of the entero-insular axis, *Diabetologia* 35:701–711.
20. Habener, J.F., 1993, The incretin notion and its relevance to diabetes, *Endocrinol. Metabol. Clin. North America* 22:775–794.
21. Thorens, B., 1992, Expression cloning of the pancreatic β cell receptor for the gluco-incretin hormone glucagon-like peptide 1, *Proc. Natl. Acad. Sci. USA* 89:8641–8645.
22. Lu, M., Wheeler, M.B., Leng, X.-H., and Boyd, A.E. 1993, The role of the free cytosolic calcium level in β-cell signal transduction by gastric inhibitory polypeptide and glucagon-like peptide I(7-37), *Endocrinology* 132:94–100.
23. Yada, T., Itoh, K., and Nakata, M., 1993, Glucagon-like peptide-1-(7-36)amide and a rise in cyclic adenosine 3′,5′-monophosphate increase cytosolic free Ca^{2+} in rat pancreatic β-cells by enhancing Ca^{2+} channel activity, *Endocrinology* 133:1685–1692.
24. Ämmälä, C., Ashcroft, F.M., and Rorsman, P., 1993a, Calcium independent potentiation of insulin release by cyclic AMP in single B-cells, *Nature* 363:356–358.
25. Mei, N., Arlhac, A., and Boyer, A., 1981, Nervous regulation of insulin release by the intestinal vagal glucoreceptors, *J. Autonom. Nerv. Syst.* 4:351–363.
26. Nakabayashi, H., Nishizawa, M., Takeda, R., and Niijima, A., 1992, A novel role of truncated glucagon-like peptide-1 in the enteroinsular axis (EIA), *Diabetes* 41(suppl.1): 101A.
27. Vale, W., Rivier, J., Vaughan, J., McClintock, R., Corrigan, A., Woo, W., Karr, D., and Spiess, J. 1986, Purification and characterization of an FSH releasing protein from porcine ovarian follicular fluid, *Nature* 321:776–779.

28. Totsuka, Y., Tabuchi, M., Kojima, I., Shibata, H., and Ogata, E., 1988, A novel action of activin A: stimulation of insulin secretion in rat pancreatic islets, *Biochem. Biophys. Res. Commun.* 156:335–339.
29. Shibata, H., Yasuda, H., Sekine, N., Totsuka, Y., and Kojima, I., 1993, Activin A increases cytoplasmic free calcium concentration in rat pancreatic islet, *FEBS Lett.* 329:194–198.
30. Yasuda, H., Inoue, K., Shibata, H., Takeuchi, T., Eto, Y., Hasegawa, Y., Sekine, N., Totsuka, Y., Mine, T., Ogata, E., and Kojima, I., 1993, Existence of activin A in A- and D-cells of rat pancreatic islet, *Endocrinology* 133:624–630.
31. Gagliardino, J.J., Borelli, M.I., Estivariz, F., Atwater, I., Boschero, A.C., and Rojas, E., 1997, Islet release of ACTH-like peptides and their modulatory effect on insulin secretion, In "Physiology and Pathophysiology of the Islets of Langerhans," B. Soria, ed., Plenum Press, New York.
32. Inagaki, N., Yoshida, H., Mizuta, M., Mizuno, N., Fujii, Y., Gonoi, T., Miyazaki, J., and Seino, S., 1994, Cloning and functional characterization of a third pituitary adenylate cyclase-activating polypeptide receptor subtype expressed in insulin secreting cells, *Proc. Natl. Acad. Sci. USA* 91:2679–2683.
33. Yada, T., Sakurada, M., Nakata, M., Yaekura, K., and Kikuchi, M., 1997, PACAP stimulates insulin release via cytosolic Ca^{2+} increase due to Ca^{2+} influx through L-type Ca^{2+} channels in pancreatic, β-cells, In "Physiology and Pathophysiology of the Islets of Langerhans," B. Soria, ed., Plenum Press, New York.
34. Yamada, Y., Post, S.R., Wang, K., Tager, H.S., Bell, G.I., and Seino, S., 1992, Cloning and functional characterization of a family of human and mouse somatostatin receptors expressed in brain, gastrointestinal tract, and kidney, *Proc. Natl. Acad. Sci. USA* 89:251–255.
35. Schuit, F. C., Derde, M.-P. , and Pipeleers, D.G., 1989, Sensitivity of rat pancreatic A and B cells to somatostatin, *Diabetologia* 32:207–212.
36. Wang, Z.-L., Bennet, W.M., Wang, R.-M., Ghatei, M.A., and Bloom, S.R., 1994, Evidence of a paracrine role of neuropeptide-Y in the regulation of insulin release from pancreatic islets of normal and dexamethasone-treated rats, *Endocrinology* 135:200–206.
37. Eriksson, J., Nakazato, M., Miyazato, M., Shiomi, K., Matsukura, S., and Groop, L., 1992, Islet amyloid polypeptide plasma concentrations in individuals at increased risk of developing type 2 (non-insulin-dependent) diabetes mellitus, *Diabetologia* 35:291–293.
38. Henquin, J.-C., 1990, Established, unsuspected and novel pharmacological insulin secretagogues, In: "New antidiabetic drugs," C.J. Bailey and P.R. Flatt, eds., pp. 93–106, Smith Gordon and Co. Ltd., London.
39. Fujitani, S., and T. Yada., 1994, A novel D-phenylalanine-derivative hypoglycemic agent A-4166 increases cytosolic free Ca^{2+} in rat pancreatic β-cells by stimulating Ca^{2+} influx, *Endocrinology* 134: 1395–1400.
40. Chan, S.L.F., Scarpello, K.E., and Morgan, N.G., 1997, Identification and characterization of non-adrenergic binding sites in insulin secreting cells with the imidazoline RX821002, In "Physiology and Pathophysiology of the Islets of Langerhans," B. Soria, ed., Plenum Press, New York.
41. Lebrun, P., Antoine, M.H., Herchuelz, A., de Tullio, P., Delarge, J., and Pirotte, B., 1997, Pyridothiadiazines as potent inhibitors of glucose-induced insulin release. In "Physiology and Pathophysiology of the Islets of Langerhans," B. Soria, ed., Plenum Press, New York.
42. Springborg, J., Gromada, J., Madsen, P., and Fuhlendorff, J., 1997, Increase in $[Ca^{2+}]_i$ and subsequent insulin release from βTC3-cells with the Ca^{2+} channel activator FRL 64176, In "Physiology and Pathophysiology of the Islets of Langerhans," B. Soria, ed., Plenum Press, New York.
43. Silva, A.M., Rosario, L.M., Santos, R.M., 1994, Background Ca^{2+} influx mediated by a dihydropyridine- and voltage-insensitive channel in pancreatic β-cells, *J. Biol. Chem.* 269: 17095–17103.

15

THE HUMAN GLUCAGON-LIKE PEPTIDE-1 (GLP-1) RECEPTOR

Cloning and Functional Expression

Joseph S. Dillon, Michael B. Wheeler, Xing-Hong Leng, B. Brooke Ligon, and Aubrey E. Boyd, III

Division of Endocrinology, Diabetes, Metabolism and Molecular Medicine
New England Medical Center
Tufts University School of Medicine
Boston, Massachusetts 02111

INTRODUCTION

At similar plasma glucose concentrations much greater insulin secretion is achieved with oral glucose than with intravenous glucose. These observations lead to the concept that gastrointestinal factors (incretins) are released by nutrients, particularly glucose, to potentiate insulin release (Creutzfeldt, 1979). The two most potent incretins, GLP-1(7-37) and its amidated form GLP-1(7-36 amide), are processed from the parent 37 amino acid GLP-1 peptide, which is produced in intestinal L-cells as a posttranslational product of preproglucagon.

Studies in isolated islets or insulin-secreting rat or hamster insulinoma cell lines (RIN and HIT) have shown that both GLP-1(7-37) and GLP-1(7-36 amide) interact with high affinity receptors on the β cell to activate adenylyl cyclase, increase cAMP and potentiate glucose-stimulated insulin secretion. In addition, these peptides increase insulin gene transcription and biosynthesis through a cAMP-dependent step. Forskolin increases cAMP levels over 50-fold in insulin-secreting cells or islets by activating adenylyl cyclase without increasing insulin release and thus cAMP is not a true "second messenger" for insulin secretion in the β cell. Our previous studies demonstrated that, in the presence of glucose, an increase in cAMP in the HIT cell potentiated insulin secretion by further opening the voltage-dependent calcium channel (VDCC) in cells depolarized by glucose thus increasing the major "second messenger" in the β cell, the free cytosolic calcium level ($[Ca^{2+}]_i$) (Rajan et al., 1989). Suspecting that this signal transduction pathway would also be utilized by GLP-1(7-37) or GLP-1(7-36 amide), we examined the effects of these incretins on HIT cells (Lu, 1993). We found a remarkable agreement between the affinity of both GLP-1 peptides to bind to the receptor on the β cell, increase cAMP and $[Ca^{2+}]_i$

Physiology and Pathophysiology of the Islets of Langerhans, edited by Soria.
Plenum Press, New York, 1997.

and potentiate glucose-stimulated insulin release. The source of the increase in $[Ca^{2+}]_i$ was extracellular with Ca^{2+} entering the cell through the VDCC. In the presence of glucose these peptides further depolarize the β cell. In dispersed rat β cells, Holz has recently shown that GLP-1(7-37) sensitizes the β cell to depolarization by inhibiting ATP-sensitive K^+ channels, the same channels which are inhibited by sulfonylureas or a change in the ATP/ADP ratio as glucose is metabolized in the β cell (Holz et al., 1993) .

There has been a great deal of excitement generated by the clinical studies on GLP-1 (7-37) and GLP-1(7-36 amide) (Gutniak et al., 1992) and features of this class of compounds suggest that they will become new therapeutic agents in diabetes. In contrast to the sulfonylureas which increase insulin secretion at any blood glucose level, potentiation of glucose-stimulated insulin secretion does not occur until the blood glucose level reaches about 5mM. Thus, there is a cut off switch that should prevent hypoglycemia with the "incretins." Our HIT cell studies explain this phenomenon. At low glucose concentrations, although GLP-1(7-37) increases cAMP levels to the same extent as seen at stimulatory glucose concentrations, there is an uncoupling between the rise in cAMP and the changes in $[Ca^{2+}]_i$. Since $[Ca^{2+}]_i$ does not rise, increases in insulin secretion do not occur. In addition, GLP-1(7-36 amide) has a potent peripheral mechanism of action potentiating glucose uptake into peripheral tissue and decreasing the amount of insulin required to achieve control of the blood glucose levels in patients with IDDM. In other studies it was shown that GLP-1(7-36 amide) was effective in patients with NIDDM who had failed sulfonylureas. This also is consistent with the differences in the signal transduction pathways utilized by GLP-1 peptides and sulfonylureas. The sulfonylureas signal by inhibiting the ATP-sensitive K^+ channels, depolarizing the β cell, opening the VDCC and increasing $[Ca^{2+}]_i$ and have no effect on cAMP levels in the β cell. Thus, the potentiation of glucose-stimulated insulin secretion by cAMP is still intact in the β cell of some patients who fail sulfonylurea therapy.

Thorens recently cloned the rat GLP-1 receptor and confirmed that this receptor signaled by increasing cAMP levels (Thorens, 1992). Using a polymerase chain reaction (PCR) generated rat GLP-1 receptor, expressed in COS-7 cells, we showed that a single recombinant receptor could activate both adenylyl cyclase and phosphoinositide turnover releasing Ca^{2+} from an intracellular pool (Wheeler et al., 1993). This latter pathway is not activated in HIT cells. Since both pathways are coupled by G-proteins to the effector systems, these findings suggest that the G-protein milieu of the cell may determine how the receptor signals.

Because of the potential therapeutic value of GLP-1 in the treatment of NIDDM, and in order to determine the regions of the human receptor that are important for signal transduction we have cloned a human pancreatic islet cDNA encoding a 463 amino acid high affinity GLP-1 receptor. Similar to the related PTH and glucagon receptors the human recombinant GLP-1 receptor is coupled to at least two G-protein coupled signaling pathways, including adenylyl cyclase and phospholipase C (PLC).

MATERIALS AND METHODS

Isolation of a cDNA Encoding the GLP-1 Receptor

A PCR generated 1401 bp cDNA fragment encoding the rat GLP-1 receptor was ^{32}P labeled by random priming (Pharmacia) and used to screen a human islet cDNA library (a gift of MA Permutt, St. Louis). After overnight hybridization at 55°C in 5× SSPE (1×

SSPE is NaCl 0.15M, NaH_2PO_4 0.01M, EDTA 1mM) the filters were washed in 5× SSC (1× SSC is NaCl 0.15M, sodium citrate 0.015M) at 55°C. We identified one positive clone in 1.0×10^6 recombinants screened. After plaque purification the cDNA was sub cloned into Bluescript II vector (Stratagene) at the Eco RI site. A series of 5′ deletions in Bluescript II were generated using Exonuclease III digestion (Promega) and these were sequenced by the dideoxy sequencing method using Sequenase (US Biochemical). The positive clone (designated HGLPR#3) was 1.9 kb in length and consisted of 0.8 kb homologous with the rat GLP-1 receptor followed by 1.1 kb of 3′ untranslated and poly A tail cDNA. Three million further clones were screened using a 0.4 kb PstI fragment of HGLPR#3 — none of the isolated plaques contained inserts of greater than 1.9 kb. In order to obtain sequence of the 5′ end of HGLPR, random hexamer primed first stand cDNA was prepared from human insulinoma total RNA and used in a PCR reaction (Perkin Elmer). PCR was performed using a primer encoding the 5′ 21 bases of the rat GLP-1 receptor and a flanking Kozak consensus sequence (5′–cccgccatggccgtcacccccagcctg–3′) (Wheeler et al., 1993) and a primer complimentary to the 5′ end of HGLPR#3 spanning a ScaI site (5′–acacagtactgcatgagcaga–3′). The PCR program included a ‘hot start’ and 3 cycles of 97°C, 60°C, and 72°C each for 1 minute followed by 35 cycles of 95°C, 60°C and 72°C each for 1 minute. A band of approximately 700 bp was excised from 1.2% low melt agarose gel and directly ligated to PCR II vector (In Vitrogen) (HGLPR#6). Subsequent sequencing of this cDNA insert confirmed its close homology to the rat GLP-1 receptor. The overlapping clones HGLPR#3 and #6 were ligated at their common ScaI site and inserted into the expression vector pcDNA1 Neo at HindIII and XhoI sites (designated HGLPR-1).

For cell transfection and binding assays COS-7 cells (4×10^6) were seeded in 10 cm dishes and cultured in DMEM supplemented with 10% fetal bovine serum. Cells were transfected with 10μg of the HGLPR-1 construction by DEAE-dextran the following day. Twenty four hours after transfection, the cells were passaged into 10 cm dishes and allowed to culture for an additional 48 hours. The cells were detached from the dishes using phosphate buffered saline with 1mM EDTA and washed three times in incubation buffer (Hanks balanced salt solution, 1% bovine serum albumin, 1mg/ml bacitracin, 25mM hepes, pH 7.4). Cells ($1–5 \times 10^5$ per tube) were incubated for 45 minutes at 37°C with radiolabeled tracer (50,000 cpm) and unlabeled peptides (human GLP-1(7-37), human glucagon and human GLP-1(1-36 amide) (Bachem, 1pM–10μM) in a final volume of 200 μl. After incubation, the cell suspensions were centrifuged at 12,000×G through an oil layer (dibutyl phthalate/mineral oil 1:3 v/v). Cell associated radioactivity in the pellet was counted. Assays were performed in triplicate. The binding data were analyzed using the Ligand program. Specific binding was defined as total cpm minus cpm in the presence of 1μM unlabeled peptide.

Synthetic human GLP-1(7-37) was radioiodinated by the chloramine T method using 4μg of peptide and 0.5mCi ^{125}Iodine. The iodination products were purified by reverse phase HPLC on a Waters μ Bondapack C18 column using a gradient of 0.1% trifluoroacetic acid in water (buffer A) and acetonitrile (buffer B) (35–55%) formed in 30 minutes at a flow rate of 2 ml/minute.

For assessment of cAMP generation COS-7 cells were passaged into 6-well plates (1×10^6), twenty four hours after transfection, and allowed to culture for an additional 48 hours. CyclicAMP was extracted with 70% ethanol (v/v) after 1 hour preincubation and 30 minutes stimulation of the cells. The samples were lyophilized and reconstituted in sodium acetate buffer (pH 6.2), and measured with a commercial radioimmunoassay kit (Biomedical Technologies, MA) as previously described (Lu, 1993).

To assess the effect of GLP-1 on $[Ca^{2+}]_i$, COS-7 cells (3 days post transfection) were loaded with the Ca^{2+} fluorophore fura-2AM (Molecular Probes, OR) in the modified KRB buffer containing 4.0mM glucose. Changes in $[Ca^{2+}]_i$ were assessed as previously described (Lu, 1993). Test agents were added from concentrated stocks. All values are expressed as means ± SE. Statistical analysis was performed using the Student's t-test for paired and unpaired values.

Nylon membranes containing 2μg of poly A RNA isolated from several rat tissues (Clontech) was used for Northern analysis. The blot was probed at high stringency with a ^{32}P labeled antisense riboprobe generated with T3 polymerase of a 349 base HincII cDNA fragment (HGLPR-1 1215-1599) in BluescriptII. The blot was hybridized at 67°C overnight and washed at 0.01× SSC at 67°C and placed on film with 2 intensifying screens for 48 hours at −80°C.

RESULTS AND DISCUSSION

The HGLPR-1 cDNA isolated was 2448 bp in length. The cDNA encodes a protein of 463 amino acids which is 89.9% homologous with the rat GLP-1 receptor (Fig. 1) using the GAP program (Genetics Computer Group, WI). Similar to the rat GLP-1 receptor, the human receptor has 7 potential transmembrane spanning domains and three N-linked glycosylation sites in the putative extracellular domains at amino acid positions 68, 88, and 120. Because the strategy for obtaining the 5′ end of the receptor involved use of the 5′ rat receptor primer it is possible that the actual human cDNA sequence might differ slightly from our sequence. This sequence deviation is likely to be minor since the rat and human receptors are so homologous throughout and the primer annealing temperature in the PCR was relatively high (60°C).

To confirm that the HGLPR-1 insert sequence was appropriately expressed in COS-7 cells, binding analysis was performed with GLP-1(7-37) and related peptides. [^{125}I]-GLP-1(7-37) bound specifically to HGLPR-1 transfected COS-7 cells (Fig. 2) with a Kd of 2.8± 0.9 nM. The binding of [^{125}I]-GLP-1(7-37) to COS 7 cells transfected with the rat GLP-1

MAVTPSLLRLALLLLG**M**VGRAGPRPQGATVSL**W**ETVQKWREYR**R**QCQR**S**L 50

TE**D**P**PP**AT**D**LFCNRTFD**E**YACWPDGEPGSFVNVSCPWYLPWASSV**P**QGHV 100

YRFCTAEG**L**WL**Q**KDNSSLPWRDLSECEESK**R**GER**S**SPEEQLL**F**LYIIYTV 150

AYALSFSALVIASAIL**LG**FRHLHCTRNYIHLNLFASFILRALSVFIKDAA 200

LKWMYSTAAQQHQWDGLLSYQDSLSCRLVFLLMQYCVAANYYWLLVEGVY 250

LYTLLAFSVFSEQ**W**IF**R**LY**V**SIGWGVPLLFV**V**PWGIVKYLYEDEGCWTRN 300

SNMNYWLIIRLPILFAIGVNFL**I**F**V**RVICVI**VS**KLKANLMCKTDIKCRLA 350

KSTLTLIPLLGTHEVIFAFVMDEHARGTLRF**I**KLFTELSFTSFQG**L**MVA**I** 400

LYCFVNNEVQ**L**EFRKSWERWRLE**H**L**H**IQRDSSMKPLKCPTSS**L**SSGAT**A**G 450

SS**M**Y**T**ATCQ**A**SCS

Figure 1. Amino acid sequence of HGLPR-1. Amino acid differences between the rat and human receptors are noted in bold. The predicted transmembrane segments are underlined.

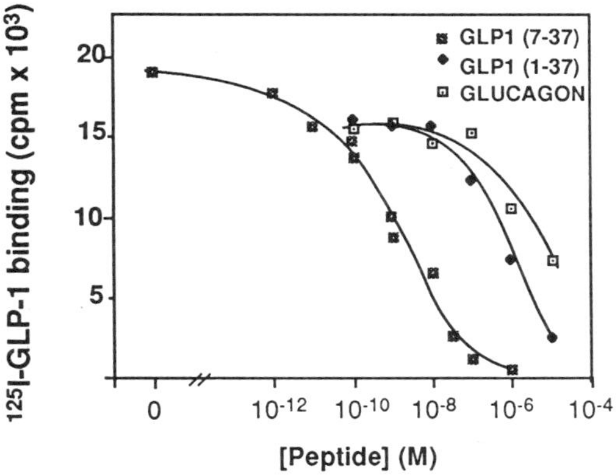

Figure 2. Displacement of ^{125}I-GLP-1(7-37) binding from HGLPR-1 transfected COS-7 cells.

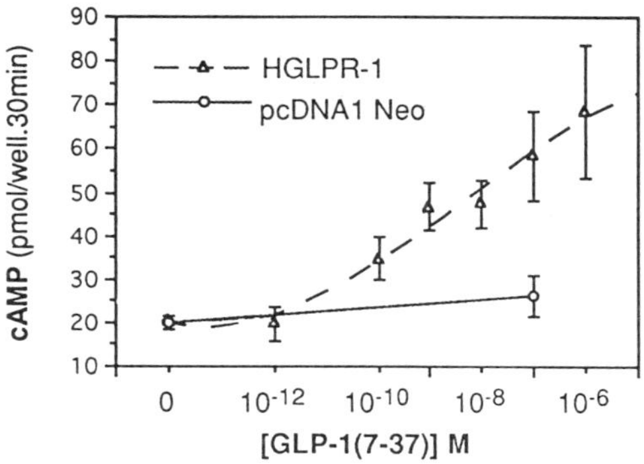

Figure 3. GLP-1(7-37) stimulated cAMP accumulation in HGLPR-1 transfected COS-7 cells.

receptor pcDNA1 construct (a gift of B Thorens) showed a similar binding curve to that of the HGLPR-1 with a Kd of 2.7±0.7 nM. There was no specific binding in COS-7 cells transfected with pcDNA1 Neo vector alone. Glucagon and GLP-1(1-36amide) displaced [^{125}I]-GLP-1 binding from transfected COS-7 cells by 32% and 55% respectively at a concentration of 10^{-6} M.

To verify that the receptor signaled through the adenylyl cyclase system, the effects of GLP-1(7-37) on intracellular cAMP in HGLPR-1 transfected COS-7 cells were examined (Fig. 3). Seventy two hours after transfection, cells were incubated for a 60 minute preincubation period in KRB buffer followed by a 30 minute stimulation period. Forskolin (10mM), a known activator of adenylyl cyclase, increased cAMP content 2.85 fold (n=6) in HGLPR-1 transfected cells. GLP-1(7-37) (100nM) increased the cellular cAMP content 2.2 fold. There was no stimulation of cAMP accumulation by GLP-1(7-37) in pcDNA1 Neo transfected cells. COS-7 cells transfected with the rat GLP-1 receptor responded to GLP-1(7-37) (100nM) with and increase of 1.8 fold in cAMP concentration.

To determine whether GLP-1 increased $[Ca^{2+}]_i$ in addition to cAMP accumulation, the effect of GLP-1 on $[Ca^{2+}]_i$ was examined using Fura 2 loaded, HGLPR-1 transfected COS-7 cells. GLP-1(7-37) (100nM) increased intracellular calcium by 31.4±7.0nM in HGLPR-1 transfected COS-7 cells (Fig 4a). In cells transfected with the rat GLP-1 receptor, GLP-1(7-37) (100nM) increased $[Ca^{2+}]_i$ by 16.3±0.4nM. There was no significant increase in $[Ca^{2+}]_i$ in cells transfected with the vector alone (1.6±1.6nM).

To examine whether the source of the increased $[Ca^{2+}]_i$ elicited by GLP-1 was from an intracellular or extracellular pool, 2.5mM EGTA was applied to the modified KRB buffer which contained 1.5 mM calcium and 4 mM glucose (Fig. 4b). Two minutes after EGTA application GLP-1(7-37) (100nM) caused a rapid rise in $[Ca^{2+}]_i$ not significantly different from that without EGTA 23.5±3.6nM. Similar to our previous work with the rat recombinant receptor the human receptor appears to signal through both adenylyl cyclase and accumulation of intracellular calcium. Thus, this receptor is similar to the PTH receptor in signaling through both phospholipase C and adenylyl cyclase in transfected COS-7 cells.

Tissue distribution of the HGLPR-1 insert sequence was assessed by Northern analysis. Northern analysis under conditions of high stringency, showed a 2.4 kb transcript in the pancreatic lane only. There were no transcripts evident in the brain, skeletal muscle, liver or lung after an exposure time of 48 hours. The rat receptor appeared to express two

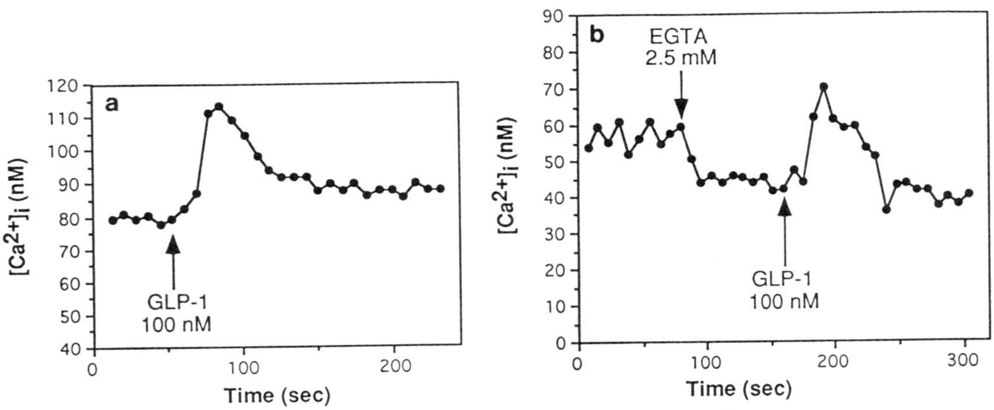

Figure 4. **(a)** Effect of GLP-1(7-37) on $[Ca^{2+}]_i$ in HGLPR-1 transfected COS-7 cells. **(b)** Cellular source of GLP-1 stimulated intracellular Ca^{2+} accumulation.

transcripts (2.4 and 3.4 kb) in our previous studies (Wheeler et al., 1993) and those of Thorens (Thorens, 1992). There was no evidence of variable transcript size in our Northern analysis of the human GLP-1 receptor expression. GLP-1 has been shown to bind a variety of animal tissues and cell lines in vitro (brain, stomach, lung) and we have shown expression of the rat receptor in these tissues (Wheeler et al., 1993). Furthermore, when administered to humans GLP-1 appears to have glucose lowering effects independent of its effect on insulin concentration (Gutniak et al., 1992), again suggesting the presence of extrapancreatic GLP-1 receptors. That we did not detect any receptor expression by Northern analysis of 2μg of poly A RNA in these tissues suggests that the receptor is present in very low abundance. The possibility that variant receptors exist which were not detected with our riboprobe exists. The riboprobe used in this study was generated from a HincII fragment of HGLPR-1 which includes the 3′ 0.2 kB of the coding region and the 5′ 0.2 kb of the 3′ untranslated region, whereas the hybridizing probe used in the rat GLP-1 receptor Northern studies was 1.4 kb in length and included the entire receptor coding region. Whether these human tissues possess this GLP-1 receptor in low abundance or another GLP-1 receptor will be determined by reverse transcription PCR and Northern analysis using riboprobes derived from different parts of the GLP-1 cDNA.

In conclusion, we have isolated a human pancreatic islet GLP-1 receptor cDNA and shown its associated second messenger pathways. Because of the importance of GLP-1 in normal glucose metabolism and its ability to normalize postprandial blood glucose in type II diabetics in a glucose dependent manner the availability of the human GLP-1 receptor cDNA and deduced protein sequence should allow for significant advances in design of receptor agonists and determination of the exact role of GLP-1 in human physiology.

ACKNOWLEDGMENTS

This work was funded by National Institutes of Health grants DK34447 and RR00054 (to A.E.B.), American Diabetes Association Mentor-Based Fellowship Awards (to J.D.) Juvenile Diabetes Foundation grant (to M.B.W. and A.E.B.). Address correspondence to J. Dillon. Tel: 617-350-8580, Fax: 617-956-4719.

REFERENCES

Creutzfeldt, W. (1979). The incretin concept today. Diabetologia, 16, 75–85.

Gutniak, M., Orskov, C., Holst, J. J., Ahren, B. and Efendic, S. (1992). Antidiabetogenic effect of glucagon-like peptide-1(7-36)amide in normal subjects and patients with diabetes mellitus. New England Journal of Medicine, 326(20), 1316–22.

Holz, G. 4., Kuhtreiber, W. M. and Habener, J. F. (1993). Pancreatic beta-cells are rendered glucose-competent by the insulinotropic hormone glucagon-like peptide-1(7-37). Nature, 361(6410), 362–5.

Lu, M. (1993) Signal transduction of the endogenous and recombinant glucagon-like peptide 1(7-37) receptor. PhD Thesis in Cell Biology, Baylor College of Medicine.

Rajan, A., Hill, R. and Boyd, A. (1989). Effect of rise in cAMP levels on Ca^{2+} influx through voltage dependent Ca^{2+} channels in HIT cells. Diabetes, 38, 874–880.

Thorens, B. (1992). Expression cloning of the pancreatic β cell receptor for the gluco-incretin hormone glucagon-like peptide 1. Proceedings of the National Academy of Sciences USA., 89(September), 8641–8645.

Wheeler, M., Lu, M., Dillon, J., Leng, X.-H., Chen, C. and Boyd, A. (1993). Functional expression of the glucagon-like peptide-1(7-37) receptor: evidence for coupling to phospholipase C as well as adenylyl cyclase. Endocrinology, 133, 57–62.

16

ISLET RELEASE OF ACTH-LIKE PEPTIDES AND THEIR MODULATORY EFFECT ON INSULIN SECRETION

Juan J. Gagliardino,[1] María I. Borelli,[1] Fernando Estivariz,[1] Illani Atwater,[2] Carlos Boschero,[2] and Eduardo Rojas[2]

[1]CENEXA-Centro de Endocrinología Experimental y Aplicada (UNLP-CONICET)
La Plata, Argentina
[2]Laboratory of Cell Biology and Genetics, NIDDK
National Institutes of Health
Bethesda, Maryland

INTRODUCTION

The B-cell secretion of insulin in response to glucose is modulated by different hormones[1,5]. Some of these hormones are produced by non-B islet cells and also by the B-cells themselves. Among these hormones, the presence of POMC[6] and some of its derivative products such as endorphin[7,8], ACTH[9] and corticotropin-like intermediate peptide[10] has been identified in the islets. It has not yet been established whether the endogenous islet POMC and its derivatives play any modulatory role in the secretion of insulin. On the other hand, it has already been reported that ACTH enhances the secretion of insulin in response to glucose[11,12]. Such effect has been attributed to its stimulation on islet adenylate cyclase[13] and to the consequent increase of 3′5′-cAMP[14] in islet content, but the mechanism by which ACTH stimulates the release of insulin is not clear.

In order to get some insight into the above mentioned unanswered questions, we have studied the release of ACTH-like peptides (ACTH-LP) from isolated islets and the effect of ACTH upon insulin secretion. In parallel, we have studied the effect of ACTH on the cytosolic Ca^{2+} concentration ($[Ca^{2+}]_i$) in islet cells, on plasma membrane Ca^{2+}-ATPase activity in isolated islets, and on B-cell membrane potential.

MATERIALS AND METHODS

Islet Isolation and Incubation

Groups of 70 rat islets isolated by collagenase digestion[15] were incubated for 15 min at 37°C in 0.6 ml of Krebs Ringer Bicarbonate buffer (KRB), ph 7.4 with 1% BSA, 400

Physiology and Pathophysiology of the Islets of Langerhans, edited by Soria.
Plenum Press, New York, 1997.

KIU/ml Trasylol (a protease inhibitor) and either 3.3 or 16.6 mM glucose[16]. At the end of the incubation period insulin and ACTH were measured in the medium by radioimmunoassay[17]. In other cases, groups of 5 isolated islets were incubated for 60 min under the same conditions but in the presence of different glucose concentrations (2 to 20 mM), polyclonal rabbit antibody (or normal rabbit serum) or corticotropin inhibiting polypeptide (CIP). The insulin released into the incubation medium was measured by radioimmunoassay[18].

Calcium Measurements

The procedure employed has been reported in detail previously[19]. In brief, calcium measurements and calibrations were performed using a method based on the procedure described by Grynkiewicz *et al.*[20] and a fluorescent inverted microscope (Diaphot-TMD, Nikon Corp. Japan) provided with two dichroic mirrors. Collagenase-isolated islets were dispersed into islet cells using versene, a Ca^{2+}-, Mg^{2+}-free saline medium and dispase. Cells were then cultured in RPMI 1640 medium supplemented with 11 mM glucose for 48 h. These cells were loaded with indo 1/AM by incubating them for 1–2 h in a solution containing 2 mM indo-1/AM, 0.023% pluronic acid and 5.6 mM glucose. After this procedure, the cells attached to a cover slip were mounted in a perifusion chamber and continuously superfused with a modified Krebs solution containing glucose and ACTH at the concentration indicated in the figures. Measurements of $[Ca^{2+}]_i$ were performed using the fluorescence inverted microscope; the intensity of the light at each wavelenght was continuously measured using a photomultiplier.

Ca^{2+}-ATPase Determination

Groups of 100 collagenase-isolated islets were incubated for 5 min in KRB buffer, ph 7.4, 1% BSA, 400 KIU/ml Trasylol and 3.3 mM glucose plus 250 pg/ml ACTH. After this incubation period, Ca^{2+}-ATPase activity was assayed by measuring ^{32}P released from $[\tau^{32}P]$ ATP by islet homogenates[21]. Protein concentration in the homogenates was determined using the procedure described by Lowry *et al.*[22]

Electrophysiology

Single islets from fasted mice were microdissected. One islet was then placed onto the soft plastic base of a chamber as described previously[23] and perifused with KRB buffer, pH 7.4 with a flow rate of 1.6 ml/min. Membrane potential was recorded between an ultra-fine high resistance (200 μΩ) intracellular microelectrode and a reference ground electrode in the bath solution. Beta cell electrical activity was printed out on a Gould chart recorder[24].

RESULTS

Incubated rat islets increased the release of insulin and ACTH-LP as a function of the glucose concentration in the incubation medium (Fig. 1).

Exogenous ACTH (50 to 500 pg/ml) enhanced the release of insulin by islets incubated in the presence of 3.3 mM glucose in a dose-dependent manner (Fig. 2a). On the other hand, the enhancing effect of ACTH (250 pg/ml) was also observed when the islets

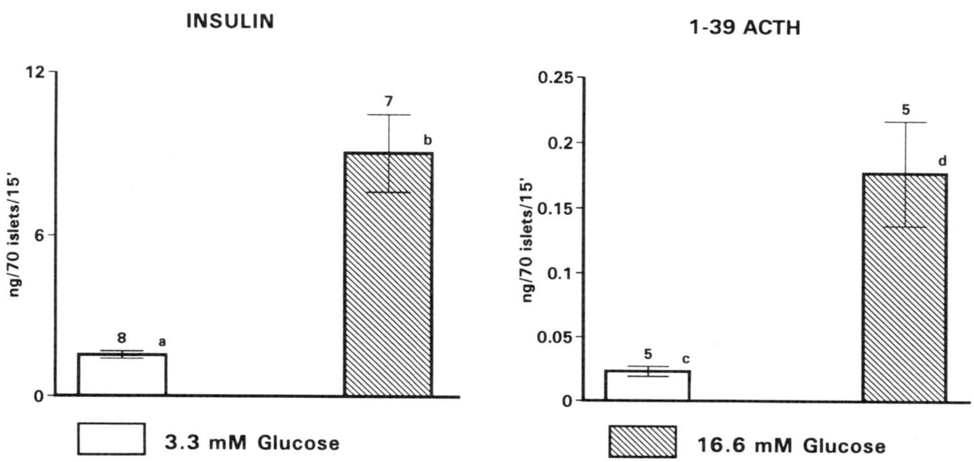

Figure 1. Secretion of insulin and ACTH-LP. Each bar represents the mean ± SEM. Number of cases above bar. **a** vs. **b**, $p < 0.001$; **c** vs. **d**, $p < 0.02$.

were incubated in the presence of increasing concentrations of glucose (4 to 16 mM) in the incubation medium. (Fig. 2b).

Isolated islets incubated in the presence of ACTH-rabbit antibody released significantly less insulin than controls in response to 16 mM glucose. Normal rabbit serum did not affect such response. A similar decrease in the glucose-induced release of insulin was obtained incubating the islets with CIP, a competitive inhibitor of ACTH biological effect (Fig. 3a and b).

The cytosolic [Ca^{2+}] increased significantly above control values under the stimulus of 500 pg/ml ACTH. This increase was evident when cytosolic Ca^{2+} concentration was continuously measured for up to a 30 min period (Fig. 4a) or determined at fixed intervals

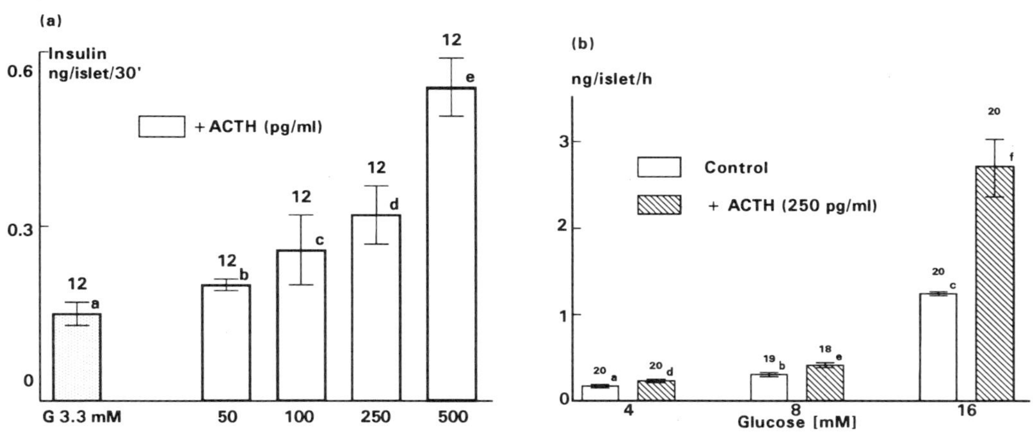

Figure 2. Effect of ACTH on insulin secretion. Each bar represents the mean ± SEM. Number of cases above bar. **(a) a** vs. **b** and **a** vs. **c**, NS; **a** vs. **d**, $p < 0.02$; **a** vs. **e**, $p < 0.001$ and **d** vs. **e**, $p < 0.025$. **(b) a** vs. **b** and **d**, NS; **d** vs. **e**, $p < 0.01$; **b** vs. **e**, $p < 0.005$; and **c** and **e** vs. **f**, $p < 0.001$.

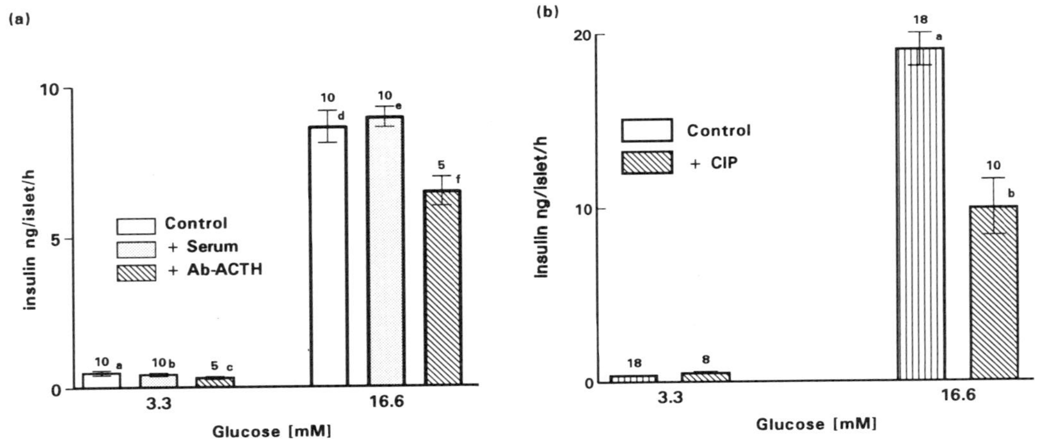

Figure 3. Effect of Ab-ACTH and CIP on insulin secretion. Each bar represents the mean ± SEM. Number of cases above bar. **(a) a** vs. **d**, **b** vs. **e**, **c** vs. **f** and **d** vs. **f**; $p < 0.001$. **(b) a** vs. **b**, $p < 0.001$.

for a 44 min period (Fig. 4b). In both cases ACTH produced a significant increase, almost double basal values, attaining the highest values between 5 and 12 minutes and remaining at that high level until the end of the sampling period (Fig. 4b). No changes in [Ca^{2+}] were detected over a similar period in the absence of ACTH.

The Ca^{2+}-ATPase activity measured in islets preincubated with 3.3 mM glucose alone significantly decreased ($p < 0.01$) when ACTH was added to the incubation medium (Fig. 5).

In the presence of 11 mM glucose, the addition of 500 pg/ml ACTH to the perifusion solution induced a slight but sustained increase in the membrane potential without significantly inhibiting the burst pattern. ACTH induced a similar hyperpolarization of about 2 mV in the presence of 5.6 mM glucose (data not shown).

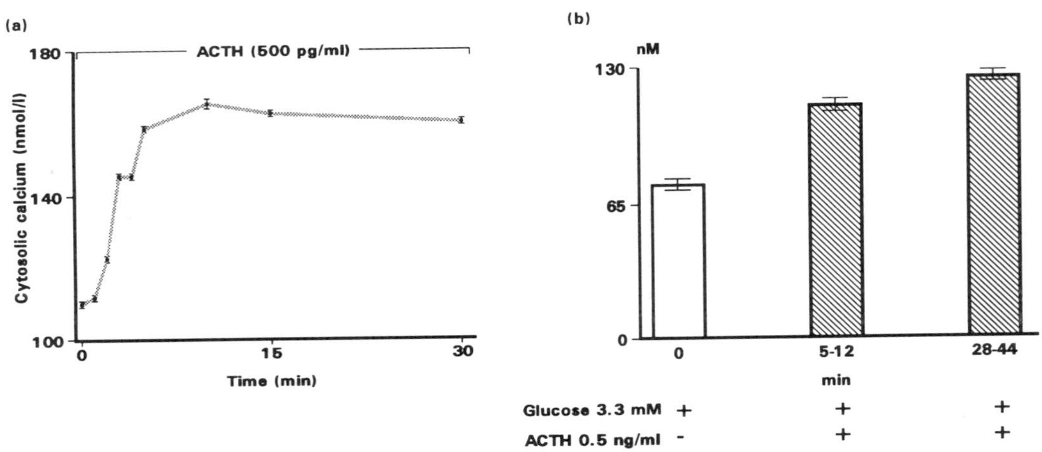

Figure 4. Effect of ACTH on cytosolic calcium in B-cells. **(a)** [Ca^{2+}] was continuously measured up to a 30 min period; **(b)** [Ca^{2+}] was determined at fixed intervals for a 44 min period. Results represent the mean of 3 experiments.

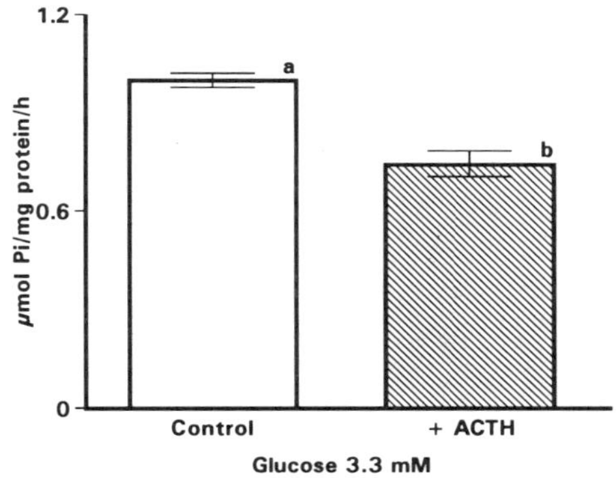

Figure 5. Effect of ACTH on islet plasma membrane Ca^{2+}-ATPase activity. Results represent the mean of 6 experiments. Each value represents the mean ± SEM. **a** vs. **b**, $p < 0.01$.

DISCUSSION

Our results show that islets isolated from normal rat pancreases increase simultaneously the release of insulin and ACTH-LP in response to high glucose. As we have previously reported, while the islets would release more of a smaller ACTH-LP when incubated with low glucose, 16 mM glucose would selectively increase the release of peptides of larger molecular size[25]. Thus, islet POMC (the ACTH-LP precursor) might be differentially processed according to the glucose concentration. These results and the reports of other authors[7,8] suggest the presence of POMC in islet cells; this conclusion is supported by the demostration of POMC-specific mRNA in the non-B cells of rat islets[6] and the changes in its production rate in response to glucose[26].

Synthetic 1-39 ACTH added to the incubation medium enhanced the release of insulin at every glucose concentration tested. Although the stimulatory effect of ACTH has been previously described by other authors[11,12,27], larger concentrations of this hormone were used in their experiments while in ours the concentration of ACTH employed was within the normal range of this peptide in rat blood[28]. On the basis of the concentration of ACTH-LP measured in the islet incubation medium and the size of the islet interstitium, we have calculated that within B-cell immediate environs these endogenous peptides may attain the concentration required to significantly stimulate insulin secretion.

Islets incubated in the presence of ACTH rabbit antibody released significantly less insulin than controls in response to 16 mM glucose. A similar decrease in the glucose-induced release of insulin was obtained incubating the islets with CIP. These results would suggest that the enhancing effect of ACTH-LP released by the islets in response to glucose would play a physiological role upon the release of insulin elicited by glucose.

We show here that ACTH also produced an increase in the cytosolic $[Ca^{2+}]$ in isolated B-cells. The magnitude of this increase was similar to the one induced by other insulin secretagogues[29] suggesting that the rise in $[Ca]_i$ could be an intracellular signal triggered by the hormone to stimulate insulin release.

The hyperpolarization of B-cell membrane induced by ACTH in mouse islets suggests that its effect on cytosolic $[Ca^{2+}]$ is not mediated through an activation of the membrane voltage-dependent Ca^{2+} channels. Conversely, the fast and significant inhibition of rat islet membrane Ca^{2+}-ATPase induced by ACTH might decrease the Ca^{2+} outflow across the plasma membrane and contribute to the increase observed in B-cells $[Ca^{2+}]_i$.

In summary, our results demonstrate that isolated rat islets release ACTH-LP simultaneously with the release of insulin; the ACTH-LP would exert a physiological positive modulation on insulin release through its inhibitory effect on cell membrane Ca^{2+}-ATPase and the consequent increase in Ca^{2+} concentration in B-cell cytosol.

ACKNOWLEDGMENTS

This work was partially supported with funds provided by National Institutes of Health of USA and CONICET of Argentina. Thanks are due to Mrs Adriana Di Maggio for excellent secretarial support and Elma E. Pérez de Gagliardino for performing the artwork.

REFERENCES

1. K. Tatemoto, S. Efendic, V. Mutt, G. Makk, G.J. Feistner, and J.D. Barrchas, Pancreastatin, a novel pancreatic peptide that inhibits insulin secretion, *Nature* 324:476 (1986).
2. I. Swenne, D.J. Hill, A.J. Strain, and R.D.J. Milner, Growth hormone regulation of somatomedin of insulin-like growth factor I production and DNA replication in fetal rat islets in tissue culture, *Diabetes* 36:288 (1987).
3. J. Knudtzon, Effects of pro-opiomelanocortin-derived peptides on plasma levels of glucagon, insulin and glucose, *Horm. Metab.Res.* 18:579 (1986).
4. D.G. Pipeleers, F.C. Schuit, P. in't Veld, E. Maes, E. Hooghe-Peters, M. van de Winkel, and W. Gepts, Interplay of nutrients and hormones in the regulation of insulin release, *Endocrinology* 117:824 (1985b).
5. F.C. Schuit, and D.G. Pipeleers, Regulation of adenosine 3′,5′-monophosphate levels in the pancreatic B-cell, *Endocrinology* 117:834 (1985).
6. H. Zuhlke, U. Lendeckel, A. Zinke, and G. Jesse, Regulation of expression of proopiomelanocortin gene in isolated islets of Langerhans, *Diabetologia* (abstract) 32:560A (1989).
7. H. Ehrenreich, and F.D. Goebel, The role of opioids in the endocrinefunction of the pancreas, *Diabetes Res.* 3:59 (1986).
8. W.R. Niendorf, and H. Zuhlke, Biosynthesis of a-endorphin in pancreatic islets of neonatal Wistar rats, *Biomed. Biochim. Acta* 44:51 (1985).
9. Sanchez, F. Franco, Y.C. Patel, and S. Reichlin, Immunoreactive adrenocorticotropin in the gastrointestinal tract and pancreatic islets of the rat, *Endocrinology* 108:2235 (1981).
10. J.B. Marshall, L.P. Kapcala, L.D. Manning, and A. McCullough, Effect of corticotropin-like intermediate lobe peptide on pancreatic exocrine function in isolated rat pancreatic lobulus, *J. Clin.Invest.* 74:1885 (1984).
11. D.L. Curry, and L.L. Bennett, Dynamics on insulin release by perfused rat pancreases: effects of hypophysectomy, growth hormone, adrenocorticotropic hormone and hydrocortisone, *Endocrinology* 93:602 (1973).
12. K.K. Sussman, and G.D. Vaughan, Insulin release after ACTH, glucagon and adenosine-3′,5′-phosphate cyclic AMP in the perfused isolated rat pancreas, *Diabetes* 16:449 (1967).
13. W.N. Kuo, D. Hodgins, and J.K. Kuo, Adenylate cyclase in islets of Langerhans, *J. Biol. Chem.* 248:2705 (1973).
14. W.J. Malaisse, F. Malaisse-Lagae, and D. Mayhew, A possible role for the adenylcyclase system in insulin secretion. *J. Clin. Invest.* 46:1724 (1967).
15. F.E. Lacy, and M. Kostianovsky, Method por the isolation of intact islets of Langerhans from rat pancreas, *Diabetes* 16:35 (1967).
16. J.J. Gagliardino, C. Nierle, and E.F. Pfeiffer, The effect of serotonin on in vitro insulin secretion and biosynthesis in mice. *Diabetologia* 10:411 (1974).
17. M. Fenger, Alpha-melanocyte-stimulating-hormone precursors in the pig pituitary, *Biochem. J.* 235:715 (1986).
18. V. Herbert, K.S. Lau, C.N. Gottlieb, and S.J. Bleicher, Coated-charcoal immunoassay of insulin, *J. Clin. Endocr. Metab.* 25:1375 (1965).
19. P. Gobbe, and A. Herchuelz, Does glucose decrease cytosolic free calcium in normal pancreatic islet cells? *Res. Commun. Chem. Pathol. Pharmacol.* 63:231 (1989).
20. G. Grynkiewicz, M. Poenie, and R.Y. Tsien, A new generation of Ca^{2+} indicators with greatly improved fluorescence properties, *J.Biol. Chem.* 260:3440 (1985).
21. J.P. Rossi, C.M. Gronda, H.N. Fernandez, and J.J. Gagliardino, Characteristics of Ca^{2+}-ATPase activity measured in islet homogenates, *Biochim. Biophys. Acta* 943:175 (1988).

22. O.H. Lowry, N.J. Rosebrough, A.L. Farr, and P.J. Randall, Protein measurement with the folin-phenol reagent, *J. Biol. Chem.*193:265 (1951).
23. I. Atwater and P.M. Beigelman, Dynamic characteristics of electrical activity in pancreatic B-cells, *J. Physiol.* 72:769 (1976).
24. I. Atwater, Control mechanisms for glucose-induced changes in the membrane potential of mouse pancreatic B-cell, *Cien. Biol. Portugal* 5:299 (1980).
25. M.I. Borelli, M.I. Morano, F.E. Estivariz, and J.J. Gagliardino, Glucose-induced secretion of ACTH-like products by rat pancreatic islets, *Arch. Internat. Physiol. Biochem.* 102:17 (1994).
26. H. Zuhlke, G. Jesse, T. Rosolsky, S. Gruska, U. Lendecker, and H. Hahn van Dorsche, Characterization of transcriptional and translational products of a-endorphin in isolated islets of Langerhans, *Diabetologia* (abstract) 31:562A (1988).
27. S. Genuth, and H.E. Lebovitz, Stimulation of insulin release by corticotropin, *Endocrinology* 76:1093 (1965).
28. F.E. Estivariz, M.I. Morano, M. Carino, S. Jackson, and P.J. Lowry, Adrenal regeneration in the rat is mediated by mitogenic N-terminal pro-opiomelanocortin peptides generated by changes in precursor processing in the anterior pituitary, *J. Endocrinol.* 116:207 (1988).
29. M. Deleers, M. Mahy, and W.J. Malaisse, Glucose increases cytosolic Ca^{2+} in pancreatic islet cells, *Biochem. Int.* 10:97 (1985).

17

CHRONIC SYMPATHETIC INNERVATION OF ISLETS IN TRANSGENIC MICE RESULTS IN DIFFERENTIAL DESENSITIZATION OF α-ADRENERGIC INHIBITION OF INSULIN SECRETION

Gerold M. Grodsky,[1] Yan Hui Ma,[1] and Robert H. Edwards[2]

[1]University of California, San Francisco
Metabolic Research Unit, HSW 1157
3rd and Parnassus, San Francisco, California 94143
[2]Department of Neurology
UCLA School of Medicine
710 Westwood Plaza, Los Angeles, California 90024-1769

SUMMARY

The effects of chronic sympathetic hyperinnervation on pancreatic β-cell insulin secretion were investigated utilizing the in vitro perfused pancreas from transgenic mice. These mice exhibit islet hyperinnervation of sympathetic neurons resulting from overexpression of nerve growth factor in their β-cells (1). The goal was to determine whether sympathetic hyperinnervation increased classic α-adrenergic inhibition of β-cell insulin secretion or, in contrast, down-regulated β-cell sensitivity to adrenergic input resulting in enhanced insulin secretion.

Both fasting and fed blood sugars and pancreatic insulin content were normal in the transgenics. Response of the transgenic perfused pancreas to low glucose (7 mM) was primarily first phase and normal whereas high glucose (22 mM) caused enhanced, rather than reduced, insulin secretion of both first and second phases. The α-antagonist, phentolamine, caused a six-fold increase in glucose-stimulated insulin secretion from the control pancreas, an effect that was blunted for the transgenic pancreas. A similarly blunted response to phentolamine occurred when this agent was superimposed on a combined glucose-forskolin stimulus. (The positive effect on insulin secretion by phentolamine in normal β-cell preparations has arguably been ascribed to non-specific ionic effects.) Therefore, as a test of possible changes in the ATP regulated K^+ channel or the linked Ca^{++} channels, glyburide was perfused during glucose stimulation. Insulin secretion in response to glyburide was increased two fold in the control pancreas. However, with the transgenic pancreas, in con-

Physiology and Pathophysiology of the Islets of Langerhans, edited by Soria.
Plenum Press, New York, 1997.

trast to the enhanced response to glucose, the effect of glyburide was almost completely inhibited. It is concluded that: 1) chronic adrenergic hyperinnervation results in enhanced glucose-stimulated insulin secretion by desensitization of a major α-adrenergic inhibitory site(s); and 2) adrenergic hyperinnervation acts directly or indirectly on ion flux to partially inhibit insulin release, an effect which is not desensitized. Since down-regulation of a single α-adrenergic receptor would be expected to desensitize both phenomena the observed differential desensitization indicates that different post receptor events or more than one adrenergic receptor are involved.

INTRODUCTION

Sympathetic neuronal input, mediated by catecholamines, provides a major regulatory function for control of the islet β-cell (2–5). Although the catecholamines stimulate β-adrenergic activity, their predominant acute effect is α-adrenergic activation via G proteins resulting in inhibition of insulin secretion (6–8).

The effect of chronic α-adrenergic hyperinnervation of the β-cell is still not established. Studies in vivo in which catecholamines are modified by diabetes-induced stress (9,10) or hypothalamic lesions (11) produce additional total body changes which preclude unequivocal interpretation. Results of prolonged exposure to "α-or β-adrenergic agents" in vivo or in vitro are also subject to misinterpretation since these agents are notoriously non-specific (12). Furthermore, their action at different levels of β-cell function (e.g. adrenergic receptors, G proteins, target pathways, etc.) can change depending on the presence of other signals regulating β-cell metabolism.

Finally, although chronic exposure of the β-cell to catecholamines would be expected to be inhibitory, it is now established that desensitization to chronically presented inhibitors, as well as stimulators, is characteristic of β-cell regulation (13–15). In other cell systems "long-term" desensitization of β- and α-adrenergic function has been demonstrated (16). Thus, down regulation of one or more of the α-adrenergic actions of the catecholamines could occur.

Recently, a non-diabetic transgenic mouse has been developed which overexpresses Nerve Growth Factor selectively in the islet β-cell (1). This results in a dramatic increase in specific innervation of the islets and not the surrounding acinar tissue. The innervation is almost exclusively sympathetic; innervation by sensory and parasympathetic neurons remains unchanged (1). This model, therefore, permits novel studies of the effect of enhanced chronic adrenergic innervation of the β-cell relatively independent of extra pancreatic influences.

In this investigation, we determined changes in regulation of insulin secretion from the perfused pancreas of this transgenic model. Results suggest existence of at least two inhibitory sites for α-adrenergic action in β-cells. Chronic α-adrenergic innervation causes differential sustained inhibition of one site, but desensitization of the other.

MATERIALS AND METHODS

Animals

Transgenic mice were those previously described and produced by the microinjection of rat insulin promoter-Nerve Growth Factor (NGF) fusion constructs into the C57BL/6 mouse germ line with expression of NGF in pancreatic β-cells (1). Heterozygous non-fasting female mice, age 2–6 months, from the RIP-NGF-2 line were used as the source of pancreases for all studies (1). For convenience, these animals will be subsequently referred to by the term, NGF transgenics. Control mice were strain, age, and sex matched.

Pancreatic Perfusion

Pancreas and the adjacent stomach, spleen, and duodenum were surgically removed from pentobarbitol-anesthetized mice (100 mg/kg body wt) as previously described for the rat or Chinese hamster pancreas (17,18). Perfusate consisting of bicarbonate-phosphate-calcium buffer containing 0.2% purified "stabilized" bovine albumin + 3% T-40 Dextran (18) was introduced into the celiac artery at 1 ml/min. Effluent was collected at 1–2 minute intervals from the portal vein after a single passage through the pancreas. As with the perfused Chinese hamster pancreatic preparation, glass was employed for the influx tubing to minimize loss of soluble oxygen during the transit time from oxygenator to pancreas. Agents (including glucose, forskolin (CalBiochem, La Jolla, Ca), phentolamine (CIBA Pharmaceutical, Summit, NJ), glyburide (Upjohn, Kalamazoo, MI), and idazoxan (Ultrafine Chemicals, Manchester, UK) were added as indicated in the individual figures. Because of limited availability of transgenic animals, these agents were usually added in sequence. However, in all cases identical perfusion patterns were employed for transgenics and controls, thereby permitting direct comparisons of responses in their given setting. At the end of each experiment, pancreatic insulin was determined by mincing the pancreas, precipitating total protein with 5% TCA, and extracting the precipitate in acid alcohol (alcohol:H_2O:conc HCl, 750:235:15 by vol), 20 ml/pancreas overnight at 4°C (19). Extraction of the precipitate was repeated two additional times and the three extracts were combined.

Hormone Assay

Insulin was assayed in perfusate or diluted pancreatic extracts of pancreas by solid phase radioimmunoassay (20), using rat insulin as reference standard and antiporcine insulin antibody (Linco Research, Eureka, MO).

Statistical Analysis

Results were analyzed by Student's "t" test for paired or unpaired values.

RESULTS

To supplement previous observations of normal fasting blood sugars in the NGF transgenics (4.3 ± 0.4 vs 4.1 ± 0.3 mM; control vs transgenic (N=12 & 5)) we also measured morning blood sugars in the fed mice. Under these conditions, which presumably represent a greater stimulatory challenge to the β-cell, blood sugars in control and transgenic animals still did not differ (10.8 ± 0.9 vs 10.7 ± 0.7 mM; control vs transgenic; N=9). Pancreatic insulin content in controls and NGF transgenics was also identical (97 ± 38 vs 100 ± 45 μg/g wet pancreas weight; control vs transgenic; N=16).

Figure 1 illustrates the design and typical pattern of insulin secretion for control pancreases perfused to evaluate responses to different concentrations of glucose, and to

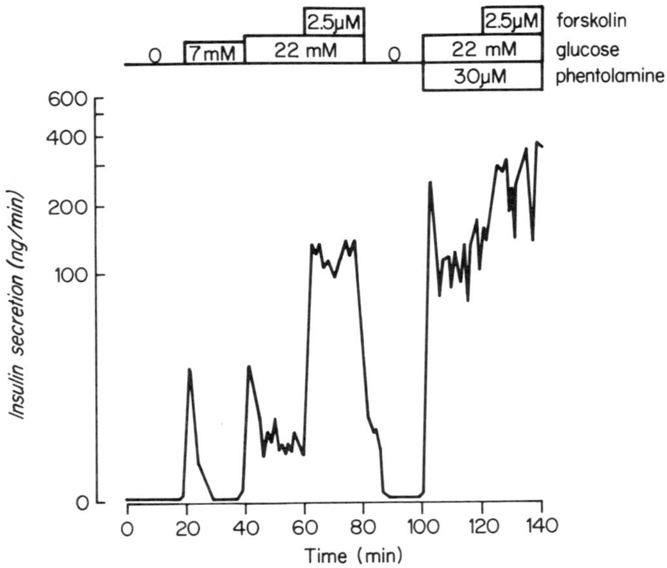

Figure 1. Example of experimental design and results showing insulin release from a control pancreas stimulated by steps of glucose onto which forskolin and phentolamine were superimposed. Note log scale. Results from groups of control and NGF-transgenic pancreas are compared in Figures 2 and 3.

forskolin or phentolamine. Quantitative comparison of results from control and transgenic pancreas is summarized in Figures 2 and 3.

The perfused pancreas responds to ascending steps of glucose in a threshold-dependent manner in which each progressive step elicits that insulin capable of being secreted by that step less that previously released at the lower concentration (21,22). In this study, typical response to low (7 mM) glucose of control mouse pancreas caused first-phase

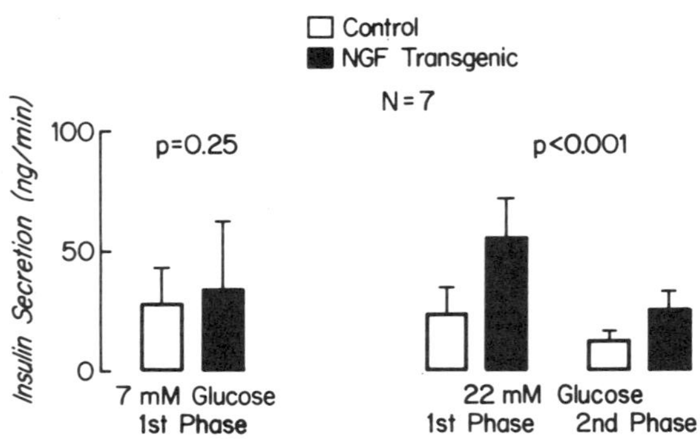

Figure 2. Effects of 7 and 22 mM sequential glucose steps on insulin release from groups of control and NGF-transgenic pancreas. Data is taken from the first 90 min of experiments using the design illustrated in Figure 1. First phase release was the mean total insulin secreted per minute during the first five min of each glucose stimulus. Second phase was the mean secretion per minute for the subsequent 15 min of stimulation. P values compare responses of control vs NGF-transgenics at each glucose concentration.

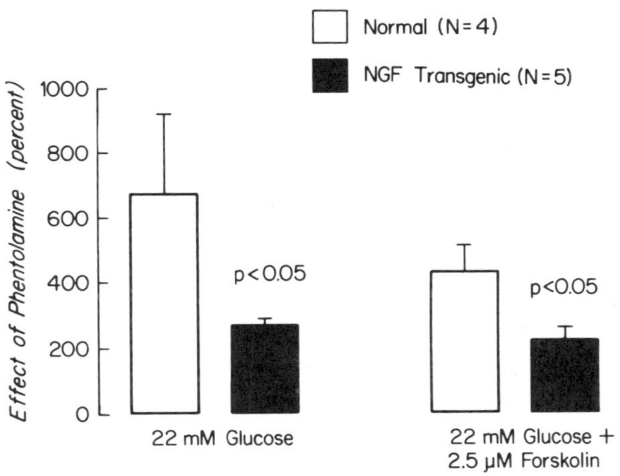

Figure 3. Effects of phentolamine on glucose or glucose + forskolin stimulation of insulin release from groups of control and NGF-transgenic pancreases. Data is taken from experiments using the design illustrated in Figure 1. Results are presented as % change evoked by phentolamine compared to internal controls of each experiment and calculated as

$$100 \times \frac{\text{insulin secreted in min } 100-120}{\text{insulin secreted in min } 40-60} \quad \text{for 22 mM glucose}$$

$$100 \times \frac{\text{insulin secreted in min } 100-140}{\text{insulin secreted in min } 60-80} \quad \text{for 22 mM glucose + forskolin}$$

release with a low second-phase secretion (Figure 1). At 22 mM glucose, second phase release was more prominent, though this is less pronounced than for the rat (23–25). Response to subsequent forskolin was about five-fold over 22 mM glucose alone. The α-antagonist, phentolamine, enhanced insulin secretion whether superimposed on glucose alone or glucose plus forskolin.

Constitutive release of insulin was undetectable in any control or transgenic animals during the non-stimulatory period of 0–20 mins.

Figure 2 shows that total insulin secretion at 7 mM glucose, though variable, was the same for control and transgenic pancreases. But at 22 mM glucose, insulin secretion from transgenic pancreases was significantly enhanced above control pancreases when either first-phase or second-phase insulin secretion were compared.

As seen in Figure 3, phentolamine caused a six or four-fold increase in secretion when added to glucose or glucose plus forskolin respectively in pancreases from control animals. This positive effect was markedly blunted by at least 50% in the transgenic pancreases in the presence of either glucose or glucose plus forskolin.

Recent studies suggested that the positive effects of phentolamine on insulin secretion were due less to its action as an α-adrenergic antagonist than to a poorly defined alternative action at the level of ion flux (26,27). Since idazoxan was claimed to be a more specific α-adrenergic agent and not to cause positive insulin secretion, we compared this agent's effect to phentolamine on control pancreas. Figure 4 shows that idazoxan also enhanced glucose-stimulated insulin secretion and was even more potent than phentolamine at an equal molar concentration. Because of idazoxan's similar action to phentolamine on control pancreas, studies with the less available NGF transgenics were not performed.

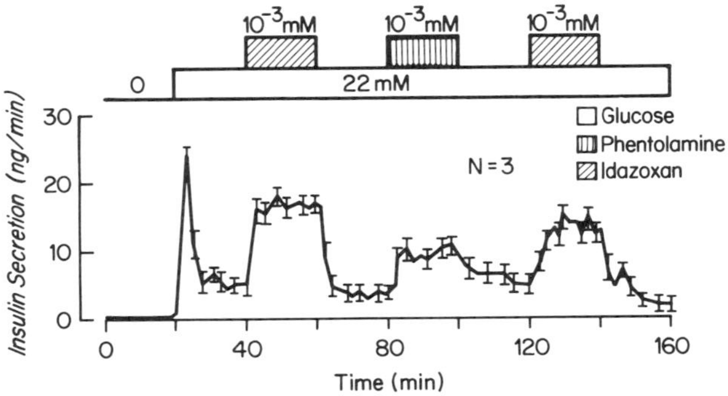

Figure 4. Effects of equal molar concentrations of phentolamine and idazoxan on glucose stimulation of insulin release from control mice pancreases.

Sulfonylureas stimulate insulin secretion by inhibiting an ATP-regulated potassium channel and thereby enhancing Ca^{++} influx (28,29). To evaluate possible changes in this ion flux caused by chronic adrenergic innervation, insulin responses to glyburide were compared in pancreases from control and NGF transgenics (Figure 5). Glyburide enhanced glucose-stimulated insulin secretion by two fold in the pancreas from control animals, whereas in transgenic pancreases, this effect of sulfonylurea was completely lost.

Planned parallel experiments using the α-agonist, clonidine, to inhibit insulin secretion were discontinued when the novel observation was made with control pancreas that clonidine at low concentrations, though inhibitory on glucose-stimulated insulin secretion, increased nsulin release in the presence of a low concentration of forskolin (to be published).

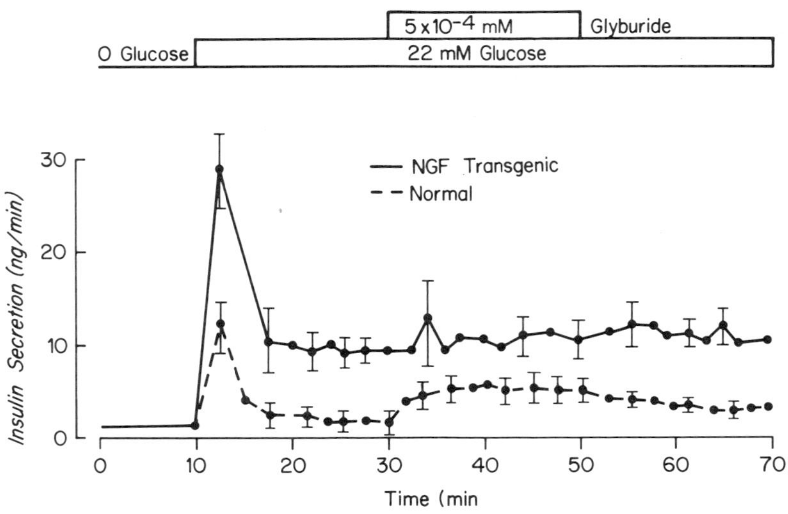

Figure 5. Effect of glyburide on glucose-stimulated insulin release from control and NGF transgenic pancreas. Statistical significance (mean insulin released/min during minutes 30–50 compared to mean insulin released/min during minutes 20–30); controls, $p < .001$; transgenics, NS.

DISCUSSION

The availability of the NGF transgenic mouse provides a unique opportunity to evaluate the effect of increased local and chronic sympathetic hyperinnervation on β-cell insulin secretion. Since catecholamines released from sympathetic nerves inhibit insulin release through their predominant α-adrenergic activity, an impairment of β-cell function could have been predicted. However, the recent demonstrations (13,14,30,31) that the β-cell down regulates to chronic glucose, other secretagogues and even inhibitors (e.g. somatostatin, verapamil) suggests that desensitization to chronic sympathetic exposure is an alternative regulatory possibility.

Our data showing that insulin release from the perfused pancreas of NGF transgenic mice in response to glucose was increased, not decreased, suggest that desensitization to inhibitory catecholamine action was a predominant result of the sympathetic hyperinnervation. Since pancreatic insulin content was the same for transgenics and controls, the increased insulin response was related to a change in stimulus-secretion signals and was not a reflection of increased insulin stores. The enhanced secretion from the perfused pancreas was not seen at 7 mM glucose but was highly significant at 22 mM demonstrating that desensitization to sympathetic innervation caused increased β-cell response to a near-maximal stimulation rather than an increase in glucose sensitivity at low levels. This normal sensitivity at moderate glucose levels can explain the normal basal fasting or fed glucose levels found in vivo.

Enhanced β-cell response to glucose after chronic sympathetic hyperinnervation could have resulted from either desensitization of catecholamine's α_2-adrenergic component, or an increase of its stimulatory β-adrenergic component. Our observation that the positive effect of the α_2-antagonist, phentolamine, was blunted suggests the enhanced response to glucose was at the level of the α-adrenergic regulatory system. This blunting of phentolamine action in the NGF transgenic pancreas also occurred when insulin secretion was massively increased by forskolin (2.5 μM), a condition where increase of c-AMP is near maximal and β-adrenergic effects to further increase this mediator (and thereby insulin secretion) would be marginal. In contrast, α-adrenergic regulation in β-cells persists despite increased c-AMP production (32,33).

There is growing evidence that α-adrenergic inhibition of insulin secretion may occur at more than one metabolic site. Inhibition of c-AMP production mediated through Gi protein is well established (34,35). In addition, steps subsequent to c-AMP or diacyl glycerol production (33,36,37), involving pathways affecting protein phosphorylation (referred to as distal inhibition (33)), may also be target sites. Finally, inhibition of secretion may also occur by direct interference in ion flux. Thus, catecholamines added to islets caused hyperpolarization (38), increased K permeability via ATP-sensitive or low-conductance channels (6,27,39) and, in HIT cells, inhibition of Ca^{++} influx through the voltage-dependent calcium channel (40). Most of these effects are mediated via pertussis-sensitive G proteins.

Since the sulfonylureas directly inhibit the ATP sensitive K^+ channel or proteins associated with it (28,29,41,42), we compared glyburide's action on control and transgenic pancreas to further test if adrenergic hyperinnervation affects this channel or the linked Ca^{++} channels. In contrast to the positive effect of glucose, we found that glyburide's effect on insulin secretion from the transgenic pancreas was almost completely blocked.

Recently it was shown that part of the increased insulin release caused by phentolamine results from a direct action on K^+ or Ca^{++} ion channels (26,27,33,38). Thus, our observed decreased sensitivity to phentolamine is consistent with the decreased sensitivity found to glyburide and supports the conclusion that hyperadrenergic innervation caused inhibition of secretion-dependent ion flux. It has been suggested that the secretion-promoting effect of phentolamine on β-cell ion channels is non-specific and independent of its antagonist action on α-adrenergic receptors. These conclusions were based on observations in vivo and in vitro that whereas phentolamine increased insulin release, the more specific α-adrenergic blocking agents, idazoxan (43) and rauwolscine (26) did not. We found, however, that in the control mouse pancreas, idazoxan at 10^{-6} M was an even more effective stimulator of insulin secretion than an equimolar concentration of phentolamine. Another "α_2-specific" adrenergic antagonist, D_6-5128, also increased insulin secretion in the perfused rat pancreas (44). Our results showing a change of phentolamine effectiveness in hyperinnervated transgenic mice indicate that the action of phentolamine to increase insulin secretion is at least partially at the level of adrenergic regulation.

An impaired Ca^{++} flux suggested by the decreased response to glyburide would cause inhibition of insulin secretion, and could not explain the increased insulin secretion during glucose stimulation from the transgenic pancreas. Assuming that part of phentolamine's action is on the classic α-adrenergic receptor(s) distal to β-cell ion flux, the decreased response to glyburide observed in this study, together with the increased response to glucose, suggest that desensitization of these normally inhibiting distal sites of α-adrenergic action has occurred. It is possible that these sites may involve protein phosphorylation similar to that implicated in β-cell desensitization induced by chronic exposure to glucose (31,45,46).

We emphasize that different sites of α-adrenergic inhibition, though perhaps interacting, may operate independently. Thus, distal inhibition by epinephrine is observed when ion levels and flux are held constant in permeabilized RIN cells (33). Conversely, patch clamp and other studies (6,38,43,47) demonstrate adrenergic impairment of ion flux can occur independent of c-AMP or diacylglycerol-mediated metabolism. Our observation that chronic exposure to adrenergic innervation in transgenic mice can inhibit one mechanism (related to ion flux) while desensitizing inhibition of another further emphasizes the relative independence of these target sites.

In conclusion, our results are consistent with the following: 1) that chronic adrenergic hyperinnervation results in enhanced glucose-stimulated insulin secretion by desensitization of an overriding, distal α-adrenergic inhibitory site(s); and 2) that chronic innervation also affects ion flux (directly or indirectly) to inhibit insulin release, an action which is not desensitized. Each of these sites may be differentially regulated by their receptors and cross-talk between their pertussis sensitive and insensitive G proteins (48,49,50). Since down regulation of a sole α-adrenergic receptor would be expected to desensitize both sites, the observed differential desensitization may reflect relatively independent post receptor events. In other cell systems similar down regulation of α-adrenergic activity has been localized directly at adenyl cyclase, or as a result of receptor phosphorylation (reviewed in 51). On the other hand it must be considered that there may be more than one α-adrenergic receptor (49,52,53) whose structure or sites on the β-cell may influence their susceptibility to desensitization.

ACKNOWLEDGMENTS

This work was supported by NIH grant DK 01410, NSF Grant BNS 9011883, and a Basil O'Connor Award from the March of Dimes. We thank Dr. Douglas Hanahan and Lena DiLacio for graciously providing the NGF-transgenic mice used in this study. We also thank Mary Ann Jones for her technical assistance and Teri Elander for assistance in preparing the manuscript.

REFERENCES

1. R.H. Edwards, W.J. Rutter, D. Hanahan, 1989, Directed expression of NGF to pancreatic β cells in transgenic mice leads to selective hyperinnervation of the islets, Cell 58:161–170.
2. H.G. Coore, P.J. Randle, 1964, Regulation of insulin secretion studied with pieces of rabbit pancreas incubated in vitro, Biochem J 93:66–78.
3. E. Cerasi, S. Efendic, R. Luft, 1969, Role of adrenergic receptors in glucose-induced insulin secretion in man, Lancet ii:301-302.
4. F. Rohner-Jearenaud, B. Jeanrenaud, 1980, Consequences of ventromedical hypothalamic lesions upon insulin and glucagon secretion by subsequently isolated perfused pancreas in the rat, J Clin Invest, 65: 902–910.
5. P.H. Smith, S.C. Woods, D Porte, 1979, Control of the endocrine pancreas by the autonomic nervous system and related neural factors. In: "Integrative Functions of the Autonomic Nervous System," C.M. Brooks, K. Koizumi, A Sato, eds, Elsevier/North-Holland, Amsterdam, Netherlands, 84–97.
6. P. Rorsman, K. Bokvist, C. Ammala, P. Arkhammar, P.-O. Berggren, O. Larsson, K. Wahlander, 1991, Activation by adrenaline of a low-conductance G protein-dependent K^+ channel in mouse pancreatic B cells, Nature, 349:77–79.
7. T. Nakaki, T. Nakadate, K. Ishii, R. Kato, 1981, Postsynaptic alpha-2 adrenergic receptors in isolated rat islets of langerhans: inhibition of insulin release and cyclic 3′,5′-adenosine monophosphate accumulation, J Pharmacol Exp Ther 216:607–612.
8. H.H. Keahey, A.E. Boyd III, D.L. Kunze, 1990, G protein-dependent modification of calcium currents in clonal pancreatic β-cells, J Physiol 257:C1171–C1176.
9. D. Porte, 1969, Sympathetic regulation of insulin secretion, Arch Intern Med 123:252–260.
10. R.P. Robertson, J.B. Halter, D. Porte, 1976, A role for α-adrenergic receptors in abnormal insulin secretion in diabetes mellitus, J Clin Invest 57:791–795.
11. L.A. Campfield, F.J. Smith, 1983, Alteration of islet neurotransmitter sensitivity following ventromedial hypothalamic lesion, Am J Physiol 244:R635–R640.
12. M.C. Michel, P.A. Insel, 1989, Are there multiple imidazoline binding sites?, TIPS 10:342–344.
13. G.M. Grodsky, 1989, A new phase in insulin secretion. How will it contribute to our understanding of B-cell function?, Diabetes 38:673–678.
14. G.M. Grodsky, J.L. Bolaffi, 1992, Desensitization of the insulin-secreting beta cells, J Cell Biochem 48:3–11.
15. G.G. Weir, J.L. Leahy, S. Bonner-Weir, 1986, Experimental reduction of β-cell mass: implications for the pathogenesis of diabetes, Diabetes Metab Rev 2:125–161.
16. W.P. Hausdorff, M.G. Caron, R.J. Lefkowitz, 1990, Turning off the signal: desensitization of β-adrenergic receptor function, FASEB J 4:2881–2888.
17. G.M. Grodsky, R. Fanska, 1974, The in vitro perfused pancreas. In "Methods in Enzymology," J.G. Hardman, B.W. O'Malley, eds., Academic Press, New York, 363–372.
18. G.M. Grodsky, A. Heldt, 1984, Methods for the in vitro perfusion of the pancreas., In "Methods in Diabetes Research," J. Larner, S.L. Pohl, eds., Wiley and Sons, New York, 137–146.
19. G.M. Grodsky, C.T. Peng, 1959, Extractable insulin measured by immuno-chemical assay: effect of tolbutamide, Proc Soc Exp Biol and Med 101:100–103.
20. G.M. Grodsky, F. Schmidt-Formby, 1985, Kinetic and quantitative relationships between insulin release and ^{65}Zn efflux from perifused islets, Endocrinology 117:704–710.
21. M.D.L. O'Connor, H. Landahl, G.M. Grodsky, 1990, Comparison of storage-and signal-limited models of pancreatic insulin secretion, Am J Physiol 238:R378–R389.
22. G.M. Grodsky, 1972, Threshold distribution hypothesis for packet storage of insulin and its mathematical modeling, J Clin Invest 51:2047–2059.
23. G.M. Grodsky, Y.H. Ma, B. Cullen, N. Sarvetnick, 1992, Effect on insulin production sorting and secretion by major histocompatibility complex class II gene expression in the pancreatic β cell of transgenic mice, Endocrinology 131:933–938.
24. S. Lenzen, 1979, Insulin secretion by isolated perfused rat and mouse pancreas, Am J Physiol 236: E391–E400.
25. O. Berglund, 1987, Lack of glucose-induced priming of insulin release in the perfused mouse pancreas, J Endocrinol 114:185–189.
26. A. Schulz, A. Hasselblatt, 1989, An insulin-releasing property of imidazoline derivatives is not limited to compounds that block α-adrenoceptors, Naunym-Schmiedebergs Arch Pharmacol 340:321–327.
27. T.D. Plant, J.C. Henquin, 1990, Phentolamine and yohimbine inhibit ATP-sensitive K^+ channels in mouse pancreatic β-cells, Br J Pharmacol 101:115–120.

28. A.E. Boyd, 1988, Sulfonylurea receptors, ion channels and fruit flies, Diabetes 37:847–850.
29. I. Niki, J.L. Nicks, S.J. Aschroft, 1990, The beta cell glibenclamide receptor is an ADP-binding protein, Biochem J 268:713–718.
30. J.L. Bolaffi, G. Rodd, Y.H. Ma, G.M. Grodsky, 1990, Effect of glucagon or somatostatin on desensitized insulin secretion, Endocrinology 126:1750–1775.
31. J.L. Bolaffi, G.G. Rodd, Y.H. Ma, D. Bright, G.M. Grodsky, 1991, The role of Ca^{++}-related events in glucose-stimulated desensitization of insulin secretion, Endocrinology 129:2131–2138.
32. W.H. Hsu, H. Xiang, A.S. Rajan, A.E. Boyd, 1991, Activation of α_2-adrenergic receptors decreases Ca^{2+} influx to inhibit insulin secretion in a hamster β-cell line: An action mediated by a guanosine triphosphate-binding protein, Endocrinology 128:958–964.
33. S. Ullrich, C.B. Wollheim, 1988, GTP-dependent inhibition of insulin secretion by epinephrine in permeabilized RINm5F cells, J Biol Chem 263:8615–8620.
34. C.B. Wollheim, M. Kikuchi, A.E. Renold, G.W.G. Sharp, 1977,Somatostatin-and epinephrine-induced modification of $^{45}Ca^{++}$ fluxes in insulin release in rat pancreatic islets maintained in tissue culture, J Clin Invest 60:1165–1173.
35. S. Ullrich, C.B. Wollheim, 1985, Expression of both α- and α_2-adrenoceptors in an insulin secreting cell line: Parallel studies of cytosolic free Ca^{++} and insulin release, Mol Pharmacol 28:100–106.
36. A. Robinovitch, E. Cerasi, G.W.G. Sharp, 1978, Adenosine 3′,5′-monophosphate-dependent and independent inhibitory effects of epinephrine on insulin release in rat pancreatic islets, Endocrinology 102:1733–1740.
37. S.J. Persaud, P.M. Jones, S.L. Howell, 1993, Activation of protein kinase C partially alleviates noradrenaline inhibition of insulin secretion, Biochem J 289:497–501.
38. S. Santana de Sa, R. Ferrer, E. Rojas, I. Atwater, 1983, Effects of adrenaline and noradrenaline on glucose-induced electrical activity of mouse pancreatic β cell, J Physiol 68:247–258.
39. G. Drews, A. Debuyser, M. Henquin, J.C. Henquin, 1990, Galanin and epinephrine act on distinct receptors to inhibit insulin release by the same mechanisms including an increase in K^+ permeability of the B-cell membrane, Endocrinology 126:1646–1653.
40. W.H. Hsu, H. Xiang, A.S. Rajan, A.E. Boyd III, 1991, Activation of α_2-adrenergic receptors decreases Ca^{2+} influx to inhibit insulin secretion in a hamster β-cell line: An action mediated by a guanosine triphosphate-binding protein, Endocrinology 128:958–964.
41. L. Siconolfi-Baez, M.A. Banerji, H.E. Lebovitz, 1990, Characterization and significance of sulfonylurea receptors, Diabetes Care 13:2–8.
42. H. Schmid-Antomarchi, J. DeWeille, M. Fosset, M. Lazdunski, 1987, The receptor for antidiabetic sulfonylureas controls the activity of the ATP-modulated K^+ channel in insulin-secreting cells, J Biol Chem 262: 15840–15844.
43. C.-G. Ostenson, A.G. Cattaneo, J.C. Doxey, S. Efendic, 1989, α-adrenoceptors and insulin release from pancreatic islets of normal and diabetic rats, Am J Physiol 257 (Endocrinol Metab 20):E439–E443.
44. G. Koh, Y. Seino, K. Tsuda, S. Nishi, H. Ishida, J. Takeda, H. Fukumoto, T. Taminato, H. Imura, 1992, Effect of the α_2-blocker DG-5128 on insulin and somatostatin release from the isolated perfused rat pancreas, Life Sciences 40:1113–1118.
45. G.M. Grodsky, J.L. Bolaffi, 1992, Desensitization of insulin-secreting beta cells, J of Cellular Biochem 48:3–11.
46. W.S. Zawalich, K.A. Zawalich, G.I. Shulman, L. Rossetti, 1990, Chronic in vivo hyperglycemia impairs phosphoinositide hydrolysis and insulin release in isolated perfused rat islets, Endocrinology 126:253–260.
47. N.G. Morgan, 1987, Regulation of insulin secretion by α_2-adrenergic agonists, TIPS 8:369–370.
48. C.M. Fraser, S. Arakawa, W.R. McCombie, J.C. Venter, 1989, Cloning, Sequence analysis, and permanent expression of a human α_2-adrenergic receptor in chinese hamster overy cells, J of Biol Chem 264:11754–11761.
49. H.R. Bourne, A.L. DeFranco, 1989, Signal transduction and intercellular messengers. In "Oncogenes and the Molecular Origins of Cancer," R. Weinberg, M. Wigler, eds., Cold Spring Harbor Laboratory Press, 97–124.
50. A. Schmidt, J. Hescheler, S. Offermanns, K. Spicher, K.-D. Hinsch, F.-J. Klinz, J. Codina, L. Birnbaumer, H. Gausepohl, R. Frank, G. Schultz, W. Rosenthal, 1991, Involvement of pertussis toxin-sensitive G-proteins in the hormonal inhibition of dihydropyridine-sensitive Ca^{2+} currents in an insulin-secretion cell line (RINm5F), J of Biol Chem 266:18025–18033.
51. J.L. Benivic, M. Bouvier, M.G. Caron, R.J. Lefkowitz, 1988, Regulation of adenyl cyclase-coupled β-adrenergic receptors, Ann Rev Cell Biol 4:405–428.
52. J. Garthwaite, 1990, Nitric oxide synthesis linked to activation of excitatory neurotransmitter receptors in the brain. In "Nitric Oxide from L-Arginine: A Bioregulatory System," Excerpta Medica, New York, 115–137.
53. L. Birnbaumer, J. Abramowitz, A. Yatani, K. Okabe, R. Mattera, R. Graff, J. Sanford, J. Codina, A.M. Brown, 1990, Roles of G Proteins in Coupling of Receptors to Ionic Channels and Other Effector Systems, Biochem and Molecular Biology 25:225–244.

18

COLOCALIZATION OF WE-14 IMMUNOSTAINING WITH THE CLASSICAL ISLET HORMONES IN THE PORCINE PANCREAS

W. J. Curry, C. F. Johnston, C. Shaw, and K. D. Buchanan

Department of Medicine
Institute of Clinical Science
The Queen's University of Belfast
Belfast, Nothern Ireland, United Kingdom

INTRODUCTION

WE-14, a tetradecapeptide possessing an N-terminal tryptophanyl (W) and a C-terminal glutamyl (E) residue, was isolated from extracts of a liver metastasis of an ileal carcinoid[1] and from a phaeochromocytoma[2]. Analysis of the chromogranin A (CGA) cDNA sequences revealed that WE-14 represents residues 322–339, 314–331, 341–358, 338–355 and 311–327 of human, bovine, rat, murine and porcine CGA, respectively[3]. Human and bovine WE-14 are of identical primary structure. The rat and murine peptides are homologous but differ from the human peptide by a single Arg/Lys conservative substitution, whilst, the porcine peptide differs by a single non-conservative Gln/Arg substitution. Each peptide is flanked by conserved pairs of basic amino acid residues. The characterisation of the novel CGA-derived peptides: B-granin[4], pancreastatin (PST)[5], chromostatin (CST)[6], vasostatin[7] and parastatin[8], in conjunction with the determination of several CGA cDNA sequences which revealed the presence of multiple proteolytic processing sites, supports the concept that CGA is a prohormone.

Light and electron microscopical studies have revealed that CGA immunoreactivity is localised to the secretory vesicles of some or all islet cells in a range of species[9]. PST has been reported in all islets cells[10–13], whilst, CST has only been observed in the human B cell population[14]. B-granin immunoreactivity was localised to a population of B and A cells[15] and, with rat PST-like immunoreactivity, in rat islets[15]. The objective of this study was to investigate the distribution of the CGA-derived peptide, WE-14, with that of the classic islet hormones in the porcine pancreas.

Physiology and Pathophysiology of the Islets of Langerhans, edited by Soria.
Plenum Press, New York, 1997.

Table 1. Primary antisera, code and working dilution

	Primary antisera	
	Code	Dilution
Guinea pig		
Insulin	005	1:1000
Somatostatin	182	1:500
WE-14	G44	1:400
Rabbit		
Glucagon	YY89	1:500
Pancreatic polypeptide	221	1:500
WE-14	814	1:200

MATERIALS AND METHODS

Antisera Production

Synthetic human WE-14 [Peninsula] (600 μg) was dissolved in phosphate-buffered saline (pH 7.2), coupled via 1% glutaraldehyde to bovi ne serum albumin [Sigma] (3 mg) and emulsified with Freund's Complete adjuvant. New Zealand white rabbits received a primary immuni sation of 200 μg/ml followed by monthly boosts of 100 μg/ml emulsified in Freund's Incomplete adjuvant. Guinea pigs received a primary immunisation of 100 μg/ml of WE-14 coupled via 1% glutaraldehyde to keyhole limpet hemocyanin [Sigma] followed by monthly boosts of 50 μg/ml. Bleeds were taken 10–14 days after boosting. Rabbit code 814 and guinea pig code G44 produced suitable antisera for immunocytochemical investigation.

Immunohistochemistry

Fresh porcine pancreatic tissues were obtained and immersed in buffered 4% paraformaldehyde (pH 7.2) at the abattoir, transported on ice and fixed for 4 h at 4°C. Cryoprotected tissue sections (15 μm) were air dried on to gelatin-coated slides and simultaneously immunostained with the primary rabbit and guinea pig antisera (Table 1) for 24 h at 4°C. After a 10 min wash in PBS the sections were incubated (30 min) with biotinylated donkey-anti-rabbit (Amersham Int., Buchinghamshire, UK), the primary rabbit antisera were reapplied to ensure that all the free Fab binding sites on the donkey-anti-rabbit were completely bound. Follow-

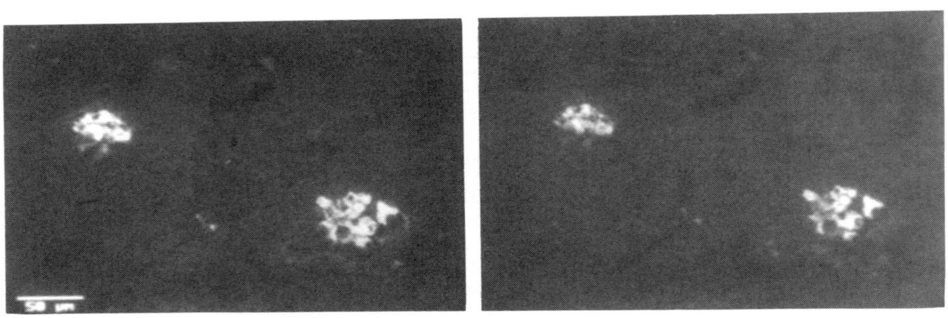

Figure 1. Confocal scanning laser micrograph of intense insulin (left) and moderate WE-14 (right) immunoreactivity of central islet cells of porcine pancreatic body.

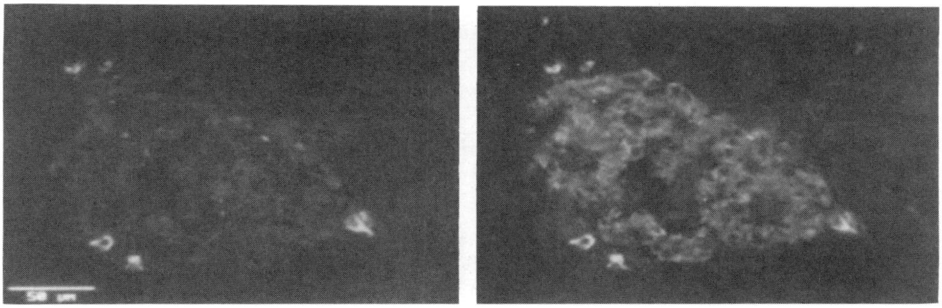

Figure 2. Intense PP (left) WE-14 (right) immunostaining of peripheral islet cells in the porcine body, with moderate WE-14 immunoreactivity in central cells.

ing a 10 min wash the sections were incubated (30 min) with Texas Red streptavidin (Amersham Int.) washed and incubated (30 min) with fluorescein-conjugated rabbit-anti-guinea pig (Dakopatts, Glostrup, Denmark). The sections were washed, mounted in 0.1 M PBS/glycerol prior to examination employing a Bio-Rad (Abingdon, UK) Lasersharp MRC 500 confocal scanning laser microscope fitted with a double channel filter block set with bright excitation lines at 488 nm and 514 nm. Control studies included the liquid-phase preadsorption of the primary antisera with synthetic peptides, the omission of the primary antisera and following the primary incubation, the section were washed for 1 h in phosphate-buffered 0.5 M NaCl to abolish any potential non-specific ionic antibody binding[16].

RESULTS

Moderate and intense WE-14 immunoreactivity was detected with both rabbit and guinea pig antisera throughout the porcine islets (Figs. 1–4). WE-14 immunostaining was localised to the B-cell population throughout the head, body and tail (Fig. 1). An additional pop ulation of WE-14 positive, insulin-negative cells were evident. All PP cells in the pancreatic head and body exhibited WE-14 immunoreactivity (Fig. 2). A population of D cells scattered throughout the pancreas (Fig. 3) and A cells in the body and tail exhibited WE-14 immunostaining (Fig. 4). WE-14 immunoreactivity was abolished by the addi-

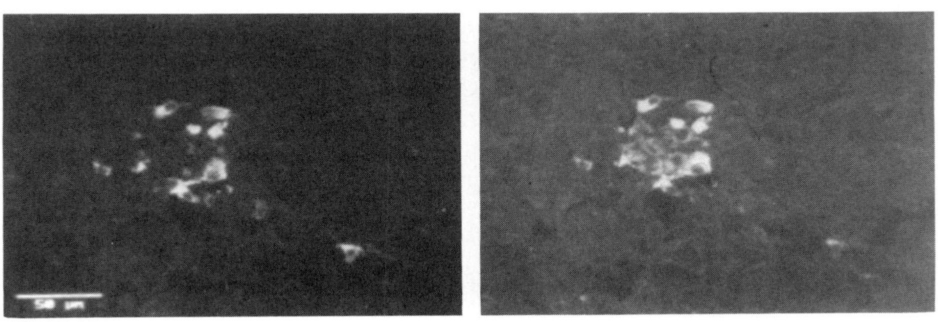

Figure 3. Peripheral islet cells in the pancreatic tail displaying intense glucagon (left) and moderate WE-14 (right) immunoreactivity.

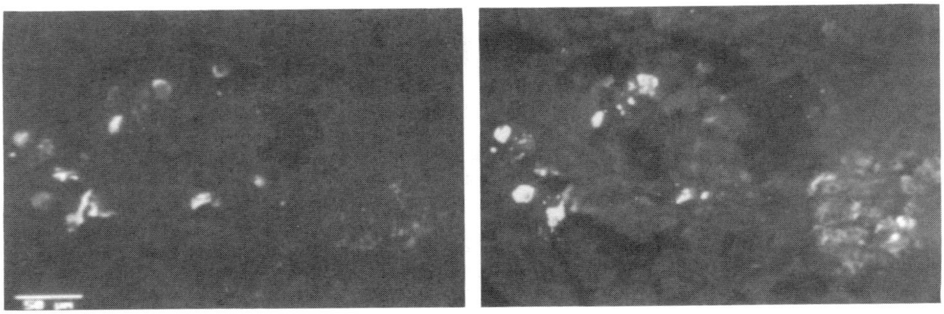

Figure 4. Intensely staining somatostatin (left) and WE-14 (right) positive cells scattered throughout an islet in the head of the pancreas.

tion of 500 ng/ml–1 μg/ml of synthetic WE-14. No immunoreactivity was evident with the omission of the primary antisera. The additional high molarity salt wash did not diminish the intensity of immunostaining of any of the antisera.

DISCUSSION

The isolation of WE-14 from two neoplastic tissue extracts has established that CGA is proteolytically-processed at the paired basic residues[1,2]. Pulse-chase tracer studies of CGA processing in the rat pancreatic islet have revealed that it is rapidly processed to an N-terminal 21 kDa peptide, a 45 kDa intervening peptide and a C-terminal 14 kDa peptide. The 45 kDa peptide is further processed to liberate two smaller peptides; a 5 kDa and 3 kDa peptide exhibiting PST and WE-14 immunoreactivity respectively[17]. A comparision of the proteolytic processing of CGA in bovine tissues revealed the presence of a heterogeneous group of pancreastatin-related peptides differentially expressed in tissues of the gastro-entero-pancreatic tract, whilst in the adrenal medulla CGA was intact[18]. However, a recent investigation of the proteolytic processing of CGA in bovine chromaffin vesicles revealed the presence of 12 cleavage sites[19]. These studies would suggest that CGA may be subject to differential tissue-specific processing and that the novel peptides expressed in each tissue may exhibit a variety of physiological roles.

The present study has demonstrated that the CGA-derived peptide,WE-14, is expressed in major population of porcine pancreatic cells.

Previous investigations employing antisera raised to intact CGA have detected immunostaining in a range of islet cell types[9]. These contradictory reports may be due to the species-specificity and regional-specificity of the CGA antisera employed. The distribution of PST immunostaining in the porcine pancreas has been reported in a range of islet cells types[10–13]. In the rat islet, intense PST-like and B-granin immunoreactivity have been detected in peripheral islet cells, central islet cells exhibit a heterogeneous immunostaining pattern[16]. In the human islet PST immunostaining was primarily detected in A and D cells[11]. CST immunoreactivity has been localised to the human pancreatic B cell[14]. In the porcine pancreas, WE-14 exhibits a similar widespread distribution to that of PST. Numerous immunocytochemical studies have established that all adrenal chromaffin cells express CGA immunostaining[9]. In a previous study employing an antisera raised to the conserved C-terminal hexapeptide of WE-14, immunostaining was observed in discrete clusters of rat adrenomedullary cells[16]. The antisera employed in this study, raised to synthetic human WE-14, exhibit a similar pattern of immunostaining in a subpopulation of chromaffin cells in a range of mammalian adrenal medullae[20]. This would suggest that under immunocytochemical conditions, these WE-14 antisera do not cross react with intact CGA. In addition, the fact that WE-14 exhibits a high degree of inter-species homology (93–100%) may preclude the aberrant immunostaining patterns which has been reported for CGA and other CGA-derived peptides. Quantative analysis have detected levels (ng/g ± SEM, n=3) of 60.1 ± 2.4 and 46.7 ± 3.0 in porcine pancreatic extracts of head and tail, respectively. In addition, soft gel permeation, reverse phase HPLC and gel permeation HPLC of porcine pancreatic extracts have resolved a peptide which co-elutes with synthetic human WE-14.[21]

CONCLUSION

Within the past decade a number of novel CGA-derived peptides have been isolated and characterised each of which have been reported to exhibit inhibitory physiological roles. The present investigation has demonstrated that CGA-derived peptide, WE-14, is generated in a major population of porcine pancreatic islet cells. This would suggest that WE-14 may be co-released with the resident peptide hormones. The potential physiological role of WE-14 as a autocrine/paracrine regulatory peptide of the endocrine pancreas remaims to be determined.

ACKNOWLEDGMENTS

W.J.C is in receipt of the British Diabetic Association, R.D. Lawrence Research Fellowship.

REFERENCES

1. W.J. Curry, C. Shaw, C.F. Johnston, L. Thim, and K.D. Buchanan, Isolation and primary structure of a novel chromogranin A-derived peptide, WE-14, from a human midgut carcinoid tumour. FEBS Lett 301: 319–321 (1992)
2. J.M. Conlon, B. Hamberger, and L. Grimelius, Isolation of peptides arising from the specific posttranslational processing of chromogranin A and chromogranin B from human phaeochromocytoma. Peptides 13: 639–644 (1992)
3. J.-P. Simon, and D. Aunis, Biochemistry of the chromogranin A protein family. Biochem. J. 262:1–13 (1989)
4. J.C. Hutton, F. Hansen, and M. Peshavaria, Beta-granin: 21kDa co-secreted peptides of the insulin secretory granule closely related to adrenal medullary chromogranin A. FEBS Lett. 188:,336–340 (1985)
5. K. Tatemoto, S. Efendic, V. Mutt, G. Makk, G.J. Feistner, and J.D. Barchas, Pancreastatin, a novel pancreatic peptide that inhibits insulin secretion. Nature 324: 476–478 (1986)
6. E. Galindo, A. Rill, M.-F. Bader, and D. Aunis, Chromostatin, a 20-amino acid peptide derived from chromogranin A, inhibits chromaffin cell secretion. Proc. Natl. Acad. Sci. USA, 88:1426–1430 (1991)
7. S. Ardal, and K.B. Helle, The vasoinhibitory activity of bovine chromogranin A fragments (vasostatin and its dependence of extracellular in isolated segments of human blood vessels. Regul Pept. 41:9–18 (1992)
8. B.H. Fasciotto, C.A. Trauss, G.H. Greeley, and D.V. Cohn, Parastatin (porcine chromogranin A 347–419), a novel chromogranin A-derived peptide, inhibits parathyroid cell secretion. Endocrinology 133:461–466 (1993)

9. B. Wiedenmann, and W.B. Huttner, Synaptophysin and chromogranins/secretogranins — widespread constitutents of distinct types of neuroendocrine vesicles and new tools in tumor diagnosis. Virchows Archiv. B. Cell. Pathol. 58:95–121 (1989)
10. M. Ravazzola, S. Effendic, C.G. Ostenson, K. Tatemoto, J.C. Hutton, and L. Orci, Localization of pancreastatin immunoreactivity in porcine endocrine cells. Endocrinology 123: 227–229 (1988)
11. W.E. Schmidt, E.G. Siegel, R. Lamberts, B. Gallwitz, and W. Creutzfeldt, Pancreastatin: Molecular and immunocytochemical characterization of a novel peptide in porcine and human tissues. Endocrinology 123: 1395–1404 (1988)
12. D. Bretherton-Watt, M.A. Ghatei, A.E. Bishop, P. Facer, M. Fahey, M. Hedges, G. Williams, K.L. Valentino, K. Tatemoto, K. Roth, J.M. Polak, and S.R. Bloom, Pancreastatin: Distribution and plasma levels in the pig. Peptides 9: 1005–1014 (1988)
13. R. Lamberts, W.E. Schmidt, and W. Creutzfeldt, Light and electron microscopical immunocytochemical localisation of pancreastatin -like immunoreactivity in porcine tissues. Histochemistry 93: 369–380 (1991)
14. Y. Cetin, D. Aunis, M.-F. Bader, E. Galindo, A. Jorns, G. Bargsten, and D. Grube, Chromostatin, a chromogranin A-derived bioactive peptide, is present in human pancreatic insulin (B) cells. Proc. Natl. Acad. Sci. USA 90:2360–2364 (1993)
15. J.C. Hutton, M. Peshavaria, C.F. Johnston, M. Ravazzola, and L. Orci, Immunolocalization of B-granin: a chromogranin A-related protein of the pancreatic B-cell. Endocrinology 122: 1014–1020 (1987)
16. W. J. Curry, C.F. Johnston, J.C. Hutton, S.D. Arden, N.G. Rutherford, C. Shaw, and K.D. Buchanan, The tissue distribution of rat chromogranin A-derived peptides: Evidence for differential tissue processing from sequence specific antisera. Histochem 96: 531–538 (1991)
17. S.D. Arden, N.G. Rutherford, P.C. Guest, W.J. Curry, E.M. Bailyes, C.F. Johnston, and J.C. Hutton, The post-translational processing of chromogranin A in the pancreatic islet: involvement of the eukaryote subtilisin PC2. Biochem. J. 298: 521–528 (1994)
18. A. Watkinson, A.-C. Jonsson, M. Davison, J.Young, C. Lee, S. Moore, and G.J. Dockray, Heterogeneity of chromogranin A-derived peptides in bovine gut, pancreas and adrenal medulla. Biochem. J. 276: 471–479 (1991)
19. M.-H. Metz-Boutigue, P. Garcia-Sablone, R. Hogue-Angeletti, and D. Aunis, Intracellular and extracellular processing of chromogranin A: Determination of cleavage sites. Eur. J. Biochem 217: 247–257 (1993)
20. C.K. Connolly, W.J. Curry, C.F. Johnston, and K.D.Buchanan, Evidence for the proteolytic processing of chromogranin A in mammalian adrenal medullae and phaeochromocytomas. Regul. Pep. 51: 279 (1994)
21. W.J Curry, C.F. Johnston, C. Shaw, and K.D. Buchanan, Characterisation of WE-14 immunoreactivity in human, porcine and rat endocrine pancreata. Regul. Pep. 51: 280 (1994)

19

PYRIDOTHIADIAZINES AS POTENT INHIBITORS OF GLUCOSE-INDUCED INSULIN RELEASE

P. Lebrun,[1] M.-H. Antoine,[1] R. Ouedraogo,[1] A. Herchuelz,[1] P. de Tullio,[2] J. Delarge,[2] and B. Pirotte[2]

[1]Laboratory of Pharmacology
Free University of Brussels, School of Medicine (CP 617)
B-1070 Brussels, Belgium
[2]Department of Medicinal Chemistry
University of Liège
Liège, Belgium

INTRODUCTION

In the last few years, great interest has been focused on drugs (diazoxide, pinacidil, cromakalim, ...) whose mechanism of action involves the activation of membrane K^+ channels (1,2). Such compounds, which may control the membrane poten- tial and the excitability of a variety of cells, constitute a new class of drugs: the "K^+ channel openers." Although the K^+ channel openers presently available display several potential clinical applications, the diversity of K^+ channels offers the possibility to develop new agents selective for specific K^+ channel types.

Recently, we have synthetized more than 60 novel pyridothiadiazine derivatives which are structural analogues of diazoxide. Some of these compounds bearing different aminoalkyl side chains in the 3-position may be regarded as sulfonylguanidines and, therefore, are also structurally related to cyanoguanidines such as pinacidil (3). The main objective of the present study was to characterize the ionic and secretory response of pancreatic islet cells to these new compounds.

MATERIALS AND METHODS

The methods used to measure ^{86}Rb (a tracer for K^+), ^{45}Ca fractional outflow rate (FOR), ^{45}Ca uptake, insulin release from rat pancreatic islets and cytosolic Ca^{2+} concentrations from single B cells have been described previously (4,5). BPDZ 44 was synthetized at the Department of Medicinal Chemistry (University of Liège, Liège, Belgium) and

Physiology and Pathophysiology of the Islets of Langerhans, edited by Soria.
Plenum Press, New York, 1997.

Table 1. Effects of pyridothiadiazine derivatives, diazoxide and pinacidil on insulin release (%)

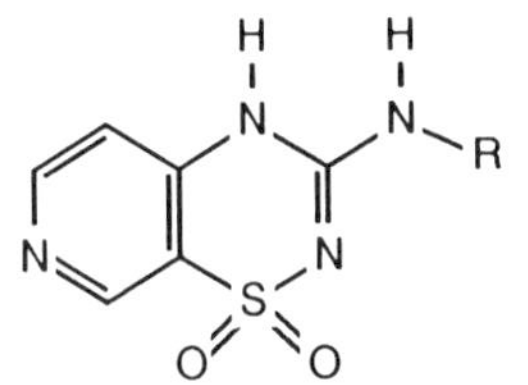

BPDZ 29-62

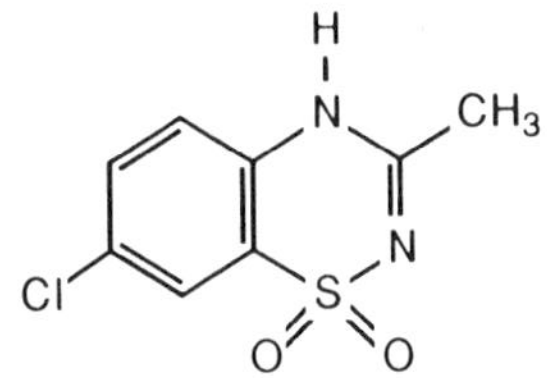

DIAZOXIDE

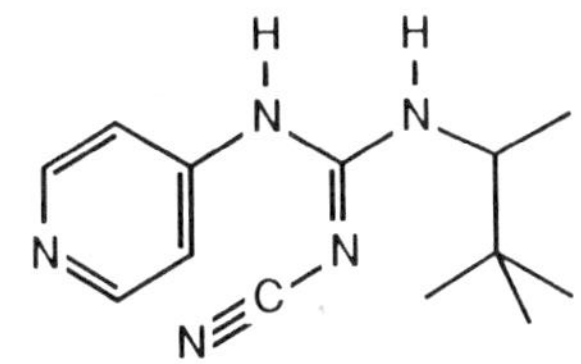

PINACIDIL

Drug	Substituent (R)	500 μM	100 μM	50 μM	10 μM	1 μM
BPDZ 29	H	---	---	104.1 ±. 6.5 (14)	---	---
BPDZ 39	$(CH_2)_2CH_3$	8.99 ± 0.99 (15)	21.9 ± 3.37 (14)	57.67 ± 3.82 (14)	87.31 ± 6.71 (15)	97.1 ± 5.89 (8)
BPDZ 40	$CH(CH_3)_2$	8.77 ± 0.88 (8)	18.43 ± 3.87 (8)	42.55 ± 6.91 (8)	55.27 ± 8.08 (8)	110.33 ± 11.33 (6)
BPDZ 41	$CH_2(CH_2)_2CH_3$	8.98 ± 1.98 (8)	32.51± 5.05 (8)	38.62 ± 5.6 (7)	82.03 ± 6.20 (8)	83.73 ± 6.22 (8)
BPDZ 42	$CH(CH_3)CH_2CH_3$	9.37 ± 2.15 (7)	7.14 ± 0.58 (8)	9.38 ± 0.87 (8)	48.97 ± 5.41 (7)	97.81 ± 9.08 (8)
BPDZ 43	$CH_2CH(CH_3)_2$	9.74 ± 0.80 (8)	10.16 ± 0.37 (8)	23.42 ± 3.12 (8)	71.84 ± 7.16 (16)	84.22 ± 10.99 (8)
BPDZ 44	$CH(CH_3)CH(CH_3)_2$	8.43 ± 0.88 (24)	8.81± 0.87 (24)	8.64 ± 0.94 (23)	13.70 ± 1.17 (23)	70.52 ± 4.42 (19)
BPDZ 45	C_5H_9(cyclopentyl)	4.41 ± 0.66 (8)	9.16 ± 0.43 (8)	31.55 ± 4.03 (7)	71.08 ± 11.24 (7)	82.77 ± 9.67 (8)
BPDZ 46	C_6H_{11} (cyclohexyl)	6.20 ± 0.48 (8)	18.36 ± 3.55 (8)	40.50 ± 4.32 (8)	64.40 ± 9.46 (7)	74.38 ± 4.46 (8)
BPDZ 47	NC_4H_8O (N-morpholinyl)	---	---	98.80 ± 3.90 (16)	---	---
BPDZ 62	$CH(CH_3)C(CH_3)_3$	6.86 ± 0.57 (20)	7.89 ± 0.42 (22)	10.27 ± 0.75 (20)	41.04 ± 2.23 (19)	69.95 ± 3.41 (24)
DIAZO		8.51 ± 0.70 (21)	14.01 ± 1.36 (21)	28.84 ± 2.45 (21)	70.02 ± 3.62 (22)	78.95 ± 3.83 (21)
PINA		22.06 ± 2.24 (19)	88.32 ± 5.80 (12)	92.72 ± 8.01 (14)	99.26 ± 8.92 (13)	110.5 ± 18.31 (6)

Rat pancreatic islets were incubated for 90 min in the presence of 16.7 mM glucose. The residual insulin release (mean values ± S.E.) was expressed in percent of the value recorded in control experiments (100 %; no added drug). Figures in parentheses are numbers of individual experiments. BPDZ = pyridothiadiazine derivatives, DIAZO = diazoxide, PINA = pinacidil).

diazoxide was obtained from Essex Labo (Brussels, Belgium). BPDZ 44 and diazoxide were dissolved in dimethylsulfoxide which was added to both control and test media at final concentrations not exceeding 0.1% (v/v). All results are expressed as the mean (± S.E.) together with the number of individual experiments.

RESULTS

The sulfonylguanidines appeared to be potent inhibitors of the insulin releasing process. Table 1 clearly indicates that the addition of micromolar concentrations of the drugs (designated as BPDZ 44, -42, etc.) to islets incubated in the presence of 16.7 mM

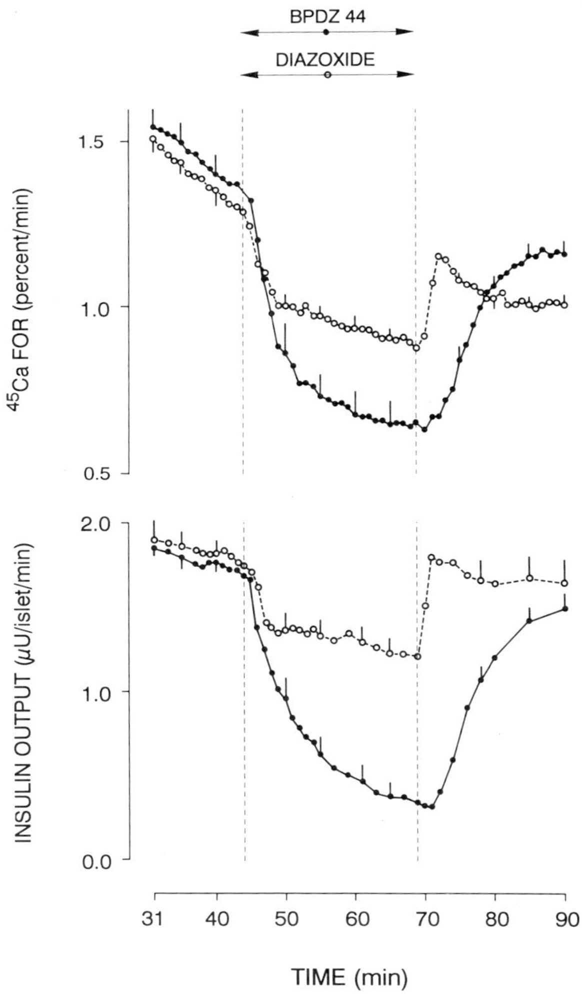

Figure 1. Effect of BPDZ 44 (●; 10 μM) and diazoxide (○; 10 μM) on ^{45}Ca outflow (upper panel) and insulin release (lower panel) from islets perifused throughout in the presence of 16.7 mM glucose. Basal media contained 2.56 mM Ca^{2+}. Mean values (± SE) refer to 4 individual experiments.

glucose provoked a dose-dependent decrease in insulin release. BPDZ 42 [3-(1′-methylpropyl)amino-4H-pyrido[4,3-e][1,2,4]thiadiazine 1,1-dioxide], BPDZ 44 [3-(1′,2′-dimethylpropyl)amino-4H-pyrido[4,3-e][1,2,4]thiadiazine 1,1-dioxide] and BPDZ 62 [3-(1′,2′,2′-trimethylpropyl)amino-4H-pyrido[4,3-e][1,2,4]thiadiazine 1,1-dioxide] were more potent than diazoxide and pinacidil in inhibiting the glucose-induced insulin release.

In another series of experiments, we determined whether the effects of BPDZ 44 and BPDZ 62 on the secretory process were related to changes in ionic movements and cytosolic Ca^{2+} concentrations. BPDZ 44 (50 μM) and BPDZ 62 (50 μM) increased the rate of ^{86}Rb outflow from prelabelled and perifused rat pancreatic islets. These stimulatory effects persisted in the absence of extracellular Ca^{2+} but were abolished by glibenclamide (10 μM). The increases in ^{86}Rb outflow provoked by the two drugs were more marked than that evoked by diazoxide. BPDZ 44 was also more potent than diazoxide in affecting ^{45}Ca outflow and short term (5 min) ^{45}Ca uptake. A low concentration of BPDZ 44 (10 μM) completely suppressed the increases in ^{45}Ca outflow and ^{45}Ca uptake mediated by a rise in the extracellular concentration of glucose (5.6 to 16.7 mM) whilst diazoxide (10 μM) failed to abolish and only reduced these cationic responses to glucose. In islets exposed throughout to 16.7 mM glucose, the addition of BPDZ 44 (10 μM) or diazoxide (10 μM) provoked a rapid and sustained inhibition of ^{45}Ca outflow and insulin release (Fig. 1). The inhibitory effects of BPDZ 44 were again more marked than those elicited by diazoxide ($P < 0.001$).

Lastly, BPDZ 44 (50 μM) failed to affect the cationic responses provoked by a rise in the extracellular concentration of K^+ (5 to 50 mM). Indeed, the drug did not affect the increase in ^{45}Ca outflow mediated by K^+ depolarization. Moreover, in single B-cells, BPDZ 44 inhibited the glucose but not the KCl-induced rise in cytosolic Ca^{2+} concentration.

CONCLUSIONS

The present data clearly show that some pyridothiadiazine derivatives are more potent than the reference molecule diazoxide in affecting the ionic and secretory events in rat pancreatic B cells. Our data also suggest that these newly synthetized pyridothiadiazine derivatives inhibit the insulin releasing process by activating ATP-sensitive K^+ channels. This K^+ channel activation will lead to a decrease in Ca^{2+} influx and cytosolic Ca^{2+} concentration. The difference in potency between diazoxide and BPDZ 44 or BPDZ 62 implies that the latter compounds could be valuable pharmacological tools for characterizing further the structural requirements for ATP-sensitive K^+ channel activation and selectivity.

REFERENCES

1. P. Lebrun, M.-H. Antoine and A. Herchuelz, Minireview: K^+ channel openers and insulin release, Life Sciences 51:795 (1992).
2. N.S. Cook and U. Quast, Potassium channel pharmacology, in: "Potassium channels, Structure, Classification, Function and Therapeutic potential", N.S. Cook, ed, Ellis Horwood Limited, Chichester, England (1990).
3. B. Pirotte, P. de Tullio, P. Lebrun, M.-H. Antoine, B. Masereel, M. Schynts, L. Dupont, A. Herchuelz and J. Delarge, 3-Alkylamino-4H-pyrido[4,3-e][1,2,4]thiadiazine 1,1-dioxides as powerful inhibitors of insulin release from pancreatic B cells, J. Med. Chem. 36:3211 (1993).
4. P. Lebrun, V. Devreux, M. Hermann and A. Herchuelz, Similarities between the effects of pinacidil and diazoxide on ionic and secretory events in rat pancreatic islets, J. Pharmacol. Exp. Ther. 250:1011 (1989).
5. M.-H. Antoine, M. Hermann, A. Herchuelz and P. Lebrun, Sodium nitroprusside inhibits glucose-induced insulin release by activating ATP-sensitive K^+ channels, Biochim. Biophys. Acta 1175:293 (1993).

20

INCREASE IN $[Ca^{2+}]_i$ AND SUBSEQUENT INSULIN RELEASE FROM βTC3-CELLS WITH THE L-TYPE Ca^{2+}-CHANNEL ACTIVATOR, FPL 64176

Janne Springborg, Jesper Gromada, Peter Madsen, Annemarie R. Varming, and Jannie Fuhlendorff*

Novo Nordisk A/S
Novo Allé, DK-2880 Bagsvaerd, Denmark

INTRODUCTION

The regulation of calcium entry is central in the control of insulin secretion from the pancreatic β-cell. Glucose is the primary physiological stimulator of insulin secretion and a principal action of glucose is consequently to depolarize the β-cell by closing K^+-channels sensitive to the ATP produced during metabolism of the sugar[1,2]. This will lead to membrane depolarization and activation of the voltage-dependent L-type Ca^{2+}-channels leading to increase in intracellular calcium concentration, $[Ca^{2+}]_i$, and insulin secretion. Pharmacological important secretagogues such as sulphonylureas (e.g. glibenclamide) close the ATP-sensitive K^+-channels leading to depolarization of the β-cell membrane, activation of voltage gated Ca^{2+}-channels by opening the channels and initiation of repetitive action potentials. The resulting calcium influx increases the $[Ca^{2+}]_i$ and thereby triggers insulin release. Compounds interfering with this process also regulate the insulin secretion and therefore the L-type Ca^{2+}-channel might, like the ATP-sensitive K^+-channel, be a suitable target for therapeutic intervention in treatment of Non-Insulin Dependent Diabetes Mellitus (NIDDM). The ligands for L-type Ca^{2+}-channels can be divided into three categories: dihydropyridines, phenylalkylamines and benzothiazepines. Bay K 8644 has become the prototype for the class of dihydropyridines. Some of the dihydropyridines are chiral and resolution of these have revealed the (–)-enantiomers as potent activators, whereas the (+)-enantiomers are weak in-activators[3]. Analysis of the calcium current activation and deactivation kinetics shows that Bay K 8644 increases the mean open time

* Author for correspondence at address β-Cell Biology 6B.3.99, Novo Nordisk, Novo Alle, DK-2880 Bagsvaerd, Denmark.

Physiology and Pathophysiology of the Islets of Langerhans, edited by Soria.
Plenum Press, New York, 1997.

while it leaves the mean closed times of the Ca^{2+}-channel unchanged[4]. While Bay K 8644 acts as an activator, other dihydropyridins such as nitrendipine and nifedipine acts as inactivators like the phenylalkylamine, verapamil. Recently, a new benzoyl pyrrole compound, FPL 64176 has been synthesized and shown to have properties consistent with Ca^{2+}-channel activation[5].

We have tested FPL 64176 for insulin release in monolayers of βTC3 cells and compared the potency with various drugs affecting L-type Ca^{2+}-channels and ATP-sensitive K^+-channels. The effect of FPL 64176 on $[Ca^{2+}]_i$ is examined by the use of the calcium fluorescent indicator fura-2/AM. Here, for the first time, we describe the action of a non-dihydropyridine Ca^{2+}-channel activator, FPL 64176, on the insulin secretion.

MATERIALS AND METHODS

Synthesis

FPL 64176 was synthesized at Novo Nordisk essential as described[6]. Bay K 8644 (RBI Research Biochemicals) was resolved by HPLC (multiple injections of 100 μg, on a column of Chiracel OD, 4.6 × 250 mm, eluted with hexane: 2-propanol (9:1), with a flow of 0.45 ml/min. and detected at 254 nm) to give (−)-(S)-Bay K 8644 and (+)-(R)-Bay K 8644 > 99.2 and 92% ee, respectively.

Cell Culture

All experiments were carried out with the insulin secreting cell line, βTC3, which was kindly provided by Cold Spring Harbor Laboratory. The βTC3 cell line is derived from insulinomas of transgenic mice that express the simian virus 40 T antigen under control of the insulin promoter[7]. Cells were plated in Nunclon culture flasks (800 ml) and grown in Dulbecco's modified Eagle's medium (5.5 mM glucose, GIBCO), (DMEM) in the presence of 10% fetal calf serum, 100 units/ml penicillin and 0.1 mg/ml streptomycin in an atmosphere of 5% CO_2 in air at 37°C. Once a week the cells were split 1:7 and the medium was changed after 4 days.

Insulin Release

The insulin release experiments were carried out in monolayer cultures in batch type incubation at 37°C. After trypsination the cells were plated in 12-wells dishes (area 4.5 cm^2/well, approximately 4×10^5 cells/well) and cultured until 70–90% confluency (2 days). The cells were washed twice to remove dead or floating cells with Hepes Krebs Ringer (Hepes K.R.) medium consisting of 10 mM Hepes, pH 7.4, 119 mM NaCl, 4.74 mM KCl, 2.54 mM $CaCl_2$, 1.19 mM $MgSO_4 \cdot 7H_2O$, 25 mM $NaHCO_3$, 0.1% human serum albumin and 0.15 mM glucose. The cells were then incubated for one hour with the medium whereafter the compounds were added in fresh Hepes K. R. medium. After another hour incubation the medium from each well was transferred to minisorb vials which were centrifuged at 190 × g for 5 min at 20°C. The supernatant was used in a double sided enzyme-linked-immunosorbant-assay (ELISA) to determine the insulin released. The wells were washed twice with PBS and added 1 ml 0.1 M NaOH. After 20 min the NaOH containing the cells were transferred to minisorb vials and the content of protein was determined using Pierce protein assay.

The insulin releasing effects of the compounds were calculated as the amount secreted in the presence of compounds over basal.

ELISA Method for Determination of Mouse Insulin

The ELISA used was a sandwich ELISA. Nunc maxisorb immuno plates were coated over night at 4°C with 10 μg/ml monoclonal-mouse-anti-human-insulin (HUI-018, Novo Nordisk) diluted in saline phosphate buffer, pH 7.4 (PBS). The plates were washed three times in tween-20:PBS, 1:2000 and were then incubated for 2 hours with standard rat insulin (Novo Nordisk) or medium from experiments. The plates were washed as above. Guinea-pig anti-human-insulin coupled to biotin was used as detecting antibody in a concentration of 5 μg/ml diluted in PBS-buffer added 0.1% human serum albumin (HSA). The plates were incubated for 1 hour. After three times wash the plates were incubated for 30 min. with horse radish avidin peroxidase (Vector) diluted 1:10,000 in PBS added 0.1% HSA. The plates were washed three times and incubated with tetramethylbenzidine dihydrochloride 17 μg/well in 3.2 mM borate acetate buffer, pH 5.0 for 15 min. The reaction was stopped by addition of 4 M phosphoric acid. The absorbance was read at 650 nm.

Measurements of $[Ca^{2+}]_i$

Changes in $[Ca^{2+}]_i$ in suspensions of βTC3 cells were measured in a Perkin-Elmer LS-5B fluorescence spectrophotometer with a thermostatically controlled cuvette[8] at 37°C. Prior to the experiments βTC3 cells were resuspended in Hepes K. R. medium and loaded for 40 min. with the fluorescent indicator fura-2/AM (3 μM). The "calcium free Hepes K. R. medium" was without calcium added and supplemented with 100 μM EGTA.

Images of $[Ca^{2+}]_i$ in single βTC3 cells were obtained by means of a fluorescence microscope and a digital image processing and analysis system[9]. Clusters of cells as used in the experiments are shown in Figure 1. The free intracellular calcium concentrations were calculated from the measurement of the ratio of fluorescence intensities according to the equation[10]:

$$[Ca^{2+}]_i = K_d\,[(R - R_{min})/(R_{max} - R)] \times (s_{f2}/s_{b2}).$$

The values obtained for the βTC3 cells: R_{max}=241. R_{min} and the proportionality constant (s_{f2}/s_{b2}) was obtained from a medium with high potassium concentration and amounted to 27 and 9.8, respectively. A K_d of 224 nM was used[10].

RESULTS

The Ca^{2+}-channel activators Bay K 8644 and (–)-Bay K 8644 was both found to stimulate the insulin secretion approximately two fold (with 97% and 84% respectively) at a concentration of 1 μM, while no stimulation was observed neither at a lower nor at a higher concentration (0.01 μM and 100 μM) of the two (Fig. 2). These results are in good agreement with experiments in rat islets[11]. The antagonist (+)-Bay K 8644 did only slightly inhibit the basal insulin release whereas the antagonist verapamil inhibited the insulin release about 50%. An inhibition of the insulin release by verapamil has earlier been seen in rat islets experiments[12].

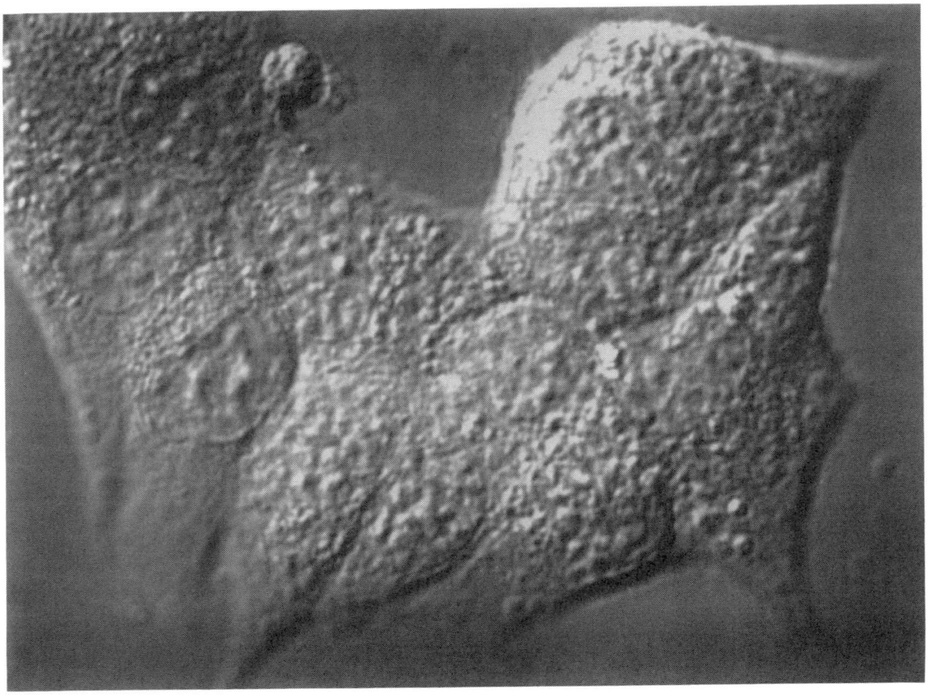

Figure 1. Differential inteference contrast microscope image of a cluster of βTC3 cells. The objective used was a Zeiss planapo 63×, 1.40.

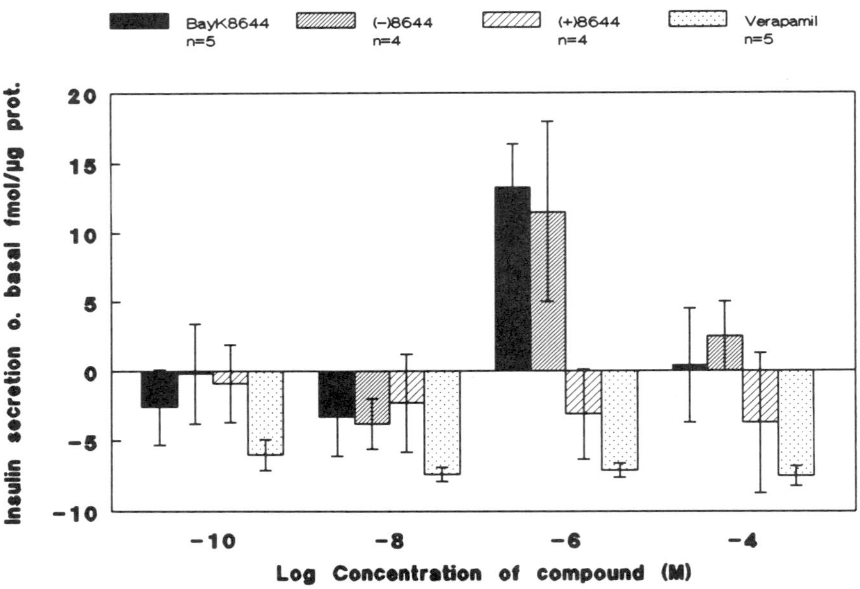

Figure 2. Insulin release from βTC3 cells when Bay K8644, (–) Bay K8644, (+) Bay K8644 and Verapamil are added in concentrations of 0.1 nM, 10 nM 1 μM and 0.1 mM.

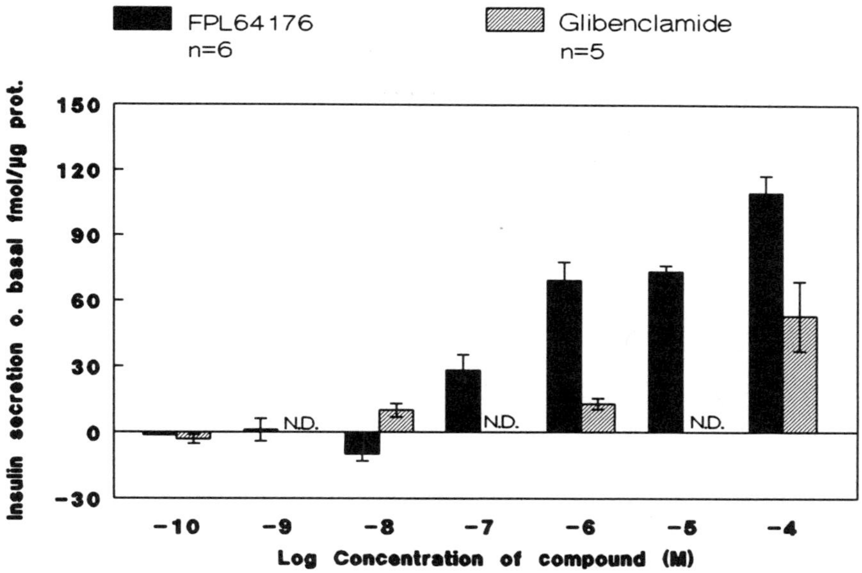

Figure 3. Insulin release fron βTC3 cells when FPL 64176 and Glibenclamide are added in concentrations of 0.1 nM, 10 nM, 1 µM, and 0.1 mM.

The K^+-channel ligand glibenclamide induced at 10 nM (Fig. 3) a two fold increase in the insulin secretion as compared to basal. An even more pronounced increase was seen for the Ca^{2+}-channel agonist FPL 64176, which increased the secretion four fold at a concentration of 100 µM.

When βTC3 cells were loaded with fura-2/AM addition of FPL 64176 induced an increased $[Ca^{2+}]_i$, an effect that was seen both in single cell measurements (1 µM) (Fig. 4) and in cell suspensions (10 µM) (Fig. 5). Subsequent stimulation with 10 µM acetylcholine (ACh) in single cell experiments caused a renewed increase in $[Ca^{2+}]_i$. We have seen heterogeneity in the single cell measurements, some cells showed a transient increase in $[Ca^{2+}]_i$ (Fig. 4) and other showed a more sustained response (data not shown). Due to this heterogeneity we only observed a slow decline towards the prestimulatory level when measuring $[Ca^{2+}]_i$ in the cell suspension (Fig. 5). A dose response relationship was measured for the change in $[Ca^{2+}]_i$ induced by FPL 64176 in the range of 50 nM to 25 µM (Fig. 6). The rise in $[Ca^{2+}]_i$ ($\Delta[Ca^{2+}]_i$) was calculated by subtracting the unstimulated $[Ca^{2+}]_i$ value from the peak $[Ca^{2+}]_i$ value. A curve was fitted to the data points using the equation:

$$\Delta[Ca^{2+}]_i = \Delta([Ca^{2+}]_i)_{max} \times [S]/(k_s + [S]),$$

where $[Ca^{2+}]_i$ is the change in $[Ca^{2+}]_i$ measured after 10 sec., $\Delta([Ca^{2+}]_i)_{max}$ is the maximal change in $[Ca^{2+}]_i$ observed, [S] is the concentration of FPL 64176 and k_s is the concentration of FPL 64176 that causes half-maximal change in $\Delta[Ca^{2+}]_i$. Addition of FPL 64176 resulted in the maximal change in $[Ca^{2+}]_i$ of 687 nM. Half-maximal change in $\Delta[Ca^{2+}]_i$ was obtained at 0.78 ± 0.21 µM FPL 64176 (Fig. 6).

Addition of 10 µM FPL 64176 in calcium free medium (Fig. 7) did not cause a change in $[Ca^{2+}]_i$. Subsequent addition of calcium to a final free concentration of 2.0 mM,

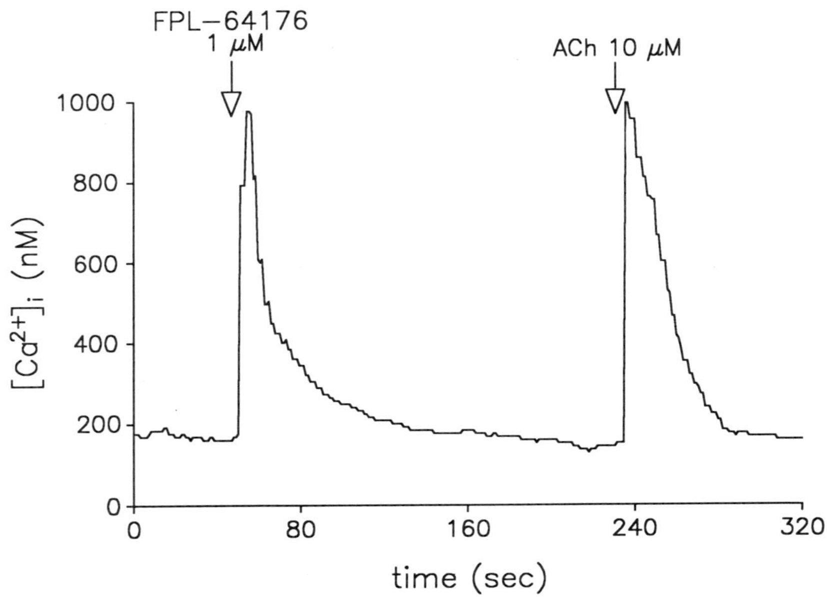

Figure 4. Single cell measurement of $[Ca^{2+}]_i$. The curve represents the signal from a single cell loaded with fura-2/AM when 1 μM FPL 64176 and 10 μM acethylcholine is added.

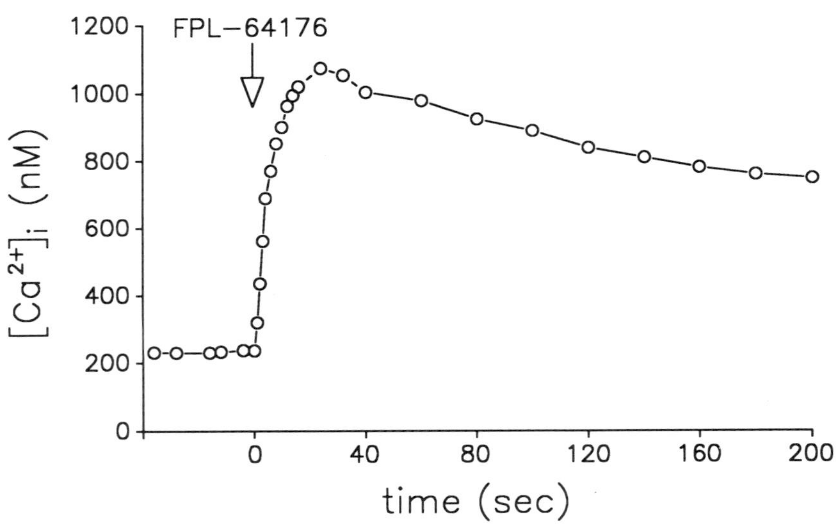

Figure 5. Fluorescence spectroscopy of βTC3 cells in suspension loaded with fura-2/AM in Hepes K.R. medium. Variation over time in $[Ca^{2+}]_i$, when 10 μM FPL 64176 was added to the medium.

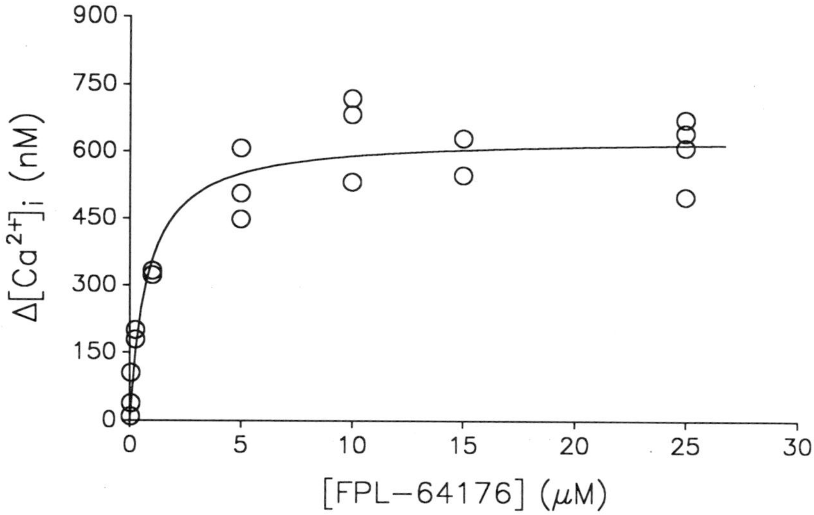

Figure 6. Dose-response relationship from suspension of βTC3 cells between the concentration of FPL 64176 and $[Ca^{2+}]_i$.

however, caused an increase in $[Ca^{2+}]_i$ from 82 to 534 nM within the first 6 seconds. In "calcium free medium" addition of calcium to a final concentration of 2.0 mM caused an increase in $[Ca^{2+}]_i$ from 102 to 300 nM within 6 seconds in the absence of FPL 64176. The effect of addition of calcium in the absence and presence of FPL 64176 was 194 and 551%, respectively.

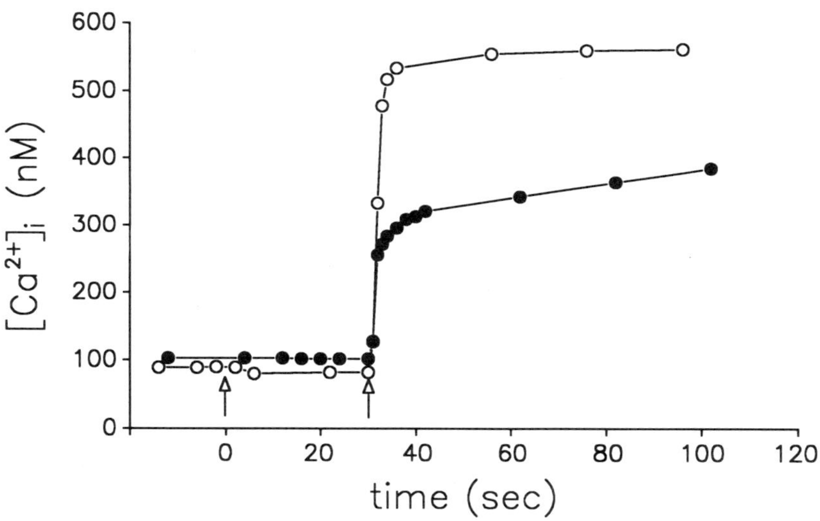

Figure 7. Fluorescence spectroscopy of suspension of βTC3 cells loaded with fura-2/AM in "calcium free" Hepes K.R. medium containing 100 μM EGTA. Variation over time in $[Ca^{2+}]_i$, when FPL 64176 and calcium was added to the medium. ● — Addition of $CaCl_2$ (at time 30 sec.) to a final free concentration of 2.0 mM $CaCl_2$. ○ — Addition of 10 μM FPL 64176 (at time 0 sec.), and subsequent addition of $CaCl_2$ (at time 30 sec.) to a final free concentration of 2.0 mM $CaCl_2$.

In single cell experiments 10 μM FPL 64176 caused an increase in $[Ca^{2+}]_i$ even in the presence of 1 μM of the Ca^{2+}-channel inactivator, verapamil (data not shown).

DISCUSSION

We have shown that FPL 64176, a non-dihydropyridine type of Ca^{2+}-channel activator very efficiently releases insulin from β-cells (βTC3). FPL 64176 is known to enhance $^{45}Ca^{2+}$ uptake in rat anterior pituitary (GH_3) cells through L-type Ca^{2+}-channels[5]. Single channel electrophysiological analyses of FPL 64176 in GH_3 cells have shown that FPL 64176 increases both the probability of channel opening and the mean opening time, the latter in a voltage dependent manner[13]. Furthermore, FPL 64176 is known to contract smooth muscles in rat tail artery strips[14,15].

When the dose-response curve for FPL 64176 was compared with the insulin secretion experiments a connection between $[Ca^{2+}]_i$ and the amount of secreted insulin was seen. Both $[Ca^{2+}]_i$ and the insulin secretion increased in the concentration range of FPL 64176 between 50 nM and 5 μM. At higher concentrations of FPL 64176 in the range of 5 μM and 25 μM, however, no increase of $[Ca^{2+}]_i$ was observed. This could indicate that FPL 64176 in addition to augment $[Ca^{2+}]_i$ also stimulates other factors that has a counter regulatory action.

In experiments performed in "calcium free medium" addition of 10 μM FPL 64176 had no effect on $[Ca^{2+}]_i$. When calcium was added to the media an increase in $[Ca^{2+}]_i$ was observed. Addition of calcium in the presence of FPL 64176 lead to a larger increase in $[Ca^{2+}]_i$ than in the absence of FPL 64176. These results clearly demonstrate that FPL 64176 stimulates the Ca^{2+}-channels and that the rise in $[Ca^{2+}]_i$ is caused by influx of calcium from the extracellular media and not by calcium released from intracellular stores.

In conclusion, Ca^{2+}-channel agonists can induce a rise in insulin secretion from βTC3-cells. Furthermore FPL 64176 gives rise to an increased $[Ca^{2+}]_i$ that is not mobilized from intracellular stores; an increase that is consistent with the observed insulin release. Whether this insulin release is glucose dependent or not need further investigation. Such experiments were not possible in the βTC3 cell line which in our hands does not respond properly on glucose stimulation.

Expression of the genes encoding the voltage dependent Ca^{2+}-channels of the L-type has been described in a variety of tissues, and evidence for alternative splicing of the transcripts of non-allelic genes has been reported[16]. This is raising the possibility that tissue specific drugs can be developed. It is tempting to speculate that Ca^{2+}-channel activators are potential drugs for treatment of NIDDM. So far, however, selective β-cell acting agonists still need to be developed.

REFERENCES

1. Ashcroft, F.M., Harrison, D.E. & Ashcroft, S.J.H.: Glucose induces closure of single potassium channels in isolated rat pancreatic β-cells. *Nature* **312** 446–448 (1984).
2. Cook, D.L. & Hales, C.N.: Intracellular ATP directly blocks K^+ channels in pancreatic B-cells. *Nature* **311** 271–273 (1984).
3. Triggle, D.J., Langs, D.A. & Janis, R.A.: Ca^{2+} Channel Ligands: Structure-Function Relationships of The 1,4-Dihydropyridines *Medicinal Research Reviews* **9** (no 2) 123–180 (1989).
4. Bechem, M. & Schramm, M.: Calcium-agonists. *J. Mol. Cell Cardiol.* **19** (Suppl. II) 63–75 (1987).
5. McKechnie, K., Killingback, P.G., Naya, I., O'Connor, S.E., Smith, G.W., Wattam, D.G., Wells, E., Whitehead, Y.M. & Williams, G.E.: Calcium channel activator properties in a novel non-dihydropyridine — FPL 64176. *Br. J. Pharmacol.* **98** 673P (1989).

6. Dalton, C.R., Kane, J.M. & Rampe, D.: An extremely short synthesis of benzoylpyrrole-type calcium channel activators. *Tet. Lett.* **33** 5713–16 (1992).
7. Efrat, S., Linde, S., Kofod, H., Spector, D., Delannoy, M., Grant, S., Hanahan, D. & Baekkeskov, S.: Beta-cell lines derived from transgenic mice expressing a hybrid insulin gene-oncogene. *Proc. Natl. Acad. Sci. USA* **85** 9037–41 (1988).
8. Nauntofte, B. & Dissing, S.: Stimulation-induced changes in cytosolic calcium in rat parotid acini. *Am. J. Physiol.* **253** G290–G297 (1987).
9. Dissing, S., Nauntofte, B. & Sten-Knudsen, O.: Spatial distribution of intracellular, free Ca^{2+} in isolated rat parotid acini. *Pflügers Arch.* **417** 1–12 (1990).
10. Grynkiewicz, G., Poenie, M. & Tsien, R.Y.: A New Generation of Ca^{2+} Indicators with Greatly Improved Fluorescence Properties. *J. Biol. Chem.* **260** 3440–3450 (1985).
11. Malaisse-Lagae, F., Mathias, P.C.F. & Malaisse, W.J.: Gating and blocking of calcium channels by dihydropyridines in the pancreatic B-cell. *Biochem. Biophys. Res. Comm.* **123** 1062–1068 (1984).
12. Bolaffi, J.L., Rodd, G.G., Ma, Y.H., Bright, D. & Grodsky, G.M.: The Role of Ca^{2+}-Related Events in Glucose-Stimulated Desensitization of Insulin Secretion. *Endocrinology* **129** 2131–2138 (1991).
13. Kunze, D.L. & Rampe, D.: Characterization of the Effects of a New Ca^{2+} Channel Activator, FPL 64176, in GH_3 Cells. *Am. Soc. Pharm. and Exp. Ther. Molecular Pharm.* **42** 666–670 (1992).
14. Zheng, W., Rampe, D. & Triggle, D.J.: Pharmacological; Radioligand Binding, and Electrophysiological Characteristics of FPL 64176, a Novel Nondihydropyridine Ca^{2+} Channel Activatot in Cardiac and Vascular Preparations. *Am. Soc. Pharm. and Exp. Ther. Molecular Pharm.* **40** 734–741.
15. Rampe, D. & Dage, R.C.: Functional Interactions between Two Ca^{2+} Channel Activators, (S)-Bay K 8644 and FPL 64176, in Smooth Muscle. *Am. Soc. Pharm. and Exp. Ther. Molecular Pharm.* **41** 599–602 (1992).
16. Perez-Reyes, E., Wei, X., Castellano, A., Birnbaumer, L.: Molecular diversity of L-type Calcium Channels. J. Biol. Chem. **265** 20430–20436 (1990).

21

IDENTIFICATION AND CHARACTERIZATION OF NON-ADRENERGIC BINDING SITES IN INSULIN-SECRETING CELLS WITH THE IMIDAZOLINE RX821002

Susan L. F. Chan, Kay E. Scarpello, and Noel G. Morgan

Cellular Pharmacology Group
Department of Biological Sciences
Keele University
Keele, Staffs., ST5 5BG, United Kingdom

INTRODUCTION

Recent studies have shown that certain compounds which possess an imidazoline moiety within their structure, are able to enhance the rate of insulin secretion, both *in vivo* and *in vitro*[1]. $^{86}Rb^{+}$ efflux experiments and electrophysiological studies[2,3] have provided evidence that this response is due to the reduction in potassium flux via ATP-regulated K^{+} channels across the islet B-cell plasma membrane, resulting in membrane depolarization. The nature of the binding site mediating the effects of imidazolines in islets is unclear but it is significant that a class of binding sites known as "imidazoline-preferring" receptors has recently been described in a wide variety of tissues[4]. However, the pharmacology of the defined I_1- and I_2-imidazoline sites does not correlate with the observed responses to imidazolines in islets, although I_2-receptors (also known as non-adrenoceptor idazoxan binding sites (NAIBS)) have been described in pancreatic islets[5] and RINm5F insulinoma cells[6]. Moreover, we have shown that the secretory response induced by the imidazoline efaroxan shows stereoselectivity and is subject to down-regulation in the presence of agonist[7]. Thus, the possibilty remains the islet imidazoline receptor may represent a novel, third type of imidazoline binding site.

RX821002, the methoxy derivative of idazoxan, is a potent and highly selective α_2-adrenoceptor antagonist that, in contrast to the parent compound, binds almost exclusively to α_2-adrenoceptors, possessing an affinity for I_2-sites at least 1000 fold lower than that of idazoxan[8]. However, RX821002 can directly potentiate insulin release in isolated rat islets. Hence, we have employed [^{3}H]-RX821002 in an attempt to label and to characterize the binding site responsible for mediating the secretagogue activity of certain imidazoline compounds. Due to the limiting availabilty of islet tissue, radioligand binding experiments were performed using the insulin-secreting cell line RINm5F.

Physiology and Pathophysiology of the Islets of Langerhans, edited by Soria.
Plenum Press, New York, 1997.

METHODS

Insulin Secretion Experiments

Islets of Langerhans were isolated from the pancreata of male Wistar rats by collagenase digestion[9]. The isolation medium was a bicarbonate-buffered physiolgical saline solution[10], pH 7.4, containing 4mM glucose and 2 mM $CaCl_2$. For islet incubations, this medium was supplemented with 1mg/ml bovine serum albumin. In static incubation experiments, groups of three isolated islets were incubated for 60 min. at 37°C with test reagents. After this time, samples of the medium were removed for measurement of their insulin content by radioimmunoassay.

Radioligand Binding Experiments

Membranes were prepared from RINm5F cells, cultured in RPMI-1640 supplemented with 10% (v/v) foetal calf serum. Briefly, cell monolayers were washed with PBS and the cells scraped in ice-cold TEM buffer (50mM Tris-HCl, pH 7.5, 1mM EDTA, 10mM $MgCl_2$) supplemented with 50μM PMSF. Following homogenization and centrifugation (40,000×g, 20 min., 4°C), the resulting pellet was resuspended in TEM buffer and re-centrifuged. The final crude membrane fraction was resuspended in the required volume of TEM and aliquots were quickly frozen and stored at –70°C. Protein content was measured by the bicinchoninic acid method[11].

Membranes (50–100μg protein), [^{3}H]-RX821002 and competing drugs were incubated in a final volume of 100μl TEM buffer for 60 min. at 25°C. The reaction was stopped by adding 3ml of ice-cold TEM buffer. Bound and free radioligand were separated by filtration through GF/B Whatman filters under vacuum. Filters were washed and their radioactivity measured after addition of scintillant.

For saturation studies, [^{3}H]-RX821002 was used over the range 1–100nM and non-specific binding was defined in the presence of 10μM phentolamine. In experiments designed to specifically study binding at the "imidazoline" site, incubations were performed in the presence of 10μM adrenaline to block α_2-adrenoceptors.

RESULTS & DISCUSSION

In isolated rat islets, RX821002 (100μM) significantly augmented the basal insulin secretion rate (Fig. 1). Furthermore, like other imidazoline compounds that can directly potentiate insulin release[1–3,12], RX821002 was able to counteract the inhibition of glucose-induced insulin secretion induced by the K^+_{ATP} channel agonist diazoxide (125μM; Fig. 1). These data confirm previous suggestions that the possible mechanism of action for the secretagogue activity of imidazoline compounds involves interaction with a regulatory component associated with ATP-sensitive potassium channels.

The binding of [^{3}H]-RX821002 to RINm5F membranes was rapid, with the steady state being reached within 20 minutes at 25°C (data not shown). When employed at concentrations between 1–10nM, [^{3}H]-RX821002 labelled a high affinity site which was saturable. However, raising the concentration of [^{3}H]-RX821002 further revealed the presence of a second binding site of much lower affinity, which remained less than fully saturated even at a radioligand concentration of 100nM. Scatchard analysis confirmed the presence of two sites. The high affinity site bound [^{3}H]-RX821002 with a K_D of 2.01

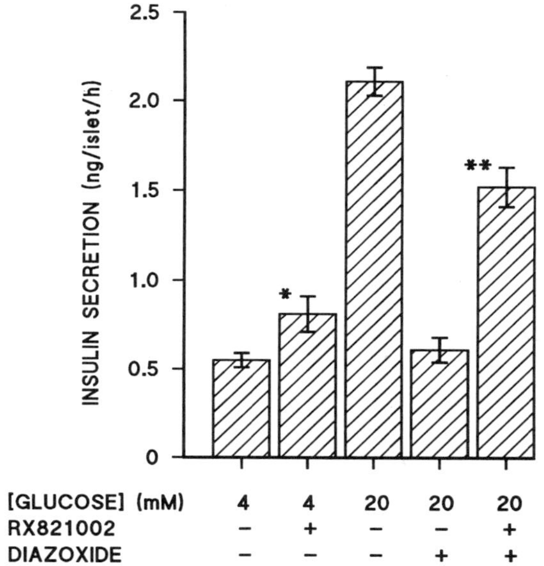

Figure 1. Effects of RX821002 on basal insulin release and on the inhibitory response to diazoxide in rat islets. Groups of three isolated islets were incubated for 60 minutes at 37°C, in the presence of test reagents as shown. After this time, samples of medium were removed for measurement of insulin content by RIA. Data are presented as mean values ± S.E. for 12–18 observations. *P<0.0125, **P<0.001; relative to incubation in the absence of RX821002.

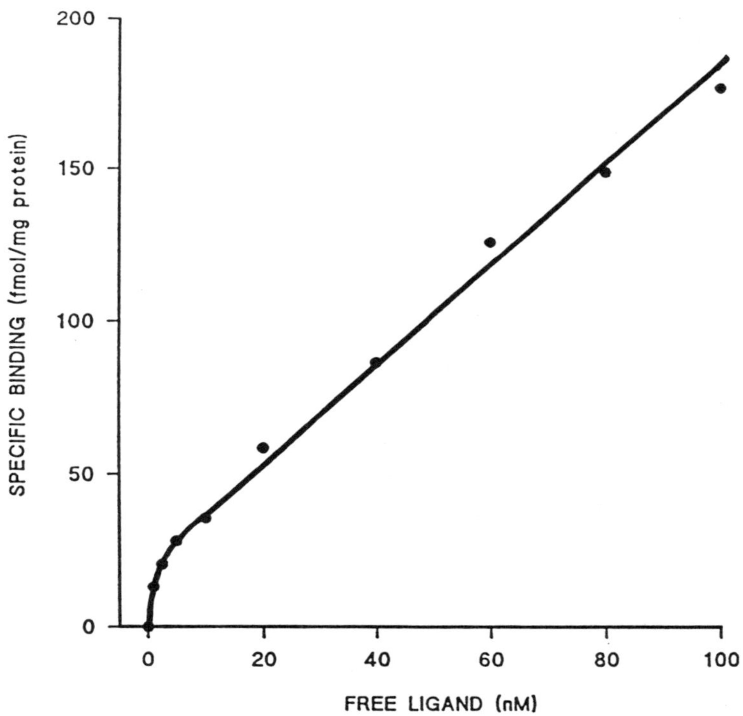

Figure 2. Specific binding of [^{3}H]-RX821002 to RINm5F membranes. RINm5F membranes were incubated with [^{3}H]-RX821002, over the concentration range 1.0–100nM, for 60 minutes at 25°C. Non-specific binding was determined in the presence of 10μM phentolamine. Shown is a representative experiment with each point determined in triplicate.

Table 1. Effects of imidazoline compounds on the binding of [^{3}H]RX821002 to the low affinity binding site in RINm5F membranes

Imidazoline (10μM)	[^{3}H]RX821002 binding (% maximal)
Idazoxan	95.2 ± 4.8
UK14,304	107.1 ± 8.1
Efaroxan	74.6 ± 4.2[b]
RX821002	76.5 ± 6.3[b]
Clonidine	86.2 ± 6.0[a]
Phentolamine	82.5 ± 5.5[a]

Competition binding studies were performed on RINm5F membranes with a single concentration (50nM) of [^{3}H]RX821002. Competing agents were present at 10μM. Adrenaline (10μM) was included in all tubes to block α_2-adrenoceptors. The data are expressed as percentages of the control binding (100%) measured in the absence of competitor, and are means ± s.e. mean for 12–18 observations. [a]$p<0.01$; [b]$p<0.001$, versus control.

± 0.7nM, consistent with interaction with α_2-adrenoceptors. By contrast, the second site exhibited an estimated K_D of 145 ± 22nM but bound [^{3}H]-RX821002 with much higher capacity (B_{max}: 364 ± 22fmol/mg protein, for 4 separate observations) than the α_2-adrenoceptor site (B_{max}: 34 ± 10.4fmol/mg protein).

Further characterization of this second low affinity site in competition/displacement binding assays employing imidazoline compounds of varying secretagogue activity was difficult, since the K_D of the site is so low. However, experiments employing 50nM [^{3}H]-RX821002 and performed in the presence of adrenaline revealed that the pharmacological profile of this site correlates well with that observed in functional secretion experiments (Table 1). Hence, efaroxan, RX821002, phentolamine and clonidine, all of which can augment insulin release[1–3,13], inhibited the specific binding of [^{3}H]-RX821002 to this low affinity "imidazoline" binding site, whereas UK14,304 and idazoxan (non-secretagogue I_2-ligands) had little effect on binding of the radioligand to this site.

These results reveal that [^{3}H]-RX821002 can label a low affinity site on RINm5F cell membranes whose pharmacology is consistent with the possibilty that it may represent the previously elusive "imidazoline" receptor responsible for regulation of B-cell K^+_{ATP} channel activity. The binding data further confirm that the site responsible for mediating the stimulation of insulin release does not correspond to NAIBS/I_2-sites. In addition, the site is unlikely to represent an I_1-imidazoline site since efaroxan is reported to act as an I_1-antagonist[14], whereas it acts agonistically on insulin secretion and ATP-sensitive potassium channel blockade and is able to down-regulate the secretory response[7]. Thus, this islet imiazoline site displays characteristics which are distinct from those of the designated I_1- and I_2-sites.

ACKNOWLEDGMENTS

We are grateful to the British Diabetic Association, the Royal Society, the MRC and the North Staffs. Hospital Trust for their financial support.

REFERENCES

1. S.L.F. Chan, Role of α_2-adrenoceptors and imidazoline-binding sites in the control of insulin secretion, *Clin. Sci.* 85: 671 (1993).
2. S.L.F. Chan, M.J. Dunne, M.R. Stillings, and N.G. Morgan, The α_2-adrenoceptor antagonist efaroxan modulates K^+_{ATP} channels in insulin-secreting cells, *Eur. J. Pharmacol.* 204: 41 (1991).
3. J.-C. Jonas, T.D. Plant, and J.C. Henquin, Imidazoline antagonists of α_2-adrenoceptors increase insulin release *in vitro* by inhibiting ATP-sensitive K^+ channels in pancreatic β-cells, *Br. J. Pharmacol.* 107: 8 (1992).
4. M.C. Michel, and P. Ernsberger, Keeping an eye on the I site: imidazoline-preferring receptors, *Trends Pharmacol. Sci.* 45: 369 (1992).
5. C.A. Brown, A.C. Loweth, S.A. Smith, and N.G. Morgan, Stimulation of insulin secretion by imidazoline compounds is not due to interaction with non-adrenoceptor idazoxan binding sites, *Br. J. Pharmacol.* 108: 312 (1993).
6. A. Remaury, and H. Paris, The insulin-secreting cell line, RINm5F, expresses an *alpha*-2D adrenoceptor and nonadrenergic idazoxan-binding sites, *J. Pharmacol. Exp. Ther.* 260: 417 (1992).
7. S.L.F. Chan, C.A. Brown, and N.G. Morgan, Stimulation of insulin secretion by the imidazoline α_2-adrenoceptor antagonist efaroxan is mediated by a novel, stereoselective, binding site, *Eur. J. Pharmacol.* 230: 375 (1993).
8. D. Langin, M. Lafontan, M.R. Stillings, and H. Paris, [^{3}H]-RX821002: A new tool for the identification of α2A-adrenoceptors, *Eur. J. Pharmacol.* 167: 95 (1989).
9. W. Montague, and K.W. Taylor, Pentitols and insulin release by isolated rat islets of Langerhans, *Biochem. J.* 109: 339 (1968).
10. G.O. Gey, and M.K. Gey, Maintenance of human normal cells in continuous culture: preliminary report; cultivation of mesoblastic tumors and normal cells and notes on methods of cultivation, *Am. J. Cancer* 27: 45 (1936).
11. P.K. Smith, R.I. Krohn, G.T. Hermanson, A.K. Mallia, F.H. Gartner, M.D. Provenzano, E.K. Fujimoto, N.M. Goeke, B.J. Olson, and D.C. Klenk, Measurement of protein using bicinchoninic acid, *Anal. Biochem.* 150: 76 (1985).
12. S.L.F Chan, M.R. Stillings, and N.G. Morgan, Mechanisms involved in stimulation of insulin secretion by the hypoglycaemic *alpha*-adrenergic antagonist, DG-5128, *Biochem. Biophys. Res. Commun.* 176: 1545 (1991).
13. A. Schulz, and A. Hassleblatt, Dual action of clonidine on insulin release: suppression but stimulation when α_2-adrenoceptors are blocked, *Naunyn-Schmiedeberg's Arch. Pharmacol.* 340: 305 (1989).
14. P.R. Ernsberger, K.L Westbrook, O. Christen, and S.G. Schäfer, A second generation of centrally acting antihypertensive agents act on putative I_1-imidazoline receptors, *J. Cardiovasc. Pharmacol.* 20: S1 (1992).

22

PACAP AS LOW AS 10^{-13} M RAISES CYTOSOLIC Ca^{2+} ACTIVITY IN PANCREATIC B-CELLS BY AUGMENTING Ca^{2+} INFLUX THROUGH L-TYPE Ca^{2+} CHANNELS TO TRIGGER INSULIN RELEASE

Toshihiko Yada,[1,*] Masaya Sakurada,[2] Masanori Nakata,[1] Kazuro Yaekura,[1] and Masatoshi Kikuchi[2]

[1]Department of Physiology
Kagoshima University School of Medicine
8-35-1 Sakuragaoka
Kagoshima 890, Japan
[2]Division of Endocrinology and Metabolism
The Institute for Adult Diseases
Asahi Life Foundation
Tokyo 160, Japan

INTRODUCTION

Pancreatic insulin secretion is under control by peptides, as well as by nutrients and other substances[1,2]. Truncated glucagon like peptide-1 (tGLP-1), gastric inhibitory peptide (GIP) and glucagon, the members of glucagon/VIP/secretin family of peptides, stimulate insulin release in a low concentration range around 10^{-9} M, and are thought to be involved in the physiological regulation of insulin release[3–5].

Pituitary adenylate cyclase activating polypeptide (PACAP), originally isolated from ovine hypothalamus, is a new member of this family[6,7]. PACAP exists as a 27- (PACAP27) or a 38-residue peptide (PACAP38)[6,8], and is present in a variety of tissue, abundant in the central nervous system, posterior pituitary, adrenal and testis[9]. A neuromodulator role for PACAP is proposed based on the finding of PACAP-containing nerve fibers[7,10]. PACAP in the range of 10^{-10}–10^{-8} M exhibits a wide spectrum of biological activities, which include hormone release from perifused pituitary cells[7,11] and adrenal chromaffin cells[12], amylase release from exocrine pancreas[13,14], and vasodilating effect[15]. PACAP signal transduction

* To whom all correspondence should be addressed. Fax: 81-992-75-5231.

involves an activation of adenylate cyclase in a variety of cell species[6,7] and an increase in the cytosolic free Ca^{2+} concentration ($[Ca^{2+}]_i$) in hippocampal neurons[16], pituitary cells[17,18] and chromaffin cells[12].

We have recently found that PACAP as low as 10^{-13} M stimulates insulin release from rat pancreatic islets and increases $[Ca^{2+}]_i$ in B-cells in a glucose-dependent manner[19]. Moreover, PACAP is localized in pancreatic nerve fibers and islets, suggesting that PACAP may serve as a physiological regulator of insulin secretion from pancreatic B-cells[19].

To explore the B-cell mechanisms underlying the strikingly potent insulinotropic action of PACAP, the present study sought to characterize the nature of the $[Ca^{2+}]_i$ increase and to examine its link to the stimulated insulin release. We report that the $[Ca^{2+}]_i$ increase induced by PACAP at 10^{-13} M is completely inhibited under a Ca^{2+}-free condition and by a Ca^{2+} channel blocker. A number of common properties observed between the $[Ca^{2+}]_i$ and insulin secretory responses to PACAP suggest that the $[Ca^{2+}]_i$ increase is the triggering signal for the PACAP-induced insulin secretion.

MATERIALS AND METHODS

Solutions and Chemicals

Insulin release experiments were carried out in KRB composed of (mM): NaCl 121.7, KCl 4.4, KH_2PO_4 1.2, $CaCl_2$ 2.0, $MgSO_4$ 1.2, $NaHCO_3$ 23.0 at pH 7.4 supplemented with 0.1% bovine serum albumin (BSA) and equilibrated against a mixture of 95% O_2–5% CO_2 at 37°C. $[Ca^{2+}]_i$ experiments in open chambers were performed in KRB containing HEPES and a reduced HCO_3^- : NaCl 129, KCl 4.7, KH_2PO_4 1.2, $CaCl_2$ 1.0, $MgSO_4$ 1.2, $NaHCO_3$ 5.0, and HEPES 10 at pH 7.4 supplemented with 0.1% BSA. PACAP27 was from American Peptide Co. (Sunnyvale, CA) and Peptide Institute (Osaka, Japan). Fura-2/acetoxymethylester were from Dojin Chemical (Kumamoto, Japan). Tolbutamide was from Nacalai Tesque (Kyoto, Japan). Nitrendipine was a gift from Yoshitomi Pharmaceutical (Osaka, Japan).

Measurement of Insulin Release

Islets of Langerhans were isolated from Wistar rats of 8–12 weeks by collagenase digestion. Islets were incubated for 60 min in the presence of a basal (2.8 mM) or an elevated glucose concentration (8.3 mM) with or without PACAP, and aliquots were assayed for insulin by radioimmunoassay. The calculated values were expressed as mean ± S.E. for the number of observations (N). Student's t test was used for statistical analysis of the results.

Preparation and Selection of B-Cells

Isolated islets were immediately dispersed into single cells in Ca^{2+}-free KRB with 1 mM EGTA. The single cells were plated on coverslips and cultured for 1–3 days in Eagle's MEM containing 5.6 mM glucose, 10% fetal bovine serum, 100 µg/ml streptomycin and 100 U/ml penicillin at 37°C in a 95% air plus 5% CO_2 atmosphere before experiments. The cells during this period responded to glucose, PACAP and tolbutamide in a consistent manner. B-cells were selected according to the previously reported proce-

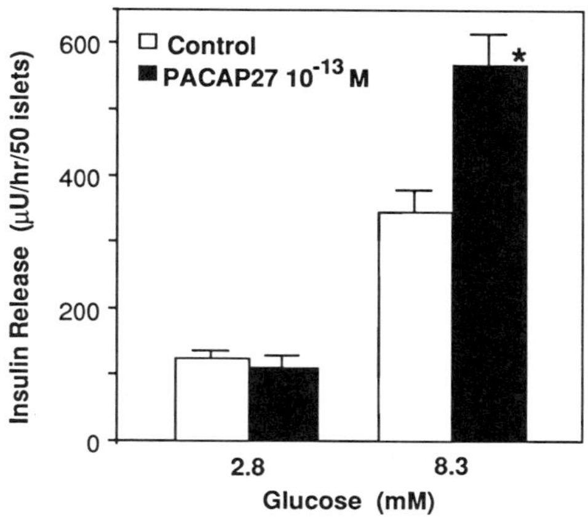

Figure 1. Glucose-dependent effect of PACAP27 to stimulate insulin release from rat islets. Insulin release from rat islets in static incubation for 60 min in KRB containing 2.8 or 8.3 mM glucose with (filled column) or without 10^{-13} M PACAP27 (open column). Each point represents the mean ± S.E. for 6 experiments. *$P<0.01$ vs. control without PACAP.

dure[20]. Briefly, when the cells with a diameter of 12.5–17.5 µm were examined, the majority of the cells responded to glucose (8.3 mM) and almost all the cells to tolbutamide (TB, 100–1000 µM) with increases in $[Ca^{2+}]_i$, the responses typical of the immunocytochemically identified B-cells[19]. Data from such glucose- and TB-responsive cells were employed.

Measurement of $[Ca^{2+}]_i$

$[Ca^{2+}]_i$ was measured according to the previously reported method[19,21]. In brief, single cells were incubated with 1 µM fura-2/acetoxymethylester[22] for 30 min at 37°C, mounted in a chamber and superfused at 1 ml/min at 37°C with KRB. The fura-2 loaded cells were excited at 340 nm and 380 nm alternately every one second, the emission signals at 510 nm were detected by a photomultiplier, and the ratio of the two signals was produced by P1 system (Nikon, Tokyo, Japan). Alternately, fura-2 fluorescence was detected every 2.5 sec by an ICCD camera, and the ratio was produced by Argus-50 system (Hamamatsu Photonics, Hamamatsu, Japan).

RESULTS AND DISCUSSION

In the presence of 8.3 mM glucose, a stimulatory concentration for insulin release, PACAP27 at 10^{-14} to 10^{-12} M stimulated insulin release from rat islets both under perifusion[19] and static incubation conditions (Fig. 1). A maximal response was obtained at 10^{-13} M of this peptide (Fig. 2). It was previously reported that PACAP27 in a relatively high range of 10^{-9}–10^{-8} M stimulated insulin release from perfused rat pancreas[23]. We observed that PACAP27 in 10^{-9}–10^{-8} M also increased insulin release but to a lesser extent than at 10^{-13} M (data not shown). In the presence of 2.8 mM glucose, a non-stimulatory concentration for insulin release, PACAP failed to alter insulin release (Fig. 1).

An outstanding finding was that PACAP27 in a concentration as low as 10^{-13} M markedly stimulated insulin release, indicating that PACAP is at least 3 log orders more potent than the known insulinotropic peptides such as tGLP-1, GIP and glucagon[3–5]. It has been demonstrated that pancreatic B-cell is the direct target of PACAP[19]. Therefore, the signal transduction mechanism in B-cells underlying the outstanding potency of PACAP is of great interest.

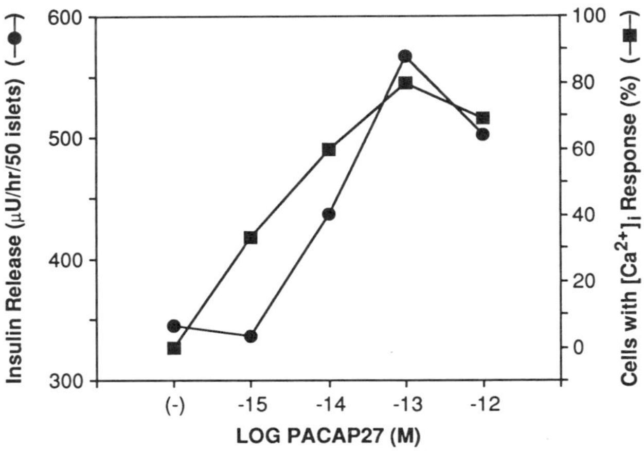

Figure 2. Concentration-dependent effect of PACAP27 to stimulate insulin release from rat islets in static incubation for 60 min (circle) and to increase $[Ca^{2+}]_i$ in single rat islet B-cells (square). Glucose concentration is 8.3 mM. Each point represents 5–20 experiments.

Since cytosolic Ca^{2+} in islet B-cells plays a crucial role in the regulation of insulin secretion[1], we examined the effect of PACAP27 on $[Ca^{2+}]_i$ in rat islet B-cells. Under superfusion condition with 8.3 mM glucose, PACAP increased $[Ca^{2+}]_i$ (Fig. 3) in a concentration-dependent manner over 10^{-15} to 10^{-12} M, and a maximal effect was obtained at 10^{-13} M (Fig. 2). The peptide at relatively high concentrations (10^{-9}–10^{-8} M) also increased $[Ca^{2+}]_i$ (data not shown). With a basal glucose (2.8 mM), PACAP at 10^{-13} M was without effect on $[Ca^{2+}]_i$ (Fig. 3).

We then asked the origin and route for the $[Ca^{2+}]_i$ increase. In the Ca^{2+}-free KRB made with 0.1 mM EGTA and no added Ca^{2+}, the $[Ca^{2+}]_i$ response to 10^{-13} M PACAP was completely inhibited in a reversible manner (Fig. 4). Nitrendipine (1 μM), a blocker of the L-type Ca^{2+} channel, also completely inhibited the $[Ca^{2+}]_i$ response to PACAP in a reversible manner (Fig. 5). These results indicate that PACAP27 stimulates Ca^{2+} influx by augmenting the activity of the dihydropyridine-sensitive L-type Ca^{2+} channel that is primarily activated by glucose[24].

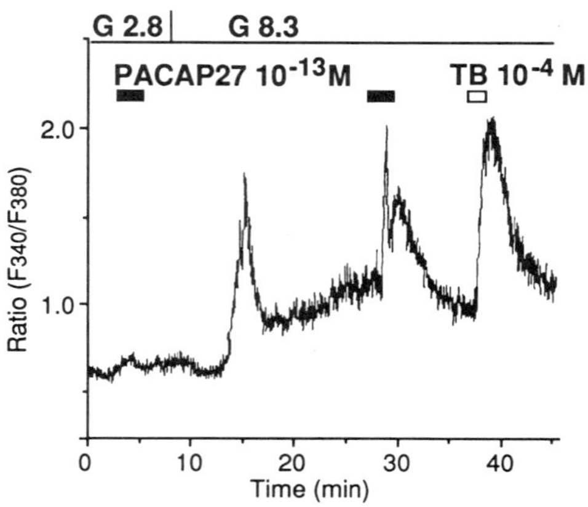

Figure 3. Glucose-dependent effect of 10^{-13} PACAP27 to increase $[Ca^{2+}]_i$ in single rat islet B-cells. The tracing is representative of four similar experiments (N=4). Thin lines and thick lines above tracings indicate the glucose concentrations and the periods of exposure to the agents, respectively.

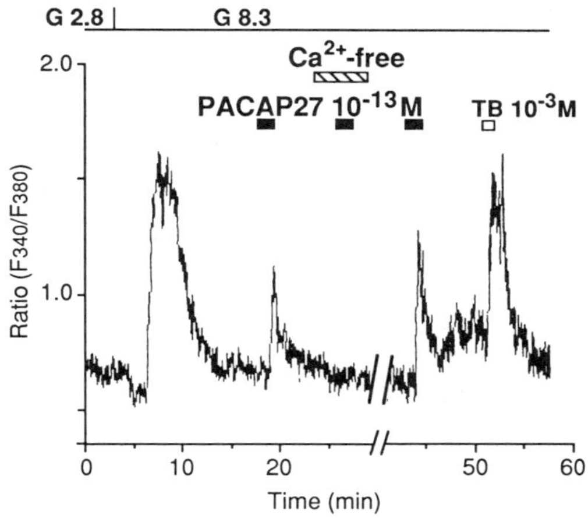

Figure 4. Complete and reversible inhibition of B-cell $[Ca^{2+}]_i$ responses to 10^{-13} M PACAP27 under Ca^{2+}-free conditions (N=4). Slanting lines indicate an omission of recording for 12 min.

The stimulation of insulin release by PACAP at 10^{-13} M was completely abolished in the Ca^{2+}-free KRB and by 1 μM nitrendipine[(19)], the conditions where the $[Ca^{2+}]_i$ response to PACAP was completely inhibited (Table 1). The strict glucose-dependency was observed commonly for the $[Ca^{2+}]_i$ and insulin responses to PACAP at 10^{-13} M (Table 1). An analysis of concentration-response relationships has demonstrated that PACAP started to raise $[Ca^{2+}]_i$ in some of individual B-cells at 10^{-15} M, whereas the stimulatory effect of this peptide on insulin release was first detected at 10^{-14} M (Fig. 2) (Table 1). Thus the $[Ca^{2+}]_i$ response took place slightly earlier than the insulin secretory response as the concentration of PACAP was raised. This suggests that the increase in $[Ca^{2+}]_i$ is not a result of insulin release, but can be qualified as a causal factor for insulin release. It has been well established that an increase in $[Ca^{2+}]_i$ is the triggering event for exocytosis in B-cells[(25,26)]. All the evidences strongly suggest that the stimulated insulin release by PACAP in sub- picomolar concentrations is initiated by the increased $[Ca^{2+}]_i$ in B-cells. PACAP-induced insulin release occurred in a biphasic manner[(19)], while the $[Ca^{2+}]_i$ increase was transient (Figs. 3, 4 and 5). It is in agreement with that a transient $[Ca^{2+}]_i$ increase could trigger a sustained insulin release[(26,27)].

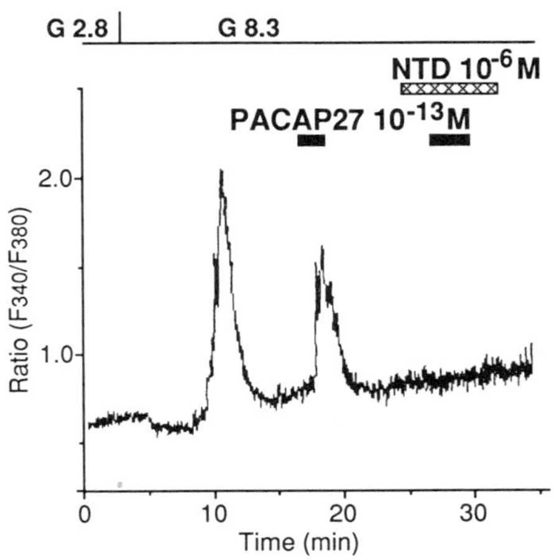

Figure 5. Complete inhibition of B-cell $[Ca^{2+}]_i$ responses to 10^{-13} M PACAP27 by 1 μM nitrendipine (NTD) (N=6). A recovery of a $[Ca^{2+}]_i$ response, obtained at around 58 min, is not presented here.

Table 1. Properties of the $[Ca^{2+}]_i$ and insulin secretory responses to PACAP27

	PACAP concentration (M)		Glucose			
	Onset	Peak	2.8 mM	8.3 mM	Ca^{2+}-free	Nitrendipine (10^{-6} M)
$\Delta [Ca^{2+}]_i$	10^{-15}	10^{-13}	–	+	–	–
Δ insulin release	10^{-14}	10^{-13}	–	+	–	–

+, response observed; –, response not observed or completely inhibited.

CONCLUSIONS

PACAP27 stimulates insulin release from rat islets and raises $[Ca^{2+}]_i$ in rat islet B-cells in a similar manner: the insulin secretory response and the $[Ca^{2+}]_i$ response are absolutely glucose-dependent, start with the peptide at 10^{-14} M and peak at 10^{-13} M. PACAP increases $[Ca^{2+}]_i$ by augmenting Ca^{2+} entry through the dihydropyridine-sensitive L-type Ca^{2+} channel that is primarily stimulated by glucose. Inhibition of the $[Ca^{2+}]_i$ response to PACAP by blocking the Ca^{2+} entry concomitantly abolished the insulin secretory response. Based on these evidences, we conclude that the stimulation of insulin release by sub-picomolar PACAP is triggered by the increased $[Ca^{2+}]_i$ in B-cells.

ACKNOWLEDGMENTS

We thank Kayoko Itoh and Kaori Yamamoto for skillful technical assistance.

This work was supported in part by grants from the Ministry of Education, Science and Culture of Japan, Kodama Foundation for Research of Medical Science and Japan Diabetes Foundation (to TY).

REFERENCES

1. Wollheim, C.B., and Sharp, G.W.G., 1981, Regulation of insulin release by calcium, *Physiol. Rev.* 61: 914–973.
2. Prentki, M., and Matschinsky, F.M., 1987, Ca^{2+}, cAMP, and phospholipid-derived messengers in coupling mechanisms of insulin secretion, *Physiol. Rev.* 67: 1185–1248.
3. Pipeleers, D., Veld, P.I., Maes, E., and Winkel, M.V.D., 1982, Glucose-induced insulin release depend on functional cooperation between islet cells, *Proc. Natl. Acad. Sci. USA* 79: 7322–7325.
4. Mojsov, S., Weir, G.C., and Habener, J.F., 1987, Insulinotropin: glucagon-like peptide 1(1–37) co-encoded in the glucagon gene is a potent stimulator of insulin release in the perfused rat pancreas, *J. Clin. Invest.* 79: 616–619.
5. Orskov, C., 1992, Glucagon-like peptide-1, a new hormone of the entero-insular axis, *Diabetologia* 35: 701–711.
6. Miyata, A., Arimura, A., Dahl, R.R., Minamino, N., Uehara, A., Jiang, L., Culler, M.D., and Coy, D.H., 1989, Isolation of a novel 38 residue-hypothalamic polypeptide which stimulates adenylate cyclase in pituitary cells, *Biochem. Biophys. Res. Commun.* 164: 567–574.
7. Arimura, A., 1992, Pituitary adenylate cyclase activating polypeptide (PACAP): discovery and current status of research, *Regul. Pept.* 37: 287–303.
8. Miyata, A., Jiang, L., Dahl, R.D., Kitada, C., Kubo, K., Fujino, M., Minamino, N., and Arimura, A., 1990, Isolation of a neuropeptide corresponding to the N-terminal 27 residues of the pituitary adenylate cyclase activating polypeptide with 38 residues (PACAP38), *Biochem. Biophys. Res. Commun.* 170: 643–648.
9. Arimura, A., Somogyvari-Vigh, A., Miyata, A., Mizuno, K., Coy, D.H., and Kitada, C., 1991, Tissue distribution of PACAP as determined by RIA: highly abundant in the rat brain and testes, *Endocrinology* 129: 2787–2789.

10. Koves, K., Arimura, A., Somogyvari-Vigh, A., Vigh, S., and Miller, J., 1990, Immunohistochemical demonstration of a novel hypothalamic peptide, pituitary adenylate cyclase activating polypeptide, in the ovine hypothalamus, *Endocrinology* 127: 264–271.
11. Goth, M. I., Lyons, C.E., Canny, B.J., and Thorner, M.O., 1992, Pituitary adenylate cyclase activating polypeptide, growth hormone (GH)-releasing peptide and GH-releasing hormone stimulate GH release through distinct pituitary receptors, *Endocrinology* 130: 939–944.
12. Isobe, K., Nakai, T., and Takuwa, Y., 1993, Ca^{2+}-dependent stimulatory effect of pituitary adenylate cyclase-activating polypeptide on catecholamine secretion from cultured porcine adrenal chromaffin cells, *Endocrinology* 132: 1757–1765.
13. Mungan, Z., Ertan, A., Hammer, R.A., and Arimura, A., 1991, Effect of pituitary adenylate cyclase activating polypeptide on rat pancreatic exocrine secretion, *Peptides* 12: 559–562.
14. Raufman, J.-P., Malhotra, R., and Singh, L., 1991, PACAP38, a novel peptide from ovine hypothalamus, is a potent modulator of amylase release from dispersed acini from rat pancreas, *Regul. Pept.* 36: 121–129.
15. Warren, J.B., Donnelly, L.E., Cullen, S., Robertson, B.E., Ghatei, M.A., Bloom, S.R., and MacDermot, J., 1991, Pituitary adenylate cyclase-activating polypeptide: a novel, long-lasting, endothelin-independent vasorelaxant, *Eur J. Pharmacol.* 197: 131–134.
16. Tatsuno, I., Yada, T., Vigh, S., Hidaka, H., and Arimura, A., 1992, Pituitary adenylate cyclase activating polypeptide and vasoactive intestinal peptide increases cytosolic free calcium concentration in cultured rat hippocampal neurons, *Endocrinology* 131: 73–81.
17. Canny, B.J., Rawlings, S.R., and Leong, D.A., 1992, Pituitary adenylate cyclase-activating polypeptide specifically increases cytosolic calcium ion concentration in rat gonadotropes and somatotropes, *Endocrinology* 130: 211–215.
18. Yada, T., Vigh, S., and Arimura, A., 1993, Pituitary adenylate cyclase activating polypeptide (PACAP) increases cytosolic-free calcium concentration in folliculo-stellate cells and somatotropes of rat pituitary, *Peptides* 14: 235–239.
19. Yada, T., Sakurada, M., Ihida, K., Nakata, M., Murata, F., Arimura, A., and Kikuchi, M., 1994, Pituitary adenylate cyclase activating polypeptide is an extraordinarily potent intra-pancreatic regulator of insulin secretion from islet β-cells, *J. Biol. Chem.* 269: 1290–1293.
20. Yada, T., Itoh, K., and Nakata, M., 1993a, Glucagon-like peptide-1-(7-36)amide and a rise in cyclic adenosine 3′-5′-monophosphate increase cytosolic free Ca^{2+} in rat pancreatic β-cells by enhancing Ca^{2+} channel activity *Endocrinology* 133:1685–1692.
21. Yada, T., Kakei, M., and Tanaka, H., 1992, Single pancreatic β-cells from normal rat exhibit an initial decrease and subsequent increase in cytosolic free Ca^{2+} in response to glucose, *Cell Calcium* 13:69–76.
22. Grynkiewicz, G., Poenie, M., and Tsien, R.Y., 1985, A new generation of Ca^{2+} indicators with greatly improved fluorescence properties *J.Biol.Chem* 260:3440–3450.
23 Kawai, K., Ohse, C., Watanabe, Y., Suzuki, S., Yamashita, K., and Ohashi, S., 1992, Pituitary adenylate cyclase activating polypeptide stimulates insulin release from the isolated perfused pancreas, *Life Sci* 50: 257–261.
24 Ashcroft, F.M., and Rorsman, P., 1989, Electrophysiology of the pancreatic β-cell, *Prog. Biophys. Mol. Biol.* 54: 87–147.
25 Penner, R., and Neher, E., 1988, The role of calcium in stimulus-secretion coupling in excitable and non-excitable cells, *J. Exp. Biol.* 139: 329–345.
26 Ämmälä, C., Eliasson, L., Bokvist, K., Larsson, O., Ashcroft, F.M., and Rorsman, P., 1993, Exocytosis elicited by action potentials and voltage-clamp calcium currents in individual mouse pancreatic B-cells, *J.Physiol.* 472: 665–688.
27 Yada, T., Russo, L.L., and Sharp, G.W.G., 1989, Phorbol ester-stimulated insulin secretion by RINm5F insulinoma cells is linked with membrane depolarization and an increase in cytosolic free Ca^{2+} concentrations, *J.Biol.Chem.* 264: 2455–2462.

23

CHARACTERIZATION OF PURINERGIC RECEPTOR-EVOKED INCREASES IN INTRACELLULAR Ca^{2+} TRANSIENTS IN ISOLATED HUMAN AND RODENT INSULIN-SECRETING CELLS

Purinergic Receptor Signalling and $[Ca^{2+}]_i$ in Human β-Cells

P. E. Squires,[1] R. F. L. James,[2] N. J. M. London,[2] and M. J. Dunne[1]

[1]Department of Biomedical Science
The University of Sheffield
Alfred Denny Building, Western Bank
Sheffield, S10 2TN, United Kingdom
[2]The University of Leicester Department of Surgery
School of Medicine
Clinical Sciences Building, Leicester Royal Infirmary
PO Box 65
Leicester, LE2 7LX, United Kingdom

INTRODUCTION

In vivo many factors determine the regulation of insulin secretion from the β-cells of the pancreatic islets of Langerhans. The most predominant influence is a rise in the concentration of plasma glucose, which will promote secretion by mechanisms associated with Ca^{2+} influx across the plasma membrane[(1)]. Insulin release is also governed by changes in the concentration of circulating amino acids, gastrointestinal hormones, neuropeptides and neurotransmitters. These influences are important avenues for β-cell regulation as they not only provide a link between the gastrointestinal tract and the pancreatic islets — *the enteroinsular axis*, but they also govern the neurohormonal control of secretion. For many years it has been recognised that extracellular ATP is a potent insulin secretagogue[(2)]. *In vitro* it has been demonstrated using rodent and clonal insulin-secreting cells that purinergic receptor activation is coupled to an increase in $[Ca^{2+}]_i$ [(3–6)]. However, few studies have examined intracellular Ca^{2+} signalling in isolated human insulin-secreting cells[(4,7–10)]. In a recent paper we have shown that ATP and other agonists of the puriner-

Physiology and Pathophysiology of the Islets of Langerhans, edited by Soria.
Plenum Press, New York, 1997.

gic receptor evoke marked increases in $[Ca^{2+}]_i$ in β-cells isolated from transplantable human islets of Langerhans[11]. In this paper we examine: (i) the purinergic receptor subtype present in human tissue, (ii) compare purinergic receptor-evoked increases in $[Ca^{2+}]_i$ in both rodent and human β-cells and (iii) demonstrate that intracellular Ca^{2+} signals can also be recorded in cryopreserved human β-cells originally isolated from cadaver organ donors.

METHODS

Cell Preparation: Human and Rodent Insulin-Secreting Cells

Studies involving human tissue were performed (with permission) on transplantable pancreatic β-cells from non-diabetic, heart beating cadaver organ donors. Islets of Langerhans were isolated using a collagenase digestion technique under aseptic conditions following similar procedures to those described previously[12]. In brief, the pancreatic duct was cannulated and the pancreas distended with 2 ml/g of collagenase solution (concentration 3 mg/ml Serva, Heidelberg, Germany). The pancreas was then placed into a stainless steel chamber and gradually warmed to 39°C whilst the chamber was gently agitated. The fluid from the chamber was sampled on a regular basis and when the presence of islets was confirmed by dithizone staining, the digest was collected. Islets were then purified from the digest using continuous gradients of BSA (bovine serum albumin) on a COBE 2991 cell processor. Purity of the preparations ranged from 60–95%. Human islets were then either placed into cryopreservation for long-term storage[13], or into standard tissue culture conditions for short-term maintenance[12]. Rodent insulin secreting cells were prepared from male Wistar rats using procedures previously described[14]. Once isolated rodent islets were placed into tissue culture conditions for maintenance. Whole islets and isolated cells were maintained for up to 16 days in RPMI 1640 tissue culture media, supplemented with 10% foetal calf serum, and 100 IU/ml penicillin and 100 μg/ml streptomycin in a humidified atmosphere of 95% O_2 and 5% CO_2 at a temperature of 37°C. Before use in experimental studies islets were hand-picked, and gentle trituration employed to dissociate them into single isolated cells, and small clusters of cells. These were then plated onto poly-D-lysine (5 μg/ml) treated coverglass for overnight attachment.

Single Cell Microfluorimetry Techniques

Experiments were performed using dual-excitation microfluorimetry techniques with fura-2-loaded cells (20 minute incubation at 37°C in 1 ml of RPMI media containing 1.5 μM fura 2-acetoxymethyl ester (Sigma, Poole, UK)). A Na^+-rich balanced salt solution was used as the standard extracellular media, containing (mM): NaCl 137, KCl 5.4, $CaCl_2$ 1.3, $MgSO_4$ 0.8, Na_2HPO_4 0.3, KH_2PO_4 0.4, $NaHCO_3$ 4.2, N-[2-hydroxyethyl] piperazine-N′-[2-ethanesulphonic acid] (HEPES) 10 and glucose 2. The pH was adjusted to 7.4 with NaOH. For 'calcium-free' experiments, $CaCl_2$ was omitted from the Na^+-rich solution, and 1 mM ethylenebis(oxonitrilo)tetraacetate (EGTA) was added; under these conditions we estimate the free Ca^{2+} concentration to be less than 10 nM[11]. The osmolality of all solutions was set at 290 ± 5 mosmol/Kg. A low-pressure, rapid superfusion system (flow rate: approximately 3–4 ml min^{-1}) was used to change solutions in the bath. All data have been expressed as a relative change in the fluorescence recorded at 350 and 380nm, and therefore represent relative changes in $[Ca^{2+}]_i$.

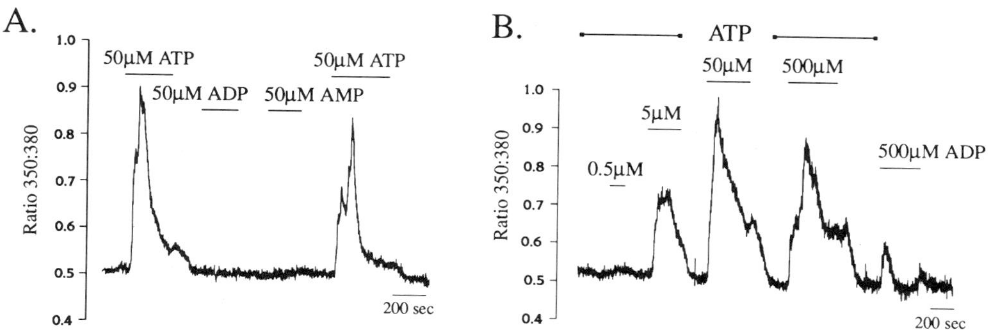

Figure 1. **A–B.** Purinergic receptor agonists elevate $[Ca^{2+}]_i$ in isolated human pancreatic β-cells. Data come from separate experiments. Data in panel A show that only 50 μM ATP but not equivalent concentrations of AMP or ADP will enhance $[Ca^{2+}]_i$. Whilst panel B shows a concentration-response relationship for ATP on $[Ca^{2+}]_i$.

RESULTS

Actions of the purinergic receptor agonists ATP, ADP, AMP and UTP on intracellular Ca^{2+} ($[Ca^{2+}]_i$) in isolated β-cells from human and rodent islets of Langerhans have been examined over the concentration range 0.05 μM–500 μM. Figure 1 shows data from two separate experiments carried out upon human β-cells which demonstrate that while 50 μM ATP will evoke repetitive Ca^{2+} signals, there was no significant action of either 50 μM ADP or 50 μM AMP under the same conditions (Fig. 1A). ADP and AMP were only able to increase $[Ca^{2+}]_i$ at a much higher concentration (500 μM) than ATP, and in general we found that the cells responded more readily to ADP than AMP. The data shown in Fig. 1B illustrates a typical ATP concentration-response relationship. At submicromolar concentrations, ATP (0.5 μM) had no significant effect on the intracellular free Ca^{2+} concentration, whilst 500 μM ATP produced a smaller increase in $[Ca^{2+}]_i$ than 50 μM ATP. Figure 2 shows that the P_2 agonist UTP also elevates $[Ca^{2+}]_i$ in human β-cells. In general, ATP-evoked increases in $[Ca^{2+}]_i$ were always greater than UTP > ADP. Suramin, the mixed P_2-receptor antagonist (10 μM–50 μM) had no significant effect upon ATP-evoked increases in $[Ca^{2+}]_i$.

In studies using rat pancreatic β-cells, responses to purinergic-receptor agonists were different to human β-cells in several respects. Firstly, the concentration-response

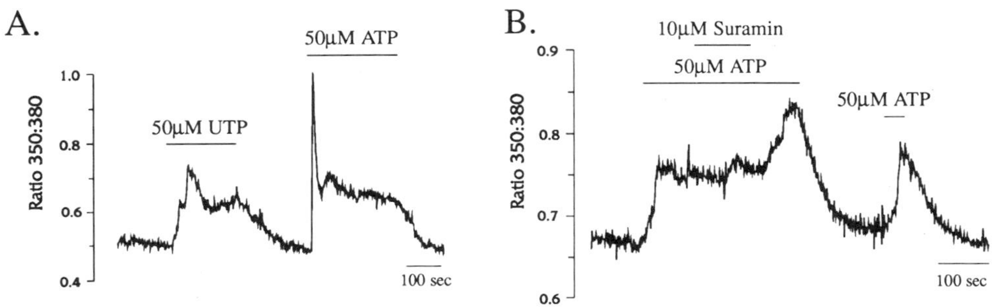

Figure 2. **A–B.** Actions of UTP and ATP on $[Ca^{2+}]_i$ in human pancreatic β-cells, as well as effects of the P_2-antagonist suramin (10 μM) on agonist-evoked increases in $[Ca^{2+}]_i$.

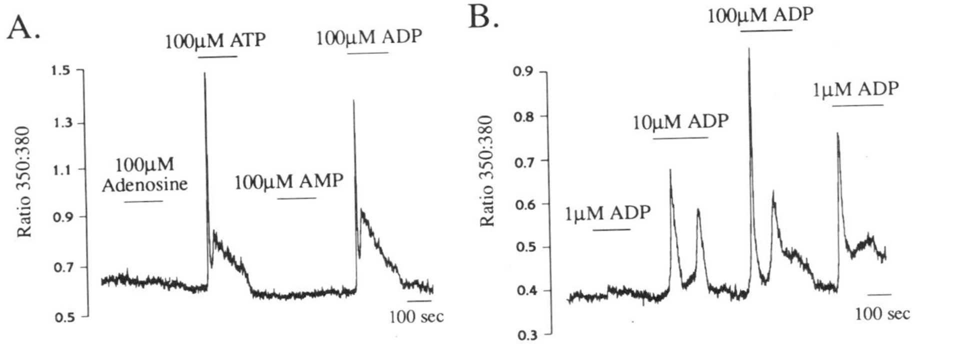

Figure 3. Comparative effects of purinergic receptor agonists upon $[Ca^{2+}]_i$ in rodent tissue. Compare the potency, and the selectivity for the P_2-receptor in rodent to human tissue (Figs 1, 2 and 4) as well as the patterns of $[Ca^{2+}]_i$ signals.

profile to ATP, ADP and AMP is different: in rodent tissue ADP produced increases in $[Ca^{2+}]_i$ that were similar in magnitude to those of ATP, Fig. 3A. Secondly, the patterns of Ca^{2+} responses were somewhat different, and were more generally preceeded by a very large, rapid but transient increase in $[Ca^{2+}]_i$, Fig. 3. Finally, in rodent β-cells UTP generally produced smaller changes in $[Ca^{2+}]_i$ than ADP. These data would tend to indicate that in rat β-cells the purinergic receptor subtype is probably of the P_{2Y} nomenclature with the profile of responses ATP ≥ ADP >> UTP; clearly different to human tissue where ATP > UTP > ADP >> AMP.

Access to acutely isolated human pancreatic β-cells is on occasions very limited, consequently we have also performed a series of experiments upon human β-cells cryopreserved for long-term maintenance. Cryopreservation of islets is increasingly more important to transplantation studies since it enables larger numbers of islets to be donated to the recipient. Despite this, little is known of the mechanisms that govern sub-cellular signal transduction events in β-cells stored in this manner. Figure 4A summarises the actions of ATP, ADP, AMP, UTP and adenosine on $[Ca^{2+}]_i$ from cryopreserved β-cells. The

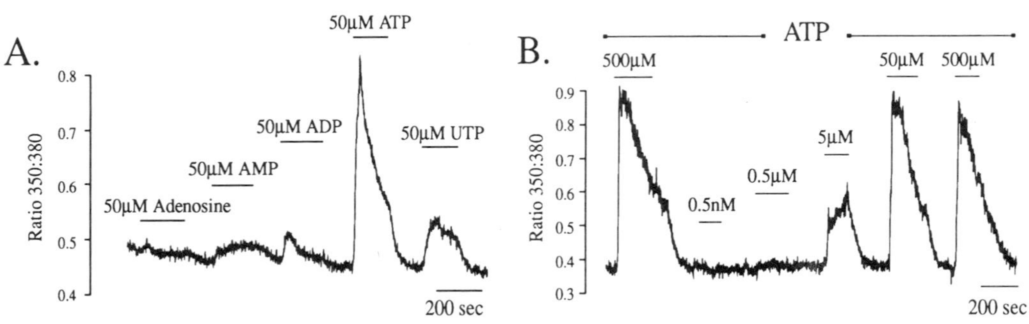

Figure 4. **A–B.** Purinergic receptor agonists elevate $[Ca^{2+}]_i$ in isolated cryopreserved human pancreatic β-cells. Data come from separate experiments. Panel A shows that only 50 μM ATP and 50 μM UTP cause any significant increase in $[Ca^{2+}]_i$, whilst 50 μM adenosine, ADP and AMP have relatively no effect upon $[Ca^{2+}]_i$. Panel B shows a concentration-response relationship for ATP on $[Ca^{2+}]_i$ in cryopreserved tissue. Compare this data to that shown in Figure 1 from non-cryopreserved human β-cells.

pattern of response is almost identical to that demonstrated in Figure 1A; ATP > UTP > ADP >> AMP, adenosine. Figure 4B shows data from a separate experiment with cryopreserved β-cells exposed to a range of concentrations of ATP. As with acutely isolated β-cells the threshold for ATP-evoked increases in $[Ca^{2+}]_i$ are approximately 5 μM, with 500 μM ATP causing no further increase in $[Ca^{2+}]_i$ than 50 μM. In a separate series of experiments we found that cryopreserved β-cells also responded to muscarinic agonists, amino acids and pharmacological agents in a similar manner to non-cryopreserved tissue.

DISCUSSION

ATP and other agonists of purinergic receptors are known to be potent stimulators of insulin secretion. These effects can be seen both *in vivo*(2), and *in vitro* using rodent(4,5) and clonal β-cells(3,4,6), but no studies have addressed in detail the role of purinergic receptor agonists in the regulation of cytosolic Ca^{2+} signals using single, isolated pancreatic β-cells from human cadaver donor tissue, either acutely isolated or cryopreserved. In acutely isolated human tissue we described elsewhere that responses to P_2-agonists increase $[Ca^{2+}]_i$ through subcellular events that regulate transmembrane Ca^{2+} influx, and mobilisation of Ca^{2+} from internal Ca^{2+} stores(11). In this paper we have demonstrated that; (i) ATP, ADP, AMP and UTP will increase $[Ca^{2+}]_i$ in human β-cells, and (ii) that both the potency series of purinergic receptor agonists, as well as the sensitivity of the receptor to ATP are remarkably similar in both cryopreserved and non-cryopreserved tissue (compare Figs. 1 and 4).

In rodent β-cells and in insulin-secreting cell lines, the purinergic receptor has been tentatively identified as a P_{2Y}-receptor based upon studies of the potency of different adenine nucleotide ligands, and through the use of specific agonists/antagonists to this receptor (*see* 6 for references). In our present studies we have largely confirmed these findings, but show also that in human β-cells the responses to P_2 agonists are different to rodent cells in several ways: i.e. ATP is much more potent than ADP, which was only moderately more effective at elevating intracellular Ca^{2+} levels than AMP (Fig. 1), whereas UTP generally gave larger increases in $[Ca^{2+}]_i$ than ADP in human but not rodent β-cells. This would therefore tend to suggest that the rank order of potency was ATP > UTP > ADP ≥ AMP; i.e. somewhat different from that expected for the P_{2Y}-receptor (ATP = ADP >> UTP) (see 15 for recent review of P-receptor physiology and pharmacology). The concentration-response relationship for the actions of ATP on changes in $[Ca^{2+}]_i$ has been examined in detail. Our major findings are, that in both human and rodent tissue, submicromolar ATP concentrations have little effect on $[Ca^{2+}]_i$, and secondly that responses to ATP are sharply attenuated at concentrations higher than 100 μM. The mixed P_2-antagonist suramin, which will influence P_{2X} and P_{2U}-receptor subtypes (15) did not significantly modulate ATP-evoked increases in $[Ca^{2+}]_i$. Together our data suggest that whilst the P_{2Y}-receptor subtype dominates in rodent β-cells, human tissue possess either a novel form of the receptor sub classification exhibiting selectivity ATP > UTP >> ADP, and/or a mixed population of P_2 receptors: P_{2Y} and P_{2U} subtypes.

Finally, several suggestions have been made to account for the physiological significance of the effects of ATP on insulin secretion. Firstly, ATP may be released, or co-released along with other neurotransmitters/neuropeptides from the nerve endings that innervate the pancreas, and thereby play an important role in the neurohormonal regulation of secretion. Alternatively, ATP may be important for the autoregulation of insulin release. Insulin-containing granules in β-cells possess relatively high amounts of ATP that will be co-released during secretion [*see* 5]. Under these conditions a stimulatory effect of ATP on plasma

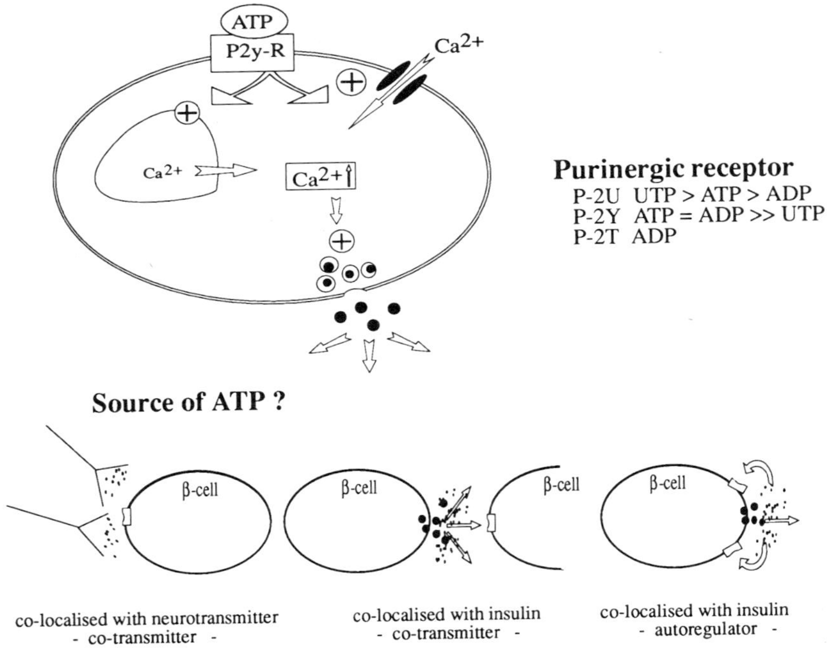

Figure 5. Model to summarise effects and possible sources of extracellular ATP on the regulation of insulin secretion.

membrane purinergic receptors could then act in the microenvironment of the β-cell to promote further release of insulin in a 'feed-forward' mode of action, Figure 5.

ACKNOWLEDGMENTS

Human insulin-secreting cell experiments were supported by the British Diabetic Association through grants to MJD and RFLJ/NJML, and by the Wellcome Trust (MJD).

REFERENCES

1. Wollheim, C,B., and Sharp, G.W.G. 1981, Regulation of insulin release by calcium. *Physiol Rev* 61: 914–973.
2. Candela, J.L.R., and Garcia-Fernandez, M.C., 1963, Stimulation of secretion of insulin by adenosine triphosphate, *Nature* 197: 1210.
3. Arkhammar, P., Hallberg, A., Kindmak, H., Nilsson, T., Rorsman. P., and Berggren, P.-O., 1990, Extracellular ATP increases cytoplasmic free Ca^{2+} concentration in clonal insulin-producing RINm5F cells, *Biochem. J.* 265: 203–211.
4. Geschwind, J.-F., Hiriart, M., Glennon, M.C., Najafi, H., Corkey, B.E., Matschinsky, F.M., and Prentki, M., 1989, Selective activation of Ca^{2+} influx by extracellular ATP in a pancreatic β-cell line (HIT), *Biochim. Biophys. Acta* 1012: 107–115.
5. Hellman, B., Gylfe, E., Wesslen, N., Hallberg, A., Grapengiesser, E., and Marcstrom, A., 1989, Plasma membrane associated ATP as a regulator of the secretory activity of the pancreatic β-cell, *Expt. Clinc. Endocrinol.* 93: 125–135.
6. Li, G., Milani, D., Dunne, M.J., Pralong, W.-F., Theler, J.-M., Petersen, O.H., and Wollheim, C.B., 1991, Extracellular ATP cause Ca^{2+}-dependent and independent insulin secretion in RINm5F cells. *J. Biol. Chem.* 266: 3449–3457.

7. Sher, E., Biancardi, E., Pollo, A., Carbone, E., Li, G., Wollheim, C.B., and Clementi, F., 1992, Omega-Conotoxin-sensitive, voltage-operated calcium channels in insulin-secreting cells. *Eur. J. Pharmacol.* 216: 407–414.
8. Pollo, A., Lovallo, M., Biancardi, E., Sher, E., Socci, C., and Carbone, E., 1993, Sensitivity to dihydropyridines, δ-conotoxin and noradrenaline reveals multiple high-voltage-activated calcium channels in rat insulinoma and human pancreatic β-cells, *Pflugers Archiv.* 423: 462–471.
9. Kindmark, H., Kohler, M., Nillsson, T., Arkhammar, P., Wiechel, K.-L., Rorsman, P., Efandic, S., and Berggren, P.-O., 1992, Measurement of cytoplasmic free Ca^{2+} concentration in human pancreatic islets and insulinoma cells, *FEBS Lett.* 291: 310–314.
10. Rojas, E., Caroll, P.B., Ricordi, C., Boschero, A.C., Stojilikovic, S.S., and Atwater, I., 1994, Control of cytosolic free calcium in cultured human pancreatic β-cells occurs by external calcium dependent and independent mechanisms, *Endocrinology* 134: 1771–1781.
11. Squires, P.E., James, R.F.L., London, N.J.M., and Dunne, M.J., 1994, ATP-induced intracellular Ca^{2+} signals in isolated human insulin-secreting cells, *Pflugers Archives* 427: 181–183.
12. London, N.J.M., James, R.F.L., and Bell, P.R.F., 1992, Islet purification. *In*: Pancreatic Islet Cell Transplantation, pp 113–123, Edited by C. Ricordi, Landes Press.
13. Rich, S.J., Swift, S., Thirdborough, S.M., Rumford, G., James, R.F.L., and London, N.J.M., 1993, Cryopreservation of rat islets of Langerhans: a comparison of two techniques, *Cryobiology* 30: 407–412.
14. Findlay, I., Dunne, M.J. and Petersen, O.H., 1985, High conductance K^+ channel in pancreatic islet cells can be activated and inactivated by internal calcium, *J. Memb. Biol.* 83: 169–175.
15. Dubyak, G.R., and El-Moatassim, C., 1993, Signal transduction via P_2-purinergic receptors for extracellular ATP and other nucleotides, *Am. J. Physiol.* 265: C577–C606.

Part IV. β-CELL METABOLISM AND $[Ca^{2+}]_i$

24

RECIPROCAL LINKS BETWEEN METABOLIC AND IONIC EVENTS IN ISLET CELLS

Their Relevance to the Rhythmics of Insulin Release

Willy J. Malaisse

Laboratory of Experimental Medicine
Brussels Free University
Brussels, Belgium

It has long been known that insulin release may occur according to a rhythmic pattern at least from the isolated perfused pancreas.[1] Likewise, it has long been questioned whether oscillations of metabolic events take place in glucose-stimulated islets and might account for the rhythmic pattern of insulin release.[2,3] The present review refers to selected observations which are considered relevant to these issues.

RHYTHMIC PATTERN OF ARGININE-STIMULATED HORMONAL RELEASE FROM THE ISOLATED PERFUSED RAT PANCREAS

Table 1 refers to a recent study[4] in which insulin, glucagon and somatostatin release was measured at 1 min intervals from the 71st to 120th min in isolated rat perfused pancreases exposed to L-arginine (5.0 mM) from the 71st min onwards. At least up to the 5th secretory peak, hormonal pulses occurred in each series of individual experiments at approximately the same time after introduction of L-arginine.

These observations not only extend from insulin and glucagon to somatostatin the concept that, under continuous stimulation, hormonal release occurs in a rhythmic fashion from the isolated perfused pancreas. Since L-arginine was used as the major secretagogue in these experiments, they also suggest that such a rhythmic pattern is not restricted to the situation in which D-glucose acts as the major stimulus for hormonal release.

Moreover, since these experiments were conducted in the isolated perfused rat pancreas, ruling out the interference of changes in circulating nutrient concentration, blood flow or central nervous system control, the findings summarized in Table 1 support — at the first glance — the concept of an intrapancreatic pacemaker. The essential question, therefore, concerns the determinism of the secretory oscillations.

Physiology and Pathophysiology of the Islets of Langerhans, edited by Soria.
Plenum Press, New York, 1997.

Table 1. Timing (min) of successive secretory peaks in insulin, glucagon and somatostatin output in pancreases exposed to L-arginine (5 mM) from the 71st min onwards

Hormone	Expt.	1st peak	2nd peak	3rd peak	4th peak	5th peak
Insulin	1	74	78	86	94	101
	2	74	79	88	96	103
	3	74	78	86	94	101
Glucagon	A	73	80	85	92	98
	B	74	80	84	91	100
	C	73	81	87	95	99
	D	74	82	86	94	98
	E	73	81	87	93	102
	F	73	81	87	92	102
Somatostatin	1	74	78 ± 1	89	83 ± 1	100 ± 1
	2	74	81	87	95 ± 1	102
	3	74	77	86 ± 1	93	103

NATURE OF THE INTRAPANCREATIC PACEMAKER

Short of alternative hypothesis, we previously proposed that the phasic pattern of insulin release may be merely accounted for by integration of secretory activity in distinct secretory units each of which is engaged in rhythmic oscillations between silent and active states.[5] Fig. 1 illustrates such a situation in groups of 40 or 180 secretory units.

This model could thus account for the oscillatory pattern seen in the whole pancreas or whenever a large number of islets or dispersed islet cells are examined. For instance, it may account for the oscillations in cytosolic Ca^{2+} concentration already encountered in the first study conducted in dispersed normal islet cells suddenly exposed to a rise in extracellular D-glucose concentration.[6]

If we accept such a view, the remaining major question concerns the determinism of oscillations in each individual secretory unit.

DO OSCILLATIONS OF GLYCOLYSIS TAKE PLACE IN SINGLE B-CELLS OR SINGLE ISLETS?

One does not need great imagination to visualize how a constant inflow signal is converted in a rhythmic pattern (Fig. 2). For instance, the bursting pattern of bioelectrical events, known to be synchronized within each islet, may involve the interplay between ATP-sensitive *versus* voltage- and/or Ca^{2+}-responsive K^+ channels, as already proposed more than a decade ago.[7] I will not elaborate on this theme, which is considered in detail elsewhere in this volume, but -instead- concentrate on a slower pattern of oscillations with a periodicity of about 6–10 min.

A current hypothesis in the latter respect relates to oscillations in metabolic events such as glycolysis. This process is best known in cytosolic muscle extracts incubated in the presence of D-glucose, ATP, NAD^+ and — most importantly — yeast hexokinase. Under these conditions, rhythmic changes are observed in the concentration of fructose-1,6-bisphosphate and NADH, which follow a synchronous pattern.[8] The NADH peaks coincide with a sudden acceleration of fructose-1,6-bisphosphate formation and further catabolism, as documented by transient increases in ^3HOH production from D-[5-^3H]glucose. They take

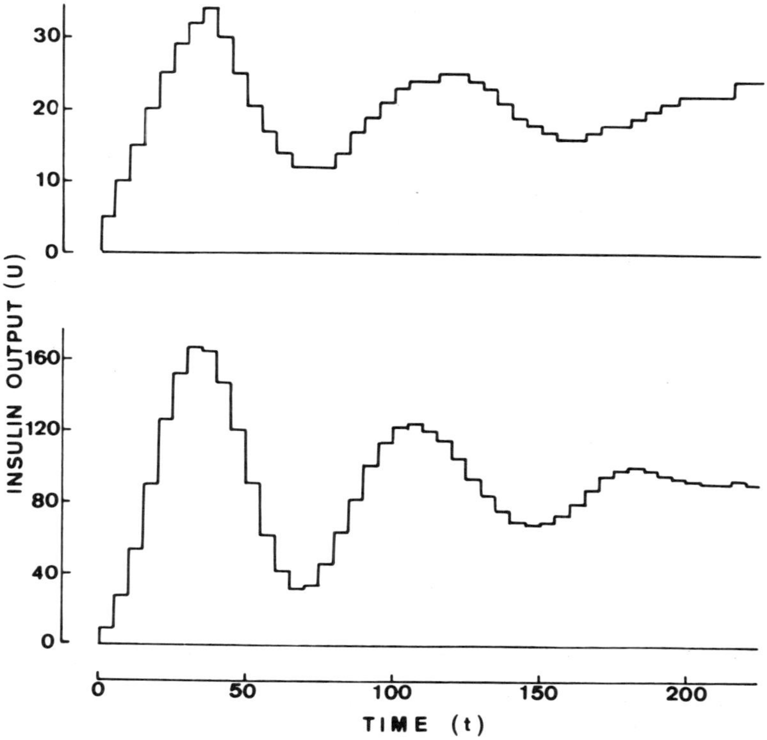

Figure 1. Time course for insulin release from 40 cells (upper panel) and 180 cells (lower panel). Throughout the period of exposure to glucose, all cells displayed a rhythmic pattern with the active and silent periods amounting to 25, 30, 35, 40 or 45 t. In the upper panel, eight cells were used for each of the latter five periodicities. In each group of eight cells, the onset of activity was delayed by steps of 5 t each, such a delay ranging from 0 to 35 t. The upper panel refers to the total output recorded in the five groups of eight cells each. In the lower panel, two further changes were introduced. First, each group involved 20 cells instead of eight cells in order to allow for a close-to-normal distribution in the onset of activity. Second, the contribution of cells with an active (or silent) period of 35 t was tripled, that of cells with an active period of either 30 or 40 t doubled and that of cells with an active period of either 25 or 45 t maintained at its single value. Hence, the lower panel refers to a total of 180 cells.

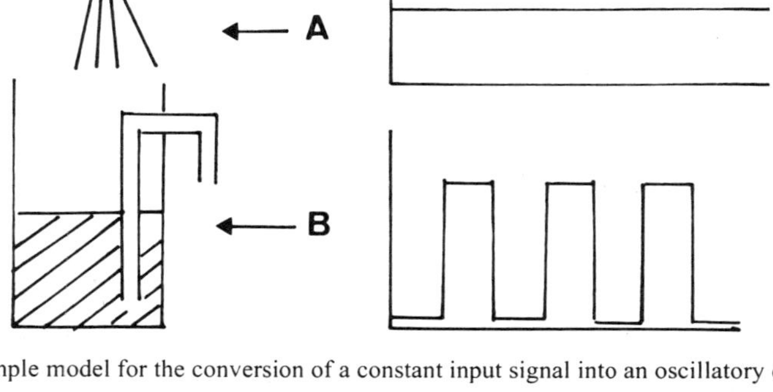

Figure 2. Simple model for the conversion of a constant input signal into an oscillatory output product.

place when the ATP concentration reaches its nadir value and, hence, when phosphofructokinase is relieved from the inhibitory action of the adenine nucleotide. The oscillations in glycolysis are indeed contemporary of oscillations in ATP concentration, with a mirror image for the concentrations of both ADP and AMP.[8]

It should be realized that this situation refers to a rather unusual system in that the presence of yeast hexokinase is imperative in two respects. First, to obtain in sustained rate of D-glucose phosphorylation, the yeast hexokinase being more resistant than mammalian hexokinase to feedback inhibition by D-glucose 6-phosphate and, second, to cause a sustained consumption of ATP which admittedly may be achieved in intact cells by specific ionic-responsive ATPases.

It is not obvious, therefore, that a comparable situation prevails in intact cells or even in extracts of other cell types. For instance, considering qualified analogies of D-glucose metabolism in B-cells and hepatocytes, we have repeated the same kind of experiments in liver extracts. At variance with the situation found in muscle extracts, no oscillation of glycolysis could be documented in liver extracts.[9]

It is quite conceivable, however, that oscillation of metabolic events nevertheless occurs in intact islet cells, in which case they may involve further regulatory mechanisms, such as a reciprocal coupling between these metabolic events and more distal ionic events in the secretory sequence.

RECIPROCAL COUPLING BETWEEN METABOLIC AND IONIC EVENTS IN THE SECRETORY SEQUENCE

It is currently assumed that, in the process of nutrient-stimulated insulin release, ionic events, e.g. changes in K^+ conductance, are tightly dependent on metabolic events, e.g. changes in cytosolic ATP concentration.[10] I wish to emphasize the opposite process in which distal ionic and functional events in the secretory sequence exert a feedback control on nutrient catabolism in islet cells.[3]

A few years ago, we reported that suppression of ATP-consuming functional events such as proinsulin biosynthesis and insulin release in islets exposed to Ca^{2+}-deprived medium and/or cycloheximide indeed results in severe alteration of D-glucose metabolism in isolated islets, culminating in a dissociation between the generation of glucose-derived acetyl residues in the reaction catalyzed by pyruvate dehydrogenase and their further oxidation in the Krebs cycle.[11]

It could be objected that the incubation of islets in Ca^{2+}-deprived media and in the presence of cycloheximide has little to do with the physiology of islet cells. However, in a more recent study, it was observed that the generation and oxidation of glucose-derived acetyl residues are indeed dissociated from one another under physiological conditions, provided that attention is paid to their respective time course.[12] This is illustrated in Fig. 3.

HETEROGENEITY AND RECRUITMENT IN THE B-CELL POPULATION

A last implication of this situation should be underlined. In a prior study, we had already expanded our mathematical model of stimulus-secretion coupling in distinct secretory units to include the phenomenon of recruitment of such secretory units at increasing

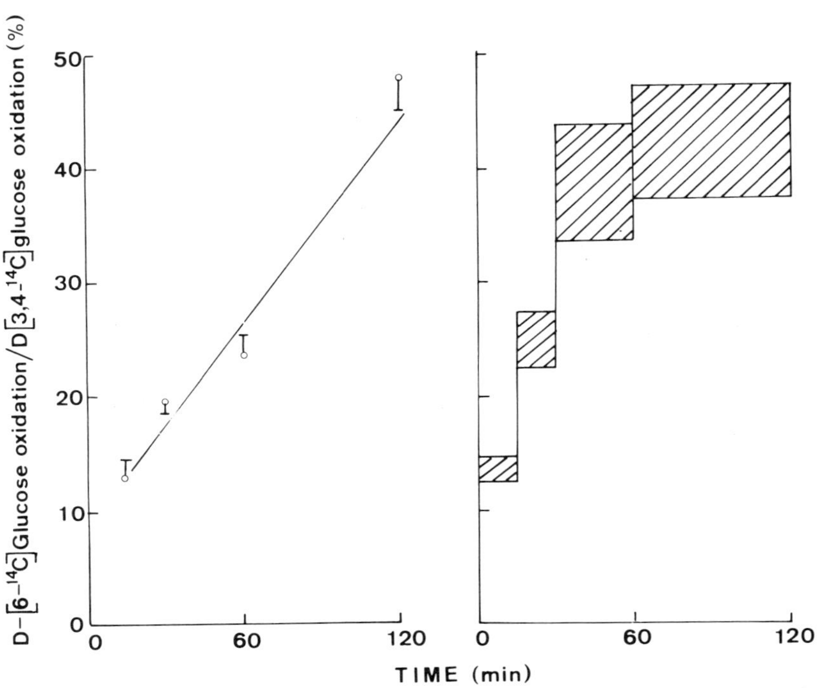

Figure 3. Mean values (± S.E.) for the ratio between D-[6-^{14}C]glucose and D-[3,4-^{14}C]glucose oxidation were judged from either the paired measurements between $^{14}CO_2$ output and ^{3}HOH generation from D-[5-^{3}H]glucose after 15, 30, 60 or 120 min incubation (left panel) of the differences between cumulative values for $^{14}CO_2$ output over each time interval (right panel). The means values for either D-[6-^{14}C]glucose or D-[3,4-^{14}C]glucose oxidation were derived from 20 individual observations at each time-point.

concentrations of D-glucose.[5] I now wish to propose that the preferential stimulation of oxidative mitochondrial events participates to this recruitment phenomenon.

The latter proposal is based on the following observation. When purified B-cells are separated into two subpopulations of so-called glucose-insensitive and glucose-sensitive cells and when the former cells are incubated at 10 mM D-glucose and the latter cells at 5 mM D-glucose in order to achieve identical rates of D-[5-^{3}H]glucose utilization, the oxidation of D-[U-^{14}C]glucose remains significantly higher in the glucose-sensitive than glucose-insensitive cells.[13] In other words, the ratio between oxidative and total glycolysis appears as one of the factors responsible for cellular heterogeneity and, hence, recruitment in the B-cell population.

CONCLUSIONS

In conclusion, two main proposals emerge from this report. First, the apparent existence of an intrapancreatic pacemaker could merely reflect the integration of independent oscillatory patterns in distinct secretory units. Second, at the level of each secretory unit, the occurrence of slow oscillations might involve a reciprocal feed-forward and feedback coupling process between metabolic and ionic events in the secretory sequence.

REFERENCES

1. V. Leclercq-Meyer, A. Herchuelz, I. Valverde, E. Couturier, J. Marchand, and W.J. Malaisse, Mode of action of clonidine upon islet function. Dissociated effects upon the time-course and magnitude of insulin release, *Diabetes* 29:193–200 (1980).
2. W.J. Malaisse, J.C. Hutton, S. Kawazu, A. Herchuelz, I. Valverde and A. Sener, The stimulus-secretion coupling of glucose-induced insulin release. XXXV. The links between metabolic and cationic events, *Diabetologia* 16:331–341 (1979).
3. W.J. Malaisse, A. Sener, A. Herchuelz, I. Valverde, J.C. Hutton, I. Atwater and V. Leclercq-Meyer, The interplay between metabolic and cationic events in islet cells : coupling factors and feedback mechanisms. *Horm. Metab. Res.* suppl. 10:61–66 (1980).
4. V. Leclercq-Meyer and W.J. Malaisse, Pulsatility of arginine-stimulated insulin, glucagon and somatostatin release, *Med. Sci. Res.* 22:151–154 (1994).
5. W.J. Malaisse and A. Owen, Mathematical modelling of stimulus-secretion coupling in the pancreatic B-cell. VI. Cellular heterogeneity and recruitment, *Appl. Math. Modelling*, 13:41–46 (1989).
6. M. Deleers, M. Mahy and W.J. Malaisse, Glucose increases cytosolic Ca^{2+} activity in pancreatic islet cells, *Biochem. Internat.* 10:97–103 (1985).
7. W.J. Malaisse and A. Herchuelz, Nutritional regulation of K^+ conductance: an unsettled aspect of pancreatic β-cell physiology, *in:* "Biochemical actions of hormones", G. Litwack, ed., Academic Press, New York, 9: 69–92 (1982).
8. G. Marynissen, A. Sener and W.J. Malaisse, Oscillations in glycolysis : multifactorial quantitative analysis in muscle extract, *Mol. Cell. Biochem.* 113:105–121 (1992).
9. G. Bernardy, A. Sener and W.J. Malaisse, Absence of glycolytic oscillation in rat liver extracts, *Med. Sci. Res.* 22:155–157 (1994).
10. W.J. Malaisse and A. Sener, Glucose-induced changes in cytosolic ATP content in pancreatic islets, *Biochim. Biophys. Acta* 927:190–195 (1987).
11. W.J. Malaisse and A. Sener, Hexose metabolism in pancreatic islets. Feedback control of D-glucose oxidation by functional events, *Biochim. Biophys. Acta* 971:246–254 (1988).
12. A. Sener, F. Malaisse-Lagae and W.J. Malaisse, Hexose metabolism in pancreatic islets : time-course of the oxidative response to D-glucose, *Biochim. Biophys. Acta* 1177:54–60 (1993).
13. W.J. Malaisse, The beta cell in non-insulin-dependent diabetes : giving light to the blind, *Diabetologia* 37 (suppl. 2):S36–S42 (1994).

25

GLYCERALDEHYDE AND THE PANCREATIC β-CELL

L. Best, A. C. Elliott, and J. Davies

Departments of Medicine and Physiological Sciences
University of Manchester
Manchester M13 9PT, United Kingdom

INTRODUCTION

D-glyceraldehyde is commonly used as a stimulus of insulin release from the pancreatic β-cell[1–3]. It is generally accepted that the triose can be metabolized in the β-cell via the glycolytic pathway, thus stimulating insulin release in a manner analogous to glucose[1–3]. In numerous studies of tumoural β-cell lines which, owing to abnormalities in glucose transport or metabolism, fail to respond to the sugar, glyceraldehyde has been employed as a 'nutrient' type stimulus[4–6]. The results of our studies on glyceraldehyde actions on the HIT-T15 cell line suggest, however, that the triose is poorly metabolized in these cells and that, unlike glucose, it stimulates the β-cell by a mechanism which does not involve its glycolytic metabolism.

MATERIALS AND METHODS

HIT-T15 cells were cultured as described previously, a standard HEPES-buffered incubation medium was used for all experiments[7]. Experimental details for the measurement of changes in membrane potential, cytosolic pH and $[Ca^{2+}]_i$, $^{86}Rb^+$ efflux, insulin release and glyceraldehyde metabolism have been previously published[7]. Uptake of D[^{14}C]-glyceraldehyde was measured using an oil filtration technique[8].

RESULTS

The addition of D-glyceraldehyde (5–20mM) to HIT-T15 cells caused a concentration-dependent depolarization, on the basis of reduced fluorescence of the dye oxonol-V (Fig. 1). This effect was accompanied by a marked intracellular acidification, a rise in $[Ca^{2+}]_i$ (assessed using the fluorescent dyes BCECF and fura-2 respectively) and up to a

Physiology and Pathophysiology of the Islets of Langerhans, edited by Soria.
Plenum Press, New York, 1997.

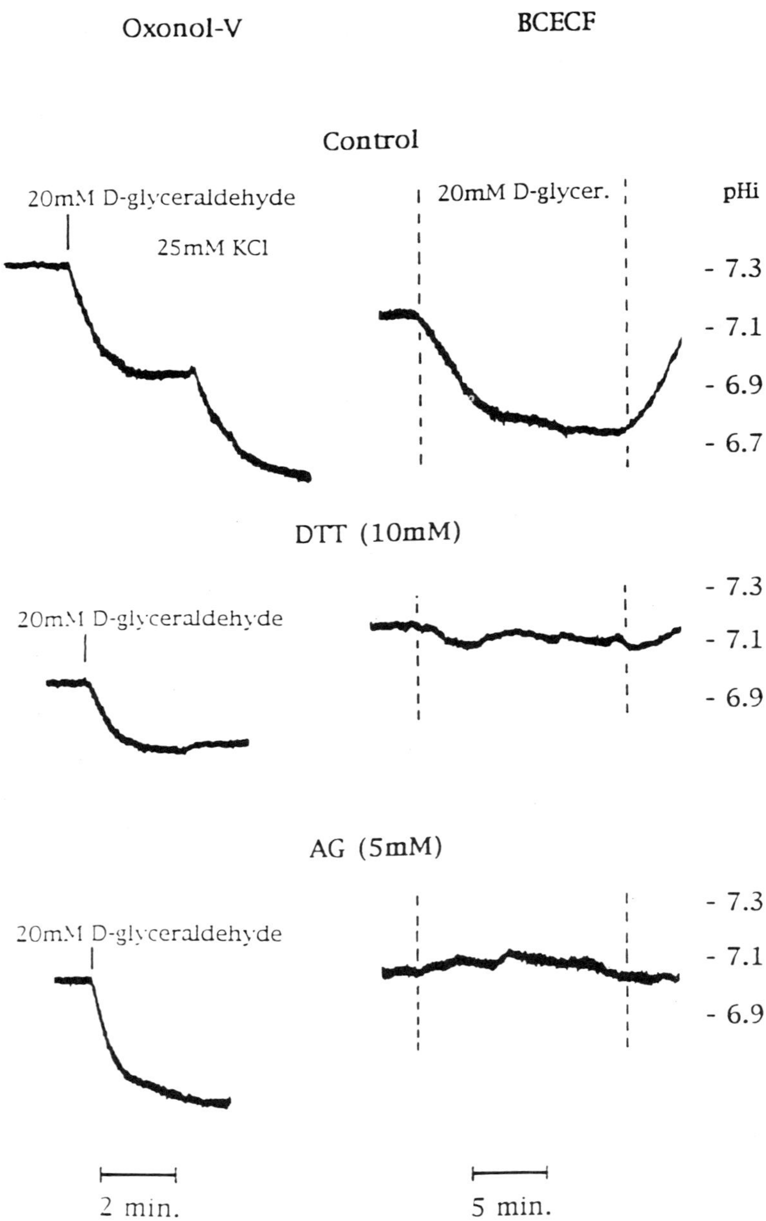

Figure 1. Effects of D-glyceraldehyde on HIT-T15 cell membrane potential (left) and intracellular pH (pHi; right) in the absence or presence of dithiothreitol (DTT) or aminoguanidine (AG).

threefold stimulation of insulin release. L-glyceraldehyde, which is supposedly less effectively metabolized than the D-enantiomer, was equally effective in eliciting the above responses. Neither D- nor L-glyceraldehyde had any apparent effect upon the rate of outflow of $^{86}Rb^+$ in preloaded cells, suggesting that the depolarization was not the result of reduced potassium permeability. The glyceraldehyde-induced intracellular acidification persisted in Na^+-free medium, although the rate and extent of depolarization appeared to be reduced in the absence of Na^+. Both the depolarization and intracellular acidification, but not the rise in $[Ca^{2+}]_i$, persisted in Ca^{2+}-free medium.

Preincubation of HIT cells with 1mM iodoacetate, a glycolytic inhibitor, failed to prevent activation of the cells by D- or L-glyceraldehyde. However, all of the responses to glyceraldehyde were inhibited by the presence of the thiol reagent N-ethylmaleimide (0.1 or 1mM). The acidification induced by glyceraldehyde was inhibited by the thiol protective agent dithiothreitol and by aminoguanidine, a compound which forms adducts with a-ketoaldehydes (Fig. 1). However, these compounds did not prevent glyceraldehyde-induced depolarization of the cells.

The rate of oxidation of 10mM D-glyceraldehyde by HIT cells, assessed by the formation of $^{14}CO_2$ from D[^{14}C]-glyceraldehyde, was extremely modest, representing approximately one sixth of the rate of oxidation of 10mM glucose. 1mM iodoacetate reduced lactate and CO_2 formation to undetectable levels, confirming its action in inhibiting glycolysis. Metabolism of glyceraldehyde via glycolysis in HIT cells was assessed by measuring the formation of L-lactate. The addition of 10mM D- or L-glyceraldehyde to HIT cells did not significantly increase L-lactate formation. The addition of 10mM glucose resulted in an approximately five-fold increase in lactate output. In contrast, the formation of D-lactate, the end product of methylglyoxal metabolism via the glyoxalase pathway, by HIT cells was greatly increased in the presence of D-glyceraldehyde.

In order to study transport of glyceraldehyde in HIT cells, uptake of D-[^{14}C] glyceraldehyde was measured using a rapid oil-filtration technique. Uptake of 20mM D-glyceraldehyde was rapid, with an initial rate of approximately 3.8 nmol/μl intracellular space per minute and reaching equilibrium within 10–15 minutes. The initial rate of transport appeared to be unsaturable within the range 1–50mM D-glyceraldehyde implying a process of passive diffusion across the cell membrane. Furthermore, uptake of D-glyceraldehyde was not inhibited by L-glyceraldehyde (Table 1). Transport was, however, inhibited by the thiol reagent N-ethyl maleimide (NEM), suggesting the involvement of a protein carrier system. Inhibitors of glucose transport (phloretin) and alanine transport (methylaminoisobutyrate) did not, however, inhibit D-glyceraldehyde uptake. The initial rate of glyceraldehyde uptake appeared to be enhanced in the presence of monensin and in citrate

Table 1. Transport of 5mM D-[^{14}C]glyceraldehyde in HIT-T15 cells

Condition	n	Glyceraldehyde uptake (nmol/μl i/c space in 5 min)
Control	55	3.20 ± 0.14
+ 20 mM L-glyceraldehyde	4	4.28 ± 0.86
+ 0.1 mM NEM	4	2.26 ± 0.08*
+ 1 mM NEM	3	0.02 ± 0.002*
+ 5 mM Phloretin	7	5.05 ± 0.97
Citrate medium	4	5.23 ± 0.33*
140 mM K^+	4	2.32 ± 0.15*

*$p<0.05$

buffer, manipulations designed to alkalinize the cell interior, and reduced in a Na^+-free medium. In addition, depolarization of the cells with high $[K^+]$ was found to diminish the initial rate of glyceraldehyde uptake, suggesting that the transport of the triose could be an electrogenic process.

DISCUSSION

The results of the present study do not support the view that glyceraldehyde stimulates the β-cell via a mechanism analogous to glucose and other 'nutrient' type stimuli, that is by generation of a metabolic signal. First, neither the D- nor the L-isomer of glyceraldehyde appeared to be metabolized to an appreciable extent, at least via the glycolytic and TCA cycle (oxidative) pathways. The finding that glyceraldehyde is a poor metabolic substrate in HIT cells probably reflects a low activity of the enzyme triokinase, as has been previously demonstrated in β-cells[9]. Furthermore, the complete inhibition of glycolysis by iodoacetate failed to prevent the stimulatory actions of glyceraldehyde on HIT cells.

The question therefore arises of how glyceraldehyde does activate the β-cell. The simplest model which could explain all of the actions of glyceraldehyde would involve electrogenic transport of the triose via a H^+- or Na^+-dependent carrier, a model analogous to the transport of certain amino-acids[10,11]. Such a mechanism would account for the rapid depolarization elicited by addition of glyceraldehyde, the subsequent entry of Ca^{2+} via voltage-sensitive calcium channels and the secretion of insulin. The triose-coupled entry of H^+ or Na^+ could also, directly or indirectly, account for the intracellular acidification accompanying the above responses. Preliminary experiments designed to investigate the modality of glyceraldehyde uptake into HIT cells suggest that transport of the triose could be linked in some way to entry of Na^+ and/or H^+ into the cell. Such a possibility would be supported by the apparent electrogenicity of glyceraldehyde uptake. How this process might be effected is at present unclear, although it is in some respects reminiscent of the Na^+-dependent alanine transport system[12]. The fact that certain other monovalent cations, including H^+, can substitute for Na^+ might explain why the effects glyceraldehyde on membrane potential and especially pHi were not completely inhibited in Na^+-free media.

Whilst formation of L-lactate, an index of glycolysis, was negligible from glyceraldehyde, it was of interest that large amounts of D-lactate could be detected following incubation of HIT cells with glyceraldehyde. This finding implies the presence of significant quantities of methylglyoxal in the triose preparation. In the light of this possibility, it was notewothy that the intracellular acidification elicited by glyceraldehyde could be inhibited by dithiothreitol and by aminoguanidine, compounds which can protect the cell against the actions of a-ketoaldehydes such as methylglyoxal. Such compounds are known to exert profound effects on certain cellular enzymes, including ATP-ases[13]. In view of this, it is of interest to note that the effects of glyceraldehyde on both pHi and membrane potential could be inhibited to some extent by dithiothreitol and aminoguanidine, two substances which form stable adducts with a-ketoaldehydes, thereby protecting cells from the actions of the latter. Whether contaminants such as methylglyoxal contribute towards the effects of glyceraldehyde on HIT-T15 cells awaits further investigation.

ACKNOWLEDGMENTS

This work was supported by the North-Western Regional Health Authority.

REFERENCES

1. B. Hellman, L.-A. Idahl, A. Lernmark, J. Sehlin and I.-B. Taljedal, The pancreatic β-cell recognition of insulin secretagogues VIII Comparisons of glucose and glyceraldehyde isomers and dihydroxyacetone. Arch.Biochem.Biophys. 162: 448–457 (1974).
2. S.J.H. Ashcroft, L.C.C. Weerasinghe and P.J.Randle, Interrelationship of islet metabolism, ATP content and insulin release. Biochem.J. 132: 223–231 (1973).
3. K. Jain, J. Logothetopoulos and P. Zucker, The effects of D- and L- glyceraldehyde on glucose oxidation, insulin release and insulin biosynthesis by pancreatic islets of the rat. Biochim.Biophys.Acta 399: 384–394 (1975).
4. S.J.H. Ashcroft, P. Hammonds and D.E. Harrison, Insulin responses of a clonal cell line of symian virus 40-transformed cells. Diabetologia 29: 727–733 (1986).
5. C.B. Wollheim, S. Ullrich and T. Pozzan, Glyceraldehyde but not cAMP-stimulated insulin release is preceded by a rise in cytosolic free Ca^{2+}. Febs Lett. 177: 17–21 (1984).
6. M.J. Dunne, I. Findlay, O.H. Peteresen and C.B. Wollheim, ATP-sensitive K^{+} channels in an insulin-secreting cell line are inhibited by D-glyceraldehyde and activated by membrane permeabilisation. J.Membr.Biol. 93: 271–279 (1986).
7. A.C. Elliott, R. Trebilcock, A.P. Yates and L. Best, Stimulation of HIT-T15 insulinoma cells by glyceraldehyde does not require its metabolism. Eur.J.Biochem. 213: 359–365 (1993).
8. L. Best, R. Trebilcock and S. Tomlinson, Lactate transport in insulin-secreting β-cells: contrast between rat islets and HIT-T15 insulinoma cells. Mol.Cell.Endocr. 86: 49–56 (1992).
9. M.J. Macdonald, Does glyceraldehyde enter pancreatic islet metabolism via both the triokinase and glyceraldehyde phosphate dehydrogenase reactions? Arch.Biochem.Biophys. 270: 15–19 (1989).
10. A.E. Lambert, Y. Kanazawa, L. Orci and H.N. Christensen, Stimulation of insulin release by natural amino acids and their non-metabolized analogues. Diabetologia 6: 635–636 (1970).
11. J. Lerner, Effectors of amino acid transport processes in animal cell membranes. Comp.Biochem.Physiol. 81: 713–739 (1985).
12. B. Hellman, J. Sehlin and I-B. Taljedal, Uptake of alanine, arginine and leucine by mammalian pancreatic β-cells. Endocrinology 89: 1432–1439 (1971).
13. M.L. Mira, F. Martinho, M.S. Azevedo and C.F. Manso, Oxidative inhibition of red blood cell ATP-ases by glyceraldehyde. Biochim.Biophys.Acta 1060: 257–261 (1991).

26

OSCILLATIONS OF CYTOSOLIC Ca^{2+} IN PANCREATIC ISLETS OF LANGERHANS

Franz Martín, Jose A. G. Pertusa, and Bernat Soria*

Center for Bioengineering, Department of Physiology
Miguel Hernandez University
Alicante, Spain

INTRODUCTION

In the last decades evidences have accumulated implicating the involvement of cytoplasmic Ca^{2+} ($[Ca^{2+}]_i$) in stimulus-secretion coupling in isolated islets of Langerhans.

The mayor physiological stimulus for insulin release is an increase in the plasma glucose concentration. The accepted model for stimulus-secretion coupling implies that glucose stimulation elicits within b-cells a complex cascade of ionic, metabolic and effector events. Briefly, glucose interacts with a tissue-specific glucose transporter [1], enters the β-cell, and is rapidly metabolized. The ATP generated by glucose metabolism blocks the ATP-dependent K^+ channels (K_{ATP} channels) which in turn depolarizes the β-cell [2]. The depolarization causes the opening of voltage-dependent Ca^{2+}-channels [3], leading to Ca^{2+} entry [4]. This Ca^{2+} entry raises $[Ca^{2+}]_i$ to the level required for activating exocytocis of secretory granules. Thus, an increase in $[Ca^{2+}]_i$ is generally accepted as the mayor triggering event that induces insulin secretion [5]. Moreover, cytosolic Ca^{2+} dependence of insulin release has been directly measured using permeabilized islets [6].

In the intact islet, glucose-induced $[Ca^{2+}]_i$ increases have been demonstrated to be organized in oscillations of $[Ca^{2+}]_i$, which are a modulated by changes in glucose concentrations [7].

In this chapter we briefly review the role of the $[Ca^{2+}]_i$ oscillations in the whole islet and their relationship with insulin release.

NUTRIENT-INDUCED $[Ca^{2+}]_i$ OSCILLATIONS IN INTACT PANCREATIC ISLETS

Glucose-Induced $[Ca^{2+}]_i$ Oscillations

It has been previously shown [7], that intermediate glucose concentrations (7–17 mM) induced two types of $[Ca^{2+}]_i$ oscillations in mouse pancreatic islets: fast (frequency of 3.1 ±

* E-mail: bernat.soria@umh.es

Physiology and Pathophysiology of the Islets of Langerhans, edited by Soria.
Plenum Press, New York, 1997.

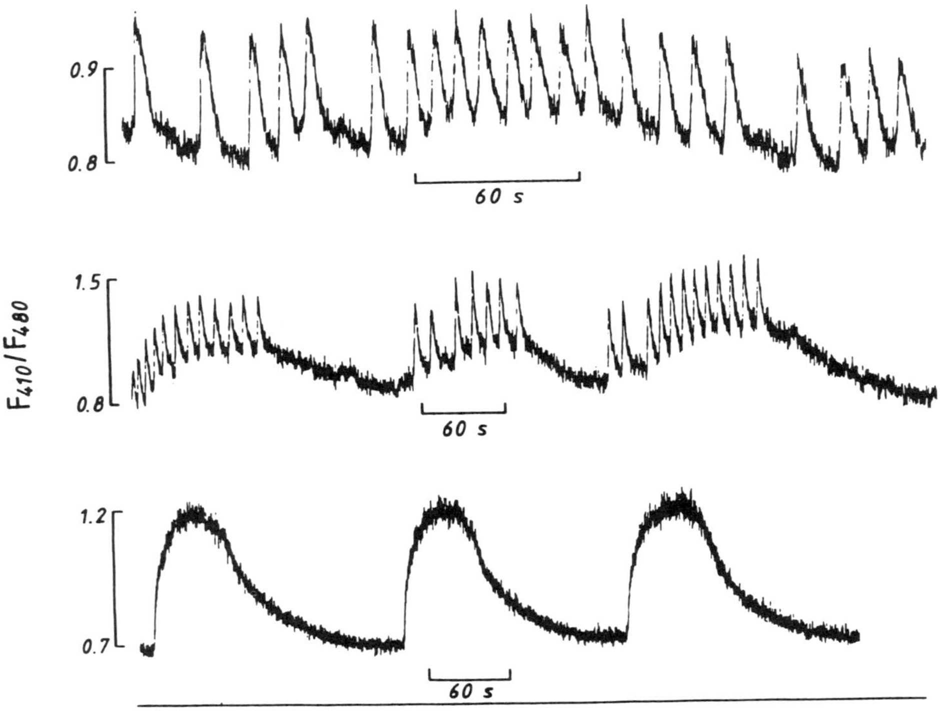

Figure 1. Two types of $[Ca^{2+}]_i$ oscillations recorded from 3 different islets in the presence of 11 mM glucose. The top panel shows a pattern of high-frequency oscillations with brief rising times ("fast" oscillations). The lower panel depicts a pure pattern of low-frequency, slowly developing ("slow") oscillations. The middle panel represents a mixed situation, with "fast" oscillations superimposing on "slow" $[Ca^{2+}]_i$ waves (taken from reference 7 with permission).

0.8 min^{-1}) and slow oscillations (frequency of 0.5 ± 0.2 min^{-1}). Fast oscillations are consistenly observed, their duration depend on glucose concentration [7] and occur synchronously in the whole islet [8, 9]. Contrariwise to that observed with the fast $[Ca^{2+}]_i$ oscillations, which have rising phases of 1–2 sec and falling phases of 10 sec, slow $[Ca^{2+}]_i$ oscillations have smooth rising phases of 0.5–0.2 min and even slower falling phases [7]. The slow $[Ca^{2+}]_i$ oscillations are found in less than 1/3 of the islets studied [7]. Two glucose-induced slow $[Ca^{2+}]_i$ oscillatory patterns are observed, the most frequent is a pure slow pattern, but occasionally a mixed pattern with fast oscillations superimposed on the top of the slow pattern is depicted [7]. In Fig. 1 we observe the different types of glucose-induced $[Ca^{2+}]_i$ oscillations.

Amino Acid-Induced $[Ca^{2+}]_i$ Oscillations. In addition to glucose, other nutrient substrates for b-cell metabolism produce a rapid reversible and dose-dependent decrease of K_{ATP} channel activity and therefore, changes in membrane potential, $[Ca^{2+}]_i$ and insulin secretion. As is the case for leucine and its deamination product alfa-ketoisocaproate (KIC). These nutrient secretagogues close K_{ATP} channels [10] and initiate electrical activity [11]. It has been recently shown that KIC, in the absence of glucose, is able to induce slow $[Ca^{2+}]_i$ oscillations with a frequency of 0.2 ± 0.13 min^{-1} [12]. This slow oscillatory pattern is preceded by a transient decrease of $[Ca^{2+}]_i$ levels [12]. Fast oscillations are frequently seen on the top of these KIC-induced slow $[Ca^{2+}]_i$ oscillations. These KIC-induced

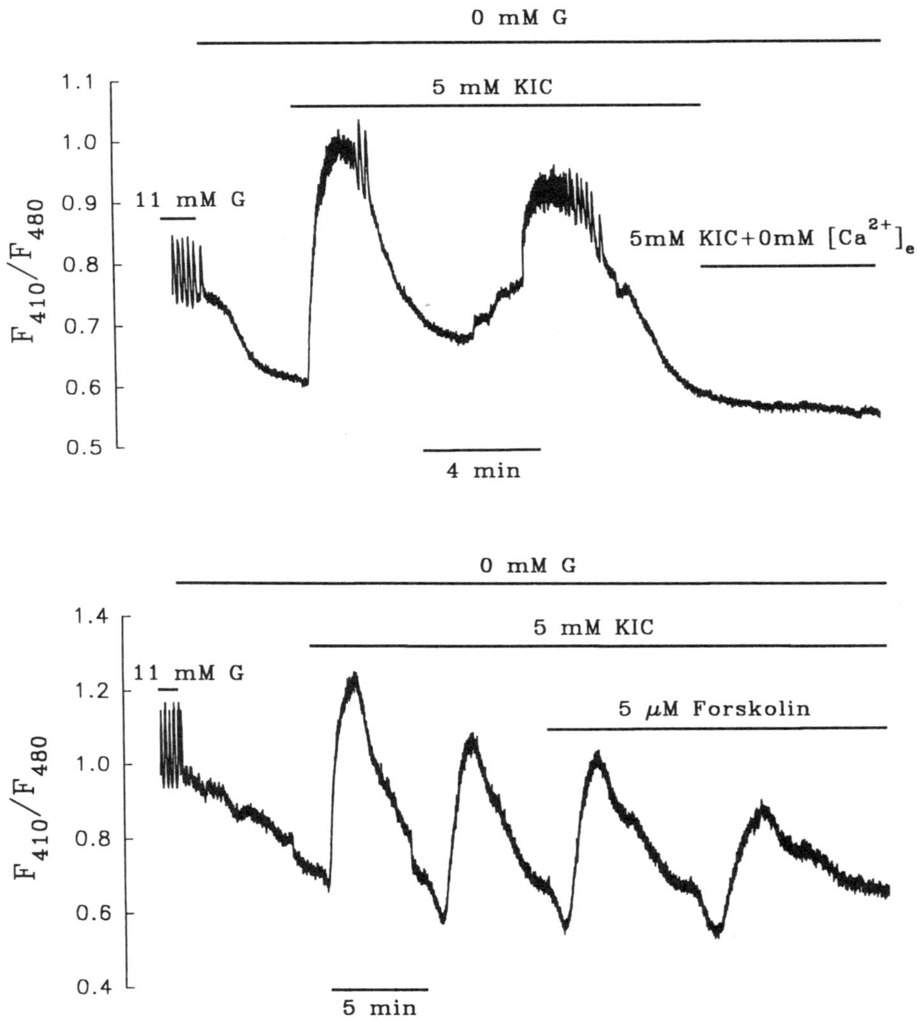

Figure 2. α-ketoisocaproate-induced slow $[Ca^{2+}]_i$ oscillations in the absence of glucose. The top panel shows 5 mM KIC-induced slow $[Ca^{2+}]_i$ oscillations in the absence of glucose and the effects of the absence of extracellular $[Ca^{2+}]_i$ on the 5 mM KIC-induced slow $[Ca^{2+}]_i$ oscillations. The lower panel represents the effects of 5 mM forskolin on 5 mM KIC-induced slow $[Ca^{2+}]_i$ oscillations (taken from reference 12 with permission).

slow $[Ca^{2+}]_i$ oscillations depend on extracellular $[Ca^{2+}]_i$ because omission of extracellular $[Ca^{2+}]_i$ abolish the KIC-induced slow $[Ca^{2+}]_i$ oscillations (Fig. 2) [12]. In addition, these slow $[Ca^{2+}]_i$ oscillations are not modulated by cAMP levels [12]. Figure 2 shows that 5 mM forskolin is unable to change the KIC-induced slow oscillatory pattern.

ORIGIN OF $[Ca^{2+}]_i$ OSCILLATIONS

Pancreatic β-cells in intact islets of Langerhans perfused with stimulatory glucose concentrations (11 mM) exhibit periodic bursting of electrical activity [13,14]. Subsequent

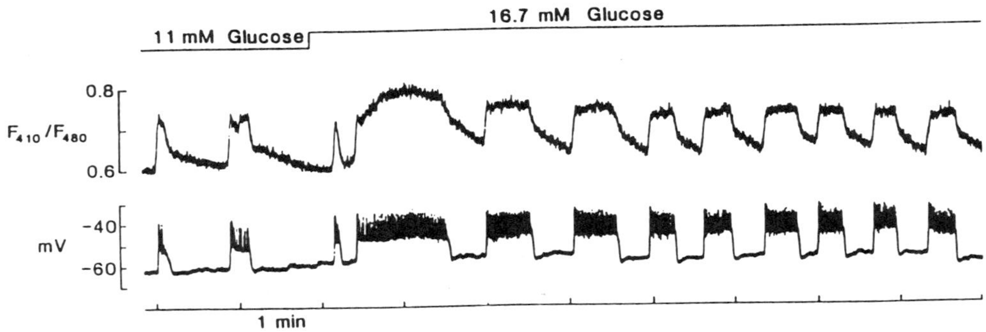

Figure 3. Modulation of β-cell membrane potential and islet $[Ca^{2+}]_i$ levels by glucose. Simultaneous measurements of the effects of increasing glucose concentration from 11 mM to 16.7 mM (step line) on $[Ca^{2+}]_i$ (top panel) and electrical activity (lower panel) (taken from reference 8 with permission).

increases in glucose concentration produce an increase in the duration of the burst and a diminution of the duration of the silent phases between bursts.

Using simultaneous measurements of membrane potential of a single β-cell and whole islet $[Ca^{2+}]_i$ levels, it has been recently reported that fast glucose-induced $[Ca^{2+}]_i$ oscillations are due to bursting of the electrical activity [8]. Moreover, raising glucose concentration from 11 mM to 16.7 mM increased the duration of the electrical bursting and of the respective $[Ca^{2+}]_i$ oscillation, remaining the amplitude of the $[Ca^{2+}]_i$ oscillation practically unchanged [8]. These results indicate that glucose regulates insulin release by a time-dependent or "duration" $[Ca^{2+}]_i$ code rather than an "amplitude" code. Figure 3 shows that fast oscillations are associated with bursting of the electrical activity.

To generate glucose-induced $[Ca^{2+}]_i$ oscillations, the β-cell must require efficient calcium removal/sequestering mechanisms, to rapidly extrude the cytosolic Ca^{2+} loads generated by the burst of electrical activity [15]. It has been proposed that the main mechanism responsible for removing cytosolic Ca^{2+} is dependent on metabolic energy and that such energy can be provided by nutrient metabolism. Such metabolic regulation is exerting its action through two mwchanisms. The first one consists in fueling the Ca^{2+}-transport mechanisms at the plasma membrane level and the Ca^{2+} pumps of intracellular stores. The second one is keeping the Na^+/Ca^{2+} exchange mechanism energized by keeping the appropiate Na+ and K^+ gradients by energizing the Na^+/K^+-ATPase. The interplay between both mechanisms may be crucial for shaping glucose-induced Ca^{2+} oscillations [16].

The mechanism responsible for slow $[Ca^{2+}]^i$ oscillations in the whole islet remains to be identified. Slow oscillations of $[Ca^{2+}]_i$ could be related to cyclic variations of the membrane potential [17], slow metabolic oscillations [18] or a so far unknown mechanism. Our recent experiments support the idea that b-cell electrical activity is one of the main mechanisms underlying slow $[Ca^{2+}]_i$ oscillations [12].

SYNCHRONIZATION OF THE CYTOPLASMIC Ca^{2+} SIGNAL

Several studies have shown a high degree of functional heterogeneity in isolated β-cells [19–21]. On the other hand, it is known that within the intact islet β-cells are coupled electrically, probably through gap junctions [22–23]. In intact islet, glucose-induced $[Ca^{2+}]_i$ response is well-organized in regular oscillations [7], suggesting that the whole

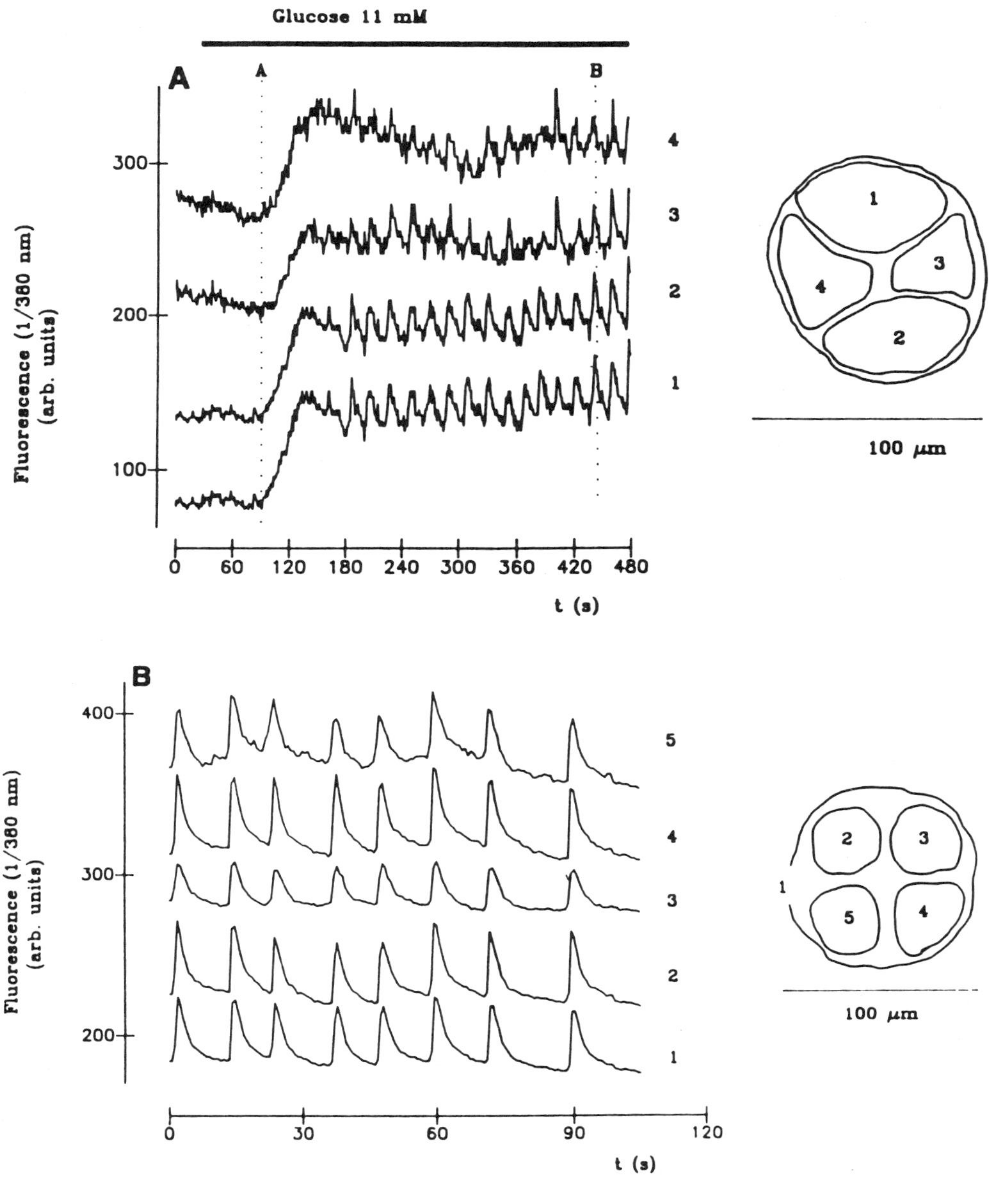

Figure 4. **A:** Initial response of an islet to a steep increase in glucose from 3 to 11 mM. The four traces represent the fluorescence signal analyzed in corresponding regions depicted on right. The 380 nm fluorescence signal was inverted, therefore an increase in fluorescence corresponds to an increase in $[Ca^{2+}]_i$. Records 2–4 have been displaced without changing the scale to facilitate comparison. **B:** $[Ca^{2+}]_i$ oscillations recorded in a different islet in the presence of 11 mM glucose. Trace 1 represents the mean fluorescence in whole islet, whereas traces 2–5 represent $[Ca^{2+}]_i$ changes in the islet regions depicted on right. Records 2–5 have been displaced without changing the scale (taken from reference 9 with permission).

islet is activated synchronously. Using fluorescence digital analysis of fura-2 loaded islets, it has been shown that glucose-induced $[Ca^{2+}]_i$ rise during the initial phase of the response, as well as $[Ca^{2+}]_i$ oscillations, are homogeneous throughout the islet (Fig. 4)[9].

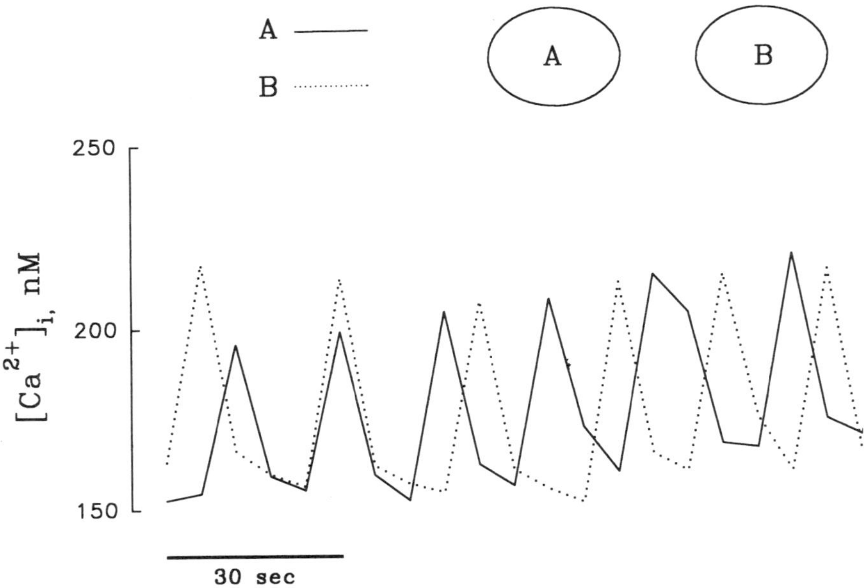

Figure 5. Simultaneous measurements of $[Ca^{2+}]_i$ oscillations in two isolated single islets. Islets were perifused with 11 mM glucose. $[Ca^{2+}]_i$ was measured 3 hours after islet isolation.

These results demonstrate that in response to glucose, the intact islet behaves as a functional syncytium and the functional heterogeneity among the β-cell population [19–21] is masked within the islet.

When analysing the mechanisms of synchrony it is essential to know how the islets interact the $[Ca^{2+}]_i$ signal with other islets inside the pancreas, to generate synchronized insulin pulses. One approach to this problem is to measure $[Ca^{2+}]_i$ in groups of isolated islets at the same time. Figure 5 shows that glucose-induced $[Ca^{2+}]_i$ oscillations measured at the same time, in two different islets are not coupled.

Our observation that isolated islets removed from the pancreatic organ and without innervation are unable of coordinate their $[Ca^{2+}]_i$ signal, together with the differences existing among the pulse periods of insulin release at different organizational levels, lead us to think that other factor plus $[Ca^{2+}]_i$ oscillations may account for the pulsatility of *in vivo* insulin secretion.

CORRELATION BETWEEN SLOW $[Ca^{2+}]_i$ OSCILLATIONS AND PULSATILE INSULIN RELEASE

Simultaneous measurements of whole islet $[Ca^{2+}]_i$ and insulin release have recently demonstrated that fast [24] and slow [12,25] $[Ca^{2+}]_i$ oscillations parallel oscillatory insulin release. This observation reinforces the point of view that $[Ca^{2+}]_i$ is a moment-to- moment regulator of insulin release. Figure 6 shows that slow $[Ca^{2+}]_i$ oscillations parallel oscillatory insulin release.

In the case of the slow $[Ca^{2+}]_i$ oscillations, this is relevant because pulsatile insulin release with periods of about 10 min have been described *in vivo* in humans [26]. Dis-

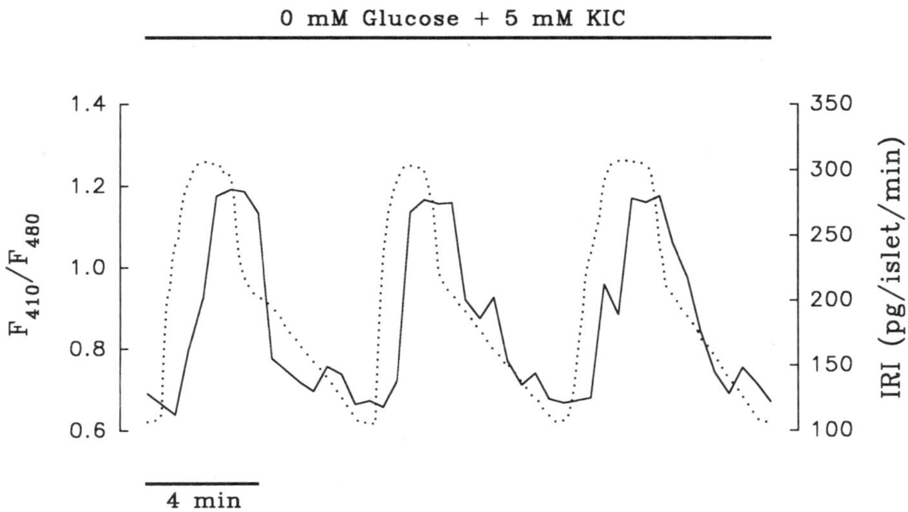

Figure 6. Simultaneous measurements of $[Ca^{2+}]_i$ oscillations and insulin release. Insulin release (—) and $[Ca^{2+}]_i$ (···) were measured simultaneously from single mouse islets. Islets were perifused with 5 mM KIC in the absence of glucose. Insulin relase record was corrected for the 20 sec delay between the chamber and the collection site. Insulin measurements (IRI) were made by triplicate. Temperature: 35 ± 1°C.

appearance of the periodic variations of the circulating insulin have been considered an early indicator of diabetes in man [27]. Furthermore, pulsed intravenously administered insulin has been shown to induce a greater hypoglycemic effect [28]. Since the slow $[Ca^{2+}]_i$ oscillations: (i) also appear when islets are incubated with other nutrient secretagogues (as leucine and KIC) [12], (ii) have periods of about 5–7 min [7,12] and (iii) do not represent a change in the total amount of released insulin (when compared with fast glucose-induced $[Ca^{2+}]_i$ oscillations), but in the dynamics of its appearance [12], we suggest that slow $[Ca^{2+}]_i$ oscillations mediate in the pulsatile insulin release observed *in vivo* under physiological conditions, when islets are exposed to a mixture of glucose and amino acids.

ACKNOWLEDGMENTS

This work was supported by Fondo de Investigaciones Sanitarias de la Seguridad Social (Grant FIS96-1994-01), Generalitat Valenciana and Commission for the European Communities (Contract ERBSC1-CT920833).

REFERENCES

1. Permutt, M.A., Korany, L., Keller, K., Lacy, P.E., Sharp, D.W., and Mueckler, M., 1989, Cloning and functional expression of human pancreatic islet glucose transporter cDNA, *Proc. Natl. Acad. Sci. USA 86*: 8688–8692.
2. Ashcroft, F.M., Harrison, D.E., and Ascroft, S.J.H., 1984, Glucose induces closure of single potassium channels in isolated rat pancreatic β-cells, *Nature 312*: 446–448.

3. Rorsman, P., and Trube, G., 1986, Calcium delayed potassium currents in mouse pancreatic β-cells under voltage clamp conditions, *J. Physiol. 374*: 531–550.
4. Valdeolmillos, M., Nadal, A., Contreras, D., and Soria, B., 1992, The relationship between glucose-induced K^+ ATP channel closure and the rise in $[Ca^{2+}]_i$ in single mouse pancreatic β-cells, *J. Physiol. 455*: 173–186.
5. Wollheim, C.B., and Pozzam, T., 1984, Correlation between cytosolic free Ca^{2+} and insulin release in an insulin-secreting cell line, *J. Biol. Chem. 259*: 2262–2267.
6. Jones, P.M., Stutchfield, J., and Howell, S.L., 1985, Effects of Ca^{2+} and a phorbol ester on insulin secretion from islets of Langerhans permeabilized by high-voltage discharges, *FEBS Lett. 191*: 102–106.
7. Valdeolmillos, M., Santos, R.M., Contreras, D., Soria, B., and Rosario, L.M., 1989, Glucose-induced oscillations of intracellular Ca^{2+} concentration resembling bursting electrical activity in single mouse islets of Langerhans, *FEBS Lett. 259*: 19–23.
8. Santos, R.M., Rosario, L.M., Nadal, A., Garcia-Sancho, J., Soria, B., and Valdeolmillos, M., 1991, Widespread synchronous $[Ca^{2+}]_i$ oscillations due to bursting electrical activity in single pancreatic islets, *Pflügers. Arch.-Eur. J. Physiol. 418*: 417–422.
9. Valdeolmillos, M., Nadal, A., Soria, B., and Garcia-Sancho, J., 1993, Fluorescence digital image analysis of glucose-induced $[Ca^{2+}]_i$ oscillations in mouse pancreatic islet of Langerhans, *Diabetes 42*: 1210–1214.
10. Ashcroft, F.M., Ashcroft, S.J.H., and Harrison, D.E., 1987, Effects of 2-keto-isocaproic acid on insulin release and single potassium channel activity in dispersed rat pancreatic β-cells, *J. Physiol. 385*: 517–529.
11. Henquin, J.C., and Meissner, H.P., 1981, Effects of amino acids on membrane potential and $^{86}Rb+$ fluxes in pancreatic β-cells, *Am. J. Physiol. 240*: E245–252.
12. Martin, F., Sanchez-Andres, J.V., and Soria, B., 1995, Slow $[Ca^{2+}]_i$ oscillations induced by ketoisocaproate in single mouse pancreatic islets, *Diabetes 44*: 300–305.
13. Dean, P.M., and Mathews, E.K., 1968, Electrical activity in pancreatic islet cells, *Nature 219*: 389–390.
14. Henquin, J.C., and Meissner, H.P., 1984, Significance of ionic fluxes and changes in membrane potential for stimulus-secretion coupling in pancreatic β-cells, *Experientia 40*: 1043–1052.
15. Sherman, A., and Rinzel, P., 1991, Model for synchronization of pancreatic β-cells by gap junction coupling, *Biophys. J. 59*: 547–559.
16. Nadal, A., Valdeolmillos, M., and Soria, B., 1994, Metabolic regulation of $[Ca^{2+}]_i$ in mouse pancreatic islets of Langerhans, *Am. J. Physiol.* 267(5): E769–E774.
17. Henquin, J.C., Meissner, H.P., and Schmeer, W., 1982, Cyclic variations of glucose-induced electrical activity in pancreatic b-cells, *Pflügers. Arch. 393*: 322–327.
18. Longo, E., Tornheim, K., Deeney, J., Varnum, B., Tillotson, D., Prentki, M., and Corkey, B., 1991, Oscillations of cytosolic free Ca^{2+}, oxygen consumption, and insulin secretion in glucose stimulated rat pancreatic islets, *J. Biol. Chem. 266*: 9314–9319.
19. Schuit, F.C., Int't Veld, P.A., and Pipeleers, D.G., 1988, Glucose stimulates proinsulin biosynthesis by a dose-dependent recruitment of pancreatic b-cells, *Proc. Natl. Acad. Sci. USA 85*: 3865–3869.
20. Salomon, D. and Meda, P., 1986, Heterogeneity and contact-dependent regulation of hormone secretion by individual β-cells, *Exp. Cell. Res. 162*: 507–520.
21. Pipeleers, D.G., 1992, Heterogeneity in pancreatic β-cells population, *Diabetes 41*: 777–781.
22. Meissner, H.P., 1974, Electrophysiological evidence for coupling between β-cells of pancreatic islets, *Nature (Lond) 262*: 502–504.
23. Eddlestone, G.T., Goncalves, A., Bangham, J.A. and Rojas, E, 1984, Electrical coupling between cells in islets of Langerhans from the mouse, *J. Membr. Biol. 77*: 1–14.
24. Gilon, P., Shepherd, R.M., and Henquin, J.C., 1993, Oscillations of secretion driven by oscillations of cytoplasmic calcium as evidenced in single pancreatic islets, *J. Biol. Chem. 268*: 22265–22268.
25. Bergsten, P., Grapengiesser, E., Gylfe, E., Tengholm, A., and Hellman, B., 1994, Synchronous oscillations of cytoplasmic Ca^{2+} and insulin release in glucose-stimulated pancreatic islets, *J. Biol. Chem. 269*: 8749–8753.
26. Lang, D.A., Matthews, D.R., Peto, J., and Turner, R.C., 1979, Cyclic oscillations of basal plasma glucose and insulin concentrations, *N. Engl. J. Med. 301*: 1023–1027.
27. O'Rahilly, S., Turner, R.C., and Matthews, D.R., 1988, Impaired pulsatile secretion of insulin in relatives of patients with non-insulin dependent diabetes mellitus, *N. Engl. J. Med. 318*: 1225–1230.
28. Matthews, D.R., Naylor, B.A., Jones, R.G., Ward, G.M., and Turner, R.C., 1983, Pulsatile insulin has greater hypoglycemic effects than continuous delivery, *Diabetes 32*: 617–621.

EFFECTS OF LOCALIZED PULSES OF HIGH K^+ AND CARBACHOL ON $[Ca^{2+}]_i$ IN PANCREATIC ISLETS OF LANGERHANS

Ana Gomis and Miguel Valdeolmillos

Departamento de Fisiología and
Instituto de Neurociencias
Facultad de Medicina
Universidad Miguel Hernandez
03080 Alicante, Spain

INTRODUCTION

Pancreatic β-cells, naturally exist aggregated forming the islet of Langerhans. Isolated β-cells show a marked variability in their response to secretagogues. The variability is found for instance in their electrical response to glucose[1], changes in intracellular calcium ($[Ca^{2+}]_i$)[2] and insulin release[3–4]. Such variability contrast with the homogeneous response of the islet of Langerhans, at least with regard to glucose-induced electrical activity[5] and $[Ca^{2+}]_i$ oscillations[6].

Experimental data shows that in the islet of Langerhans, β-cells are electrically[8] and dye coupled[9–10] by gap-junctions. Furthermore, the establishment of gap-junctions, made of a protein of the conexin family called Cx43[11] increases insulin secretion[12]. Work in hepatocytes has shown that gap-junctions (formed by the conexin Cx32) are permeable to $[Ca^{2+}]_i$ and other second messengers[13]. Therefore, junctional communication between β-cells may explain the observed synchronous response of the islets. Recent mathematical models[14] incorporating a realistic junctional conductance[15] between heterogeneous cells, can reproduce the synchronous oscillatory pattern recorded experimentally. Besides to gap-junctions, other factors like the observed oscillatory changes in extracellular potassium[16] may contribute to synchronize the islet response[17].

In this work we have examined the effects of pulses of high potassium and of the muscarinic agonist carbachol delivered to one pole of the islet and analyzed the effect on $[Ca^{2+}]_i$ in other regions of the islet. Our aim was to test if junctional communication between β-cells allows the spreading of Ca^{2+} signals.

Physiology and Pathophysiology of the Islets of Langerhans, edited by Soria.
Plenum Press, New York, 1997.

MATERIALS AND METHODS

Mouse islets of Langerhans were isolated by collagenase digestion as previously described[18]. Once isolated the islets were kept at 25°C in modified Krebs medium. $[Ca^{2+}]_i$ was monitored from single islets by measuring the fluorescence emitted by fura-2[19]. Islets were loaded with fura-2 by incubation with 2 μM of fura-2/AM (Molecular Probes, Junction City, OR) for 30 min at room temperature in standard incubation medium of the following composition (mM): 120 NaCl; 5 KCl; 25 $NaCO_3H$; 2.5 $CaCl_2$ and 1.1 $MgCl_2$. The medium was constantly gassed with 95% O_2/5% CO_2 for a final pH of 7.4. Loaded islets were transferred to an incubation chamber whose bottom was a cover slip treated with polilysine to improve their adherence. The chamber was placed on the microscope (Nikon Diaphot) stage and thermostated to 37°C. Perfusion (2–4 ml/min) with gassed solutions was started by gravity feed from reservoirs 1m above the microscope stage.

The islets were epi-illuminated alternately at 340 and 380 nm using a filter wheel with the adequate interference optical filters. Light emitted above 520 nm was amplified with an image intensifier (Hamamatsu), recorded by a CCD camera (DAGE MTI72) and analyzed using a M4 system (Imaging Res. Inc., Ontario, Canada). Fluorescence measurements were corrected for background fluorescence and dark camera current . Four video frames at each wavelength were averaged, with an overall time resolution of 3s for each pair of images at alternative wavelengths. The resulting images were rated (340/380) pixel by pixel to produce ratio images and $[Ca^{2+}]_i$ was calculated by interpolation into a look-up table constructed by imaging fura-2 solutions with known Ca^{2+} concentrations using the same microscope objective (Nikon, fluorite 40×, oil). The focal plane was intended to be equatorial, obtained by focusing the islets with its maximal diameter and sharper edges.

The solution with high potassium or carbachol was pressure-injected through a wide-bore patch pipette positioned close to one pole of the islet and oblique to the main flow, as schematically represented in Figure 1A. The islets were digitally divided into 4 square zones of 30x30 μm, as indicated in the diagram. In all the experiments, zone 1 is the more close to the patch pipette. The pulses were delivered by means of a Picospritzer and ranged in duration from 0.5 to 20 seconds.

RESULTS AND DISCUSSION

Figure 1B shows the effect of a pulse of 40 mM K^+ and 5 seconds of duration on $[Ca^{2+}]_i$ in the regions of the islet depicted in Figure 1A. The largest Ca^{2+} peak is localized in the region closer to the patch pipette and gradually decreases in amplitude in more distal zones. In all the regions of the islet the $[Ca^{2+}]_i$ peak takes place simultaneously. Essentially the same results were obtained with shorter (down to 0.5 s) pulses. Figure 1C shows a plot of the $[Ca^{2+}]_i$ peak in each zone of the islet (filled circles) normalized with respect to the change obtained in zone 1. In parallel experiments the distribution of the injected solution was monitored by loading the patch pipette with a standard solution containing fluorescein. At the wavelengths used, the injection of fluorescein decreases the fluorescence of fura-2 loaded islets. Figure 1C (hollow triangles) shows the normalized decrease in fluorescence produced by the injection of fluorescein in the same regions of the islet. The decrease in fluorescence produced by fluorescein has a similar distribution than the Ca^{2+} peaks produced by the high K^+ solution, suggesting that the changes in $[Ca^{2+}]_i$ observed with the K^+ solution reflects the distribution of extracellular K^+ in the different areas of the islet. In the experiments with high K^+ pulses, we never saw peaks of high

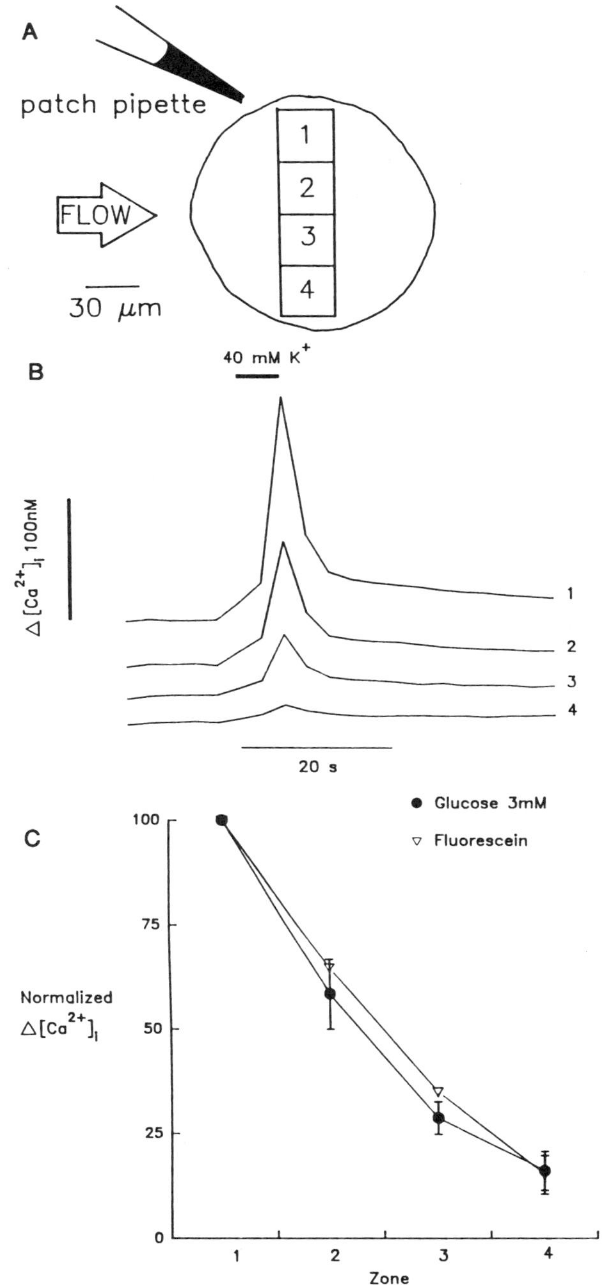

Figure 1. **A:** Schematic diagram showing the regions in which the islets of Langerhans were divided. Each zone corresponds to a square of 30 × 30 μm. The position of the injecting patch pipette was oblique to the main solution flow. **B:** Effect of a 40 mM K^+ pulse of 5 seconds of duration on $[Ca^{2+}]_i$ in the regions of the islet indicated in figure1A. Records 2–4 have been displaced without changing the scale to facilitate comparison, the same applies for the rest of the figures. The glucose concentration in this experiment was 3 mM. **C:** Changes in $[Ca^{2+}]_i$ in the different zones of the islet produced by the K^+ pulse and normalized with respect to zone 1 (filled circles). The graph also shows (hollow triangles) normalized changes in fluorescence produced by the injection of fluorescein dissolved in standard solution (5 mM K^+), and reflects the distribution of the injected solution in the vicinity of the islet. The data represents the mean ± S.E. of 12 pulses for glucose and 4 in the case of fluorescein.

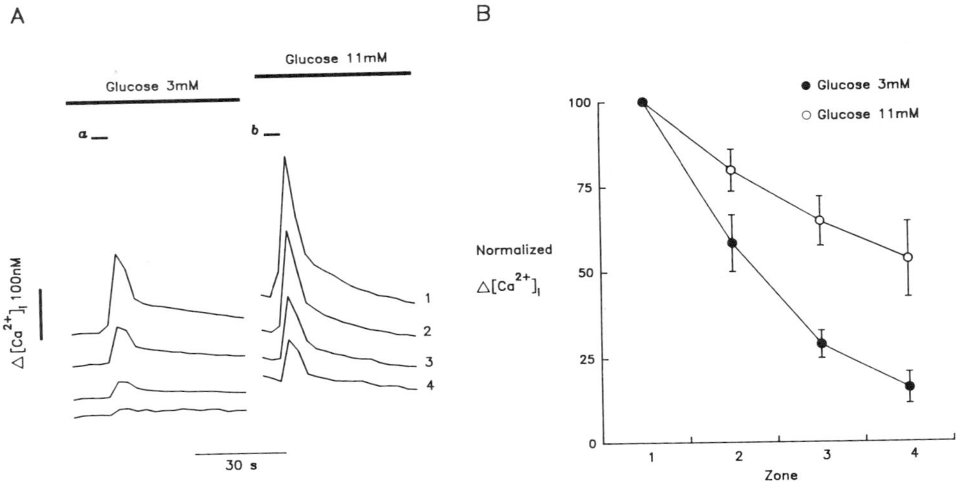

Figure 2. **A:** Effect of an increase in glucose concentration from 3 to 11 mM on the $[Ca^{2+}]_i$ peak produced by 40 mM K^+ pulses ("*a*" and "*b*", indicated by the short bars above the records) in the different regions of the islet. The gap between the two records represents an interval of 10 minutes. The increase in the resting levels of $[Ca^{2+}]_i$ in each area of the islet in 11 mM glucose with respect to 3 mM glucose is genuine. **B:** Normalized changes in $[Ca^{2+}]_i$ in the indicated zones of the islets in 3 mM glucose (filled circles) and 11 mM glucose (hollow circles). The data represents the mean ± S.E. of 7 different islets.

$[Ca^{2+}]_i$ after the cessation of the stimulus. Such "secondary peaks" would be expected if β-cells gap-junctions were permeable to Ca^{2+}, allowing the permeation of the cation with a certain delay, as has been shown in hepatocytes[13].

Previous work in islets of Langerhans measuring the electrical coupling with two microelectrodes[8] has shown that the coupling ratio (estimated by measuring the change in voltage in one cell due to current injection in another cell) increases with the concentration of glucose in the range from 0 up to 22 mM. The precise mechanism by which glucose increases junctional coupling is unknown. Figure 2A shows the effect of increasing glucose from 3 to 11 mM on K^+-induced $[Ca^{2+}]_i$ transients. The K^+ pulse in "*a*" shows the effect in the different regions of the islet in the presence of 3 mM glucose, producing Ca^{2+} peaks similar to the ones shown in Figure 1B. When glucose was increased to 11 mM, this leads to an increase in $[Ca^{2+}]_i$ in all the regions. Now, a high K^+ pulse (pulse "*b*") produced a higher Ca^{2+} peak in all the regions. When the data is normalized with respect to zone 1, as shown in Figure 2B, the more distal zones to the K^+ injection shown a relative increase in their Ca^{2+} peak. The relative increase in Ca^{2+} may be produced by several mechanisms. It is possible that the increased electrical coupling due to glucose, leads to a more effective propagation of the depolarization induced in zone 1 to the other zones. It is also possible that the depolarization produced by glucose will change the degree of activation of the Ca^{2+} channels. Given the non-linear current-voltage relationship of the Ca^{2+}-channels, now the same pulse of K^+ will produce a different change in the magnitude of the Ca^{2+} peak in the different regions of the islet. To distinguish between such possibilities we used diazoxide, a drug that directly activates the ATP-dependent K^+-channel[20], preventing the depolarization produced by glucose.

Figure 3A shows the effect of diazoxide on K^+-induced Ca^{2+} transients. The pulse labeled "*a*" was delivered under control conditions (glucose 3 mM).

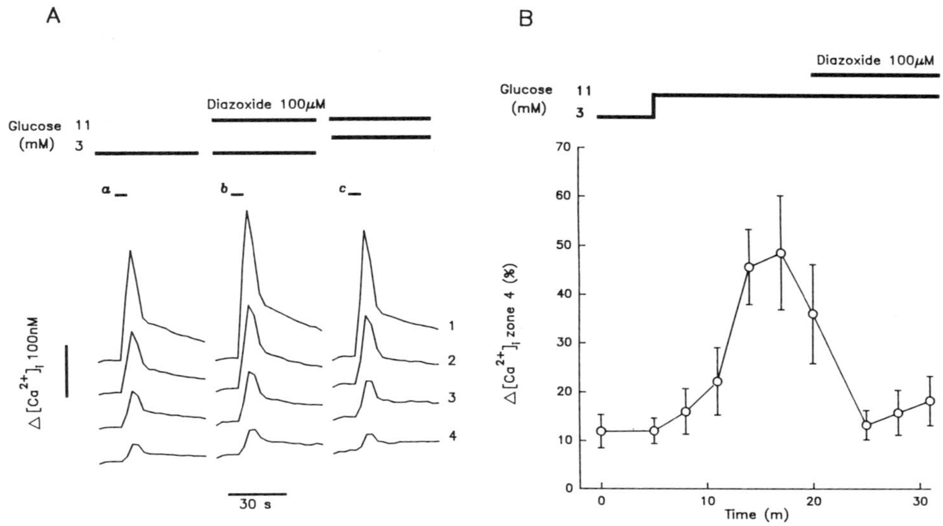

Figure 3. **A:** Effects of diazoxide on the $[Ca^{2+}]_i$ peak induced by 40 mM K^+ pulses ("*a*", "*b*" and "*c*") at different glucose concentrations. The addition of diazoxide and the change in glucose concentration are indicated by the bars at the top of the record. The gaps between the records correspond to 5 and 10 minutes respectively. **B:** Time course of the changes in $[Ca^{2+}]_i$ obtained in region 4 (normalized with respect to region 1) induced by 40 mM K^+ pulses produced by increasing glucose from 3 to 11 mM and then adding diazoxide (indicated by the bars on top of the record). The data represents the mean ± S.E. of 6 different islets.

Pulse "*b*" was delivered in the presence of 100 μM diazoxide. Here the increase in Ca^{2+} in the different zones is slightly larger than in the control situation, however, on average such increase is not significative. When in the continuous presence of diazoxide, glucose is increased from 3 to 11 mM, there are not changes in the resting levels of $[Ca^{2+}]_i$, as expected by the action of diazoxide. Furthermore, now a K^+ pulse ("*c*") does not induce the increase in the Ca^{2+} peaks observed in the absence of diazoxide (see Figure 2A). Figure 3B shows data from similar experiments but performed in the reverse order. For clarity, here only one of the zones (zone 4, where the effect of glucose is more prominent, see Figure 2B) is shown. The results are expressed as the percentage of increase in $[Ca^{2+}]_i$ obtained in zone 4 normalized with respect to zone 1. In the presence of 3 mM glucose, the Ca^{2+} transient measured in zone 4, represents approximately 10% of the transient elicited in zone 1. The increase in glucose leads to an increase in the relative peak up to approximately 50%. Now, adding diazoxide reverses the effect of glucose and decreases the relative Ca^{2+} peak toward resting values. These results suggest that the increase in the Ca^{2+} peaks observed in the presence of elevated levels of glucose are due to the membrane depolarization produced in all the regions of the islet and not by an increase in the coupling ratio.

Work in hepatocytes has shown that Inositol 1,4,5-trisphosphate (IP3) can permeate through gap-junctions[13]. Pancreatic β-cells posses cholinergic muscarinic receptors whose activation leads to an increase in the levels of IP_3 and the release of Ca^{2+} from intracellular stores[21]. The activation of such receptors also produce membrane depolarization[22].

In other group of experiments, we investigate the effect of carbachol (Cch) on Ca^{2+}. Figure 4A compares the effect of a K^+ pulse (upper panel) with a 5 seconds pulse of Cch (lower panel) in different regions of the same islet.

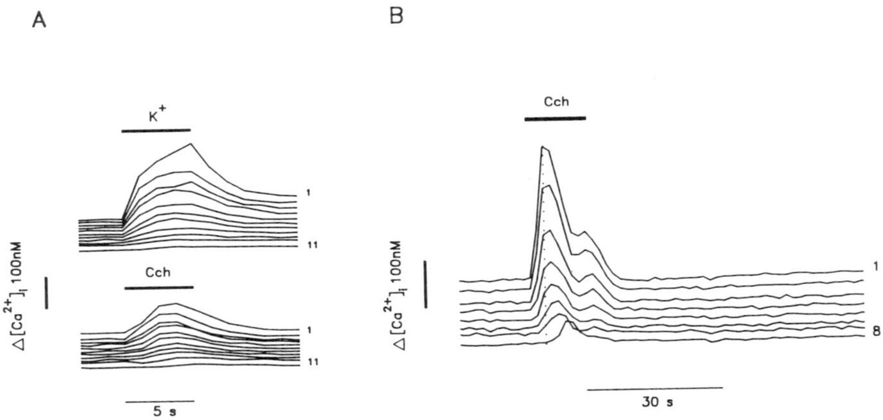

Figure 4. **A:** Comparison of the effects of a pulse of 40 mM K^+ (upper panel) and 1 mM carbachol (lower panel), both of 5 seconds of duration, on $[Ca^{2+}]_i$. In this experiment the islet (diameter=150 mm) was divided in 11 zones. **B:** Effect of a pulse of carbachol (1 mM) of 15 seconds of duration on $[Ca^{2+}]_i$. The islet (diameter=130 mm) was divided in 8 consecutive zones. Experiment representative of 16 pulses of Cch in 5 islets.

Cch produces a Ca^{2+} peak of decreasing amplitude as the distance of the region with respect to the pipette increases. However the peak occur simultaneously in all the areas. No secondary peaks were seen after the cessation of the Cch pulse. Figure 4B shows the effect of a longer pulse (15 seconds) of Cch. Here the shape of the Ca^{2+} transient is different, consisting of a first peak followed by a sustained Ca^{2+} plateau. The peak in the most distal areas (zone 8) with respect to the patch pipette is clearly delayed with respect to the closer ones (zone 1), as indicated by the dotted line in the figure. Such delay could be due to a propagated signal. However, given the fact that once the pulse ends, no delayed Ca^{2+} peaks were seen, we rather think that the delay is due to the lower Cch concentration reached in the distal areas of the islet, requiring therefore more time to attain a stimulatory concentration.

In conclusion, our results indicate that a rise in $[Ca^{2+}]_i$ produced by K^+ depolarization in a restricted area of the islet is not propagated to distal zones. In the case of carbachol, the $[Ca^{2+}]_i$ peaks in different zones does not occur simultaneously, suggesting that it may be a propagated signal. However, this result can also be explained taken into account the concentration gradients around the islets as a consequence of the localized pulse of Cch. We have been unsuccessful in recording spreading Ca^{2+} signals induced by K^+ pulses. This may be due to technical limitations, as we are measuring changes in fluorescence of zones which are to same degree contaminated by the fluorescence of neighbor areas. However, the fact that under some experimental conditions, for instance with Cch pulses, we can record delayed Ca^{2+} peaks, argues against such possibility. More likely, the absence of Ca^{2+} spreading signals may be due to the fact that under our experimental conditions, the active (depolarized) cells are in contact with the large conductance load that represents the inactive cells that act as a current sink.

ACKNOWLEDGMENTS

This work was supported by Grant (94/1345) from the Fondo de Investigaciones Sanitarias de la Seguridad Social (Spain). The authors thanks to A. Perez Vergara and S. Moya for expert technical help.

REFERENCES

1. Smith, P., Ashcroft, F. M. & Rorsman, P. (1990) Simultaneous recording of glucose-dependent electrical activity and ATP^+-regulated K^+-currents in isolated mouse pancreatic β-cells. FEBS Lett. 261, 187–190.
2. Hellman,B., Gylfe, E., Grapengiesser, E., Lund, P-E. & Berts, A. (1992) Cytoplasmic Ca^{2+} oscillations in pancreatic β-cells. Biochem. Biophys. Acta 1113: 295–305.
3. Salomon, D. & Meda, P. (1986) Heterogeneity and contact-dependent regulation of hormone secretion by individual β-cells. Exp. cell. Res. 162: 507–520.
4. Hiriart, M. & Matteson, D.R. (1988) Na channels and two types of Ca-channels in rat pancreatic β-cells identified by the reverse hemolytic plaque assay. J. Gen. Physiol. 91: 617–639.
5. Meissner, H. P. (1976) Electrophysiological evidence for coupling between beta cells of pancreatic islets. Nature 262: 502–504.
6. Santos, R.M., Rosario, L.M., Nadal, A., García-Sancho, J., Soria, B. & Valdeolmillos, M. (1991) Widespread synchronous $[Ca^{2+}]_i$ oscillations due to bursting electrical activity in single pancreatic islets. Pflügers Arch. 418: 417–422.
7. Valdeolmillos, M., Nadal, A., Soria, B. & García-Sancho, J. (1993) Fluorescence digital image analysis of glucose-induced $[Ca^{2+}]_i$ oscillations in mouse pancreatic Islets of Langerhans. Diabetes 42: 1210–14.
8. Eddlestone, G.T., Gonçalves, A., Bangham, J.A. & Rojas, E. (1984) Electrical coupling between cells in Islets of Langerhans from mouse. J. Membrane Biol. 77: 1–14.
9. Michaels, R.L., and Sheridan, J.D. (1981) Islets of Langerhans: Dye coupling among immunocytochemicaly distinct cell types. Science 214: 801–803.
10. Meda, P., Santos, R.M., and Atwater, I. (1986) Direct identification of electrophysiologically monitored cells within intact mouse islets of Langerhans. Diabetes 35: 232–236.
11. Meda, P., Bosco, D., Giordano, E., and Chanson, M., (1991) Junctional coupling modulation by secretogogues in two-cell pancreatic systems, In: "Biophysics of Gap Junction Channels." C. Peracchia, ed. CRC Press, Boca Raton.
12. Bosco D., Orci, L., Meda, P., (1989) Homologous but not heterologous contact increases the insulin secretion of individual pancreatic β-cells. Exp. Cell Res. 184: 72–80.
13. Saez, J.C., Connor, J.A., Spray, D., and Bennett, M.V.L. (1989) Hepatocyte gap junctions are permeable to the second messenger inositol 1,4,5,-triphosphate, and to calciumions. Proc. Natl. Acad. Sci. USA 86:2708–2712.
14. Smolen, P., Rinzel, J., and Sherman, A., (1993) Why pancreatic islets burst but single β cells do not. Biophys. J. 64: 1668–1680.
15. Perez-Armendariz, M., Roy, D.C., Spray, D.C. and Bennett, M.V.L., (1991) Biophysical Properties of gap junctions between freshly dispersed pairs of mouse pancreatic beta cells. Biophys. J. 59: 76–92.
16. Perez-Armendariz, M., and Atwater, I., (1986) Glucose-evoked changes in $[K^+]$ and $[Ca^{2+}]$ in the intercellular space of the mouse Islet of Langerhans. In: Biophysics of the Pancreatic B-cell. Atwater, I., Rojas, E., and Soria, B., eds. Plenum Press Publishing Corp. NY, pp. 31–51.
17. Stokes, C.L., and Rinzel, J. (1993) Diffusion of extracellular K+ an synchronize bursting oscillations in a model Islet of Langerhans. Biophys. J. 65: 597–607.
18. Lenmmark, A. (1974) The preparation of, and studies on, free cell suspensions from nouse pancreatic islets. Diabetologia 10: 431–438.
19. Grynkiewicz, G., Poenie, M., and Tisen R.Y. (1985) A new generation of Ca^{2+} indicators with greatly improved fluorescence properties. J. Biol. Chem. 260: 3440–3450.
20. Trube, G., Rorsman, P., and Ohno-Shosaku, T. (1986) Opposite effects of tolbutamide and diazoxide on the ATP-dependent K+ channel in mouse pancreatic β-cells. Pflügers Arch. 407: 493–499.
21. Gylfe, E. (1991) Carbachol induces sustained glucose-dependent oscillations of cytoplasmic Ca^{2+} in hyperpolarized pancreatic β-cells. Pflügers Arch. 419: 639–643.
22. Santos, R.M., and Rojas, E. (1989) Muscarinic receptor modulation of glucose-induced electrical activity in mouse pancreatic β-cells. FEBS Lett. 249: 411–417.

CYCLIC AMP, A MEDIATOR OF GLP-1, ACTS IN CONCERT WITH GLUCOSE AND TOLBUTAMIDE TO INCREASE CYTOSOLIC Ca^{2+} IN PANCREATIC B-CELLS

Kazuro Yaekura,[1,2] Masanori Nakata,[1] Hiromitsu Tanaka,[2] and Toshihiko Yada[1,*]

[1]Department of Physiology
[2]First Department of Internal Medicine
Kagoshima University School of Medicine
8-35-1 Sakuragaoka, Kagoshima 890, Japan

INTRODUCTION

Cyclic AMP (cAMP) plays an important role in the regulation of islet B-cell function and stimulates insulin release in a glucose-dependent manner[1]. Several physiologic peptides such as truncated glucagon-like peptide-1 (GLP-1), gastric inhibitory peptide (GIP) and glucagon are known to elevate cAMP level in islets and stimulate insulin release also in a glucose-dependent manner[1–4]. It has been recently shown that both a rise in cAMP and these peptides increase the cytosolic free Ca^{2+} concentration ($[Ca^{2+}]_i$) in pancreatic B-cells[3–7], the key intracellular signal that triggers exocytosis of insulin[8,9]. The increase in $[Ca^{2+}]_i$ is also glucose-dependent[6] and is tightly linked to insulin release[3]. However, the mechanisms for the glucose-dependent action of cAMP to increase $[Ca^{2+}]_i$ is not well understood. Whether cAMP increases $[Ca^{2+}]_i$ via specific cooperation with glucose, a fuel secretagogue, or also with other types of insulin secretagogues is of particular importance. Whether the glucose-dependent action of the peptides to increase $[Ca^{2+}]_i$ is mediated by a rise in cAMP is not thoroughly determined.

In the present study, we measured $[Ca^{2+}]_i$ in single rat pancreatic B-cells by dual-wavelength fura-2 microfluorometry and investigated the effects of the agents that raise cAMP and GLP-1 in combination with glucose, tolbutamide and high K^+. We found that both cAMP and GLP-1 acted in synergism with glucose or tolbutamide but not with high K^+ in increasing $[Ca^{2+}]_i$ in B-cells.

* To whom all correspondence should be addressed. Fax: 81-992-75-5231.

Physiology and Pathophysiology of the Islets of Langerhans, edited by Soria.
Plenum Press, New York, 1997.

MATERIALS AND METHODS

Solutions and Chemicals

Measurements were carried out in Krebs Ringer bicarbonate buffer (KRB) solution composed of 129 mM NaCl, 5.0 mM $NaHCO_3$, 4.7 mM KCl, 1.2 mM KH_2PO_4, 1.0 mM $CaCl_2$, 1.2 mM $MgSO_4$ and 10 mM HEPES at pH 7.4 supplemented with 0.1% bovine serum albumin. Fetal bovine serum was from Flow Laboratories. Fura-2, fura-2/acetoxymethylester and EGTA were from Dojin Chemical (Kumamoto, Japan). Dibutyryl-adenosine-3′,5′-monophosphate (db-cAMP) was from Boehringer. Forskolin and 3-isobutyl-1-methyl-xanthine (IBMX) were from Sigma. GLP-1(7-36)amide was from Peninsula Lab. (Belmont, CA). Tolbutamide (TB) was from Nacalai Tesque (Kyoto, Japan).

Preparation and Selection of Islet B-Cells

Islets of Langerhans were isolated from Wistar rats aged 8–12 weeks by collagenase digestion and immediately dispersed into single cells in Ca^{2+}-free KRB with 1 mM EGTA. The single cells were plated on the coverglass and cultured for 1–3 days in Eagle's MEM containing 5.6 mM glucose supplemented with 10% fetal bovine serum, 100 μg/ml streptomycin and 100 U/ml penicillin at 37°C in a 95% air plus 5% CO_2 atmosphere before experiments. The cells during this period responded to glucose, db-cAMP, GLP-1 and tolbutamide in a consistent manner. B-cells were selected according to the previously reported procedure[6]. Briefly, when the cells with a diameter of 12.5–17.5 μm were examined, the majority of the cells responded to glucose (8.3, 16.7 mM) and almost all the cells to tolbutamide (300 μM) with increases in $[Ca^{2+}]_i$, the responses typical of B-cells[10]. Data from such glucose- and TB-responsive cells were analyzed.

Measurement of $[Ca^{2+}]_i$

$[Ca^{2+}]_i$ was measured by a dual-wavelength microfluorometry[11] according to the previously reported method[10,12]. In brief, the single cells were incubated with 1 μM fura-2/acetoxymethylester for 30 min at 37°C in KRB containing 2.8 mM glucose. The cells were then mounted in a chamber and superfused using a peristaltic pump (Watson Marlow, Cornwall, United Kingdom) at 1 ml/min at 37°C with KRB with basal (2.8 mM) or elevated glucose concentrations (8.3 and 16.7 mM). The fura-2 loaded cells were excited at 340 nm and 380 nm alternately every one second, the emission signals at 510 nm were detected by a photomultiplier, and the ratio of the two signals was produced by P1 system (Nikon, Tokyo, Japan). Alternately, fura-2 fluorescence was detected every 2.5 sec by an intensified charge coupled device (ICCD) camera, and the ratio was produced by Argus-50 system (Hamamatsu Photonics, Hamamatsu, Japan).

RESULTS AND DISCUSSION

Effects of a Rise in cAMP and GLP-1 in Combination with Glucose, Tolbutamide and High K^+ on $[Ca^{2+}]_i$ in Pancreatic B-Cells

In the presence of a basal glucose concentration (2.8 mM), 5 mM db-cAMP failed to alter the resting $[Ca^{2+}]_i$ level. An elevation of the glucose concentration from 2.8 to 8.3 mM, a stimulatory concentration for insulin release, elicited an initial small decrease

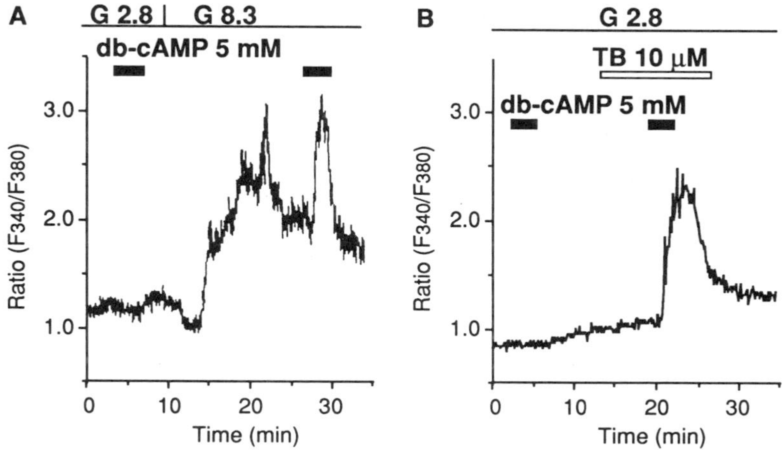

Figure 1. **A.** Effects on $[Ca^{2+}]_i$ in single pancreatic B-cells of 5 mM db-cAMP at 2.8 mM glucose, an elevation of the glucose concentration to 8.3 mM, and subsequent administration of 5 mM db-cAMP with 8.3 mM glucose. The tracing is representative of three similar experiments. **B.** Effects of 5 mM db-cAMP, 10 μM tolbutamide (TB), and 5 mM db-cAMP plus 10 μM TB on $[Ca^{2+}]_i$ at 2.8 mM glucose. N=7. Thin lines and thick lines above tracings indicate the glucose concentrations and the periods of exposure to the agents, respectively.

followed by a large increase in $[Ca^{2+}]_i$ as reported previously(12). In the presence of 8.3 mM glucose and on the moderately elevated level of $[Ca^{2+}]_i$, 5 mM db-cAMP produced a further increase in $[Ca^{2+}]_i$ (Fig. 1A).

In the presence of 2.8 mM glucose, neither db-cAMP (5 mM) nor tolbutamide (10 μM) alone altered $[Ca^{2+}]_i$, however, db-cAMP together with tolbutamide produced a large increase in $[Ca^{2+}]_i$ (Fig. 1B). With 2.8 mM glucose, a depolarizing concentration of K^+ (15–25 mM) rapidly increased $[Ca^{2+}]_i$. On the sustained and moderate elevation of $[Ca^{2+}]_i$ db-cAMP failed to further increase $[Ca^{2+}]_i$, whereas it subsequently increased $[Ca^{2+}]_i$ with 8.3 mM glucose (Fig. 2). Essentially the same effects were obtained with 1 mM db-cAMP plus 0.3 mM IBMX, 10 μM forskolin, and 10 μM forskolin plus 0.3 mM IBMX. Responses were elicited most efficiently by 10 μM forskolin plus 0.3 mM IBMX.

GLP-1(7-36)amide at 10^{-10} M elicited an increase in $[Ca^{2+}]_i$ in the presence of 8.3 mM glucose, whereas it was ineffective in 2.8 mM glucose (Fig. 3A). GLP-1(7-36)amide even at 10^{-8} M failed to alter $[Ca^{2+}]_i$ with 2.8 mM glucose (data not shown). In B-cells in which 10 μM tolbutamide alone was inadequate to increase $[Ca^{2+}]_i$ at 2.8 mM glucose, GLP-1(7-36) amide administered together with tolbutamide produced an increase in $[Ca^{2+}]_i$ (Fig. 3B). In contrast, GLP-1(7-36)amide, when administered in combination with 25 mM KCl, was unable to further increase $[Ca^{2+}]_i$ (data not shown).

Lack of Effect of GLP-1 in the Presence of Agents that Raise cAMP and Common Nature for GLP-1- and cAMP-Induced Increases in $[Ca^{2+}]_i$

In the continuous presence of 10 μM forskolin and 0.3 mM IBMX and after the transient $[Ca^{2+}]_i$ increase induced by them, GLP-1(7-36)amide was administered but it failed to increase $[Ca^{2+}]_i$. After removal of forskolin and IBMX, the second challenge with GLP-1(7-36)amide induced a clear increase in $[Ca^{2+}]_i$ (Fig. 4). The result may indicate that cAMP-dependent processes in B-cells were already maximally activated by forskolin plus

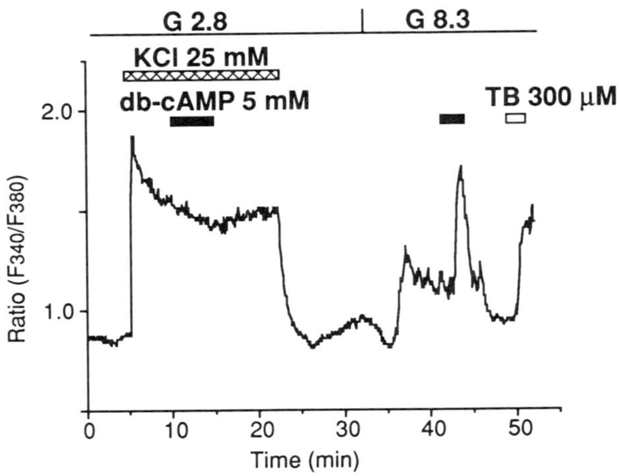

Figure 2. Effects on $[Ca^{2+}]_i$ of 25 mM KCl, 25 mM KCl plus 5 mM db-cAMP at 2.8 mM glucose, 8.3 mM glucose, and 5 mM db-cAMP at 8.3 mM glucose. N=6.

IBMX, so that GLP(7-36)amide, which acts by producing cAMP, could not evoke any further effect. In addition, remarkably common properties have been found between the GLP-1-induced and cAMP-induced increases in $[Ca^{2+}]_i$: (1) both GLP-1(7-36)amide and a rise in cAMP were able to increase $[Ca^{2+}]_i$ only when they acted in collaboration with glucose or tolbutamide but not with high K^+; and (2) the increases in $[Ca^{2+}]_i$ induced by GLP-1 and cAMP were both completely inhibited by nitrendipine, a blocker of the L-type Ca^{2+} channel[6]. GLP-1(7-37)-induced production of cAMP and its link to the $[Ca^{2+}]_i$ increase

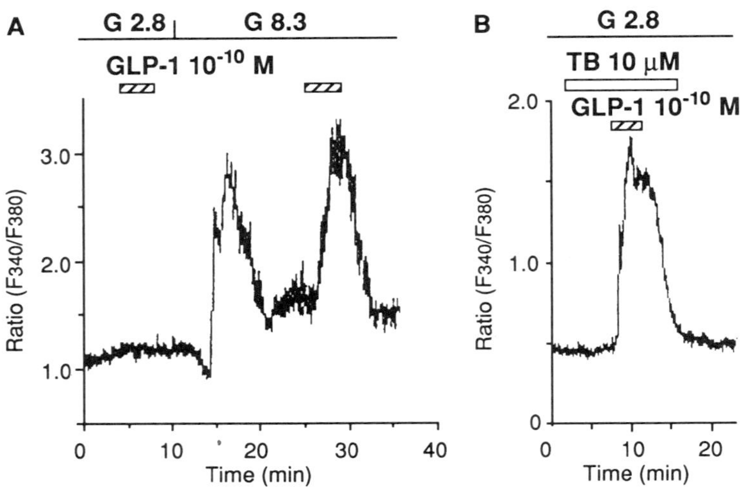

Figure 3. **A.** Effects on $[Ca^{2+}]_i$ of 10^{-10} M GLP-1(7-36)amide (GLP-1) at 2.8 mM glucose and subsequently at 8.3 mM glucose. N=4. **B.** Effects on $[Ca^{2+}]_i$ of 10 μM TB and 10^{-10} M GLP-1 together with 10 μM TB at 2.8 mM glucose. N=3.

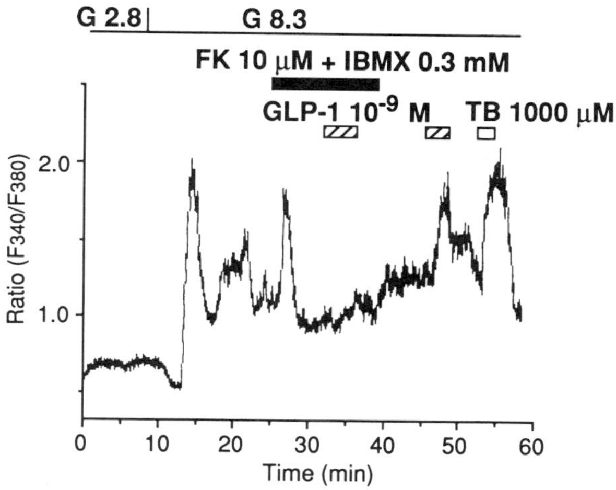

Figure 4. In the continuous presence of 10 μM forskolin and 0.3 mM IBMX and after the transient $[Ca^{2+}]_i$ increase produced by them, 10^{-9} M GLP-1 failed to increase $[Ca^{2+}]_i$. After washing out the agents that raise cAMP, the second challenge with GLP-1 increased $[Ca^{2+}]_i$. N=5.

was demonstrated in HIT insulinoma cells[3]. All the evidences favor that the GLP-1 action to increase $[Ca^{2+}]_i$ is mediated by a rise in cAMP in B-cells.

Action Sites of cAMP to Lead to $[Ca^{2+}]_i$ and Insulin Secretory Activities

The present study of $[Ca^{2+}]_i$ measurements demonstrated that cAMP and GLP-1(7-36)amide acted in cooperation with glucose and tolbutamide, the agents that inhibit the ATP-sensitive K^+ channels[13], but not with high K^+. It suggests that cAMP may influence the ATP-sensitive K^+ channel in such a manner that glucose and tolbutamide could more efficiently inhibit the channel. In support of this idea, it was recently shown that cAMP and GLP-1(7-37), when administered with glucose, led to an inhibition of the ATP-sensitive K^+ channel in B-cells which had been originally glucose-unresponsive[14]. An alternate possibility is that cAMP could modulate the voltage-dependent Ca^{2+} channel so that a mild depolarization by glucose or tolbutamide can activate the channel more effectively.

The effect of cAMP and GLP-1 to increase $[Ca^{2+}]_i$ in B-cells took place with 8.3 mM glucose or higher, stimulatory glucose concentrations for insulin release, but not with a non-stimulatory glucose concentration (2.8 mM). It appears that the glucose-dependent action to increase $[Ca^{2+}]_i$ accounts for the potentiation of the glucose-induced insulin release by cAMP and GLP-1. It was shown that the glucose-dependent increase in $[Ca^{2+}]_i$ was causally related to the insulin release in response to GLP-1 and GIP in HIT insulinoma cells[3]. On the other hand, a study of capacitance measurements recently demonstrated that cAMP potentiates the exocytosis induced by Ca^{2+} [15,16]. Therefore, it is likely that cAMP amplifies the glucose-induced insulin release both by augmenting the $[Ca^{2+}]_i$ increase and by sensitizing the exocytotic machinery of B-cells to Ca^{2+}.

CONCLUSIONS

In rat pancreatic B-cells, both cAMP and GLP-1(7-36)amide increase $[Ca^{2+}]_i$ in selective synergism with glucose and tolbutamide, the agents that act through inhibiting the

ATP-sensitive K^+ channel. The GLP-1-induced increase in $[Ca^{2+}]_i$ is mediated by a rise in cAMP. The glucose-dependent action of cAMP and GLP-1 to increase $[Ca^{2+}]_i$ accounts for, in part, their potentiation of the glucose-induced insulin release.

ACKNOWLEDGMENTS

We thank Kayoko Itoh for skillful technical assistance.

This work was supported in part by grants from the Ministry of Education, Science and Culture of Japan and from the Ichiro Kanehara Foundation (to TY).

REFERENCES

1. Sharp, G.W.G., 1979, The adenylate cyclase-cyclic AMP system in islets of Langerhans and its role in the control of insulin release, *Diabetologia* 16:287–296.
2. Orskov, C., 1992, Glucagon-like peptide-1, a new hormone of the entero-insular axis, *Diabetologia* 35: 701–711.
3. Lu, M., Wheeler, M.B., Leng, X.-H., and Boyd, A.E., 1993, The role of the free cytosolic calcium level in β-cell signal transduction by gastric inhibitory polypeptide and glucagon-like peptide I(7-37), *Endocrinology* 132:94–100.
4. Wang, J.L., Corbett, J.A., Marshall, C.A., and McDaniel, M.L., 1993, Glucose-induced insulin secretion from purified β-cells. A role for modulation of Ca^{2+} influx by cAMP- and protein kinase C-dependent signal transduction pathways, *J. Biol. Chem.* 268:7785–7791.
5. Grapengiesser, E., Gylfe, E., and Hellman, B., 1991, Cyclic AMP as a determinant for glucose induction of fast Ca^{2+} oscillations in isolated pancreatic β-cells, *J. Biol. Chem.* 266:12207–12210.
6. Yada, T., Itoh, K., and Nakata, M., 1993, Glucagon-like peptide-1(7-36)amide and a rise in cyclic adenosine 3′,5′- monophosphate increase cytosolic free Ca^{2+} in rat pancreatic β-cells by enhancing Ca^{2+} channel activity, *Endocrinology* 133:1685–1692.
7. Cullinan, C.A., Brady, E.J., Saperstein, R., and Leibowitz, M.D., 1994, Glucose-dependent alterations of intracellular free calcium by glucagon-like peptide-1(7-36amide) in individual ob/ob mouse β-cells, *Cell Calcium* 15:391–400.
8. Penner, R., and Neher, E., 1988, The role of calcium in stimulus-secretion coupling in excitable and non-excitable cells, *J. Exp. Biol.* 139:329–345.
9. Ämmälä, C., Eliasson, L., Bokvist, K., Larsson, O., Ashcroft, F.M., and Rorsman, P., 1993, Exocytosis elicited by action potentials and voltage-clamp calcium currents in individual mouse pancreatic B-cells, *J. Physiol.* 472:665–688.
10. Yada, T., Sakurada, M., Ihida, K., Nakata, M., Murata, F., Arimura, A. and Kikuchi, M., 1994, Pituitary adenylate cyclase activating polypeptide is an extraordinarily potent intra-pancreatic regulator of insulin secretion from islet β-cells, *J. Biol. Chem.* 269:1290–1293.
11. Grynkiewicz, G., Poenie, M., and Tsien, R.Y., 1985, A new generation of Ca^{2+} indicators with greatly improved fluorescence properties, *J. Biol. Chem.* 260:3440–3450.
12. Yada, T., Kakei, M., and Tanaka, H., 1992, Single pancreatic β-cells from normal rats exhibit an initial decrease and subsequent increase in cytosolic free Ca^{2+} in response to glucose, *Cell Calcium* 13:69–76.
13. Ashcroft, F.M., and Rorsman, P., 1989, Electrophysiology of the pancreatic β-cell, *Prog. Biophys. Molec. Biol.* 54:87–147.
14. Holz, G.G., Kuhtreiber, W.M., and Habener, J.F., 1993, Pancreatic beta-cells are rendered glucose-competent by the insulinotropic hormone glucagon-like peptide-1(7–37), *Nature* 361:362–365.
15. Ämmälä, C., Ashcroft, F.M., and Rorsman, P., 1993, Calcium-independent potentiation of insulin release by cyclic AMP in single B-cells, *Nature* 363:356–358.
16. Ämmälä, C., Eliasson, L., Bokvist, K., Berggren, P.-O., Honkanen, R.E., Sjöholm, A., and Rorsman, P., 1994, Activation of protein kinases and inhibition of protein phosphatases play a central role in the regulation of exocytosis in mouse pancreatic β cells, *Proc. Natl. Acad. Sci.* 91:4343–4347.

29

METABOLISM OF PHOSPHATIDYLCHOLINE IN MOUSE PANCREATIC ISLETS

K. Capito, S. E. Hansen, C. J. Hedeskov, and P. Thams

Department of Medical Biochemistry and Genetics
The Panum Institute, Blegdamsvej 3
DK-2200 Copenhagen N
Denmark

INTRODUCTION

Phosphatidylcholine (PC) is the most abundant phospholipid in pancreatic islets. "*De novo*" synthesis of islet PC has been shown to be enhanced by glucose[1] and PC is degredated during glucose stimulation of insulin secretion[2] thus implicating PC turnover as a regulatory event in glucose-induced insulin secretion. The aim of the present investigation was to evaluate the effect of insulin secretagogues on degradation of islet PC as measured by the formation of water soluble choline-containing metabolites of PC in mouse pancreatic islets.

METHODS

Islets were prepared by collagenase (Boehringer) digestion of the pancreases of male albino mice (NMRI) fed *ad libitum* on a standard laboratory diet.

For investigation of PC-degradation in intact islets, the isolated islets were kept in tissue culture for 1–4 days in TCM 199 culture medium containing 2.5 μCi/ml [^{3}H-methyl]-choline (Amersham) to obtain radioactive labeling of endogenous PC. After the labeling period, the islets were washed twice in Krebs-buffer containing 1 mM choline to remove excess ^{3}H-choline and then incubated in 250 μl Krebs-buffer in the presence of various agents for 0–120 min. Metabolism was arrested by addition of 630 μl icecold methanol/HCl (100:1). Separation of water- and lipid-soluble choline-metabolites was obtained by a 30 min extraction by 620 μl chloroform followed by addition of 310 μl H_2O and centrifugation for 5 min at 5000 rpm. The water soluble choline-metabolites were further separated by ion exchange chromatography on Dowex-50-W-H^+ columns[3] or by thinlayer chromatography[4]. Separation of PC and lyso-PC was obtained by thinlayer chromatography in $CHCl_3$:MeOH:NH_4OH:H_2O (16:13:1:3).

Physiology and Pathophysiology of the Islets of Langerhans, edited by Soria.
Plenum Press, New York, 1997.

For measurement of PC-metabolizing enzymes islets were homogenized in 100 mM Tris buffer pH 7.5 containing 1 mM EGTA and 0.1 mM PMSF. Subcellular fractions were further obtained by centrifugation at 27.000 g for 1 hr. The homogenate and subcellular fractions (approx. 20 μg of islet protein) were incubated for 2 hrs in 250 μl of Tris buffer pH 7.4 containing [^{3}H-methyl]-dipalmitoylPC (1 mCi/mmol; Amersham) or endogenously [^{3}H-choline]-labeled PC. After incubation lipid extraction and separation of water-soluble choline metabolites were performed as described above.

RESULTS AND DISCUSSION

The distribution of radioactivity in islet choline metabolites during the culture period is shown in Fig. 1. Isotopic equilibrium of ^{3}H-PC was obtained after 3 days incubation with ^{3}H-choline. The total incorporation of ^{3}H-choline at this timepoint was 7357 ± 648 cpm/islet (10) (mean ± sem (n)), 45% of which was present in PC. Labeling of the pool of phosphorylcholine reached a relative maximum already after 1 day, where it accounted for 47% of the labeling. Since less than 1% of the radioactivity was found in CDP-choline, this confirms the rate limiting function of CTP:phosphorylcholine cytidyltransferase in PC synthesis[5]. Radioactive labeling of islet lysoPC increased slowly during the culture period, probably reflecting the activity of islet phospholipase A_2. At day 4 approximately 6% of the radioactivity was found in lysoPC. The amount of radioactivity in choline and glycerophosphorylcholine (GlyPCho) amounted to 2–3% and was stable during the culture period. Labeling of other choline metabolites was negligible.

After 3 days of culture, islets were transferred from the culture medium to Krebs buffer supplemented with 3.3 mM glucose and either incubated for 0–120 minutes at 37°C to study metabolism of PC at basal conditions, or incubated for 30 min in the presence of insulin secretagogues.

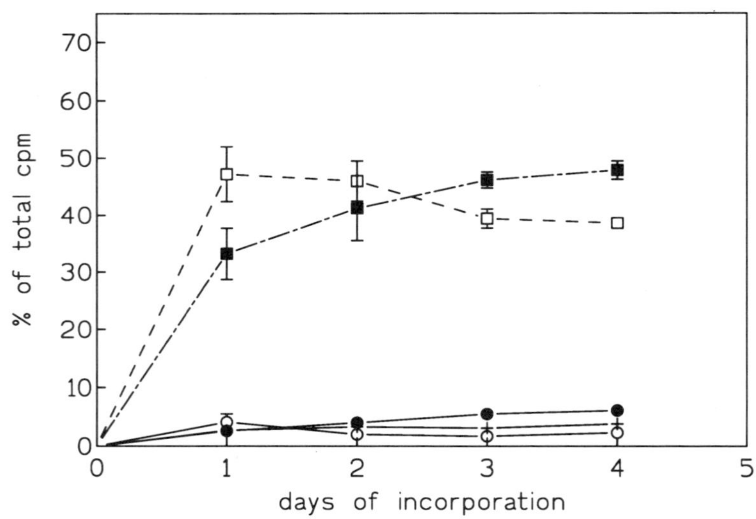

Figure 1. Incorporation of ^{3}H-choline in intact islets. Islets were kept in TCM 199 tissue culture medium for 1–4 days. After culture the distribution of ^{3}H-radioactivity in the islets was determined. PC —■—; Phosphorylcholine —□—; LysoPC —●—; GlyPCho —○—; Choline —+—.

Table 1. Production of ^{3}H-choline in prelabeled islets[a]

Additions	% ^{3}H-choline
3.3 mM glucose	5.1 ± 0.8 (10)
+ 10 μM $AlCl_3$, 10 mM NaF	9.1 ± 0.7 (9)*
20 mM glucose	4.7 ± 0.4 (13)
+ 0.16 μM TPA	6.3 ± 0.6 (13)**
+ 5 μM A23187	4.2 ± 0.4 (6)
+ 25 μM Forskolin	5.6 ± 0.9 (5)

[a]Groups of 20 islets, prelabeled with ^{3}H-choline for 3 days, were incubated in Krebs buffer for 30 min in the presence of the indicated agents. The results are given as percent of total islet radioactivity and represent mean ± sem, with the number of determinations in parentheses.
*$p < 0.001$ vs. 3.3 mM glucose; **$p < 0.05$ vs. 20 mM glucose.

Before this short time incubation, 38.6 ± 0.6% (8) of islet ^{3}H-choline labeling was found in phosphorylcholine. The amount of ^{3}H-phosphorylcholine was not changed significantly during 2 hrs incubation in 3.3 mM glucose and was also not affected by exposure for 30 min to insulin stimulatory concentrations of glucose, carbachol, TPA, forskolin and the ionophore A23187. This seems to indicate that PC-specific phospholipase C is not present in mouse islets.

During 2 hrs incubation of islets in 3.3 mM glucose the production of ^{3}H-choline increased linearly from 3.2 ± 0.3% (11) to 8.0 ± 1.2% (2) of total islet radioactivity. 30 min incubation with glucose, carbacholine, A23187 or forskolin, had no effect on production of ^{3}H-choline. However, the phorbol ester TPA and fluoride increased choline production 35% and 80% respectively (Table 1).

Theoretically, ^{3}H-choline may be produced by hydrolytic cleavage of either ^{3}H-phosphorylcholine or ^{3}H-PC. However, since no change was observed in the content of ^{3}H-phosphorylcholine during this short time incubation, the observed production of ^{3}H-choline most likely reflects phospholipase D activity. This assumption is in agreement with previous demonstrations of TPA- and fluoride-activated phosphatidic acid production from PC in rat islets[6].

During 2 hrs incubation of islets with 3.3 mM glucose the amount of ^{3}H-GlyPCho was raised from 2.0 ± 0.3% (11) to 3.7 ± 0.4% (2) of total islet radioactivity. Incubation with 20 mM glucose increased the production of ^{3}H-GlyPCho 40%, and in the presence of 20 mM glucose + 0.1 mM ATP the production of ^{3}H-GlyPCho was more than doubled, whereas the diacylglycerol lipase inhibitor, RHC 80267, inhibited ^{3}H-GlyPCho production totally (Table 2). None of the other applied insulin secretagogues affected the production of ^{3}H-GlyPCho.

The activity of hydrolytic enzymes acting on PC was further investigated in homogenates or in 27.000 g subcellular fractions employing either [^{3}H-choline]-dipalmitoyl-PC or endogenously synthesized [^{3}H-choline]-PC as substrate. These substrates were added in concentrations from 1 μM to 1 mM and several different detergents were added in order to solubilize enzymes from the membranes. It was, however, not possible to demonstrate any PC-specific phospholipase D or phospholipase C activity at any of these assay conditions. In contrast, both islet homogenate and a 27.000 g supernatant fraction catalyzed the production of ^{3}H-GlyPCho from ^{3}H-PC. Thus, at 16 μM ^{3}H-dipalmitoyl-PC, 0.66 ± 0.05% (n=6) of PC was converted to GlyPCho per 2 hrs per μg protein. This reaction was Ca^{2+}-independent and was almost totally inhibited in the presence of the diacylglycerol lipase

Table 2. Production of ^{3}H-glycerophosphorylcholine in intact islets[a]

Additions	% ^{3}H-GlyPchol
3.3 mM glucose	2.2 ± 0.3 (11)
+ 10 μM $AlCl_3$, 10 mM NaF	2.6 ± 0.5 (8)
20 mM glucose	3.1 ± 0.2 (11)*
+ 0.1 mM ATP	4.8 ± 0.4 (4)**
+ 35 μM RHC 80267	1.7 ± 0.2 (4)**
+ 5 μM A23187	2.8 ± 0.2 (6)
+ 25 μM Forskolin	3.3 ± 0.2 (5)
+ 0.16 μM TPA	3.2 ± 0.2 (11)

[a]Groups of 20 islets, prelabeled with ^{3}H-choline for 3 days, were incubated in Krebs buffer for 30 min in the presence of the indicated agents. The results are given as percent of total islet radioactivity and represent mean ± sem, with the number of determinations in parentheses.
*$p < 0.05$ vs. 3.3 mM glucose; **$p < 0.005$ vs. 20 mM glucose.

inhibitor RHC 80267 (35 μM) (data not shown). If endogenously labeled [^{3}H-choline]-PC was isolated from islets and used as substrate at a calculated concentration of 20 μM PC, the production of ^{3}H-GlyPCho was increased approx. 400%. In the 27.000 g membrane fraction no significant degradation of PC was observed.

The identity of the enzymatic activity that catalyzes the production of GlyPCho from PC has not been disclosed, but may be due either to the activity of a lysophospholipase transacylase, or to the combined action of phospholipase A_1 and phospholipase A_2. The enzyme activity is stimulated by glucose and may therefore be of importance in regulation of glucose-induced insulin secretion.

Hydrolysis of the C2-ester linkage of islet phospholipids has previously been shown to be stimulated by glucose, and it has been suggested that arachidonic acid produced by a calcium-dependent phospholipase A_2[7], or by a calcium-independent phospholipase A_2 activity[8] may be a coupling factor in glucose-induced insulin secretion. In those experiments identification of phospholipase A_2 was based on measurement of the hydrolyzed fatty acid, whereas determination of the other product, a lysophospholipid, was not attempted.

The increased labeling of lysoPC during choline incorporation (Fig. 1) seems to indicate that mouse islets do contain a phospholipase A_2 activity which acts on PC. However, the present finding that glucose enhances the production of GlyPCho from PC and the previous observation that islet lysoPC actually falls during glucose stimulation[2], seems to indicate that glucose also stimulates a lysoPC hydrolase or a lysoPC transacylase, or that glucose-activated phospholipase A_2 also displays lysophospholipase activity. The enzyme(s) responsible for production of GlyPCho in the present experiments is calcium-independent and may therefore be identical to the ATP-stimulated calcium-independent phospholipase A_2 described by Gross et al[9]. The functional importance of production of GlyPCho is not evident. If the production is catalyzed by a lysoPC transacylase the reaction may simply be a fast way of resynthesizing PC. However, although the present data are not inconsistent with the hypothesis that glucose activation of arachidonic acid production is a regulatory event in glucose-induced insulin secretion, the possibility, that not only arachidonic acid, but also GlyPCho may play a role in regulation of glucose-induced insulin secretion, should be further investigated.

In the present experiments it was not possible to demonstrate any glucose stimulation of phospholipase D. However since choline production was stimulated by TPA, phospholipase D, and its reaction product phosphatidic acid, may be involved in TPA-stimulated insulin secretion as previously suggested[6].

In conclusion, the present results demonstrate that in mouse pancreatic islets, PC may be degredated by phospholipase D, phospholipase A_2 and by a further enzymatic activity which produces GlyPCho by removal of two fatty acids from PC. The latter enzymatic activity may be a putative glucose sensor, since it is activated by glucose, and its possible significance in regulation of glucose-induced insulin secretion should be further investigated.

ACKNOWLEDGEMENTS

The technical assistance of Anita Sommerfeldt is gratefully acknowledged. The investigation was supported by the Danish Diabetes Association, The Nordisk Insulin Foundation and by Bernhard and Marie Kleins Foundation.

REFERENCES

1. Hoffmann, J.M., and Laychock, S.G., 1988, Choline turnover in phosphatidylcholine of pancreatic islets, *Diabetes* 37:1489–1498.
2. Turk, J., Wolf, B.A., Lefkowith, J.B., Stump, W.T. and McDaniel, M.L., 1986, Glucose-induced phospholipid hydrolysis in isolated pancreatic islets: quantitative effects on the phospholipid content of arachidonate and other fatty acids, *Biochim. Biophys. Acta* 879:399–409.
3. Cook, S.J. and Wakelam, J.O., 1989, Analysis of the water-soluble products of phosphatidylcholine breakdown by ion-exchange chromatography, *Biochem. J.* 263:581–587.
4. Wolf, B.A., Easom, R.A., Hughes, J.H., McDaniel, M.L. and Turk, J., 1989, Secretagogue-induced diacylglycerol accumulation in isolated pancreatic islets. Mass spectrometric characterization of the fatty acyl content indicates multiple mechanisms of generation, *Biochemistry* 28:4291–4301.
5. Tijburg, L.B.M., Geelen, M.J.H. and Von Golde, L.M.G., 1989, Regulation of the biosynthesis of triacylglycerol, phosphatidylcholine and phosphatidylethanolamine in the liver, *Biochim. Biophys. Acta* 1004:1–19.
6. Dunlop, M. and Metz, S.A., 1989, A phospholipase D-like mechanism in pancreatic islet cells: stimulation by calcium ionophore, phorbol ester and sodium fluoride, *Biochem. Biophys. Res. Commun.* 163:922–928.
7. Laychock, S.G., 1982, Phospholipase A_2 activity in pancreatic islets is calcium-dependent and stimulated by glucose, *Cell Calcium* 3:43–54.
8. Ramanadham, S., Gross, R.W., Han, X. and Turk, J., 1993, Inhbition of arachidonate release by secretagogue-stimulated pancreatic islets suppresses both insulin secretion and the rise in β-cell cytosolic calcium ion concentration, *Biochemistry* 32:337–346.
9. Gross, R.W., Ramanadham, S., Kruszka, K.K., Han, X. and Turk, J., 1993, Rat and human pancreatic islet cells contain a calcium ion independent phospholipase A_2 activity selective for hydrolysis of arachidonate which is stimulated by adenosine triphosphate and is specifically localized to islet β-cells, *Biochemistry* 32:327–336.

Phe–Met–Arg–Phe–NH_2 (FMRFa)-RELATED PEPTIDES INHIBIT Na/Ca EXCHANGE IN PANCREATIC B CELLS

F. Van Eylen,[1] P. Gourlet,[2] A. Vandermeers,[2] P. Lebrun,[1] and A. Herchuelz[1]

[1]Laboratory of Pharmacology
[2]Laboratory of Biochemistry and Nutrition
Brussels Universit y School of Medicine
Route de Lennik 808, Bâtiment GE (CP 617), B-1070 Brussels, Belgium

INTRODUCTION

Two processes located at the cell plasma membrane appear to mediate Ca^{2+} extrusion from cells: the Ca^{2+} ATP ase and the process of Na/Ca exchange [1,2]. In the heart, Na/Ca exchange appears to be the predominant mechanism for Ca^{2+} extrusion, being able to restore and control basal Ca^{2+} level on a beat-to-beat basis [3]. Although the existence of a process of Na/Ca exchange in the pancreatic B cell has been postulated for many years, the process was only recently characterized and shown to regulate cytosolic free Ca^{2+} concentration within the physiological range. One major factor that has hindered rapid progresses in our knowledge of the process of Na/Ca exchange is the lack of specific inhibitors of the exchange. Recently, opioïd analogs (e.g. naloxone) were shown to inhibit Na/Ca exchange in cardiac sarcolemmal vesicles [4]. Likewise, peptides related to Phe–Met–Arg–Phe–NH_2 (FMRFa) with naloxone-like activity were observed to induce complete inhibition of Na/Ca exchange [5]. In addition, it was suggested that endogenous analogs of FMRFa may exert some of their physiological modulatory role by inhibiting Na/Ca exchange [5]. FMRFa is a molluscan peptide with potent effects on heart, as well as on other muscles and nerves of molluscs. FMRFa-related peptides have also been localized in several mammalian tissues and appear to exert various actions in cluding antagonism to opioïd analgesia [6,7]. The aim of the present study was to examine the effects of FMRFa-related peptides on Na/Ca exchange in rat pancreatic islet cells.

MATERIALS AND METHODS

Na/Ca exchange was measured as Na_i^+-dependent Ca_o^{2+} uptake as previously described [8]. The peptide FMRFa was obtained from Sigma. The three other peptides VMRFa (Val–

Physiology and Pathophysiology of the Islets of Langerhans, edited by Soria.
Plenum Press, New York, 1997.

Met–Arg–Phe–NH_2), HMRFa (His–Met–Arg–Phe–NH_2) and FLRFa (Phe–Leu–Arg–Phe–NH_2) were synthesized by solid phase methodology with an Automated 431A Applied Biosystem apparatus (Foster City, CA, USA) using the Fmoc strategy: a 4-(2′,4′-dimethoxy-phenylfluoren-9-yl-methoxycarbonyl-aminomethyl)phenoxyresin and fluoren-9-yl-methoxy-carbonyl-labelled amino acids activated with N-hydroxybenzotriazole and benzotriazol-1-yloxytris (dimethyl amino) phosphonium hexafluorophosphate were used [9]. The peptides were purified by HPLC and their conformity established by both total amino acid composition and Edman degradation in a 477A sequencer (Applied Biosystems). All reagents for peptide synthesis were purchased from Novabiochem (Laüfelfingen, Switzerland).

RESULTS

In the presence of 2.8 mM glucose, FMRFa failed to inhibit Na/Ca exchange in rat pancreatic islet cells. Related peptides such as HMRFa (His–Met–Arg–Phe–NH2), VMRFa (Val–Met–Arg–Phe–NH2) and FLRFa (Phe–Leu–Arg–Phe–NH2) were more potent than FMRFa but their inhibitory effects were far less pronounced in pancreatic B cells (36% inhibition at 100 μM) than in cardiac sarcolemmal vesicles (50% inhibition at 1–2 μM). Since membrane potential is known to affect Na/Ca exchange activity, the effects of the two most active peptides (HMRFa and VMRFa) were examined under depolarizing conditions (16.7 mM glucose + 20 mM TEA or glucose + TEA + 1 μM BAY K 8644). Exposure of the islet cells to the peptides under depolarizing condition greatly enhanced the inhibitory activity on Na/Ca exchange of the two most potent peptides, HMRFa and VMRFa (Fig. 1). In contrast to their effect on Na/Ca exchange, HMRFa and VMRFa failed to affect voltage-sensitive Ca^{2+} channels and the Na^+-K^+-ATPase. However, in the presence of glucose (16.7 mM) the peptides exerted a modest inhibitory effect on ^{86}Rb outflow.

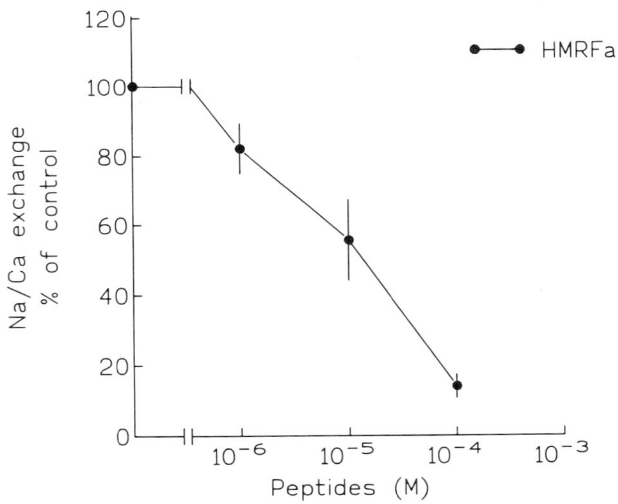

Figure 1. Effect of HMRFa on Na_i^+-dependent $^{45}Ca_o$ uptake in intact islet cells (reverse Na/Ca exchange) exposed to glucose (16.7 mM), TEA (20 mM) and BAY K 8644 (1 μM). Data are expressed in % of control values found at 0 mM extr acellular Na^+ in the absence of the peptides, after subtraction of basal uptake measured at 139 mM extracellular Na^+. Mean ± SEM refer to at least 22 individual samples. Basal uptake and control uptake averaged 183 ± 12 (n=22) fmol Ca/1000 cells and 310 ± 6 (n=24) fmol Ca/1000 cells, respectively.

CONCLUSIONS

Our data indicate that FMRFa-related peptides are weak and non-specific inhibitors of Na/Ca exchange in intact B cells. The data do not confirm the view that the peptides may exert some of their physiological role by inhibiting Na/Ca exchange.

REFERENCES

1. E. Carafoli, Membrane transport of calcium: an overview. Methods in Enzymology 157:3 (1988).
2. M.P. Blaustein, Sodium/Calcium exchange and the control of contractility in cardiac muscle and vascular smooth muscle. J. C ardiovasc. Pharmacol. 12 (suppl.5):S56 (1988).
3. D.M. Bers, Species differences and the role of Sodium-Calcium exchange in cardiac muscle relaxation. in: "Sodium-Calcium exc hange: proceedings of the second international conference", Blaustein, M.P., DiPolo, R., Reeves, J.P. Eds. Ann. NY Acad. Sci. 639: 375 (1991).
4. D. Khananshvili, and Y. Sarne, The effect of opiate agonists and antagonists on Na^+–Ca^{2+} exchange in cardiac sarcolemmal vesicles. Life Sci. 51:275 (1992).
5. D. Khananshvili, D.C. Price, M.J. Greenberg, and Y. Sarne, Phe–Met–Arg–Phe–NH_2 (FMRFa)-related peptides inhibit Na^+ –Ca^{2+} exchange in cardiac sarcolemmal vesicles. J. Biol. Chem. 268:200 (1993).
6. D.C. Price, and M.J. Greenberg, The hunting of the FaRPs: the distribution of FMRFamide-related peptides. Biol. Bull. 177:19 8 (1989).
7. R. Raffa, The action of FMRFamide (Phe–Met–Arg–Phe–NH_2) and related peptides on mammals. Peptides 9:915 (1988).
8. P.O. Plasman, P. Lebrun, and A. Herchuelz, Characterization of the process of sodium/calcium exchange in pancreatic islet cells. Am. J. Physiol. 259:E844 (1990).
9. A. Fournier, W. Dahno, and A.M. Felix, Applications of BOP reagent in solid phase peptide synthesis. III. Solid phase peptide synthesis with unprotected aliphatic and hydroxyamino acids using BOP reagent, Int. J. Pept. Protein Res. 33:133–139 (1989).

31

CELL CULTURE CONDITIONS INFLUENCE GLUCOSE-INDUCED $[Ca^{2+}]_i$ RESPONSES IN ISOLATED RAT PANCREATIC B CELLS

M.-H. Antoine, P. Lebrun, and A. Herchuelz

Laboratory of Pharmacology
Brussels University, School of Medicine
Route de Lennik 808, Bâtiment GE (CP 617)
B-1070 Brussels, Belgium

INTRODUCTION

An increase in the cytosolic free Ca^{2+} concentration ($[Ca^{2+}]_i$) in the pancreatic B cell is thought to represent a key event in the process of glucose-induced insulin release. The availability of fluorophores like Quin 2, Fura 2 and Indo 1 has recently allowed to demonstrate this increase both in intact pancreatic islets and in isolated B cells from different species. The pattern of $[Ca^{2+}]_i$ changes found in intact islets in response to glucose appears consistent among different studies and consists in fast Ca^{2+} oscillations that parallel the oscillatory bursts of electrical activity. In intact B cells, different patterns of $[Ca^{2+}]_i$ changes have been observed consisting either in discrete and regular spikes arising from a constant basal level (frequency: 0.2 to 0.5/min) [1] or in sinusodal oscillations [2,3] (frequency 2 to 3/min) observed on top of an elevated level of $[Ca^{2+}]_i$.

The latter differences may result from differences in experimental conditions (e.g. length and conditions of cell culture, Fura 2 concentration, cell photodamage, ...) or origin of the cells examined (e.g. rat, mouse, ob/ob mouse). In the present study we have examined the influence of cell culture conditions, namely length of culture and glucose concentration on $[Ca^{2+}]_i$ responses to glucose in isolated rat pancreatic B cells.

MATERIALS AND METHODS

Isolated rat pancreatic islet cells were cultured for 24 h, 48 h and 72 h at 3 different glucose concentrations (11.1 mM, 16.7 mM and 22.2 mM) before $[Ca^{2+}]_i$ measurements. The culture medium consisted in RPMI 1640 supplemented with new born calf serum, glutamine and antibiotics. After culture, the cells were loaded with Fura 2 and fluorescence was measured using dual-excitation microfluorimetry with a Spex photometric sys-

Physiology and Pathophysiology of the Islets of Langerhans, edited by Soria.
Plenum Press, New York, 1997.

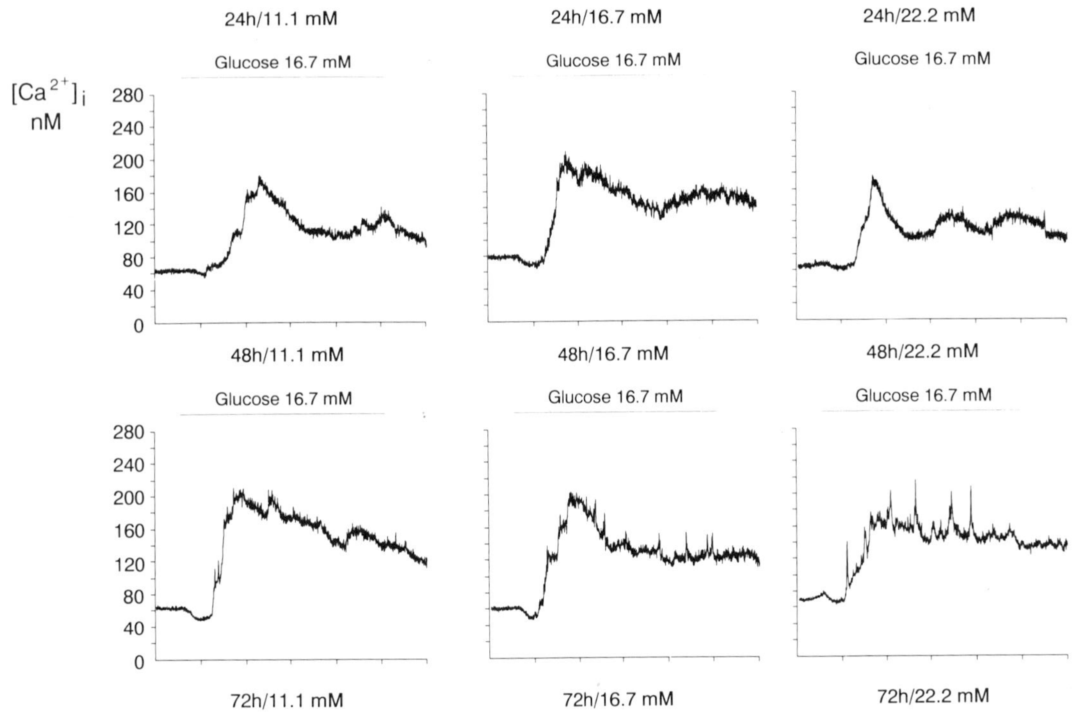

Figure 1. Effect of glucose (16.7 mM) on $[Ca^{2+}]_i$ in single B cells after culture under 9 different conditions. Data are presented as mean of 5 to 6 different experiments in each case.

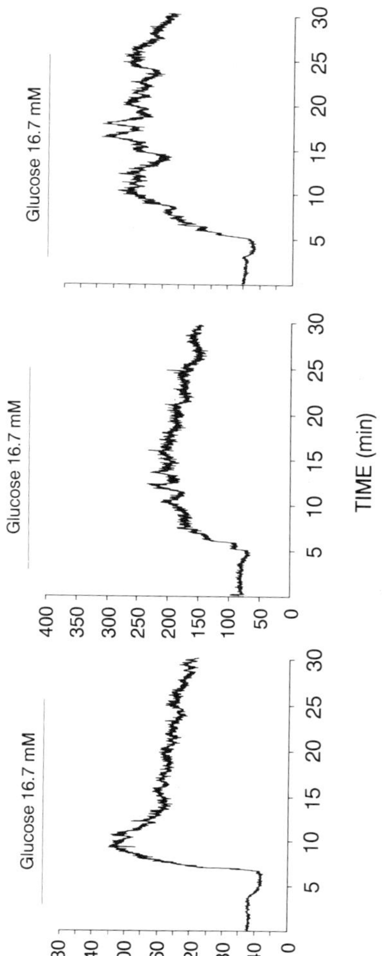

Figure 1. *(continued)*

tem [2]. Fura 2 loading and the intensity of the excitation light was kept to the minimum in order to maximally reduce $[Ca^{2+}]_i$ buffering and potential cell photodamage. The study was completely controlled so that cells from the same cellular preparation were examined under the 9 experimental conditions (6 cells/condition).

RESULTS

Fig. 1 illustrates mean increases in $[Ca^{2+}]_i$ observed in response to 16.7 mM glucose under the 9 experimental conditions. In the 54 cells tested, there was 1 experimental failure (broken coverslip). Of the 53 remaining cells, 50 (94%) responded to glucose by showing a distinct increase in $[Ca^{2+}]_i$. The absence of response was observed in cells cultured for only 24h either at 11.1 mM glucose (1 cell) or at 22.2 mM glucose (2 cells).

In most cases, the increases consisted in square wave or biphasic increases in $[Ca^{2+}]_i$ onto which fast oscillations were sometimes superimposed [3]. In four cases, regular spikes (type-a oscillations according to Hellman et al.) were observed, three after 24 h of culture (1 at each glucose concentration) and 1 after 48 h of culture at 11.1 mM glucose.

In several cells, a modest initial decrease in $[Ca^{2+}]_i$ was observed that preceeded the increase in $[Ca^{2+}]_i$. The inhibitory effect of glucose was most evident after 48 h and 72 h of culture at 11.1 mM glucose. It was less frequent and of smaller magnitude after culture at 16.7 mM and 22.2 mM glucose.

CONCLUSIONS

The present data show that cell culture conditions may influence $[Ca^{2+}]_i$ responses to glucose in isolated rat B cells. Differences in cell culture conditions may explain, in part at least, the differences in $[Ca^{2+}]_i$ responses to glucose observed in several previous studies.

REFERENCES

1. B. Hellman, E. Gylfe, E. Grapengiesser, P.-E. Lund and A. Berts, Cytoplasmic Ca^{2+} oscillations in pancreatic B cells, Biochim. Biophys. Acta 1113:295 (1992).
2. A. Herchuelz, R. Pochet, C. Pastiels and A. Van Praet, Heterogeneous changes in $[Ca^{2+}]_i$ induced by glucose, tolbutamide and K^+ in single rat pancreatic B cells, Cell Calcium 12:577 (1991).
3. M.J. Berridge and A. Galione, Cytosolic calcium oscillators, FASEB J. 2:3074 (1988).

32

STIMULATION OF INSULIN RELEASE *IN VIVO* BY THE METHYL ESTERS OF SUCCINIC ACID AND GLUTAMIC ACID

Isabel Valverde,[1] David Vicent,[1] Marisa L. Villanueva-Peñacarrillo,[1] Francine Malaisse-Lagae,[2] and Willy J. Malaisse[2]

[1]Fundacion Jimenez Diaz
Madrid, Spain
[2]Laboratory of Experimental Medicine
Brussels Free University
Brussels, Belgium

INTRODUCTION

It is currently believed that, in non-insulin-dependent diabetes mellitus, the pancreatic islet B-cell suffers from a kind of blindness to D-glucose. The secretory response of the B-cell to the hexose indeed appears to be more severely affected than that evoked by other nutrient or non-nutrient secretagogues.

Over recent years, several site-specific defects in the early steps of D-glucose handling and metabolism in the B-cell have been proposed to account for such a preferential impairment of glucose-stimulated insulin release. They include underexpression of the glut-2 gene, mutation of the glucokinase gene, hyperactivity of glucose-6-phosphatase and an inherited or acquired defect of the mitochondrial FAD-linked glycerophosphate dehydrogenase.[1] Moreover, the secondary phenomenon of so-called B-cell glucotoxicity seems attributable, in part at least, to the accumulation of glycogen in the B-cell and, hence, interference of glycogenolysis with glycolysis in response to changes in extracellular D-glucose concentration.[2]

These proposals suggest that stimulation of both proinsulin biosynthesis and insulin release in type-2 diabetes could be achieved by using non-glucidic nutrient secretagogues which would be able to bypass the above-mentioned defects in D-glucose transport, phosphorylation and further catabolism.

It is precisely in this perspective that we have recently concentrated our attention to the methyl esters of succinic acid and glutamic acid.[3–5] The selection of these esters is motivated mainly by the three following considerations. First, whereas succinic acid and glutamic acid penetrate poorly into islet cells and are virtually devoid of insulinotropic action, their methyl esters are efficiently taken up by the islet cells in which they undergo hydrolysis, so that either succinic acid or glutamic acid becomes readily available for mitochondrial

Physiology and Pathophysiology of the Islets of Langerhans, edited by Soria.
Plenum Press, New York, 1997.

catabolism. Second, by increasing O_2 uptake by islet cells, the esters of succinic acid and glutamic acid may increase both proinsulin biosynthesis and insulin release. This situation differs from that found with most pharmacological agents used for the treatment of type 2 diabetes. Thus, agents such as hypoglycemic sulfonylureas stimulate insulin release but not proinsulin biosynthesis, at least in isolated islets.[6] Third, the methyl esters of succinic and glutamic acid are indeed likely to bypass anomalies in the early steps of D-glucose metabolism in the B-cell.

Several recent findings provide further support to the potential use of the esters of succinic or glutamic acid as novel therapeutic tools in animal models of type 2 diabetes. First, the esters of succinic acid are devoid of glucagonotropic action whether *in vivo* or *in vitro*.[7,8] Second, they protect the B-cell against cytotoxic aggressions such as those caused by either streptozotocin[9] or interleukin-1.[10] Third, they exert a long-term favourable effect upon the secretory potential of the endocrine pancreas in situations such as glucopenia or starvation.[11] Fourth, they increase insulin release even at high concentrations of D-glucose[8] Fifth, under suitable experimental conditions, they enhance both the insulinotropic and hypoglycemic action of sulfonylurea.[7,12] Last, they are still able to stimulate insulin release in experimental models of B-cell glucotoxicity, under conditions in which the endocrine pancreas displays paradoxical insulin responses to rapid changes in extracellular D-glucose concentration.[13]

The methyl esters of succinic acid and glutamic acid display insulinotropic action both *in vitro* and *in vivo*. The aim of the present report is to briefly review the insulinotropic action of the monomethyl ester of succinic acid (SAM), the dimethyl ester of succinic acid (SAD) and the dimethyl ester of glutamic acid (GME) as documented in experiments conducted *in vivo*.

IN VIVO EXPERIMENTS

It was first shown that the intravenous administration of either the monomethyl ester of succinic acid (SAM) or the dimethyl ester of succinic acid (SAD), given in an amount of 1.0 μmol/g body weight to fasted and anesthetized rats, provokes an immediate increase in plasma insulin concentration.[14] On a molar basis, the response to SAM or SAD was higher than that evoked by D-glucose. In this pilot study, a positive insulin secretory response to SAM was also observed after intraperitoneal injection to fed and conscious rats.

It was then observed that, in fasted and anesthetized rats, SAM or SAD augment the insulinotropic action of glibenclamide (0.1 nmol/g body wt.) when both the methyl ester and hypoglycemic sulfonylurea were injected together intravenously.[7]

Comparable experiments were then conducted, after a 6–8 h fasting period, in both control rats and animals injected with streptozotocin during the neonatal period (STZ rats). The secretory response to SAM was much lower in STZ than control rats.[15]

In the latter study, iterative intraperitoneal administration of SAM (1.0 μmol/g body wt.) thrice daily for 7–10 days to either the control or STZ rats failed to enhance the secretory response of the endocrine pancreas to either D-glucose or glibenclamide. Incidentally, the repetitive intraperitoneal pulse dispensing of SAM (2.2 μmol/g body wt.) for one week to adult rats which had been injected with streptozotocin (20–40 mg/kg body wt.) 5 days before SAM treatment also failed to affect to any marked extent the secretory capacity of either the isolated perfused pancreas[13] or isolated pancreatic islets.[16]

In fed anesthetized rats, the intravenous administration of the dimethyl ester of glutamic acid (GME; 1.0 μmol/g body wt.) again caused an immediate increase in plasma insulin concentration, but failed to enhance the insulinotropic action of glibenclamide.[17] In fasted rats, however, GME potentiated the secretory response to glibenclamide.[18] On a molar basis, GME was less efficient than D-glucose in stimulating insulin release. A comparable hierarchy in the secretory response to GME and/or glibenclamide was observed in STZ rats.

Further work indicated that, at least in the case of SAD, the ester, even when administered enterally, reaches the bloodstream and exerts an insulinotropic action comparable to that observed after intravenous administration.[19]

CONCLUSION

The experiments briefly reviewed in this report indicate that the methyl esters of succinic acid and glutamic acid display efficient insulinotropic action *in vivo*. On a molar basis, the immediate secretory response of the B-cell is not vastly different in animals injected with either D-glucose or these esters. In the case of SAD, the ester evokes comparable increases in plasma insulin concentrations after either intravenous or enteral administration.

In the light of these findings, we have now undertaken further work to explore the insulinotropic action of other esters of these dicarboxylic acids. The methyl esters when administered *in vivo* may indeed lead to the undesirable generation of methanol. A preliminary work indicates that both the 6-O-D-glucosyl and 6-O-(3-O-methyl-D-glucosyl) ester of succinic acid monomethyl ester display insulinotropic action both *in vitro* and *in vivo*.[20] It is conceivable, therefore, that a suitable ester of either succinic or glutamic acid may be designed so that it would still display insulinotropic potency, that its hydrolysis would not lead to the generation of an undesirable alcohol, and that it would remain efficient as an insulinotropic agent when administered enterally.

Once such an agent is made available, long-term experiments could be undertaken in animal models of type 2 diabetes to investigate whether the prolonged availability of such an ester to the pancreatic B-cell may improve the secretory potential of the endocrine pancreas, including possibly its secretory responsiveness to D-glucose.

REFERENCES

1. W.J. Malaisse, Alteration of pancreatic B-cell D-glucose metabolism in type 2 diabetes: The G quintet, *Endocrinologia* 40: 309 (1993).
2. W.J. Malaisse, C. Maggetto, V. Leclercq-Meyer, and A. Sener, Interference of glycogenolysis with glycolysis in pancreatic islets from glucose-infused rats, *J. Clin. Invest.* 91: 432 (1993).
3. W.J. Malaisse, J. Rasschaert, M.L. Villanueva-Peñacarrillo, and I. Valverde, Respiratory, ionic and functional effects of succinate esters in pancreatic islets, *Am. J. Physiol.* 264: E428 (1993).
4. W.J. Malaisse, and A. Sener, Metabolic effects and fate of succinate esters in pancreatic islets, *Am. J. Physiol.* 264: E434 (1993).
5. A. Sener, I. Conget, J. Rasschaert, V. Leclercq-Meyer, M.L. Villanueva-Peñacarrillo, I. Valverde, and W.J. Malaisse, Insulinotropic action of glutamic acid dimethyl ester, *Am. J. Physiol.*: in press (1994).
6. J. Levy, and W.J. Malaisse, The stimulus-secretion coupling of glucose-induced insulin release. XVII. Effects of sulfonylureas and diazoxide on insular biosynthetic activity, *Biochem. Pharmacol.* 24: 235 (1975).
7. V. Leclercq-Meyer, and W.J. Malaisse, Enhancement by succinic acid dimethyl ester of insulin release evoked by D-glucose and glimepiride in the perfused pancreas of normoglycemic and hyperglycemic rats, *Biochem. Pharmacol.* 47: 1519 (1994).
8. D. Vicent, M.L. Villanueva-Peñacarrillo, I. Valverde, and W.J. Malaisse, Enhancement of the insulinotropic action of glibenclamide by succinic acid methyl esters in anaesthetised rats, *Med. Sci. Res.* 21: 517 (1993).

9. A.G. Akkan, and W.J. Malaisse, Protective effect of succinic acid monomethylester against streptozotocin-induced diabetes mellitus, *Med. Sci. Res.* 21: 647 (1993).
10. D.L. Eizirik, N. Welsh, A. Niemann, L.A. Velloso, and W.J. Malaisse, Succinic acid monomethyl ester protects rat pancreatic islet secretory potential against interleukin-1β (1L-1β) without affecting glutamate decarboxylase expression or nitric oxide production, *FEBS Letters* 337: 298 (1994).
11. I. Conget, T.-M. Zhang, D.L. Eizirik, and W.J. Malaisse, SAM prevents impairment of glucose-stimulated insulin secretion caused by hexose deprivation or starvation, *Am. J. Physiol.* 268: E580–E587 (1995).
12. W.J. Malaisse, P. Lebrun, and A. Sener, Modulation of the insulinotropic action of glibenclamide and glimepiride by nutrient secretagogues in pancreatic islets from normoglycemic and hyperglycemic rats, *Biochem. Pharmacol.* 45: 1845 (1993).
13. A.G. Akkan, and W.J. Malaisse, Iterative pulse administration of succinic acid monomethyl ester to streptozotocin diabetic rats, *Diab. Res.* 23: 55–63 (1993).
14. D. Vicent, M.L. Villanueva-Peñacarrillo, F. Malaisse-Lagae, V. Leclercq-Meyer, I. Valverde, and W.J. Malaisse, *In vivo* stimulation of insuln release by succinic acid methyl esters, *Arch. Int. Pharmacodyn. Ther.* 327: 246–250 (1994).
15. D. Vicent, M.L. Villanueva-Peñacarrillo, I. Valverde, and W.J. Malaisse, Impaired in vivo insulin secretion in response to non-glucidic secretagogues in adult rats after neonatal streptozotocin, *Acta Diabetol.* 31: 133–137 (1994).
16. D. Abazie, F. Malaisse-Lagae, I. Conget, A. Sener, V. Leclercq-Meyer, and W.J. Malaisse, Repetitive pulse dispensing of succinate methyl ester to streptozotocin-injected rats, *Med. Sci. Res.* 21: 667 (1993).
17. D. Vicent, J.A. Garcia-Martinez, M.L. Villanueva-Peñacarrillo, I. Valverde, and W.J. Malaisse, Insulinotropic action of the dimethyl ester of glutamic acid in anaethetised rats, *Med. Sci. Res.* 22: 299 (1994).
18. J.A. Garcia-Martinez, D. Vicent, M.L. Villanueva-Peñacarrillo, I. Valverde, and W.J. Malaisse, Insulinotropic action of the dimethyl ester of glutamic acid in anaesthetized rats, *Diabetologia* 37 (Suppl 1): A109 (1994).
19. F. Malaisse-Lagae, T.-M. Zhang, A. Bakkali Nadi, and W.J. Malaisse, Insulinotropic efficiency of enterally administered succinic acid dimethyl ester, *Med. Sci. Res.* 22: 365 (1994).
20. W.J. Malaisse, T.-M. Zhang, V. Leclercq-Meyer, A. Sener, and F. Björkling, Insulinotropic action of the D-glucosyl and 3-O-methyl-D-glucosyl monomethyl esters of succinic acid, *Diab. Res.* 25: 93–105 (1994).

33

GLUCOSE METABOLISM REGULATES CYTOSOLIC Ca^{2+} IN THE PANCREATIC β-CELL BY THREE DIFFERENT MECHANISMS

Angel Nadal and Bernat Soria*

Center for Bioengineering, Department of Physiology
Miguel Hernandez University
Alicante, Spain

INTRODUCTION

The main stimulus to promote insulin release is an increase in the extracellular glucose concentration. It has been repeatedly shown that glucose and other secretagogues induced an increase in cytosolic Ca^{2+} ($[Ca^{2+}]_i$). The sequence of events linking exposure to stimulatory glucose concentrations with the release of insulin has been established [1]. Glucose-induced $[Ca^{2+}]_i$ increase is a consequence of glucose metabolism, ATP generation and blockade of ATP-dependent K^+ channels [2,3] which in turn depolarize the cell and activate voltage-dependent Ca^{2+} channels [4]. According to this mechanism it was demonstrated that glucose-induced $[Ca^{2+}]_i$ oscillations [5] are due to bursting of the electrical activity [6]. Moreover, simultaneous measurement of K_{ATP} channel activity and $[Ca^{2+}]_i$ in isolated β-cells showed that blockade of K_{ATP} always precedes $[Ca^{2+}]_i$ increase and that there is a strict correlation between spike frequency and Ca^{2+} increase [7]. All this body of theory was in apparent contradiction with other results which indicate that under certain conditions glucose *decreased* $[Ca^{2+}]_i$ [8]. It should be noted that the physiological effect of glucose on $[Ca^{2+}]_i$ is neither a decrease nor a steady-state increase in $[Ca^{2+}]_i$ but the induction of well-shaped $[Ca^{2+}]_i$ oscillations in islet cells. A detailed description of such oscillations is given in Chapter 26.

The aim of this chapter is to discuss the mechanisms of glucose-induced $[Ca^{2+}]_i$ oscillations, its relationship with electrical activity and with calcium removal and sequestering. Here we will show that: (i) glucose-induced $[Ca^{2+}]_i$ oscillations match and are due to bursting of the electrical activity, (ii) Ca^{2+} extrusion is governed by Na^+/Ca^{2+} exchange and by Ca^{2+} pumping outside the cytosol and (iii) the main mechanism underlying both functions is directly dependent on metabolism. Furthermore, we will show that under some circumstances, glucose is able to decrease $[Ca^{2+}]_i$, probably by filling a calcium store which in turn modulates plasma membrane calcium permeability [9].

---

* E-mail: bernat.soria@umh.es

Physiology and Pathophysiology of the Islets of Langerhans, edited by Soria.
Plenum Press, New York, 1997.

THE RELATIONSHIP BETWEEN $[Ca^{2+}]_i$ AND ELECTRICAL ACTIVITY: Ca^{2+} PERMEABILITY DURING ELECTRICAL BURSTING

It has been demonstrated that in the presence of intermediate glucose concentrations (7–11 mM), $[Ca^{2+}]_i$ oscillates with a well-defined pattern [5]. Furthermore, simultaneous recording of the membrane potential of an islet β-cell and $[Ca^{2+}]_i$ from the whole islet showed that glucose-induced oscillations are due to bursting of electrical activity [6].

In order to asses the plasma membrane Ca^{2+} permeability we have used the Mn^{2+} quenching technique [11]. Simultaneous measurements of $[Ca^{2+}]_i$ and Mn^{2+} quenching can be achieved using the ratio F410/F480 to follow $[Ca^{2+}]_i$ and F_{total} = F410 + F480 for Mn^{2+} quenching. F_{total} will be independent of $[Ca^{2+}]_i$. Before starting the experiment, we gave a small depolarizing pulse with 15 mM K^+, adjusting both wavelengths to the point where the increase in fluorescence at 410 nm was cancelled by the decrease in fluorescence at 480 nm. An in vitro calibration curve was produced under the same experimental conditions, estimated values of $[Ca^{2+}]_i$ are presented in the figure legends.

Figure 1 shows the effect of 11 mM glucose on $[Ca^{2+}]_i$. As previously reported, $[Ca^{2+}]_i$ undergoes oscillations (A, upper panel) due to bursts of electrical activity. The lower panel in A shows the total fluorescence (410 + 480 nm). Figure 1B shows the effect

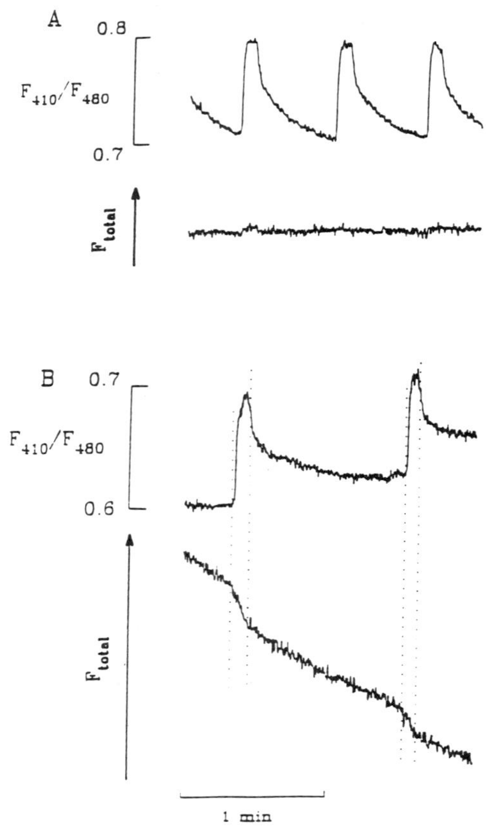

Figure 1. Effect of glucose 11 mM on the indo-1 fluorescence ratio (F410/F480) as a measure of $[Ca^{2+}]_i$ and on total fluorescence (F_{total} = F410 + F480). **A:** Upper panel: $[Ca^{2+}]_i$ oscillations recorded under steady conditions. Lower panel: Total fluorescence after correcting for photobleaching. Photobleaching represents less than 2% of total fluorescence and was constant at this time scale. **B:** Effect of adding 50 μM Mn^{2+} to the superfusion solution. The record in B is the continuation of A and was taken 3 min. after adding Mn^{2+}. The lower panel shows the total fluorescence only corrected for photobleaching applying the same constant than in A. The dotted lines have been drawn through the begining and the end of the active phase of the $[Ca^{2+}]_i$ oscillation and coincides with changes in the rate of fluorescence quenching.

of adding 50 μM Mn^{2+}. This produces a small increase in the fluorescence ratio 410/480 nm. However, the time course of the oscillations remains practically unchanged. The lower panel of Fig. 1B shows the effect of Mn^{2+} on total fluorescence. It is clear that when Mn^{2+} is added, the rate of fluorescence quenching is increased, during the inter-oscillatory periods and to a greater extent during the active phase. During the active phase, the increase in the slope of Mn^{2+} quenching, as expected, coincides with the increase in R(410/480), due to the activation of voltage-dependent calcium channels. On the other hand, the end of the oscillation — when the ratio starts to decrease — coincides with a decrease in Mn^{2+} permeability. At this point, Ca^{2+} removal and sequestering mechanisms are should be active in decreasing $[Ca^{2+}]_i$ levels.

METABOLIC REGULATION OF $[Ca^{2+}]_i$ HANDLING: EXTRUSION AND SEQUESTERING

An essential requirement for generating oscillations in cytosolic calcium is that $[Ca^{2+}]_i$ regulatory mechanisms in the B-cell have to be efficient enough to rapidly remove the cytosolic Ca^{2+} loads generated by the bursts of electrical activity [10,11]. Despite the importance of $[Ca^{2+}]_i$ handling for insulin release, our knowledge of the mechanisms implicated in $[Ca^{2+}]_i$ regulation is only fragmentary. Efflux of Ca^{2+} through the plasma membrane seems to occur by two mechanisms: (i) a Na^+/Ca^{2+} exchange driven by the Na^+ electrochemical gradient [12,13,14] and (ii) Ca^{2+} efflux through an energy dependent Ca^{2+} pump [15]. In addition to these extrusion mechanisms, cytosolic Ca^{2+} may be sequestered into intracellular organelles. In a recent work we have studied the metabolic regulation of cytosolic Ca^{2+} in mouse islets of Langerhans [16]. The effect of Na^+ omission and metabolic inhibition was studied on the recovery from K^+ induced Ca^{2+} loads. Our results suggest that both Na^+/Ca^{2+} exchange and cellular metabolic energy play a role in calcium homeostasis in islets of Langerhans, but metabolic-dependent regulation seems to be of primary importance. In the next series of experiments, we explore the role of glucose metabolism in $[Ca^{2+}]_i$ homeostasis.

Glucose Effects Independent of Membrane Potential

The direct role of glucose metabolism in $[Ca^{2+}]_i$ homeostasis is difficult to study due to the effects of glucose on membrane potential. Therefore, we used the K^+-channel opener diazoxide in order to overcome these problems. When100 μM diazoxide was present and after 15 min in the absence of glucose, addition of 3 mM glucose produced a small decrease in the basal $[Ca^{2+}]_i$ level; this effect was more noticeable when the concentration was stepped to 11 mM and appeared to saturate at this concentration, as increasing glucose concentration to 16 mM did not produce a further decrease in $[Ca^{2+}]_i$. We have previously shown [16] (see also Fig. 4A) that in the absence of glucose, adding diazoxide did not decrease $[Ca^{2+}]_i$, indicating that hyperpolarization alone is not able to decrease $[Ca^{2+}]_i$ levels. These results, obtained in cells in which their membrane potential was "clamped" to a value close to the K^+ equilibrium potential, explain the apparent contradiction pointed before.

Previous observations pointed out that glucose has a dual effect on cytosolic Ca^{2+} [8]. According to that $[Ca^{2+}]_i$ increase and decrease will cancel each other except if they occurs at different times and/or at different locations. Both seem to be true in the β-cell. Under physiological conditions, glucose both (i) increases Ca^{2+} influx through voltage-activated Ca^{2+} channels ($[Ca^{2+}]_i$ increase) and (ii) promotes Ca^{2+} sequestration into intracellular stores as well as Ca^{2+} pumping outside the cell by activating Ca^{2+}-ATPases. Both mechanisms are operative around physiological $[Ca^{2+}]_i$ (80–100 nM). When $[Ca^{2+}]_i$ reaches certain values (> 100–200 nM) energy-dependent extrusion mechanisms operate. Glucose provides energy to fuel ion pumps. While Ca^{2+}-pumps extrude Ca^{2+} from cytosolic pool, Na^+-pumps lower cytosolic Na^+ allowing Na^+/Ca^{2+} exchange to operate. Glucose-induced $[Ca^{2+}]_i$ increase seems to be unique to the β-cell (and perhaps other glucose-sensing cells) and needs 60–120 s to develop. In the opposite, glucose-induced $[Ca^{2+}]_i$ decrease needs less than 30 s to appear and *has been observed in other living cells* [17,18]. It probably constitutes a more ubiquitous system to mantain Ca^{2+} lower in the cytosol of living cells.

These experiments indicate that the main mechanism(s) responsible for calcium homeostasis in pancreatic B-cells is directly related to glucose metabolism. However, the effect of metabolism on calcium handling may not only be mediated by direct energization of Ca^{2+}-pumps. This point is analyzed in the next section.

CONTROL OF THE RESTING PERMEABILITY OF THE PLASMA MEMBRANE

A further important aspect of the regulation of $[Ca^{2+}]_i$ is the control of the resting Ca^{2+} permeability of the plasma membrane. In a wide variety of cells, a complex interrelationship between the filling status of intracellular calcium stores and the plasma membrane calcium permeability has been found [17,18]. Such a mechanism seems also to be operating in β-cells.

Stimulation of islets of Langerhans by muscarinic agonist such as carbachol (CCh) activates a phospholipase C, leading to a generation of inositol (1,4,5)triphosphate (IP3) and diacylglycerol. The intracellular free calcium concentrations response in β-cells is a $[Ca^{2+}]_i$ transient followed by a maintained plateau that disappears in the absence of extracellular calcium and is therefore attributable to entry of Ca^{2+} through the surface membrane. Entry of Ca^{2+} in the plateau phase can be detected using external Mn^{2+} as Ca^{2+} surrogate; Mn^{2+} entry is detected independently of intracellular Ca^{2+} release from the fluorescence quenching of the Ca^{2+} indicators Indo-1 or fura-2 [19]. This influx of calcium may be mediated by different mechanisms. carbachol (100 μM) induces an increase in the

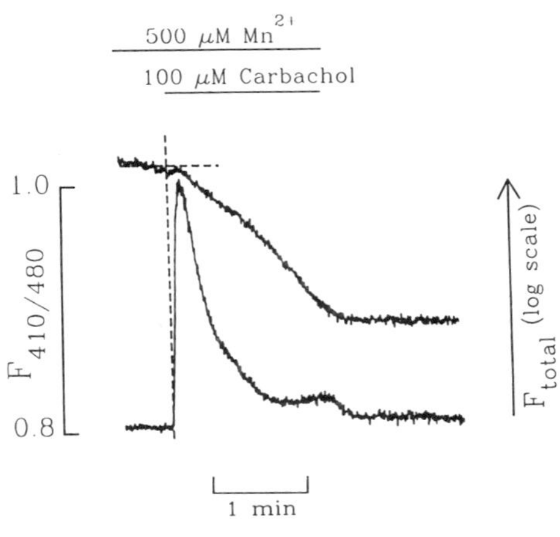

Figure 2. Applying 100 μM carbachol in the presence of 500 μM external Mn^{2+}, produces a fast increase in the ratio of fluorescence (F410/F480) (lower trace) and a slow decrease in F_{TOTAL}, due to Mn^{2+} influx (top trace). These efffects are present throughout the time that CCh is stimulating the cell. The effect is reversible and repeatable in the same cell.

rate of Mn^{2+} quenching, consistentwith an increase in Ca^{2+} permeability (Fig. 2). We shall see how this increase in Mn^{2+} quenching was also found in those situations that led to emptyng intracellular stores of calcium.

The Effect of Glucose on Resting Ca^{2+} Permeability

A standard maneuver to deplete intracellular stores consists in incubating the cells in solutions containing different Ca^{2+} concentrations. Figure 3 shows the effect of changing the degree of Ca^{2+} filling of intracellular stores on Mn^{2+} permeability. At the point indicated by the arrow, 500 μM Mn^{2+} was added to the medium in control conditions. Fluorescence quenching here was not very high. After removing Mn^{2+}, the islet was incubated in the absence of extracellular Ca^{2+} (1 mM EGTA added) for a 30 minutes period

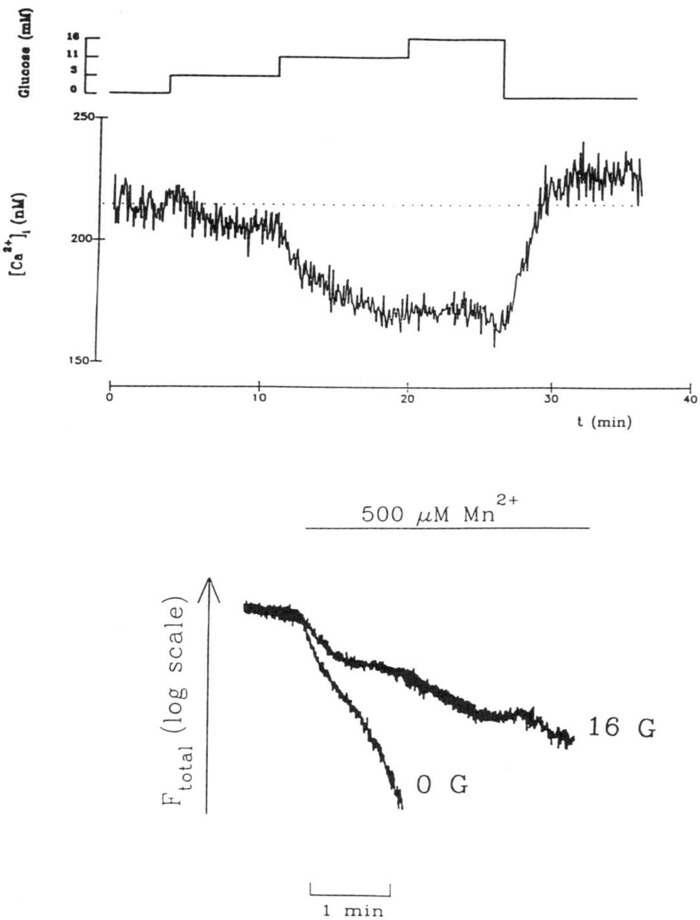

Figure 3. Effect of glucose on in the presence of 100 μM diazoxide. **Upper panel:** effect on $[Ca^{2+}]_i$. After 15 min in the absence of glucose, addition of 3 mM glucose produces a small decrease in the basal $[Ca^{2+}]_i$ level, the effect is more noticeable when the concentration was stepped to 11 mM and appeared to saturate at this contration. **Lower panel:** Mn^{2+} quenching of the total fluorescence (F_{TOTAL}). Glucose (16 mM) produces a decrease in the slope of fluorescence quenching. Upper part: Taken from ref. 16, with permission.

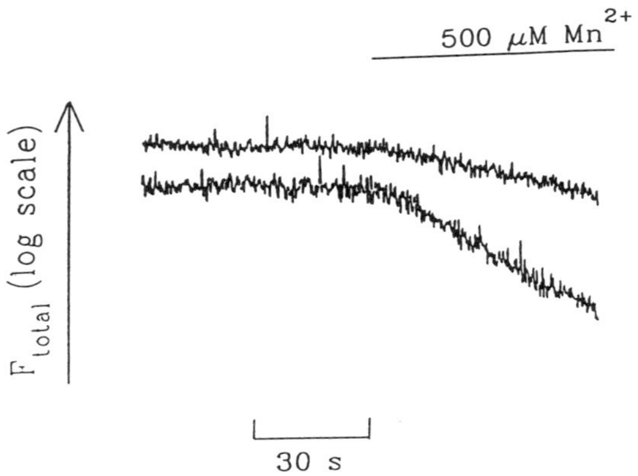

Figure 4. Effects of incubation in different extracellular calcium concentration on total fluorescence Mn^{2+} quenching. In the control (upper record) 500 Mn^{2+} were added at the point indicated by the arrow. After Mn^{2+} removal, the islet was incubated for 30 minutes in the absence of extracellular calcium (1 mM EGTA added) and then for 3 minutes in the control calcium solution. At this time, 500 μM Mn^{2+} were added (lower control). The traces have been superimposed in order to facilitate comparison.

and then for 3 minutes in the presence of standard extracellular Ca^{2+}. At this point Mn^{2+} (500 μM) was added to the superfusion solution, obtaining a substantial increase in fluorescence quenching, indicating a high plasma membrane Ca^{2+} permeability. When the experiment was done in the reverse order, essentially the same results were obtained. It seems therefore that the degree of calcium loading by the stores has an effect on membrane calcium permeability.

As previously discussed, when depolarization is prevented (clamping the cell membrane potential close to the K^+ equilibrium potential) glucose is able to decrease $[Ca^{2+}]_i$. (Figure 4) Such an effect can be the result of an increase in the rate of Ca^{2+} pumping out from the cell or pumping into an intracellular compartment. The experiment shown in Figure 4 suggest that the later seems to be the case. In this experiment, increasing the glucose concentration in the presence of 100 μM diazoxide, decreases $[Ca^{2+}]_i$. The lower panel of the figure shows the total fluorescence. Here, increasing glucose concentration decreased the rate of fluorescence quenching. This result can be interpreted as glucose pumping Ca^{2+} inside some reservoir and filling it up and consequently decreasing resting Ca^{2+} membrane permeability. Although the exact mechanisms that couples the filling status of the store and the membrane permeability is not known, there is evidence suggesting a role for phosphatidyl inositides [20], as well as the state of the cytochrome P-450 [21]. It is important however to stress that the characteristics of the coupling mechanisms and the associated Ca^{2+} permeability may be substantially different in different cells. The biophysical properties of this current, also called I_{CRAC} (calcium release activated currents), are unknown. In addition to Mn^{2+} and Ca^{2+}, other ions as Na^+ could permeate them. Such a permeability may explain the complex effects ot muscarinic agonists on β-cell membrane potential and cytosolic Ca^{2+} [9,23,24].

THE MODEL

The results presented in this paper demonstrate the multiple role played by glucose metabolism on $[Ca^{2+}]_i$ regulation in pancreatic islets of Langerhans. In addition to the well known effect of glucose metabolism on K_{ATP} closure and Ca^{2+}-channel activation, here we also describe two other effects. First, it seems clear that their are mainly two mechanisms responsible for calcium homeostasis, one of them is energy dependent and directly related to glucose metabolism, the other one is the Na^+/Ca^{2+} exchange. On the other hand, plasma

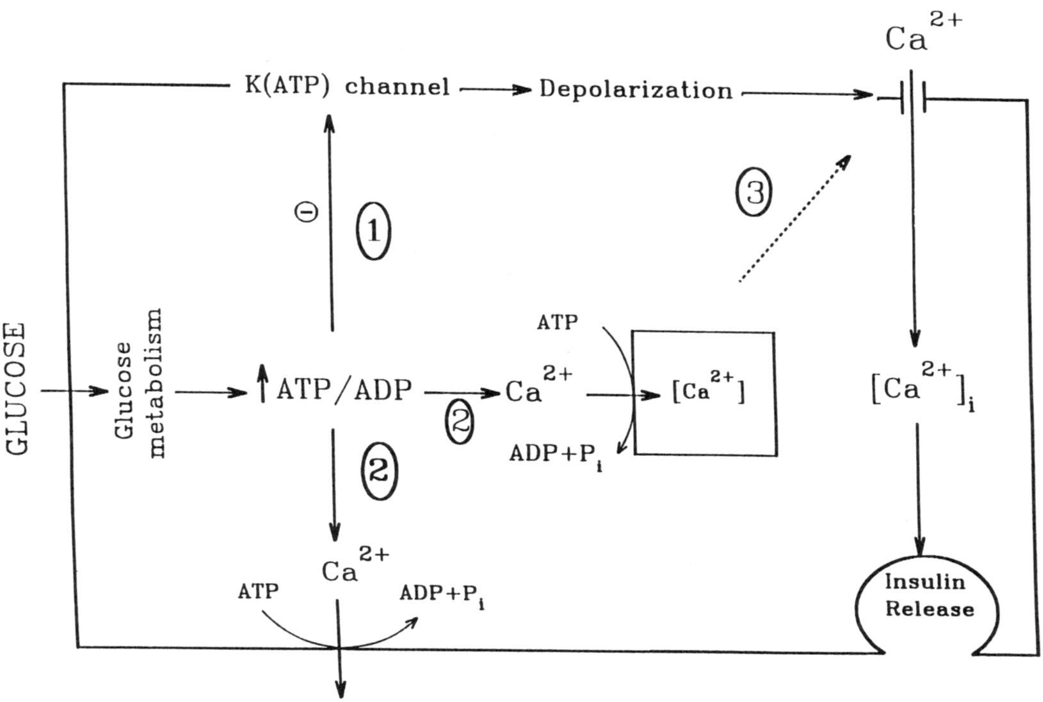

Figure 5. Schematic representation of the different ways by which glucose metabolism can control $[Ca^{2+}]_i$. See text for an explanation.

membrane calcium permeability seems to be primarily modulated by the filling status of some intracellular store which in turn may be directly dependent on the metabolic status of the cell.

Much attention has been paid to the role of K_{ATP} channels in stimulus-secretion coupling in these cells. Such an effect would be the primary target of glucose metabolism (represented as arrow 1 in Figure 5), leading through membrane depolarization to calcium channel activation and a rise in $[Ca^{2+}]_i$. However, this is not the only effect of glucose metabolism on $[Ca^{2+}]_i$. Glucose metabolism is critically affecting the regulation of $[Ca^{2+}]_i$ by a second metabolic effect wich tends to counteract with the first mechanism. This metabolic regulation exerts its action through two mechanisms. The first consists in fuelling the Ca^{2+}-transport mechanisms, both at the plasma membrane level and the Ca^{2+}-pumps of intracellular stores (marked as 2 in the diagram). On the other hand, glucose keeps the Na^+/Ca^{2+} exchange mechanism active by maintaining the apropriate Na^+ and K^+ gradients by energizing the Na^+-K^+ ATPase. The interplay between mechanisms 1 and 2 may be crucial for shaping glucose-induced $[Ca^{2+}]_i$ oscillations. The third mechanism by which glucose maintains an adequate Ca^{2+} distribution is an indirect one, through the control of the degree of filling of intracellular stores. This in turn controls calcium membrane permeability (arrow 3 in the scheme). This control may be important in regulating calcium-dependent insulin release by mechanisms other than metabolic, e.g. purinergic and cholinergic stimulation.

In summary, the model proposed suggest that glucose controls $[Ca^{2+}]_i$ in pancreatic islet cells by three different mechanims: (i) depolarizing cell membrane (and opening voltage dependent Ca^{2+} channels) as a consequence of K_{ATP} blockade, (ii) energitizing those mechanisms which are responsible for $[Ca^{2+}]_i$ homeostasis (e.g. Ca^{2+} pumps), and (iii) filling-up a Ca^{2+} reservoir that in turn controls membrane Ca^{2+} permeability.

ACKNOWLEDGMENTS

These studies have been supported by Grants from FIS (96-1994-01), Generalitat Valenciana (GV-3117/95) and the European Union (ERBSC1-CT920833). A. Nadal was a recipient of a Fellowship from the FPI (DGICYT). The skillful technical assistance of Rosa García Velasco, Simon Moya and Alfonso Perez is gratefully acknowledged.

REFERENCES

1. Ashcroft FM, Rorsman P (1991) Electrophysiology of the pancreartic β-cell. *Progress in Biophysics and Molecular Biology 54*, 87–147.
2. Cook DL, Hales CN (1984) Intracellular ATP directly blocks K^+ channels in pancreatic β-cells. *Nature 311*, 271–273.
3. Ashcroft FM, Harrison DE, Ashcroft SJH (1984) Glucose induces closure of single potassium channels in isolated rat pancreatic β-cells. *Nature 312*, 446–448.
4. Rorsman P, Trube G (1986) Calcium and delayed potassium currents in mouse pancreatic β-cells under voltage-clamp conditions. *J. Physiol. 374*, 531–550.
5. Valdeolmillos M, Santos R, Contreras D, Soria B, Rosario LM (1989) Glucose-induced oscillations of intracellular Ca^{2+} concentration resembling bursting electrical activity in single mouse islets of Langerhans. *FEBS Letters 259*, 19–23.
6. Santos RM, Rosario LM, Nadal A, García-Sancho J, Soria B, Valdeolmillos M (1991) Widespread synchronous $[Ca^{2+}]_i$ oscillations due to bursting electrical activity in single pancreatic islets. *Pflügers Archiv 418*, 417–422.
7. Valdeolmillos M, Nadal A, Contreras D, Soria B (1992) The relationship between glucose-induced K(ATP) channel closure and the rise in $[Ca^{2+}]_i$ in single mouse pancreatic B-cells. *Journal of Physiology 455*, 173–186.
8. Gylfe E (1988) Nutrient secretogogues induce bimodal early changes in cytoplasmic calcium of insulin-releasing ob/ob mouse β-cells. *Journal of Biological Chemistry 263*, 13750–13754.
9. Bertram R, Smolen P, Sherman A, Mears D, Atwater I, Martin F, Soria B (1995) A role for calcium release activated current (CRAC) in cholinergic modulation of insulin secretion. *Biophys. J. 68*, 2323–2332.
10. Chay TR, Keizer J (1983) Minimal model for membrane oscillations in the pancreatic B-cell. *Biophys. J. 42*, 181–190.
11. Sherman A, Rinzel P (1991) Model for synchronization of pancreatic B-cells by gap junction coupling. *Biophys. J. 59*, 547–559.
12. Herchuelz A, Sener A, Malaisse WJ (1980) Regulation of calcium fluxes in rat pancreatic islets: calcium extrusion by sodium-calcium countertransport. *Journal of Membrane Biology 57*, 1–12.
13. Siegel EG, Wollheim CB, Renold AE (1980) Evidence for the involvement of Na^+/Ca^{2+} exchange in glucose-induced insulin release from rat pancreatic islets. *Journal of Clinical Investigation 66*, 996–1003.
14. Plasman PO, Lebrun P, Herchuelz A (1990) Characterization of the process of sodium-calcium exchange in pancreatic islets: calcium extrusion by sodium-calcium countertransport. *J. Memb. Biol. 57*, 1–12.
15. Pershadsing HA, McDaniel ML, Landt M, Bry CG, Lacy PE, McDonal JM (1980) Ca^{2+}-activated ATPase and ATP-dependent calmodulin-stimulated Ca^{2+} transport in islet cell membrane membranes. *Nature 288*, 492–495.
16. Nadal A, Valdeolmillos M, Soria B (1994) Metabolic regulation of $[Ca^{2+}]_i$ in mouse pancreatic islets of Langerhans. *Amer. J. Physiol. 267(5)*, E769–E774.
17. Putney JW (1991) Capacitative calcium entry revisited. *Cell Calcium 11*, 611–624.
18. Putney J, Bird GSt (1993) The signal for capacitative calcium entry. *Cell 75*, 199–201.
19. Jacob R (1990) Agonist-stimulated divalent cation entry into single cultured human umbilical vein endothelial cells. *J. Physiol. 421*, 55–77.
20. Berridge MJ (1993) Inositol triphosphate and calcium signalling. *Nature 362*, 315–325.

21. Alvarez J, Montero M, García-Sancho J (1991) Cytochrome P-450 may link intracellular Ca^{2+} stores with plasma membrane Ca^{2+} influx. *Biochemical Journal 274*, 193–197.
22. Randiamamprita C, Tsien RY (1993) Emptying of intracellular Ca^{2+} stores releases a novel small messenger that stimulates Ca^{2+} influx. *Nature 364*, 809–814.
23. Sanchez-Andrés JV, Ripoll C, Soria B (1988) Evidence that muscarinic potentiation of insulin release is initiated by an early calcium entry. *FEBS Lett. 231*, 144–147.
24. Sanchez-Andrés JV, Nadal A, Martin F, and Soria B (1994) Sequential effects of muscarinic agonists on glucose-induced electrical activity and cytosolic $[Ca^{2+}]_i$ in the pancreatic B-cell. In: "*Frontiers in B-Cell Research.*" Smith Gordon and Co. Ltd. London (P. Flatt, S. Lenzen; eds.) pp. 353–358.

Part V. β-CELL HETEROGENEITY: BUILDING AN HOMOGENEOUS RESPONSE FROM AN HETEROGENEOUS POPULATION

34

HETEROGENEITY OF β-CELL SECRETION

Possible Involvement of K-ATP Channels

M. Faehling and F. M. Ashcroft

University Laboratory of Physiology
Parks Road
Oxford OX1 3PT, United Kingdom

INTRODUCTION

Studies of secretion using the reverse haemolytic plaque assay have revealed a marked heterogeneity in the response of individual β-cells to a given secretagogue concentration (Salomon & Meda, 1986; Hiriart & Matteson, 1988; Hiriart & Ramirez-Medeles, 1991). A similar heterogeneity is also found for the increase in intracellular Ca^{2+} evoked by glucose (Pralong et al., 1990; Hellman et al., 1992). The rise in $[Ca^{2+}]_i$ which stimulates insulin secretion is brought about by activation of voltage-gated Ca^{2+} channels, as a consequence of the membrane depolarisation which is produced by glucose-induced closure of ATP-sensitive K^+ channels (Ashcroft & Rorsman, 1989). Thus, one possible explanation for the heterogeneity observed in both the Ca^{2+} and the secretory responses of the β-cell to glucose is that they arise from variability in the extent of inhibition of the ATP-sensitive K^+ channel (K-ATP channel) by glucose metabolism. No difference in the maximum amplitude of K-ATP currents in β-cells with low and high secretory activity, identified by small and large plaque formation in the reverse haemolytic plaque assay, was found using the standard whole-cell patch-clamp method (Soria et al., 1991). However, these experiments measured the total K-ATP current in the absence of ATP, and did not address the question of whether heterogeneity in the metabolic regulation of the K-ATP channel might underlie the observed secretory variability. In this study, we have used the perforated patch configuration, in which metabolism is preserved, to examine this possibility.

METHODS

Mouse pancreatic islets were isolated by collagenase digestion and dispersed into single β-cells using Ca^{2+}-free solution (Smith et al., 1993). Secretion from individual

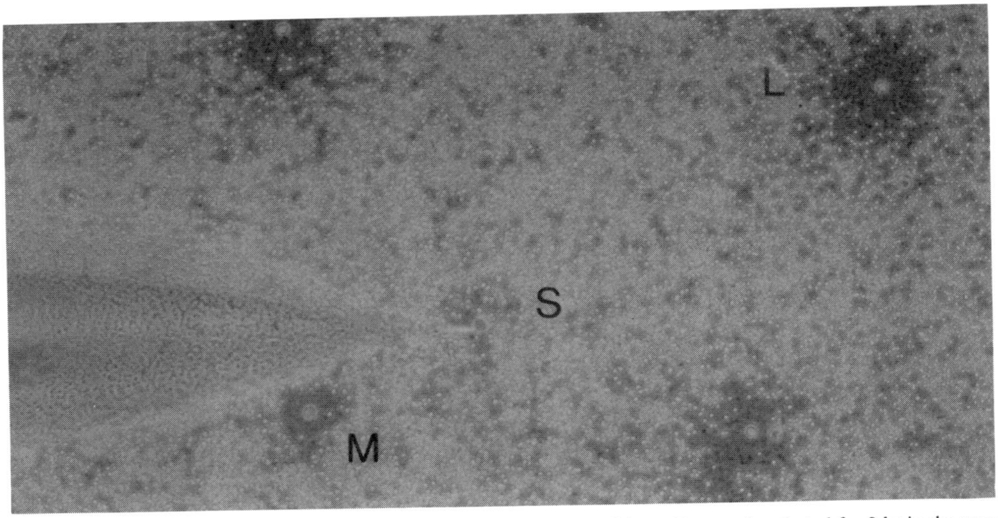

Figure 1. Pancreatic β-cells differ in their ability to secrete insulin. Islet cells were incubated for 2 hr in the presence of 10 mM glucose. Under this condition we observed small (S), medium (M) and large (L) plaques. The shadow of the patch pipette can be seen in the photograph.

β-cells was assessed using the reverse haemolytic plaque assay as described by Lewis et al. (1988), with minor modifications. Briefly, the plaque assay was carried out on polylysine coated glass coverslips attached to the bottom of 35mm petri dishes, at 37°C in an incubator gassed with 95% O_2/5% CO_2. Protein A-conjugated erythrocytes and freshly prepared β-cells were mixed, plated onto the coverslips and allowed to attach for 1 h. Secretion was then elicited by stimulation with 10 mM glucose for 2 hr in the presence of anti-C-peptide antibody. After stimulation, the cells were incubated for a further 30 min in glucose-free solution supplemented with complement to induce lysis of erythrocytes which had bound insulin. Solutions were added to one side of the coverslip using a Finn pipette and removed from the other side by gentle suction with a pipette. Following the plaque assay, cells were maintained at 37°C in RPMI 1640 tissue culture medium supplemented with 10% foetal calf serum, 10 U/ml penicillin and 10 μg/ml streptomycin and gassed with 95% O_2/5% CO_2. Patch clamp experiments were carried out within 48 hr of the plaque assay.

Whole-cell K-ATP currents were studied using the perforated patch configuration of the patch-clamp technique (Smith et al., 1993). The standard extracellular (bath) solution contained (in mM) 140 NaCl, 5.6 KCl, 1.2 $MgCl_2$, 2.6 $CaCl_2$, 10 HEPES (adjusted to pH 7.4 with NaOH). Glucose was added as indicated in the text. The pipette solution contained (in mM): 70 K_2SO_4, 10 KCl, 10 NaCl, 1.0 $MgCl_2$, 1 EGTA, 10 HEPES (adjusted to pH 7.2 with KOH) and 50–200 μg/ml nystatin in 0.1–0.2% DMSO. Experiments were carried out at 30°C.

Currents were recorded using an EPC-7 patch-clamp amplifier (List Electronic, Darmstadt, FRG), digitised and stored on video tape for later analysis. The reference potential for all measurements was the zero current potential of the pipette before establishment of the seal. The cell was held at –70 mV and alternate hyperpolarizing and depolarizing pulses of 10 mV amplitude and 200 ms duration were applied at a frequency of 0.5 Hz. Most of the resulting current during these pulses flows through K-ATP channels

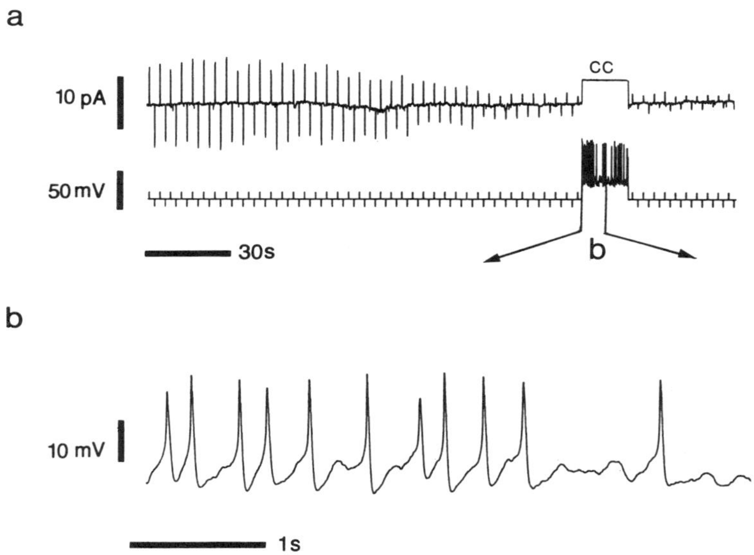

Figure 2. **(a)** Membrane potential (below) and whole-cell K-ATP currents (above) recorded under voltage-clamp using the perforated patch configuration. The cell was held at −70 mV and ±10 mV pulses of 200 ms duration were applied every 2 s. Glucose (10 mM) was added about 30 s before the start of the record. The cell was switched to current-clamp recording during the period indicated CC. **(b)** Expanded section of the membrane potential recording shown in (a) to illustrate β-cell electrical activity in the presence of glucose.

(cf. Trube et al., 1986); however, there may also be a small contribution from seal and ionic leak currents. Results have been normalised to the cell capacitance to take account of differences in cell size: the mean capacitance was 4.7 ± 0.6 pF (n=13). Data are given as mean ± S.E.M.

RESULTS

The secretory response to 10 mM glucose varied between β-cells, with cells producing plaques of different sizes (Fig. 1).

Whole-cell currents were recorded from β-cells identified using the reverse haemolytic plaque assay. Cells were classified into those forming large, medium and small plaques. A representative experiment on a large plaque-forming β-cell is shown in Fig. 2. In the absence of glucose, the β-cell was electrically silent with a resting potential of around −65 mV and a resting K-ATP current of 5.5 pA, corresponding to a conductance of 0.6 nS. Glucose produced a decrease in the amplitude of the K-ATP current which was associated with electrical activity in current-clamp recordings. These data confirm that perforated-patch recording retains β-cell metabolism (Smith et al., 1990) and indicate that our cells remain metabolically viable following the plaque assay.

Mean values for the resting K-ATP current and conductance, from all cells, were 31.3 ± 7.5 pA and 3.1 ± 0.8 nS (n=13), respectively. The mean values are in reasonable agreement with those previously reported for intact β-cells in glucose-free solution (Smith et al., 1990; Cohen et al., 1990; Smith, 1988). Comparison with the maximal K-ATP

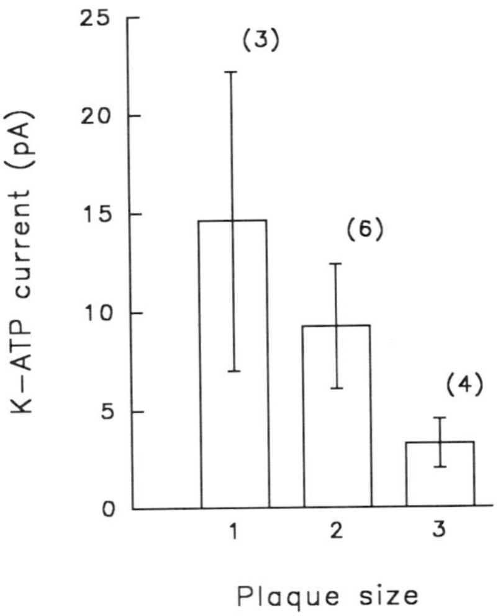

Figure 3. Cells which form larger plaques have smaller resting K-ATP currents. Mean whole-cell K-ATP currents recorded using the perforated patch configuration in glucose-free solution, from β-cells forming small (1), medium (2) or large plaques (3). The number of cells is indicated next to the error bar.

current observed following washout of ATP in standard whole-cell recordings (about 20 nS, Rorsman & Trube, 1985), suggests that >80% of the K-ATP current may be inhibited under resting conditions.

The relationship between the amplitude of the K-ATP current in glucose-free solution and the plaque size is given in Fig. 3. There was an inverse correlation in K-ATP current amplitude with plaque size, with cells forming large plaques having smaller resting K-ATP currents.

The effect of 20 mM glucose was tested on β-cells identified using the plaque assay. As found for glucose-free solutions, whole-cell K-ATP currents recorded in the presence of 20 mM glucose were smaller in β-cells with large plaques (Fig. 4A). The mean current in 20 mM glucose was 12.3 ± 4.2 pA (n = 13) which corresponds to 38% of the current recorded in glucose-free solution. This is much smaller than that predicted on the basis of single channel experiments (Ashcroft et al., 1988) for reasons we do not understand.

No consistent dependence on plaque size was found when K-ATP currents in 20 mM glucose were normalised with respect to their amplitude in glucose-free solution (Fig. 4B). Although the percentage inhibition was less for cells with small plaques than those with medium sized plaques, cells forming large plaques showed an intermediate degree of inhibition.

DISCUSSION

Our results show that the whole-cell K-ATP current of β-cells forming large plaques was smaller than that found for β-cells with small plaques, in both the presence or absence of glucose. This indicates that K-ATP channel activity is lower in cells with high insulin secretory activity, either as a result of a smaller number of K-ATP channels or a reduced channel open probability. The latter possibility seems more likely since the maximal K-ATP current measured in the absence of ATP is independent of β-cell secretory activity (Soria et al., 1993). The magnitude of the K-ATP current determines the β-cell membrane potential and thereby may regulate both electrical activity and insulin secretion. Thus the inverse correlation between plaque size and K-ATP current amplitude we observed in the presence of

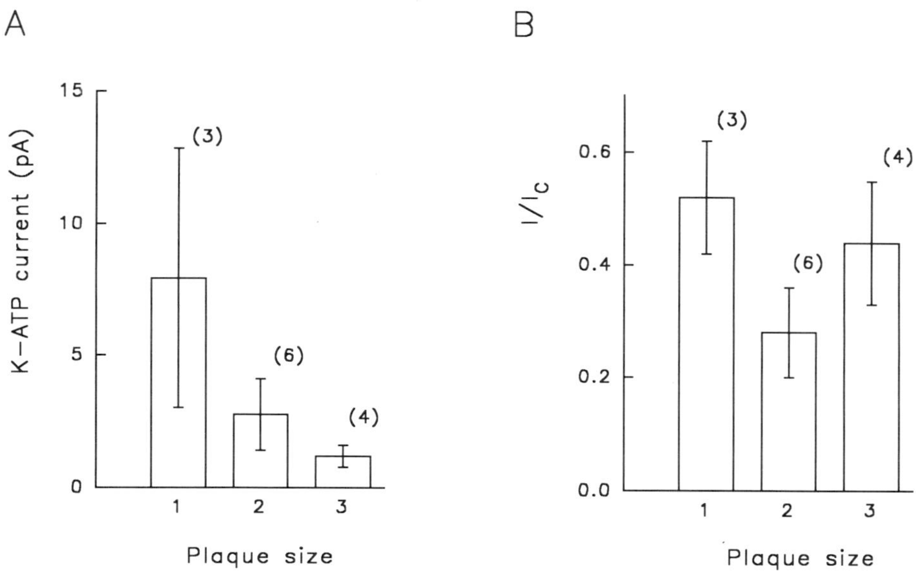

Figure 4 **A.** Cells which form large plaques have smaller K-ATP currents in the presence of glucose. Mean K-ATP currents recorded using the perforated patch configuration in response to 20 mM glucose, from β-cells forming small (1), medium (2) or large plaques (3). T he number of cells is indicated next to the error bar. Same cells as in Fig. 3. **B.** The K-ATP current recorded in 20 mM glucose solution (I), expressed as a fraction of its value in glucose-free solution (I_c) in the same cell, does not vary consistently with plaque size.

glucose suggests that at least part of the heterogeneity of insulin secretion found for individual β-cells results from differences in the magnitude of the K-ATP current.

We did not observe a correlation between plaque size and the percentage inhibition of the K-ATP current produced by 20 mM glucose. This suggest that the smaller K-ATP currents observed in β-cells with large plaques result principally from the smaller resting K-ATP currents they possess, and not from heterogeneity in the glucose-sensitivity of the K-ATP current. However, the data should be interpreted with care as the number of cells is small, especially in the large and small plaque categories. Furthermore, it is difficult to measure the glucose-induced change in current amplitude in cells forming large plaques, as these cells had small resting K-ATP currents initially. Although it may be argued that the β-cell changes its secretory response to glucose during the period between the plaque assay and the patch clamp experiment, the correlation between K-ATP current amplitude and plaque size suggests that this is not the case.

One possible explanation for the variability in resting K-ATP currents is that it results from a difference in the resting metabolic activity, and thus resting ATP levels, of individual β-cells. For example, the smaller K-ATP currents found in β-cells showing high secretory activity might result from an increased supply, or availability, of endogenous nutrients in these cells. Indeed, differences in biosynthetic activity of β-cells (Schuit et al., 1988) and in their metabolic responses to glucose (reviewed in Pipeleers, 1992) have been reported. However, the K-ATP channel is regulated by many cytoplasmic factors (Ashcroft & Rorsman, 1989), and we cannot exclude the alternative possibility that an additional regulator of the K-ATP current (other than ATP) is present, or active, to a varying extent in different β-cells.

In conclusion, our results suggest that the variability in plaque size may be due to individual differences in size of the β-cell K-ATP current. They may also explain the fact that glucose produces a dose-dependent increase in the number of plaque-forming β-cells (Hiriart & Matteson, 1988), since the threshold for electrical activity and insulin secretion will also be a function of the K-ATP current amplitude. Since different β-cells vary in the amplitude of their resting K-ATP currents, providing individual β-cells have similar glucose sensitivities (which appears to be the case), they will reach threshold at different sugar concentrations; and more cells will be recruited as glucose is increased and the K-ATP current further inhibited.

ACKNOWLEDGMENTS

We thank the British Diabetic Association, the Wellcome Trust and the Rhodes Trust for financial support. We thank Drs. A. Clark, C.E. Lewis and J. Morris for help in setting up the plaque assay method and providing the antibody.

REFERENCES

Ashcroft F. M. and Rorsman P. (1989) Electrophysiology of the pancreatic β-cell. Prog. Biophys. Molec. Biol. 54: 87–143.

Ashcroft F.M. Harrison D.E. and Ashcroft S. J.H. (1988) Properties of single potassium channels modulated by glucose in rat pancreatic β-cells. J. Physiol. 400: 501–527.

Cohen A. S., Matteson D. R., Parsey R. V. and Sala S. (1990) Ionic currents in rat pancreatic β-cells recorded with the perforated patch technique. Biophys. J. 57: 509a.

Hellman B., Gylfe E., Grappengeisser E., Lund P. E. and Marcström A. (1992) Cytoplasmic calcium and insulin secretion. In Nutrient Regulation of Insulin Secretion. Ed. P. Flatt. pp. 213–246.

Hiriart M. and Matteson D. R. (1988) Na channels and two types of Ca channels in rat pancreatic β-cells identified with the reverse haemolytic plaque assay. J. Gen. Physiol. 91: 617–639.

Hiriart M. and Ramirez-Medeles M. C. (1991) Functional subpopulations of individual pancreatic β-cells in culture. Endocrinol. 128: 3193–3198.

Lewis C., Clark A., Ashcroft S. J. H., Cooper G. J. S. and Morris J. F. (1988) Calcitonin gene-related peptide and somatostatin inhibit insulin release from individual rat β-cells. Mol. Cell. Endocrinol. 57: 41–49.

Pipeleers D., Kiekens R, and In't veld P. (1992) Morphology of the pancreatic β-cell. In Insulin : Molecular Biology to Pathology. Ed. Ashcroft F. M. and Ashcroft S. J. H. pp. 5–33.

Pralong W. F., Bartley C. and Wollheim C. B. (1990) Single islet beta-cell stimulation by nutrients: relationship between pyridine nucleotides, cytosolic Ca^{2+} and secretion. EMBO J. 9: 53–60.

Rorsman P. and Trube G. (1985). Glucose-dependent K^+ channels in pancreatic β-cells are regulated by intracellular ATP. Pflügers Arch. 405: 305–309.

Salomon D. and Meda P. (1986) Heterogeneity and contact-dependent regulation of hormone secretion by individual β-cells. Exp. Cell. Res. 162: 507–520.

Schuit F. C., In't Veld P.A., Pipeleers D.G. (1988) Glucose stimulates proinsulin biosynthesis by a dose-dependent recruitment of p ancreatic β-cells. Proc. Natl Acad. Sci. U.S.A. 85: 3865–3869.

Soria B., Chanson M., Giordano E., Bosco D. and Meda P. (1991) Ion channels of glucose-responsive and un-responsive cells. Diabetes 40: 1069–1078.

Smith P. A., Rorsman P. and Ashcroft F. M. (1990) Simultaneous recording of glucose-dependent electrical activity and ATP-regulated K^+-currents in isolated mouse pancreatic β-cells. FEBS Lett. 261: 187–190.

Smith P. A. (1988) Electrophysiology of β-cells from pancreatic islets of Langerhans. Ph.D. thesis, University of East Anglia.

Smith P. A., Ashcroft F. M. and Fewtrell C. M. S. (1993) Permeation and gating properties of the L-type calcium channel in mouse pancreatic β-cells. J. Gen. Physiol. 101: 767–797.

Trube G., Rorsman P. and Ohno-Shosaku T. (1986). Opposite effects of tolbutamide and diazoxide on the ATP-dependent K^+ channel in mouse pancreatic β-cells. Pflügers Arch. 407: 493–499.

35

HETEROGENEITY OF β-CELL Ca^{2+} RESPONSES TO GLUCOSE

P. Smith,[1] P. J. Millard,[2,*] C. M. S. Fewtrell,[2] and F. M. Ashcroft[1]

[1]University Laboratory of Physiology
Parks Road
Oxford OX1 3PT, United Kingdom
[2]Department of Pharmacology
Cornell University
Ithaca, New York 14853

INTRODUCTION

Insulin secretion is initiated by an increase in the cytoplasmic calcium concentration. Glucose metabolism stimulates this rise in $[Ca^{2+}]_i$ by closing ATP-sensitive K-channels in the plasma membrane, thereby producing membrane depolarisation, activation of voltage-gated Ca^{2+} channels and influx of extracellular Ca^{2+} (Ashcroft & Rorsman, 1989). Electrical activity, and thus Ca^{2+} influx, occurs in bursts and gives rise to synchronous oscillations in $[Ca^{2+}]_i$ (Santos et al., 1991; Valdeolmillos et al., 1989). Considerable heterogeneity in the $[Ca^{2+}]_i$ oscillatory behaviour of single β-cells has been reported (Pralong et al., 1991; Hellman et al., 1992). However, within an islet (which contains >1000 β-cells) the cells appear to oscillate in synchrony (Valdeolmillos et al., 1993), a feature which no doubt results from the well-established electrical coupling between β-cells (Eddlestone et al., 1984). Most previous studies have focused on the response of the β-cell or islet to a single glucose concentration. In this paper, therefore, we have examin ed the relationship between glucose and intracellular Ca^{2+} over a wide range of glucose concentrations, using imaging techniques to record simultaneous responses from a population of β-cells.

METHODS

Pancreatic islets from Smith-Webster mice were isolated by collagenase digestion and dispersed into single β-cells using Ca^{2+}-free Hank's solution (Smith et al., 1993). The

[*] Current address: Molecular Probes, P.O. Box 22010, Eugene, Oregon 97402-0414, USA.

cells were plated onto glass coverslips and cultured overnight at 37°C in RPMI 1640 medium supplemented with 11mM glucose, 10% heat-inactivated foetal calf serum and 50 μg/ml gentamycin.

Immediately before an experiment the coverslips were gently rinsed in Hank's solution supplemented with 3 mM glucose and 0.1% BSA. Cells were loaded with fura-2 by incubating the coverslip in supplemented Hank's solution plus 1 μM fura-2 acetoxymethyl ester for 30 min at room temperature. The coverslip was then mounted in a flow-through chamber and maintained at 37°C on the microscope stage. Unincorporated dye and non-adherent cells were then washed away using an external solution containing (mM) 138 NaCl, 5.6 KCl, 10 HEPES (pH 7.4 with NaOH), 2.6 $CaCl_2$, 1.1 $MgCl_2$ and 3 mM glucose before beginning the experiment. The glucose dose-response relationship was measured by perfusion with external solution containing increasing concentrations of glucose (3, 5, 8, 11, 16, and 22 mM). Data acquisition began 5 mins after each solu-

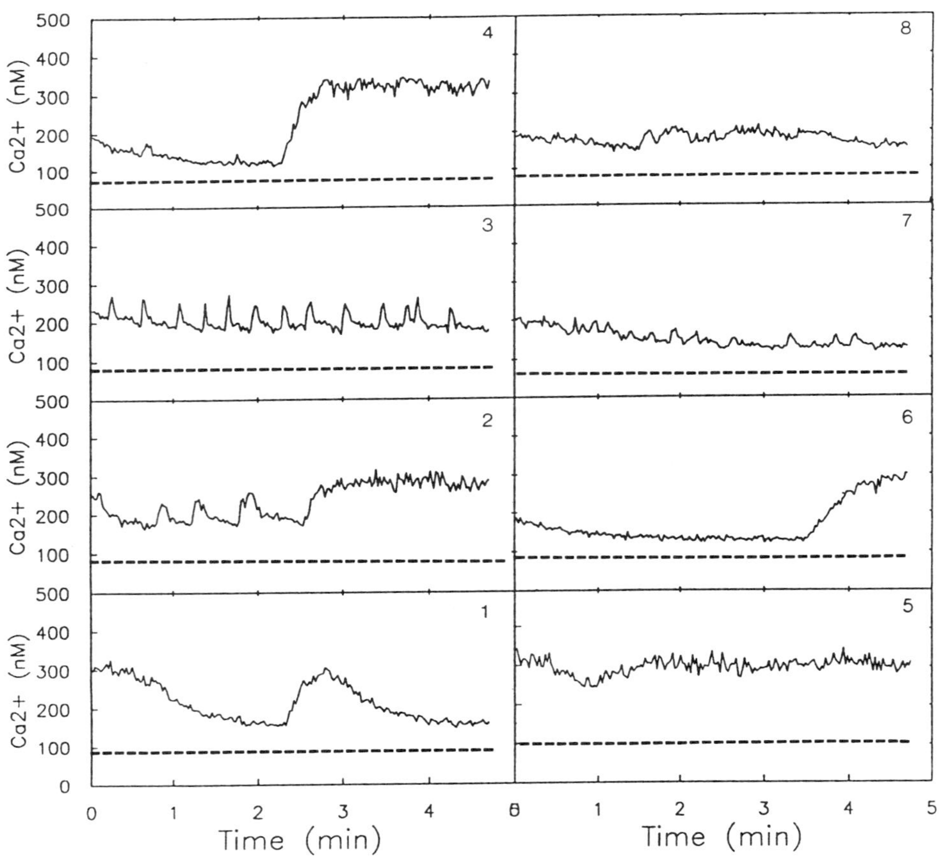

Figure 1. $[Ca^{2+}]_i$ responses of β-cells in the presence of 11 mM glucose. Each record shows the response of a single β-cell (records 4–8) or a cluster of β-cells (records 1–3) from the same field. The cells were exposed to glucose for 5 mins before the data were recorded. The dashed line in each record indicates the $[Ca^{2+}]_i$ in each cell or cluster under resting conditions (3 mM glucose).

tion change and the cells were exposed to each glucose concentration for a total period of 10 mins.

Cell fluorescence was imaged as described (Cleveland et al., 1993). Image pairs were acquired every 1.4 s and stored on a high resolution optical disc recorder. After the experiment the images were digitised and the appropriate background subtraction, thresholding and ratio imaging was carried out. Generation of ratio images and quantification of $[Ca^{2+}]_i$ in each cell (or group of cells) was performed as described previously (Millard et al., 1989). The Ca^{2+} concentrations given here are calculated as the average $[Ca^{2+}]_i$ across the whole cell; that beneath the membrane may be much higher.

In this paper we refer to single β-cells. However, we cannot be absolutely certain that these correspond to single cells as we did not identify individual cells unequivocally using a nuclear stain. It is therefore possible that some of our single β-cells may in fact be doublets. However, this does not alter our conclusions.

RESULTS

Figure 1 shows the intracellular Ca^{2+} recorded simultaneously from 3 clusters of β-cells (records 1–3) and 5 single β-cells (records 4–8) exposed to 11 mM glucose. The cells in each cluster oscillated in synchrony, as previously described (Gylfe et al., 1992). Both single β-cells and clusters of cells show a marked heterogeneity in their response to glucose, and both slow (4,8) and fast (3) oscillations in $[Ca^{2+}]_i$ are observed.

We examined the glucose-dependence of the Ca^{2+} response by exposing the cells to a range of increasing glucose concentrations, and calculating the average $[Ca^{2+}]_i$ during a 5 min period for each cell or group of cells. Fig. 2a plots the mean glucose dose-response curve obtained by including data from both single β-cells and β-cell clusters. The individual dose-response curves for the single β-cells are shown in Fig. 2b and those for the β-cell clusters in Fig. 2c. There is a marked variation in the threshold glucose concentration required to elicit an increase in $[Ca^{2+}]_i$ in single β-cells, and the glucose concentration for half-maximal response is also different.

It is clear from this experiment that whereas there is considerable heterogeneity in the glucose-sensitivity of single β-cells, there is little difference between that of clusters. Moreover the individual dose-response curves for the β-cell clusters lie very close to that of the mean data (dashed line). These results cannot be attributed to the position of the cells in the field since cells and clusters were randomly distributed. Rather they suggest that β-cell clustering produces an averaged glucose-sensitivity.

DISCUSSION

Our results indicate that individual β-cells exhibit a marked heterogeneity in the relationship between glucose and intracellular Ca^{2+}. This variability probably underlies the heterogeneous secretory response measured for single β-cells using the reverse haemolytic plaque assay (Salomon & Meda, 1988; Hiriart & Matteson, 1988). Although the oscillatory responses of clusters of cells are also quite heterogeneous (Fig. 1), the clusters appear to exhibit less variability in their response to various concentrations of glucose (Fig. 2). This is presumably because cells in clusters are electrically coupled and therefore give an averaged response which is closer to the mean of the entire population.

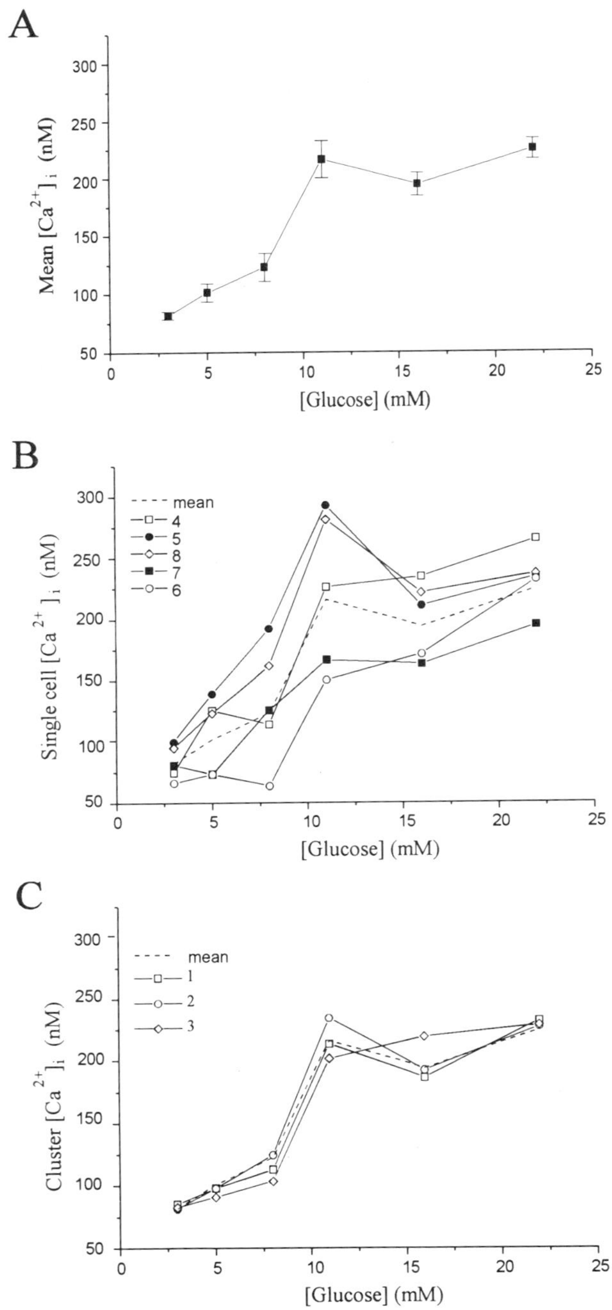

Figure 2. Effect of increasing glucose concentration on the time-averaged $[Ca^{2+}]_i$ responses of individual β-cells and clusters of β-cells. **A.** Mean response of all cells and clusters shown in Fig.1. **B, C.** Individual responses of single cells (B; records 4–8, Figure 1) or cell clusters (C; records 1–3, Figure 1). Each data point represents the average $[Ca^{2+}]_i$ in a cell or group of cells recorded over a period of 4.7 min and is the mean of 200 measurements taken at 1.4 s intervals. The cells were exposed to each glucose concentration for 5 min before the data were recorded. The dashed line shows the mean dose-response curve.

ACKNOWLEDGMENTS

We thank the British Diabetic Association, the Wellcome Trust, the Royal Society, the National Institutes of Health and the National Science Foundation for financial support.

REFERENCES

Ashcroft F. M. and Rorsman P. (1989) Electrophysiology of the pancreatic β-cell. Prog. Biophys. Molec. Biol. 54: 87–143.

Cleveland P. L., Millard P. J., Showell H. J. and Fewtrell C. M. S. (1993) Tenidap: a novel inhibitor of calcium influx in a mast cell line. Cell Calcium 14: 1–16.

Eddlestone G. T., Gonçalves A., Bangham J. A. and Rojas E. (1984) Electrical coupling between cells in islets of Langerhans from mouse. J. Memb. Biol. 77: 1–14.

Hellman B., Gylfe E., Grappengeisser E., Lund P. E. and Marcström A. (1992) Cytoplasmic calcium and insulin secretion. In Nutrient Regulation of Insulin Secretion. Ed. P. Flatt. pp. 213–246.

Hiriart M. and Matteson D. R. (1988) Na channels and two types of Ca channels in rat pancreatic β-cells identified with the reverse haemolytic plaque assay. J. Gen. Physiol. 91: 617–639.

Millard P. J., Ryan T. A., Webb W. W. and Fewtrell C. (1989) Immunoglobulin E cross-linking induces oscillations in intracellular free ionized calcium in individual tumor mast cells. J. Biol. Chem. 264: 19730–19739.

Pralong W. F., Bartley C. and Wollheim C. B. (1990) Single islet beta-cell stimulation by nutrients: relationship between pyridine nucleotides, cytosolic Ca^{2+} and secretion. EMBO J. 9: 53–60.

Salomon D. and Meda P. (1986) Heterogeneity and contact-dependent regulation of hormone secretion by individual B-cells. Exp. Cell. Res. 162: 507–520.

Santos R. M., Rosario L. M., Nadal A., Garcia-Sancho J., Soria B. and Valdeolmillos M. (1991) Widespread synchronous $[Ca^{2+}]_i$ oscillations due to bursting elecrical activity in single pancreatic islets. Pflügers Arch 418: 417–244.

Smith P. A., Ashcroft F. M. and Fewtrell C. M. S. (1993). Permeation and gating properties of the L-type calcium channel in mouse pancreatic β-cells. J. Gen. Physiol. 101: 767–797.

Valdeolmillos, M., Santos R. M., Contreras D., Soria B. and Rosario LM (1989) Glucose-induced oscillations of intracellular Ca^{2+} concentration matching bursting electrical activity in single mouse islets of Langerhans. FEBS Lett. 259: 19–23.

Valdeolmillos M., Nadal A., Soria B., Garcia-Sancho J. (1993) Fluorescence digital image analysis of glucose-induced $[Ca^{2+}]_i$ oscillations in mouse pancreatic islets of Langerhans. Diabetes 42: 1210–1214.

36

GLUCOSE-INDUCED B-CELL RECRUITMENT AND THE EXPRESSION OF HEXOKINASE ISOENZYMES

Frans C. Schuit,* Anick De Vos, Karen Moens, Erik Quartier, and Harry Heimberg

Department of Biochemistry
Diabetes Research Center
Vrije Universiteit Brussel
Laarbeeklaan 103, B-1090 Brussels, Belgium

B-CELL RECRUITMENT

The balanced release of insulin and glucagon by the endocrine pancreas is an important feature of glucose homeostasis in mammals. Adaptation of hormonal output from the endocrine pancreas to physiological demands is thought to depend on a glucose sensor — also called glucostat — which not only measures the prevailing extracellular glucose concentration but also ensures the signal transduction mechanisms required for appropriate glucagon and insulin release by A-cells and B-cells respectively (1–4). The scope of this paper is restricted to review some recent research concerning glucose sensing in B-cells, neglecting the glucose sensor in glucagon-producing A-cells about which relatively little is known.

Most knowledge about the nature of the glucose sensor in B-cells is based upon *in vitro* rodent models such as pancreatic tissue slices (5), isolated islets of Langerhans (6) and purified B-cells (7). Glucose is a potent and physiologically important stimulus for several steps in mammalian insulin gene expression (8) and the sugar stimulates insulin release by promoting the exocytosis of mature secretory granules (1–4). Importantly, the observed dose response curves for glucose-stimulated B-cell function normally display a sigmoidal shape with little or no change in biological response at glucose concentrations below 3 mM or above 20 mM and with maximal sensitivity to glucose levels between 5 and 10 mM. Consequently, glucose sensing acquires its maximal sensitivity in the physiological range of plasma glucose concentrations. It was believed for some time that such sigmoidal glucose dose-responsiveness is based upon a common phenotype of all individual B-cells. *In vitro*

* To whom correspondence should be addressed. Tel. 32-2-4774470; Fax 32-2-4774000.

Physiology and Pathophysiology of the Islets of Langerhans, edited by Soria.
Plenum Press, New York, 1997.

measurements of glucose-induced insulin biosynthesis (9) and insulin release (10) from single B-cells indicate that this assumption is wrong. Rather than smoothly activating proinsulin biosynthesis in all cells alike, glucose recruits dose- dependently cells which differ in their threshold sensitivity for the sugar (9). When glucose reaches the threshold level for insulin biosynthesis of a particular B-cell, translational activity is switched on with large increase in activity (9). Heterogenous threshold sensitivity to glucose of the total cell population therefore leads to a dose-dependent recruitment of cells into biosynthetic and secretory activity. Further increase of the glucose stimulus above the threshold concentration leads to amplification of the response of the recruited cells (9–11) suggesting that B-cells are not solely functioning at the level of "all-or-none."

The functional heterogeneity of rat pancreatic B-cells has subsequently been correlated with intercellular differences in glucose-induced redox state which was measured as increased NAD(P)H autofluorescence (12,13). This correlation not only supported the view that glucose-induced B-cell function is the consequence of the metabolic flux generated when glucose is used as a substrate (14,15); the observation also resulted in the introduction of a new experimental model to investigate the molecular constituents of the glucose sensor in B-cells. Autofluorescence-activated cell sorting was used to purify islet B-cells from rat islets (16). The purified cells were then separated according to their metabolic redox state at 7.5mM glucose. In this condition approximately 50% of the cells exhibited elevated NAD(P)H levels; the subpopulation of "high" B-cells was sorted from "low" B-cells which had maintained basal NAD(P)H levels in the 7.5 mM glucose condition (13). The sorted subpopulations were labelled with ^{3}H-tyrosine at various glucose levels to measure total protein and (pro)insulin biosynthesis. It was observed that translation of preproinsulin and non-insulin proteins occurred at least 3-fold more rapidly in high B-cells than in low B-cells at all glucose concentrations that were tested (13,17). Perifusion studies with low and high B-cells indicated that glucose dose-dependently recruits B-cells both to secretory and biosynthetic activity (18).

METABOLIC HETEROGENEITY AMONG B-CELLS

The molecular basis of B-cell recruitment was then investigated. Glucose metabolism was measured both by conversion of D-[5-^{3}H]glucose into tritiated water and via $^{14}CO_2$ production from [U-^{14}C] labeled D-glucose. At different glucose concentrations the rates of glucose utilisation and glucose oxidation by the high responsive B-cells were more than two-fold higher than those observed in the low B-cells (17). Non-specific metabolic malfunctioning of low B-cells or cellular damage due to islet cell isolation were excluded by the similar rates of amino acid oxidation in low and high B-cells and the high vitality and normal cellular ultrastructure of both cell populations.

Heterogeneity in glucose-specific catabolism could be the result of intercellular differences in the expression level of proteins involved in the proximal part of glycolysis. We concentrated on proteins involved in glucose transport and phosphorylation, particularly on the glucose transporter isoform GLUT2 and the hexokinase type IV isoenzyme (from now on called glucokinase). Both proteins were proposed as candidate glucose sensing proteins because of the following arguments: (i) restricted tissue distribution and expression in pancreatic B-cells; (ii) low affinity for glucose, compatible with a dose-related flux in the millimolar range of substrate levels, and (iii) the observed parallel changes in expression level of these proteins and the glucose sensitivity of the B-cells (19,20). The technical possibility to separate B-cell subpopulations which differ in their biological glucose responsiveness (13) allowed us to examine if heterogeneity in glucose transporter or hexokinase gene expression is correlated to the phenomenon of glucose-induced B-cell recruitment.

The process of 3-O-methyl glucose (3-OMG) uptake was extremely rapid in B-cells, even when it was studied at low temperature. Indeed, as was reported before (21,22), the calculated rate of glucose uptake in B-cells exceeded the mean rate of glucose metabolism by almost two orders of magnitude. Since the initial velocity of 3-OMG uptake was similar in low and high B-cells, it seems unlikely that intercellular differences in glucose transporter gene expression is the molecular basis for glucose-induced B-cell recruitment. This assumption was verified by Northern and Western blots using probes and antibodies specifically recognising GLUT2. The two subpopulations indeed displayed the same degree of GLUT2 gene expression, both at at the mRNA and at the protein level (17). GLUT2 expression is therefore homogeneously distributed over high and low B-cell subpopulations. The extremely high uptake capacity ensures a rapid equilibration between extracellular and intracellular glucose concentration, so that true extracellular glucose levels can be accurately sensed in the cytosol of all B-cells.

In contrast to the transport step, rates of glucose phosphorylation were comparable to the observed overall glycolytic flux in intact cells (17). Furthermore, both at 1 and at 20 mmol/l substrate, the rate of glucose phosphorylation was more elevated in the high B-cells than in the low B-cells. Glucose phosphorylation was measured radiometrically, both in the absence or presence of excess glucose-6-phosphate (Glc-6P), in order to distinguish between low-Km Glc-6P suppressible hexokinases I-III and high-Km Glc-6P insensitive glucokinase. Glucose phosphorylation via glucokinase proceeded 60 percent more rapidly in the high responsive B-cells than in the low-responsive B-cells (17). This difference in enzyme activity was associated with a 2-fold more elevated glucokinase mRNA abundance (17) and a twofold higher glucokinase protein content per cell (23) in the high B-cells as compared to the low B-cells. Heterogeneous distribution was also observed for hexokinase(s), since low-Km Glc-6P-suppressible enzyme activity was only measured in extracts from high-responsive B-cells (17). It is difficult to exclude that this activity is caused by a cell type selectively contaminating the high B-cells. Studies examining this possibility by FACS-analysis are in progress. No hexokinase I, II or III mRNA or protein has been detected so far on Northern or Western blots, but this may be due to limitations in the sensitivity of these techniques. Hexokinase I mRNA could indeed be detected after reverse-transcription and cDNA amplification using degenerate and isoform-specific primers (23).

HEXOKINASE ISOENZYME EXPRESSION AND B-CELL GLUCOSE RESPONSIVENESS

Glucokinase has been considered as a crucial protein in the process of glucose sensing in B-cells (20). Several features distinguish this enzyme from the other hexokinases. First, glucokinase is selectively expressed in the liver and pancreatic B-cells (24), whereas the other hexokinases are much more widely distributed. Recently, expression of the glucokinase gene was described in some neuroendocrine cells of gut and brain which may also be involved in glucose sensing (25). Second, glucokinase has a low affinity for its substrate ($S_{0.5}$ of approximately 8 mM), while low-Km hexokinases are already saturated with 1 mM glucose (26). Together with its sigmoidal concentration-dependency, this kinetic property results in catalytic activities that can be altered substantially within the physiologic range of plasma glucose levels (20). Third, again in contrast to the other hexokinases, glucokinase is not subject to feedback inhibition by glucose-6-phosphate (26), allowing sustained elevation of catalytic flux in conditions of stimulated insulin secretion.

In addition to our own data from B-cell subpopulations with differential glucose sensitivity (17), other direct experimental evidence has supported the role of glucokinase in the glucose sensor. It has been proposed that glucokinase catalyses the rate-mimiting step of glycolysis in B-cells. The Vmax of glucokinase-mediated glucose phosphorylation in isolated islets of Langerhans parallelled the activity of glucose-inducible functions (27, 28) and is much lower than the activities of phophofructokinase-1 and pyruvate kinase, two highly regulated enzymes of glycolysis (29). In mice expressing a glucokinase antisense transgene coupled to a ribozyme element, suppression of 70% of glucokinase enzyme activity was reported. Glucose-induced insulin release in these animals was significantly disturbed, strongly suggesting that the remaining 30% of glucokinase mRNA was not sufficient to sustain normal glucose sensing in B-cells (30). The potential medical relevance of these animal studies is supported by some recent observations in human diabetes. Mutations in the human glucokinase gene have been identified in kindreds with the rare disease maturity-onset diabetes of the young, which is inherited in an autosomal dominant way (31). The endocrine pancreas of heterozygous patients displays more than 50% reduction of insulin release during a euglycemic or hyperglycemic glucose clamp (32), suggesting that the glucose sensor of B-cells is disturbed. Mutant forms of the gene were isolated and expressed in *E. coli*, so that the catalytic properties of the recombinant proteins could be analysed. At least ten different missense mutations were found causing either dramatic decrease in Vmax or increase in the Km for glucose (33,34).

Rat liver glucokinase is controlled posttranslationally via a 62 kDa regulatory protein which binds stoichiometrically to the enzyme and which decreases the affinity of glucokinase for glucose (35). Binding of fructose 6-phosphate to the regulatory protein promotes this inhibition, while suppression is relieved by fructose 1-phosphate (35). Purified rat liver regulatory protein interacts with partially purified rat islet glucokinase (36), leaving open the interesting possibility that glucose sensing in B-cells can also be modulated via the expression level of the glucokinase regulatory protein.

Invariably, 50% or more of total glucose phosphorylation by islet homogenates can be attributed to low-Km hexokinases (27,37). The biologic importance of the expression of these enzymes for the pancreatic B-cell is not fully understood. The steady state glucose 6-phosphate concentration in islets (0.4–0.6 mM) is thought to inhibit more than 75% of low-Km hexokinase activity *in situ* (37), while leaving glucokinase undisturbed. Furthermore, part of the low-Km hexokinase activity disappears during islet culture (27). It is not clear if this loss is solely due to altered gene expression in B-cells or also caused by death of contaminating non-endocrine cells during tissue culture. The presence of hexokinase in B-cells is supported by the fact that low-Km enzyme activity was measured in homogenates from purified cell preparations (37). The enzymatic activity co-segregates uniquely with the high-responsive B-cells after cell sorting in 7.5 mM glucose (17). As mentioned before, it should be excluded that this enzyme activity is caused by the 5% or less contaminating non-B cells. Since low-Km hexokinases appear to be abundant in tumoral B-cells (38), it is conceivable that hexokinase expression is a physiological marker for dedifferentiated B-cells or replicating B-cell precursors. In the adult rat B-cell population, approximately 3% or less cells are believed to be part of the replicative compartment (39). A similar percentage of cells is triggered to protein synthesis by 1 mmol/l glucose (9). A third possibility is that the co-expression of low-Km hexokinases contributes — together with high-Km glucokinase — to the threshold glucose sensitivity of differentiated B-cells. It is possible that B-cells which are actively recruited to induced protein synthesis by 1mM glucose (9) are abundant in hexokinase I-III, as opposed to the majority of B-cells which solely express glucokinase. The physiologic role of the low-Km hexokinase-containing B-cells could be the maintenance of a basal level of pancreatic insulin output even in conditions of fasting and hypoglycemia. The overall calibration of the pancreatic glucose sensor may therefore be the result of the hexokinase/glucokinase expression ratio in the B-cell population. With constant glucokinase gene expression, physiological or pathological change in hexokinase expression is expected to recalibrate the glucose sensor. Evidence for this possibility was provided in transgenic mice expressing the yeast hexokinase B gene in the pancreatic B-cells (40). In contrast to rat hexokinases, this enzyme is not inhibited by glucose 6-phosphate. Insulin release (40) and proinsulin biosynthesis (41) from transgenic islets were stimulated by lower glucose concentrations than control islets, suggesting that hexokinase upregulation shifts the overall dose-response curve of the pancreas to the left via a more pronounced B-cell recruitment at low glucose levels. In agreement with these observations, transfection of neonatal rat B-cells with a insulin II promoter/hexokinaseI transgene markedly shifted the glucose sensitivity of B-cells to the left, while no major alteration in glucose sensing was achieved after transfecting the insulin II promoter/GLUT1 transgene (42). The same conclusion was drawn from studies with pancreatic B-cell lines. Phenotypes with functional and metabolic glucose-sensitivity similar to that of normal islets of Langerhans display a high glucokinase over hexokinase gene expression ratio (43–45). Increase of low-Km hexokinase enzyme activity with passage number (44) or by transfection with a hexokinase I expression vector (46) shifts the dose response curves of glucose-induced insulin secretion to the left. In contrast, transfection of the glucose transporter GLUT1 had no effect (46), again indicating that glucose phosphorylation rather than glucose transport determines the rate of overall glucose metabolism in B-cells (17).

Newgard and collaborators conferred biological glucose responsiveness to the non-B-cell line AtT-20ins by adenovirus-mediated gene transfer of the GLUT2 gene (47). Interestingly, this change in phenotype could be dissociated from the enhanced glucose transport per se, since GLUT1 gene transfer also increased transport capacity but the transfected cells remained glucose-unresponsive (48). Increased glucokinase activity has been reported by the same authors in GLUT2-transfected RIN cells (49). The results indicate that GLUT2 may — in addition to its properties as transport protein — influence glucose sensing via additional functions. Binding of glucokinase or another glucose-sensing protein to GLUT2 have been proposed as possible mechanisms explaining these observations.

CONCLUSIONS

A number of recent *in vitro* and *in vivo* studies in animal models strongly indicate that the overall glucose sensitivity of the endocrine pancreas is intimately correlated to the expression level of hexokinase isoenzymes in the total B-cell population. *In vitro* studies using isolated rat islet cells indicate that individual B-cells markedly differ in their threshold sensitivity of glucose-induced biological activity and that this functional heterogeneity is correlated to intercellular differences in hexokinase isoenzyme activity. Further studies are required to assess if heterogeneous glucose responsiveness also exists in human B-cells and — if so — whether human B-cell recruitment is correlated to intercellular differences in glucose phosphorylation.

ACKNOWLEDGMENTS

Part of the work reviewed in this paper was supported by grants from the Belgian Fund for Medical Scientific Research (FGWO grants 3.0013.89 and 3.0127.93), the Belgian Programme on Interuniversity Poles of Attraction initiated by the Belgian State (IUAP 15) and from the Research Council of the Vrije Universiteit Brussel.

REFERENCES

1. C.J. Hedeskov, Mechanism of glucose-induced insulin secretion, *Physiol. Rev.* 60:442–509 (1980).
2. C.B. Wollheim and G.W.G. Sharp, Regulation of insulin release by calcium, *Physiol. Rev.* 61:914–973 (1981).
3. M. Prentki and F.M. Matschinski, Ca^{2+}, cAMP, and phospholipid-derived messengers in coupling mechanisms of insulin secretion, *Physiol. Rev.* 67:1185–1248 (1987).
4. J.C. Henquin, Cell biology of insulin secretion, In: Joslin's Diabetes Mellitus, eds. C.R. Kahn, G.C. Weir, Lea & Febiger, Pennsylvania (1994).
5. H.G. Coore and P.J. Randle, Regulation of insulin secretion studied with pieces of rabbit pancreas incubated *in vitro*, *Biochem. J.* 93: 66–78 (1964).
6. C. Hellerström, Effects of carbohydrates on the oxygen consumption of isolated pancreatic islets of mice, *Endocrinology* 81: 105–112 (1967).
7. D. Pipeleers, P. In 't Veld, E. Maes and M. Van De Winkel, Glucose-induced insulin release depends on functional cooperation between islet cells, *Proc. Natl. Acad. Sci. (USA)* 79:7322–7325 (1982).
8. D.F. Steiner, G.I. Bell and H.S. Tager, Chemistry and biosynthesis of pancreatic protein hormones, In: L.J. De Groot, ed. Endocrinology, 2nd Ed., Vol 2 Philadelphia, W.B. Saunders 1263–1289 (1989).
9. F.C. Schuit, P.A. In 't Veld and D.G. Pipeleers, Glucose stimulates proinsulin biosynthesis by a dose-dependent recruitment of pancreatic beta cells, *Proc. Natl. Acad. Sci. (USA)* 85:3865–3869 (1989).
10. D. Salomon and P. Meda, Heterogeneity and contact-dependent regulation of hormone secretion by individual B cells, *Exp. Cell Res.* 162:507–520 (1986).
11. M. Hiriart and M.C. Ramirez-Medeles, Functional subpopulations of individual pancreatic B-cells in culture, *Endocrinology* 128:3193–3198 (1991).
12. M. Van De Winkel and D. Pipeleers, Autofluorescence-activated cell sorting of pancreatic islet cells: purification of insulin-containing B-cells according to glucose-induced changes in cellular redox state, *Biochem. Biophys. Res. Commun.* 114:835–542 (1983).
13. R. Kiekens, P. In 't Veld, T. Mahler, F. Schuit, M. Van De Winkel and D. Pipeleers, Differences in glucose recognition by individual rat pancreatic B cells are associated with intercellular differences in glucose-induced biosynthetic activity, *J. Clin. Invest.* 89:117–125 (1992).
14. W.J. Malaisse, A. Sener, A. Herchuelz and J.C. Hutton, Insulin release: the fuel hypothesis, *Metabolism* 28:373–386 (1979).
15. M.J. MacDonald, Elusive proximal signals of β-cells for insulin secretion, *Diabetes* 39:1461–1466 (1990).
16. M. Van De Winkel, E. Maes and D. Pipeleers, Islet cell analysis and purification by light scatter and autofluorescence, *Biochem. Biophys. Res. Commun.* 107:525–532 (1982).
17. H. Heimberg, A. De Vos, A. Vandercammen, E. Van Schaftingen, D. Pipeleers and F. Schuit, Heterogeneity in glucose sensitivity among pancreatic β-cells is correlated to differences in glucose phosphorylation rather than glucose transport, *EMBO J.* 12:2873–2879 (1993).
18. C.F.H. Van Schravendijk, R. Kiekens and D.G. Pipeleers, Pancreatic β cell heterogeneity in glucose-induced insulin secretion, *J. Biol. Chem.* 267:21344–21348 (1992).
19. R.H. Unger, Diabetic hyperglycemia: link to impaired glucose transport in pancreatic β cells, *Science* 251:1200–1205 (1991).
20. F. Matschinsky, Y. Liang, P. Kesavan, L. Wang, P. Froguel, G. Velho, D. Cohen, M.A. Permutt, Y. Tanizawa, T.L. Jetton, K. Niswender and M.A.Magnuson, Glucokinase as pancreatic β cell glucose sensor and diabetes gene, *J. Clin. Invest.* 92:2092–2098 (1993).
21. B. Hellman, J. Sehlin and I.B. Täljedal, Evidence for mediated transport of glucose in mammalian pancreatic β-cells, *Biochim. Biophys. Acta* 241:147–154 (1971).
22. F.K. Gorus, W.J. Malaisse and D.G. Pipeleers, Differences in glucose handling by pancreatic A- and B-cells, *J. Biol. Chem.* 259:1196–1200 (1984).

23. H. Heimberg, A. De Vos, A. Vandercammen, E. Van Schaftingen, D. Pipeleers and F. Schuit, Intercellular differences in glucose phosphorylation can explain the heterogeneity in glucose sensitivity of rat pancreatic β-cells, *Diabetologia* 36:119 (1993).
24. P.B. Iynedjian, G. Möbius, H.J. Seitz, C.B. Wollheim and A.E. Renold, Tissue-specific expression of glucokinase: Identification of the gene product in liver and pancreatic islets, *Proc. Natl. Acad. Sci. USA* 83: 1998–2001 (1986).
25. T.L. Jetton, Y. Liang, C.C. Pettepher, E.C. Zimmerman, F.G. Cox, K. Horvath, F.M. Matschinsky and M.A. Magnuson, Analysis of upstream glucokinase promoter activity in transgenic mice and identification of glucokinase in rare neuroendocrine cells in the brain and gut, *J. Biol. Chem.* 269:3641–3654 (1994).
26. P.B. Iynedjian, Mammalian glucokinase and its gene, *Biochem. J.* 293:1–13 (1993).
27. Y. Liang, H. Najafi and F.M. Matschinsky, Glucose regulates glucokinase activity in cultured islets from rat pancreas, *J. Biol. Chem.* 265:16863–16866 (1990).
28. F. Purrello, M. Buscema, A.M. Rabuazzo, V. Caltabiano, F. Forte, C. Vinci, M. Vetri and R. Vigneri, Glucose modulates glucose transporter affinity, glucokinase activity, and secretory response in rat pancreatic β-cells, *Diabetes* 42:199–205 (1993).
29. M.D. Trus, W.S. Zawalich, P.T. Burch, D.K. Berner, V.A. Weill and F.M. Matschinsky, Regulation of glucose metabolism in pancreatic islets, *Diabetes* 30:911–922 (1981).
30. S. Efrat, M. Leiser, Y.J. Wu, D. Fusco-Demane, O.B. Emran, M. Surana, T.L. Jetton, M.A. Magnuson, G. Weir and N. Fleischer, Ribozyme-mediated attenuation of pancreatic β-cell glucokinase expression in transgenic mice results in impaired glucose-induced insulin secretion, *Proc. Natl. Acad. Sci. USA* 91:2051–2055 (1994).
31. N. Vionnet, M. Stoffel, J. Takeda, K. Yasuda, G.I. Bell, H. Zouali, S. Lesage, G. Velho, F. Iris, P. Passa, P. Froguel and D. Cohen, Nonsense mutation in the glucokinase gene causes early-onset non-insulin-dependent diabetes mellitus, *Nature* 356:721–722 (1992).
32. G. Velho, P. Froguel, K. Clement, M.E. Pueyo, B. Rakotoambinina, H. Zouali, P. Passa, D. Cohen and J.J. Robert, Primary pancreatic beta-cell secretory defect caused by mutations in glucokinase gene in kindreds of maturity onset diabetes of the young, *Lancet* 340:444–448 (1992).
33. M. Gidh-Jain, J. Takeda, L.Z. Xu, A.J. Lange, N. Vionnet, M. Stoffel, P. Froguel, G. Velho, F. Sun, D. Cohen, P. Patel, Y.M.D. Lo, A.T. Hattersley, H. Luthman, A. Wedell, R. St Charles, R.W. Harrison, I.T. Weber, G.I. Bell and S.J. Pilkis, Glucokinase mutations associated with non-insulin-dependent (type 2) diabetes mellitus have decreased enzyme activity: implications for structure/function relationships, *Proc. Natl. Acad. Sci. USA* 90:1932–1936 (1993).
34. J. Takeda, M. Gidh-Jain, L.Z. Xu, P. Froguel, G. Velho, M. Vaxillaire, D. Cohen, F. Shimada, H. Makino, S. Nishi, M. Stoffel, N. Vionnet, R. St. Charles, R.W. Harrison, I.T. Weber, G.I. Bell and S.J. Pilkis, Structure/function studies of human β-cell glucokinase, *J. Biol. Chem.* 268:15200–15204 (1993).
35. E. Van Schaftingen, M. Detheux and M.V. Da Cunha, Short-term control of glucokinase activity: role of a regulatory protein, *FASEB J.* 8:414–419 (1994).
36. W.J. Malaisse, F. Malaisse-Lagae, D.R. Davies, A. Vandercammen and E. Van Schaftingen, Regulation of glucokinase by a fructose-1-phosphate sensitive protein in pancreatic islets, *Eur. J. Biochem.* 190: 539–545 (1990).
37. M-H. Giroix, A. Sener, D.G. Pipeleers and W.J. Malaisse, Hexose metabolism in pancreatic islets, *Biochem. J.* 223:447–453 (1984).
38. U. Vischer, B. Blondel, C.B. Wollheim, W. Höppner, H.J. Seitz and P.B. Iynedjian, Hexokinase isoenzymes of RIN-m5F insulinoma cells, *Biochem. J.* 241:249–255 (1987).
39. I. Swenne, Effects if ageing on the regenerative capacity of the pancreatic B-cell of the rat, *Diabetes* 32:14–19 (1983).
40. P.N. Epstein, A.C. Boschero, I. Atwater, X. Cai and P.A. Overbeek, Expression of yeast hexokinase in pancreatic β cells of transgenic mice reduces blood glucose, enhances insulin secretion, and decreases diabetes, *Proc. Natl. Acad. Sci. USA* 89:12038–12042 (1992).
41. M.E. Voss-McCowan, B. Xu and P.N. Epstein, Insulin synthesis, secretory competence, and glucose utilization are sensitized by transgenic yeast hexokinase, *J. Biol. Chem.* 269:15814–15818 (1994).
42. M.S. German, Glucose sensing in pancreatic islet beta cells: The key role of glucokinase and the glycolytic intermediates, *Proc. Natl. Acad. Sci. USA* 90:1781–1785 (1993).
43. M. Asafari, D. Janjic, P. Meda, G. Li, P.A. Halban, C.B. Wollheim, Establishment of 2-mercaptoethanol-dependent differentiated insulin-secreting cell lines, *Endocrinology* 130:167–178 (1992).
44. S. Efrat, M. Leiser, M. Surana, M. Tal, D. Fusco-Demane, N. Fleischer, Murine insulinoma cell line with normal glucose-regulated insulin secretion, *Diabetes* 42:901–907 (1993).
45. H. Ishihara, T. Asano, K. Tsukuda, H. Katagiri, K. Inukai, M. Anai, M. Kikuchi, Y. Yazaki, J.I. Miyazaki and Y. Oka, Pancreatic beta cell line MIN6 exhibits characteristics of glucose metabolism and glucose-stimulated insulin secretion similar to those of normal islets, *Diabetologia* 36:1139–1145 (1993).

46. H. Ishihara, T. Asano, K. Tsukuda, H. Katagiri, K. Inukai, M. Anai, M. Kikuchi, Y.Yazaki, J.I. Miyazaki and Y. Oka, Overexpression of hexokinase I but not GLUT1 glucose transporter alters concentration dependence of glucose-stimulated insulin secretion in pancreatic β-cell line MIN6, *J. Biol. Chem.* 269:3081–3087 (1994).
47. C.B. Newgard, Cellular engineering and gene therapy strategies for insulin replacement in diabetes, *Diabetes* 43:341–350 (1994).
48. S.D. Hughes, C. Quaade, J.H. Johnson, S. Ferber and C.B. Newgard, Transfection of AtT-20_{ins} cells with GLUT-2 but not GLUT-1 confers glucose-stimulated insulin secretion, *J. Biol. Chem.* 268:15205–15212 (1993).
49. S. Ferber, H. BeltrandelRio, J. Johnson, R.J. Noel, L.E. Cassidy, S. Clark, T.C. Becker, S. Hughes and C.B. Newgard, GLUT-2 gene transfer into insulinoma cells confers both low and high affinity glucose-stimulated insulin release, *J. Biol. Chem.* 269:11523–11529 (1994).

PHYSIOLOGICAL BEHAVIOR OF FUNCTIONAL SUBPOPULATIONS OF SINGLE PANCREATIC β-CELLS

Marcia Hiriart,[1] Ma. Teresa Martinez,[1] and Ma. del Carmen Ramírez-Medeles[2]

[1]Department of Bioenergetics
Instituto de Fisiología Celular
Universidad Nacional Autónoma de México
[2]Department of Biological Systems
Universidad Autónoma Metropolitana
Xochimilco, D.F., Mexico

INTRODUCTION

Single pancreatic β-cells are heterogeneous, the following are observations of β-cell variability: insulin content and biosynthesis of individual β-cells (Pipeleers, 1987; Schuit et al., 1988), glucose transport (Tominaga et al.,1986), electrical activity (Dean and Mattews, 1970; Ashcroft et al., 1987) and insulin secretion (Salomon and Meda, 1986; Hiriart and Matteson, 1988; Hiriart and Ramirez-Medeles, 1991; Van Schravendijk et al., 1992).

We have described functional adult β-cell subpopulations that differ in: a) insulin secretion rate, b) glucose threshold (Hiriart and Ramirez-Medeles, 1991) and c) secretory response to the muscarinic agonist, carbachol (Hiriart and Ramirez-Medeles, 1993). It is not clear if adult β-cell functional subpopulations are determined by differences in the metabolic state, in the maturation stage, or if they are genetically defined.

In this study we characterized the secretory response of single fetal β-cells to glucose and carbachol and explored if heterogeneity is present since this developmental stage.

The amount of insulin secreted by β-cells is the result of complex mechanisms implicated in stimulus-secretion coupling. During this process, the activity of different types of ionic channel is involved. We have previously demonstrated that sodium channel activation is important for glucose stimulated-insulin secretion in single rat pancreatic β-cells (Hiriart and Matteson, 1988). In this study we have explored if the heterogeneous secretion rate of adult β-cell subpopulations could be due, in part, to differences in sodium channel density between adult β-cells.

Physiology and Pathophysiology of the Islets of Langerhans, edited by Soria.
Plenum Press, New York, 1997.

METHODS

Animals and Pancreatic Islet Cell Cultures

Young adult male Wistar rats, (200–250 g), or pregnant rats in the 18th day of gestation, were obtained from the local animal facility. Adult and fetal pancreatic islet cells were isolated as described previously (Hiriart and Ramirez-Medeles, 1991), with minor modifications. First, pancreatic islets were separated from the acinar tissue by collagenase digestion and a Ficoll gradient centrifugation, clean islets were hand-picked. Dissociation of the cells was achieved by incubating the cells in a shaker bath, for 10 minutes, at 37°C in calcium-free Spinner's solution, with 15.6 mM glucose, 0.5 BSA and 0.01% trypsin, followed by mechanical disruption. Isolated islet cells were cultured in RPMI 1640, supplemented with 1 or 10% fetal bovine serum, 100 U/ml penicillin, 100 μg/ml streptomycin and 0.25 μg/ml fungizone. Cells were used after one day in culture.

Reverse Hemolytic Plaque Assay (RHPA)

Insulin secretion from individual beta cells was analyzed with a reverse hemolytic plaque assay (RHPA) (Neill and Frawley, 1983), as described previously (Hiriart and Matteson, 1988). The immunoplaques revealed insulin secreted by single β-cells during 1 h in the presence of different glucose concentrations with or without CCh 10 μM. At least 60 cells were counted per experimental point, and all experiments were carried out by duplicate.

The overall secretory activity of β-cells under a given experimental condition was expressed as a secretion index, which was calculated by multiplying the average plaque area by the percentage of plaque-forming cells.

As previously described (Hiriart and Ramirez-Medeles, 1991), β-cell subpopulations were classified according to the amount of insulin secreted by single cells, as follows: small plaque-forming cells (*SP*), plaque area < 2000 μm^2; medium plaque-forming cells (*MP*) plaque area between 2000 and 4000 μm^2 and large plaque-forming cells (*LP*) plaque area > 4000 μm^2.

Patch-Clamp Recording

Whole-cell recordings were performed using conventional patch-clamp techniques with an Axopatch 200 amplifier. Patch pipettes were made from Kimax-51 glass (Kimble products, USA) and were insulated with Sylgard 184 (Dow Co., Pomona, CA). Pipette resistances were 1.5 to 2 MΩ. The capacitive transients were subtracted from the records and series resistance compensation was used to compensate for some of the access resistance.

External solution contained (mM): 130 NaCl, 5 KCl, 5 $CaCl_2$, 2 $MgCl_2$, 10 HEPES and 10 glucose, pH 7.35, 300 mOsm. Internal solution contained (mM): 120 Cesium Aspartate, 10 CsCl, 10 CsF, 10 BAPTA, 10 HEPES, 2 MgATP, pH 7.3, 280 mOsm. In some experiments 15 mM NaCl was also included.

The temperature was maintained at 20 ± 1°C with a bipolar temperature controller.

RESULTS

Single Fetal β-cells Response to Glucose

It has been generally accepted that fetal islet cells do not discriminate between different extracellular glucose concentrations (see Ammon et al., 1989). We characterized the

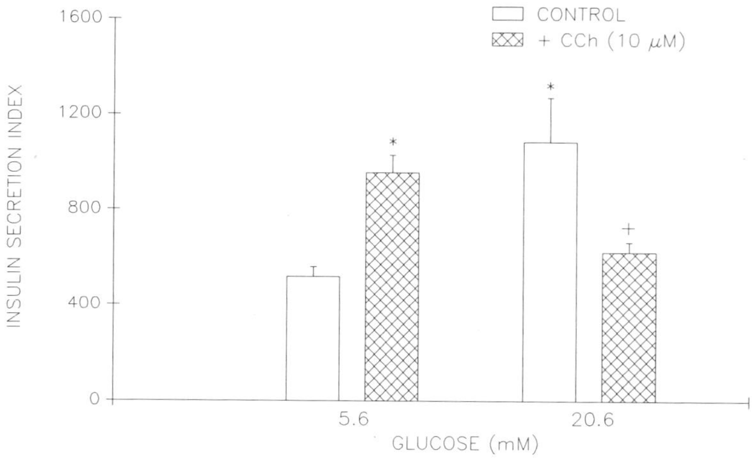

Figure 1. Single fetal β-cells respond to glucose and CCh. Insulin secretion index in single fetal β-cells (18 i.u.) increased by 2-fold in 20.6 mM glucose with respect to basal glucose concentration (5.6 mM). In 5.6 mM glucose CCh stimulated by 2-fold, insulin secretion in fetal β-cells. In contrast, in 20.6 mM glucose CCh decreased insulin secretion. These results resemble to those obtained in adult cells; however, the total amount of insulin secreted by fetal cells was nearly one half of that observed in single adult β-cells. *denotes significant level with respect to control in 5.6 mM glucose, $p < 0.01$. $^{+}$denotes significant level with respect to control in 20.6 mM glucose, $p < 0.05$.

response of single fetal β-cells to glucose and explored the possibility that the predominant subpopulation at this developmental stage would be the low-rate secreting β-cells (SP cells), as it has been observed that the functional subpopulations with the higher secretion rate (MP and LP cells) are more responsive to glucose than SP cells (Hiriart and Ramirez-Medeles, 1991).

Single fetal β-cells do discriminate between different glucose concentrations. The secretory response of fetal β-cells to 20.6 mM glucose is 2 fold higher than in 5.6 mM glucose (Figure 1). In high glucose, the mean plaque area increased by 69% and the percentage of plaque-forming cells increased by 21%, compared to 5.6 mM glucose (Table 1).

It is interesting that, even at this developmental stage, the three functional β-cell subpopulations were detected (Figure 2), although in different proportions than in adult cells. For example, when adult β-cells were exposed to 20.6 mM glucose, 13% of large-plaque forming cells were detected, whereas LP cells comprise only a 3% of total fetal β-cells. In addition, near 50% of total secreting cells formed small plaques in both glucose concentrations (5.6 mM and 20.6 mM). In contrast, medium-plaque forming cells increased by 4-fold in high glucose, compared with basal glucose level.

Table 1

	Plaque area (μm^2)	% of plaque forming-cells	Secretion index	n
Glucose 5.6 mM	952 ± 73	55 ± 1	519 ± 42	10
+ CCh	1443 ±104*	66 ± 1	956 ± 75*	9
Glucose 20.6 mM	1608 ± 210*	66 ± 2.7	1086 ± 187*	9
+ CCh	1054 ± 53**	59 ± 3	623 ± 42**	6

*denotes significant level with respect to control in 5.6 mM glucose, $p < 0.01$.
**denotes significant level with respect to control in 20.6 mM glucose, $p < 0.05$.

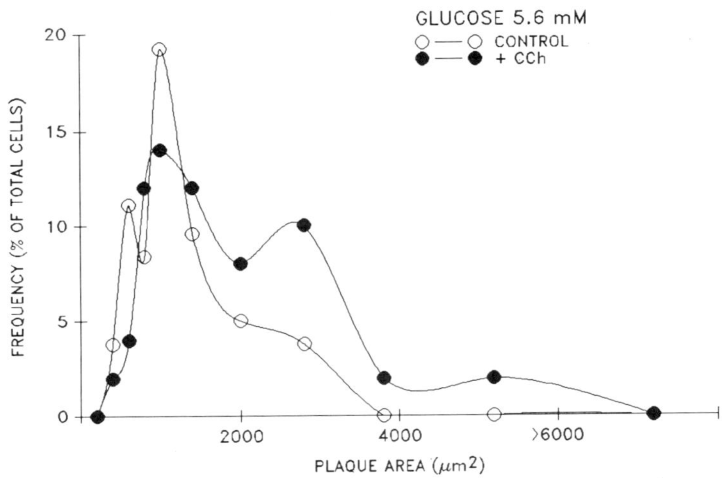

Figure 2. Functional fetal β-cell subpopulations. β-cell subpopulations were classified according to the amount of insulin secreted by single cells, as follows: small plaque-forming cells (*SP*), plaque area < 2000 μm^2; medium plaque-forming cells (*MP*) plaque area between 2000 and 4000 μm^2 and large plaque-forming cells (*LP*) plaque area > 4000 μm^2. Functional β-cell subpopulations are present at this developmental stage, but in different proportions compared to adult β-cells. Around 50% of the cells have low secretion rate (SP). In this case, the percentage of β-cells with medium secretion rate (MP) increased in the presence of high glucose and also with CCh in 5.6 mM glucose. The percentage of fetal β-cells with the highest secretion rate (LP) was very low. *denotes significant level with respect to control in 5.6 mM glucose, $p < 0.01$.

Cholinergic Modulation of Insulin Secretion in Functional β-Cell Subpopulations

Single fetal β-cells response to CCh depends on extracellular glucose concentration, similarly to the response of single adult β-cells, previously observed (Hiriart and Ramirez-Medeles, 1991). In 5.6 mM glucose, CCh (10 μM) increased the insulin secretion index by 1.8-fold (Figure 1) and both, the insulin secreted by individual cells and the percentage of plaque-forming cells increased by 52 and 21%, respectively (Table 1). CCh effects were blocked by atropine (data not shown). In 20.6 mM glucose, CCh decreased insulin secretion index by 43%, as shown in Figure 1.

In 5.6 mM glucose, CCh increased by 4-fold the percentage of medium plaque-forming cells (MP cells), without affecting the percentage of small-plaque forming cells (SP), as shown in Figure 2. In contrast, the effect of CCh on adult β-cell, predominated on LP cells. However, as this subpopulation only constitute a 3% of total fetal β-cells, it is not surprising that the subpopulation with highest secretion rate in fetal β-cells (MP cells), is the one that is principally affected by the muscarinic agonist.

On the other hand, in 20.6 mM glucose, the percentage of MP cells decreased 76% (Figure 2), in parallel with the reduction on the insulin secretion index.

Sodium Current Density in Adult Functional Subpopulations of β-cells

We have previously shown that rat adult β-cells have TTX-sensitive, voltage-dependent sodium channels that are functionally important for stimulus-secretion coupling at high glucose concentrations (Hiriart and Matteson, 1988). We examined the possibility that sodium channel expression could contribute to explain the functional heterogeneity among β-cells.

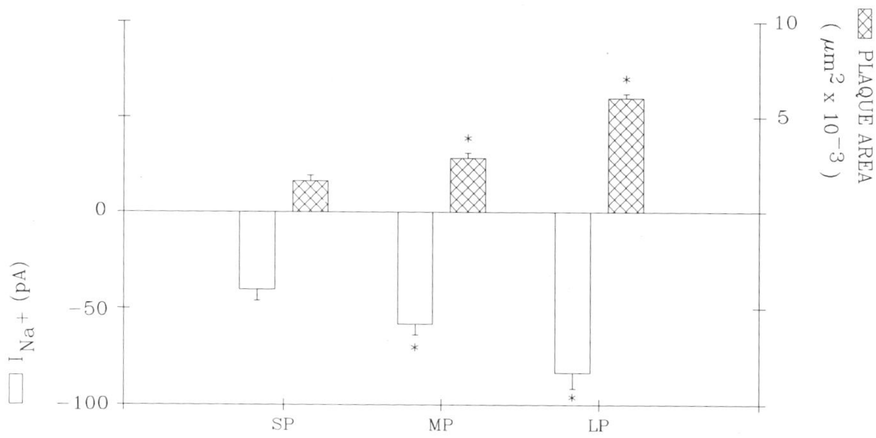

Figure 3. Peak sodium current is related to the amount of insulin secreted by single β-cells. Insulin secretion of adult β-cells was measured with the reverse hemolytic plaque assay (RHPA), in 20.6 mM glucose. Sodium current was recorded in the previously RHPA-identified cells, with the whole cell variant of the patch clamp technique. Plaque area is proportional to the amount of insulin secreted by the single cell. Maximum sodium current (measured at +10 mV) was higher in the cells that secreted more insulin. *denotes significant level with respect to control in 5.6 mM glucose, $p < 0.01$.

Sodium current in β-cells rapidly activates to peak and then inactivates during maintained depolarization. As previously described (Hiriart and Matteson, 1988), in all the β-cells studied, the current activates near −30 mV, reaches a maximum near +10 mV, and is blocked by TTX (100 nM).

The average maximum sodium current in the functional β-cell subpopulations was of: 29.5 ± 3.9 pA in SP cells (n=17), 51.3 ± 5.3 pA in MP cells (n=29), and 76.7 ± 8.6 pA in LP cells (n=19). As shown in Figure 3, the relative amount of insulin secreted by β-cells from each subpopulations, (size of plaque area) is correlated to the maximum sodium current (measured at +10 mV).

Differences in sodium current amplitude could not be attributed to variations in cell surface area, as the capacitance among β-cells subpopulations was not different. The peak current (normalized by the capacitance)-voltage relationship for 6 cells of each subpopulation is shown in Figure 4. Maximum sodium current density was of 3.7 ± 0.7, 6.8 ± 1.3 and 8.9 ± 1.5 pA/pF, respectively for SP, MP and LP cells.

Since sodium channels in rat β-cells could be involved in membrane depolarization in stimulus-secretion coupling, the differences in sodium current density can partially explain the differences in insulin secretion rate among β-cell subpopulations.

DISCUSSION

Single Fetal β-Cells Response to Glucose and Carbachol

Single fetal β-cells increased by 2-fold insulin secretion in response to 20.6 mM glucose stimulation (compared to basal secretion in 5.6 mM glucose), and also in response to CCh (10 μM, in 5.6 mM glucose). This results are comparable to those observed in single adult β-cells (Hiriart and Ramirez-Medeles, 1991 and 1993), although fetal β-cells secretion was considerably lower than secretion of adult B-cells in all conditions tested.

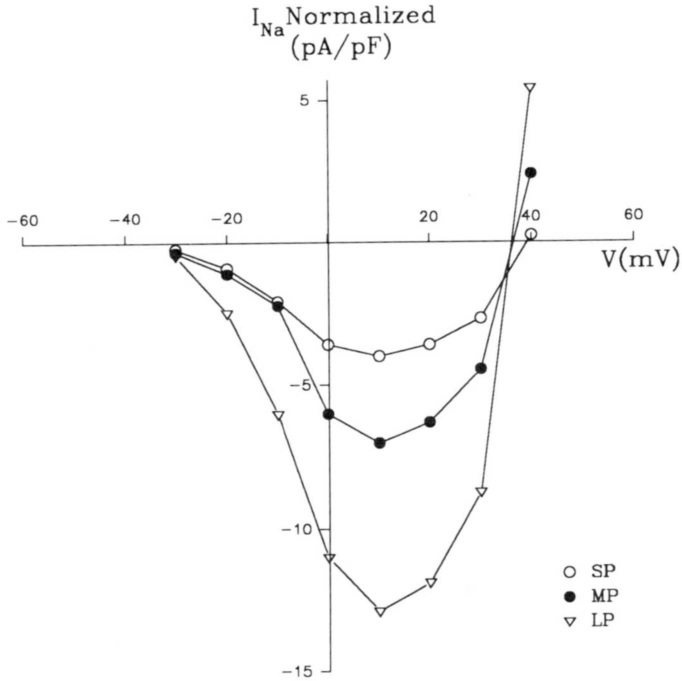

Figure 4. Sodium current density differs in β-cell functional subpopulations. Sodium I-V relationship (normalized by cell capacitance) of β-cell functional subpopulations (n = 6 for each case). Differences between sodium current size could not be attributed to variations in cell surface area, as the capacitance among β-cells subpopulations were not different.

The differences observed between the amount of insulin secreted by fetal and adult β-cells, are due to the lower secretion rate of fetal cells (indicated by the size of the insulin plaque), as the percentage of plaque forming-cells in the different conditions are very similar in both, fetal and adult cells.

It is interesting to note that in 20.6 mM glucose, CCh decreases the insulin secretion index by 43% in fetal β-cells, analogous to the 47% inhibition observed in adult β-cells under the same condition. This could be due to desensitization by the combination of secretagogues (Hiriart and Ramirez-Medeles, 1993).

Insulin secretion in fetal β-cells is also heterogeneous, and cells can be grouped according to their insulin secretion rate, as the adult β-cells. Nearly 50% of the total fetal cells display a low secretion rate (SP cells) in all the conditions tested. This percentage is 25% higher than in adult β-cells.

The β-cell subpopulation with the highest secretion rate (LP cells) only constitute around 3% of total fetal cells. This observation is important because adult LP-cells are more suitable to be modulated by secretagogues than the other two subpopulations and consequently are the cells responsible for most of the insulin secreted (Hiriart and Ramirez-Medeles, 1993).

On the other hand, in fetal β-cells the medium secretion rate-cells (MP cells), constitute the subpopulation that predominantly determines the total amount of insulin secreted in a given condition. For example, it can be observed that the percentage of MP cells detected in high glucose concentration and in CCh was in both cases, 4-fold higher compared to basal glucose concentration.

Sodium Current Density in Adult β-Cell Subpopulations

Sodium current density in adult β-cells is correlated with the amount of insulin secreted by single cells. We have shown that high and medium rate secretors (LP and MP cells) express a higher sodium channel density than the low rate-secretors (SP cells), without changing the voltage dependence of the current. Similar results were observed in functional subpopulations of rat lactotropes (Horta et al., 1991). It is then possible that differences in secretion rate between functional β-cell subpopulations could be related to distinct sodium channel density.

The functional role of β-cell subpopulations *in vivo* is unknown, it is possible that the cells that exhibit a high insulin secretion rate, the lowest glucose threshold, and the highest sodium channel density, could be the first cells to be recruited by secretagogues. Then the response of the whole islet, including less responsive cells, could involve intercellular communication.

ACKNOWLEDGMENTS

We thank Carmen Sánchez-Soto for her expert technical assistance in some experiments.

Supported by DGAPA, UNAM grant: IN206291, Mexico.

REFERENCES

Ammon, H.P.T., Glocker, C., Waldner, R.G., and Wahl, M.A., 1989, Insulin release from pancreatic islets of fetal rats mediated by leucine b-BCH, tolbutamide, glibenclamide, arginine, potassium chloride, and theophylline does not require stimulation of Ca^{2+} net uptake, Cell Calcium 10:441–450.

Ashcroft, F.M., Harrison, D.E., Ashcroft, S.J.H., 1987, A potassium channel modulated by glucose metabolism in rat pancreatic B-cells, in "Biophysics of the Pancreatic B-Cells," I. Atwater, E. Rojas, B. Soria, eds., Plenum Press, New York.

Dean, P.M., and Mattews, E.K., 1970, Glucose-induced electrical activity in pancreatic islet cells, J. Physiol 210: 255–264.

Hiriart, M. and M.C. Ramírez-Medeles, M.C., 1991, Functional subpopulations of individual pancreatic B-cells in culture, Endocrinology 128: 3193–3198.

Hiriart, M., and Ramírez-Medeles, M.C., 1993, Muscarinic modulation of insulin secretion by single pancreatic B-cells, Mol. and Cellular Endocrinology 93: 63–69.

Hiriart, M., and Matteson, D.R., 1988, Na channels and two types of Ca channels in rat pancreatic B cells identified with the reverse hemolytic plaque assay, J. Gen. Physiol. 91: 617–639.

Horta, J., Hiriart, M. and Cota, G. , 1991, Differential expression of Na channels in functional subpopulations of rat lactotropes, Am. J. Physiol. 261: C865–C871.

Neill, J.D., and Frawley, L. S., 1983, Detection of hormone release from individual cells in mixed populations using a reverse hemolytic plaque assay, Endocrinology 112: 1135–1137.

Pipeleers, D., 1987, The biosociology of pancreatic B cells, Diabetologia 30:277–291.

Salomon, D., and Meda, P., 1986, Heterogeneity and contact-dependent regulation of hormone secretion by individual B cells, Exp. Cell. Res. 162:507–520.

Schuit, F.C., In'tVeld, P.A., and Pipeleers, D.G., 1988, Glucose stimulates proinsulin biosynthesis by a dose-dependent recruitment of pancreatic beta cells, Proc. Natl. Acad. Sci. USA. 85: 3865–3869.

Tominaga, M., Komiya, I., Johnson, J.H., Inman, L., Alam, T., Moltz, J., Crider, B., Stefan, Y., Baetens, D., McCorkle, K., Orci, L., and Unger, R.H., 1986, Loss of insulin response to glucose but not arginine during the development of auto immune diabetes in BB/W rats: relationships to islet volume and glucose transport rate, Proc. Natl. Acad. Sci. USA. 83:9749–9753.

Van Schravendijk, C.F.H., Kiekens, R., and Pipeleers, D.G., 1992, Pancreatic β cell heterogeneity in glucose-induced insulin secretion, J. Biol. Chem. 267: 21344–21348.

38

COMPUTER MODELING OF HETEROGENEOUS β-CELL POPULATIONS

Arthur Sherman and Paul Smolen

Mathematical Research Branch
National Institutes of Health
Bethesda, Maryland

1. INTRODUCTION

β-cells differ significantly with respect to their electrical and secretory properties (Pipeleers, 1992), leading us to consider whether heterogeneity may have functional significance for the behavior of β-cell populations, such as the natural unit, the islet of Langerhans. On the other hand, β-cells in islets behave essentially synchronously, at least with regard to electrical activity (Eddlestone et al., 1984) and cytosolic Ca^{2+} levels (Santos et al., 1991). Several questions arise:

- How does the islet synchronize? Are the reported size and density of gap junctional connections adequate to produce synchrony?
- What is the role of cell heterogeneity? Is it important for building the graded response to glucose or merely an obstacle that must be overcome in order to achieve coordinated behavior?
- Does glucose increase insulin secretion by recruiting more cells (Pipeleers, 1992) into activity or by increasing the output of each cell (Beigelman et al., 1977)?
- How is the oscillatory activity of the islet generated in the absence of a pacemaker?

We have explored these questions by computer simulations of cell clusters (ca. 100–1000 cells), each represented by differential equations of the Chay-Keizer family for ionic channel kinetics and Ca^{2+} handling.

Physiology and Pathophysiology of the Islets of Langerhans, edited by Soria
Plenum Press, New York, 1997

2. MATERIALS AND METHODS

There is yet no consensus on the correct ionic model for β-cell bursting electrical activity, which may well depend on currents not yet identified (Satin and Smolen, in press). A number of models have been proposed, all following the scheme of Chay and Keizer (1983) and, with respect to issues of synchronization and heterogeneity, all essentially equivalent.

The minimal features are (1) an equation for the balance of ionic currents that determines the membrane potential (Kirchhoff's Law) (2) a Ca^{2+} balance equation, that includes at least influx and efflux across the plasma membrane, and (3) a slow variable that modulates the voltage equation. An example is:

$$\frac{dV_m}{dt} = -I_{\mathrm{Ca}} - I_{\mathrm{K(V)}} - I_{\mathrm{slow}}(S) \tag{1}$$

$$\frac{d[\mathrm{Ca}^{2+}]_i}{dt} = \alpha I_{\mathrm{Ca}} - k_{\mathrm{Ca}}[\mathrm{Ca}^{2+}]_i \tag{2}$$

$$\frac{dS}{dt} = (S_\infty(V,R) - S)/\tau_s \tag{3}$$

Additional auxiliary variables (not shown) represent channel gating kinetics. The fast currents, I_{Ca} and $I_{\mathrm{K(V)}}$, generate the spikes while S, with a long time constant τ_s, acts through I_{slow} to switch the cell between the spiking and silent phases. The two main variants within this class have a K^+ current that is slowly activated (Chay and Keizer, 1983; Smolen and Keizer, 1992) during the spiking phase or a Ca^{2+} current that is slowly inactivated (Chay and Cook, 1988; Keizer and Smolen, 1991). The simulations for Figs. 2, 4, and 5 were carried out with the Smolen-Keizer model, in which S is ADP concentration and activates $I_{\mathrm{K(ATP)}}$. There, S_∞ depends on $[\mathrm{Ca}^{2+}]_i$ rather than V_m. R is the glucose-sensing parameter (see below).

In order to simulate an islet, we couple the cells into a 5x5x5 cube by adding a term to Eq. (1) to represent the coupling current that flows between neighboring cells:

$$-I_{\mathrm{coup}} = -\sum_j g_{c,j}(V_m - V_j).$$

Cell parameters are varied randomly according to a normal distribution with a 10–20% standard deviation. We also vary the coupling conductance between cell pairs according to the histogram of Perez-Armendariz et al. (1991); not every pair need be connected. See Smolen et al. (1993) for details. Single cells can be studied with an ordinary PC, while for serious study of multi-cell preparations we used a Cray YMP supercomputer (Mendota Heights, MN, USA).

3. RESULTS AND DISCUSSION

We next review the principles of bursting foı single cells, showing that this leads to a natural class of mechanisms for glucose-sensing, and then consider synchronization and glucose-sensing in heterogeneous populations.

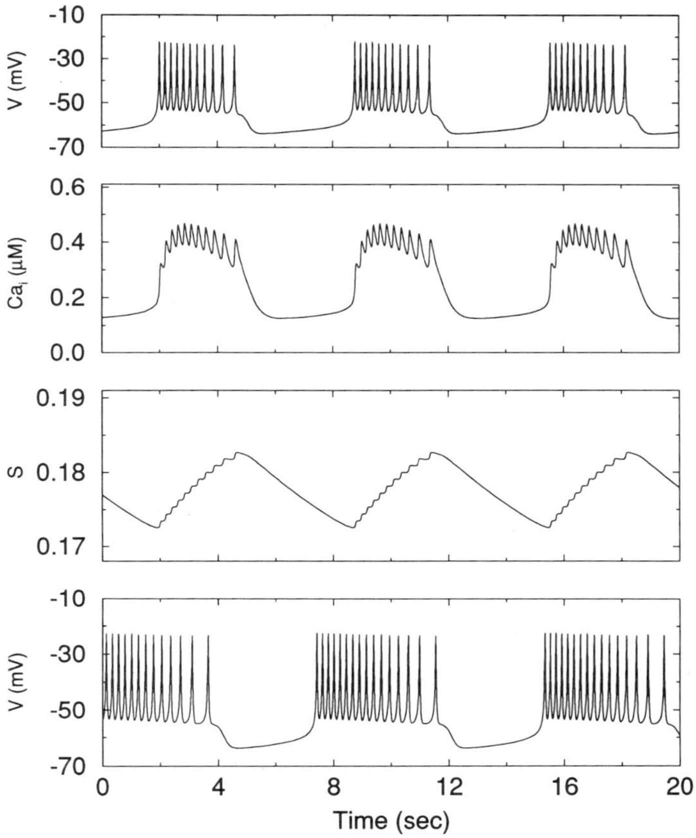

Figure 1. Generic bursting model (from Sherman and Rinzel, 1992; R is V_s) Top panel shows membrane potential; second panel shows $[Ca^{2+}]_i$; third panel shows a generic slow variable, S, which switches the cell between silent and active phases. Bottom panel: Increasing R increases plateau fraction. See text.

3.1. Bursting

Plasma glucose is regulated by negative feedback. A rise in glucose increases insulin secretion, which lowers the glucose. This is analogous to a household thermostat which responds to an increase of temperature by turning on the air conditioner. Both systems respond to an increased challenge by increasing the duty-cycle, or fraction of time active ("plateau fraction" for the islet). Maximum output is achieved when the system is continuously active. The thermostat also has an internal negative feedback system. When activated, some internal parameter, such as the bending of a bar, slowly changes until it shuts the system off. Similarly, models for bursting in the islet postulate that some correlate of activity (V_m or $[Ca^{2+}]_i$) slowly changes a parameter (S) that terminates the active phase. At a given value of S, the system may either be active or silent, depending on whether S is rising or falling (Fig. 1). This is called *bi-stability*. Some neurons burst by mechanisms other than bi-stability (Rinzel, 1987), but all β-cell models to date rely on it. Bi-stability implies that adequate, brief perturbations of membrane potential should be able to reset the islet from the active to the silent phase or vice-versa. This has been demonstrated by Cook et al. (1981), although with some anomalies. (See Smolen and Sherman, in press.) Oscillations in V_m (Smith et al., 1990) and $[Ca^{2+}]_i$ (Gylfe et al., 1991) in single cells have been identified with islet bursting; this could be tested by resetting.

3.2. Glucose-Sensing

Increasing the parameter R in Eq. (3) increases the plateau fraction by slowing the rise of S toward its maximum switch point and accelerating its decline toward the minimum (Fig. 1, bottom panel). Since the fast spiking mechanism is not altered, there is no change in spike amplitude or frequency or silent phase potential, in agreement with experiment. Further increases in R induce continuous spiking, while reduction takes the cell below threshold for bursting. For any postulated slow variable it is possible to devise a parameter that gives the desired behavior, though some are more physiologically plausible than others.

Since $[Ca^{2+}]_i$ follows V_m, an increase in glucose is transduced into an increase in mean $[Ca^{2+}]_i$ averaged over a burst period rather than a change in the absolute silent and active phase levels. Along with other possible glucose-dependent factors (Gembal et al., 1992), this leads to increased insulin secretion. Thus, glucose-sensing with a threshold and a graded response, emerges naturally from the ionic mechanisms that determine bursting. To the extent that isolated cells can burst, then, the response to glucose is a property of individual cells.

3.3. Heterogeneity and Recruitment

We were motivated in part by the observation that bursting models are sensitive to parameter variation to ask how the islet is able to "find" the right parameters. Figure 2 shows the result of randomly distributing the parameters of a model (Smolen and Keizer, 1992). Before coupling there is a broad range of intrinsic behaviors at a fixed value of the glucose-sensing parameter, R, here related to the rate of ATP production. For the case shown, only a handful of cells burst, with the rest split evenly between tonically silent and tonically spiking. When the cells are coupled electrically by gap junctions, however, their intrinsic properties are masked and the bursts (though not the spikes) are synchronous. The population can burst, roughly, if its mean parameters are in the correct range, even if none of the individual cells' parameters are appropriate. Indeed, it would be difficult to determine what the intrinsic (isolated) response of a given cell would be from its behavior in the islet. As R is changed, different cells enter into bursting (see Fig. 4 below), but only when coupled can they all burst at the same value of R.

We now consider the collective response of a simplified caricature incorporating the variable responsiveness of isolated cells, some secreting at basal glucose, others at higher levels. According to the recruitment hypothesis (Pipeleers, 1992), as glucose increases more cells join in. If the response thresholds are normally distributed, the average secretion per cell will be sigmoidal (Fig. 3). Here cells are recruited by the stimulus; interaction between cells is neglected. As we saw above, however, a synchronous population may behave approximately like a single cell with average parameters. In this caricature, the response would be a sigmoid with the average threshold (Fig. 3). In some cases this can be shown to hold exactly. In some versions of the recruitment hypothesis, the cells are assumed to have an all-or-none response. Then, the uncoupled response would be graded, but the response of an exactly synchronized population would be all-or-none. We have tested the above caricature with the islet model of Fig. 2, computing average response per cell for both non-interacting and interacting populations. Since secretion is not included in the model, we used plateau fraction or mean $[Ca^{2+}]_i$ level as a surrogate. With no electrical coupling the dose response curve

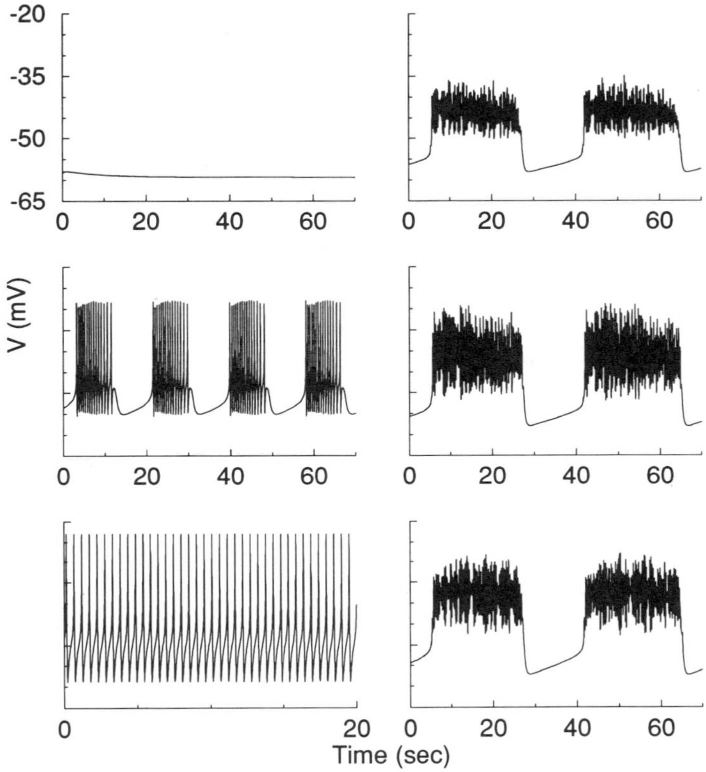

Figure 2. Heterogeneous model islet (125 cells). Left panels: Three representative cells with randomly distributed parameters, uncoupled. Right panels: Same cells with electrical coupling. Redrawn from Smolen et al., 1993 and Sherman, in press.

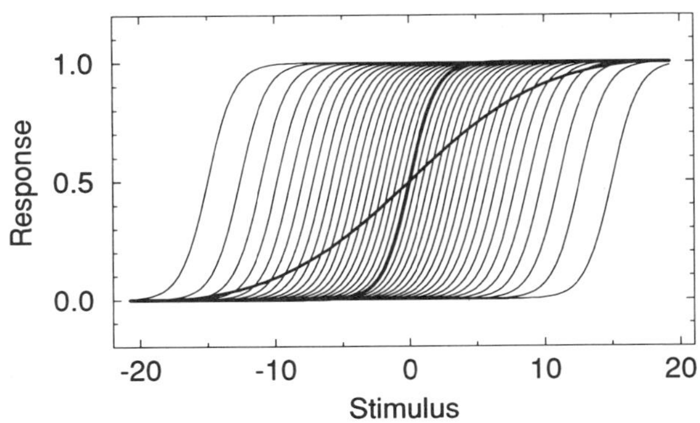

Figure 3. Caricature of a population glucose response (arbitrary units). Thin curves: hypothetical sigmoidal responses of individual cells with normally distributed thresholds. Shallow thick curve: summed activity of non-interacting cells. Steep thick curve: collective response assuming perfect synchrony.

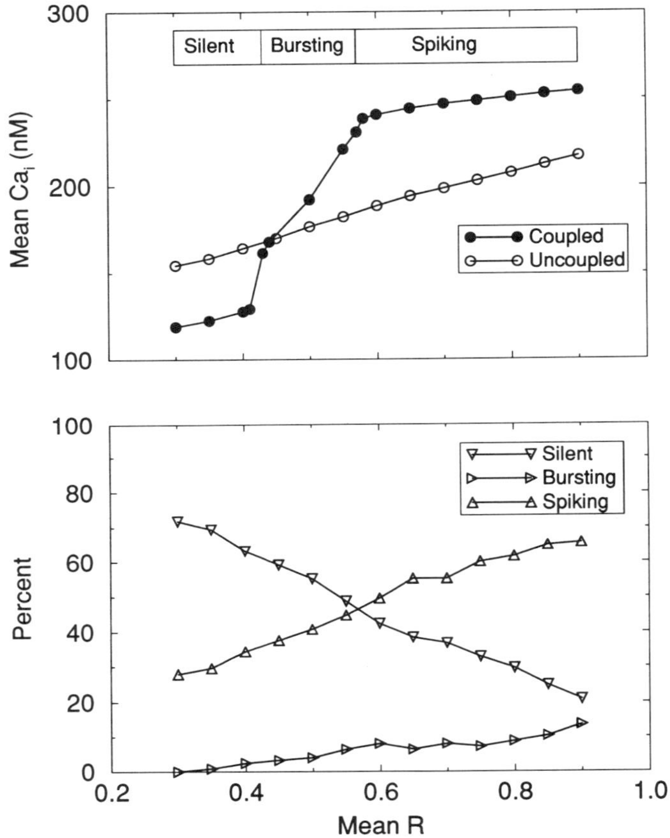

Figure 4. Glucose dose response curves for the heterogeneous islet model. Top panel: Mean $[Ca^{2+}]_i$ averaged over a burst vs. glucose (mean population R) with and without coupling. Silent, bursting, and spiking regimes for coupled islet are indicated. Bottom panel: Proportion of cells silent, bursting, and spiking as a function of glucose when uncoupled. Redrawn from Sherman, in press.

is shallow, while with coupling the curve is steep (Fig. 4, top panel). The bottom panel of Fig. 4 shows how this works. As glucose increases, it recruits more cells into spiking. The response of the coupled population depends on the balance of intrinsic spikers and silent cells. At any glucose level, there are a few intrinsic bursters, but these are negligible. The coupled population has a threshold: a critical number of intrinsically active cells is needed to recruit the rest of the cells to burst. As the proportion of intrinsically active cells increases, the population plateau fraction increases towards 100%. The conversion is non-linear due to the non-linear membrane properties of the cells. Although the exact response of individual cells in the coupled islet varies, at each value of glucose they essentially are all silent, all bursting, or all spiking continuously. Each cell's plateau fraction and $[Ca^{2+}]_i$ increase with glucose. The detailed islet model behaves like the cartoon of Fig. 3, except that the coupled response is not quite that of a cell with the average parameters (Smolen et al., 1993). Both illustrate two distinct possible roles for heterogeneity. With no cell-to-cell interactions, heterogeneity broadens the population response and can make it graded even if the individual cell responses are all-or-none. On the other hand, if the isolated cells have a graded response (owing to their burst dynamics), cell interactions can overcome the heterogeneity and produce a coordinated response with a common threshold. A third possibility arises if one considers a population of cells, none of which can burst for any value of the glucose-sensing parameter. Then the cells' electrical response is all-or-none: silent or continuously spiking. With, and only with, coupling such a population can burst. See Sherman and Rinzel (1992) for an example with two identical cells. The effect becomes more robust if the cells are heterogeneous and if population size is increased (unpublished simulations). Thus, it is possible for each cell to respond in an all-or-none manner when isolated, but in a graded way in the islet. All of the above simulations only take into account the electrical behavior of cells. Molecules diffusing through gap junctions or the intercellular space could lead to other biochemical or metabolic effects. The latter, and not electrical coupling, may for example underlie the results of Meda et al. (1991) showing synergy in secretion when two cells are coupled. We also have not modeled possible paracrine effects from non-β-cells in the islet.

3.4. Pacemaking

Bursting oscillations are generated in the heterogeneous islet model by cooperation of the tonically active and silent active sub-populations, neither of which is able to dominate. The active cells tend to initiate the active phase, while the silent cells initiate the silent phase. This differs from the situation in the heart where a spatially and electrically localized group of fast pacemaker cells drive the rest of the cells, which have slower intrinsic frequencies. Simulations (Smolen et al., 1993) show that because the islet is three dimensional, it is very difficult for a small group of active cells to drive the population. Even if they are spatially localized, they are electrically close to a large conductance load. They cannot activate the rest of the cells unless they are already close to threshold.

Similarly, it seems unlikely that coupling could account for the increased frequency of oscillations of Ca^{2+} and V_m seen in islets compared to isolated cells (Gylfe et al., 1991). The fastest cells would not drive the slow, but rather the population would oscillate at an intermediate frequency. Because of special features of the burst mechanism, coupling can *slow down* the population below the intrinsic frequency of the individual cells (Sherman and Rinzel, 1991, 1992), but we have never seen the reverse.

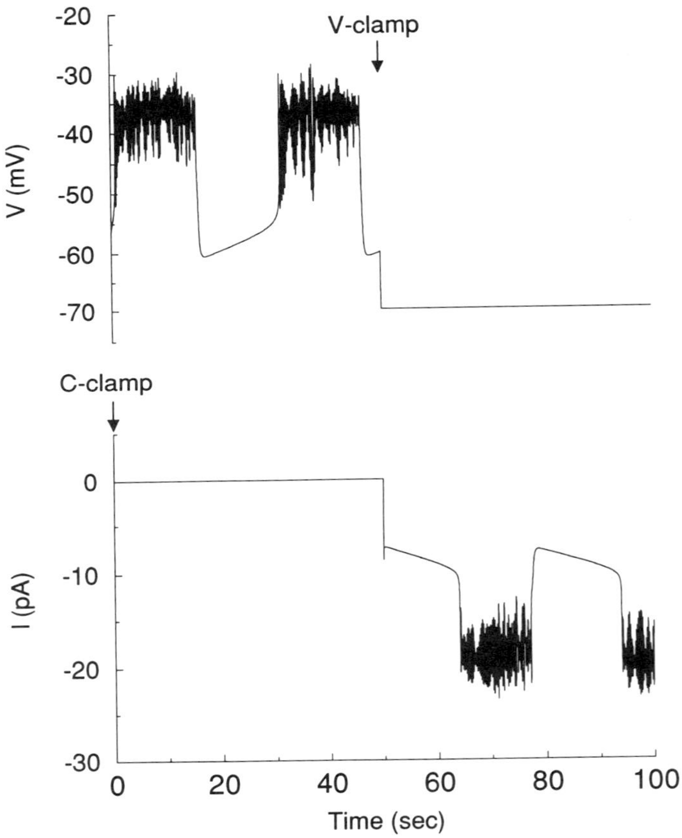

Figure 5. Simulated current- and voltage-clamp currents in an islet with a single cell clamped. In zero-current current clamp, normal bursting activity is observed. After switching to voltage-clamp, invading burst currents, reflecting the activity of unclamped neighbors, can be used to estimate gap-junctional conductance.

3.5. Are Gap Junctions Enough?

It is clear that sufficiently strong gap-junctional coupling would be able to synchronize the islet, but is there in fact enough coupling to do the job? What other mechanisms might be involved? Dye-coupling experiments indicate that coupled domains are rather small, on average a few cells (Meda et al., 1986). Under some conditions, such as pre-exposure to prolactin (Sheridan et al., 1986), dye-coupling is much more extensive. Direct electrical measurements have been made on pairs of cells that remain attached to each other when islets are dissociated. Perez-Armendariz et al (1991) found a broad distribution of coupling conductance (215 ± 110 pS), with 65% of pairs showing some coupling. Similar experiments by Meda et al. (1991) found only 20% of pairs coupled. In the simulations for Fig. 2 we assigned coupling conductances according to the histogram of Perez-Armendariz et al and easily attained synchrony. Reducing the probability of pair-wise connection to 20%, however, prevented synchrony. Thus, the experiments to date are quantitatively inconclusive. Also, it is possible that dissociation breaks or weakens connections. Simulations (Sherman et al., submitted) of the protocol of Rojas et al. (submitted) for voltage-clamping β-cells within an intact islet have suggested a method to measure the coupling conductance g_c *in situ*. Figure 5 shows a bursting cell in a model islet under (zero-current) current clamp. When that cell is voltage-clamped to -70 mV, its neighbors continue bursting, manifest as invading inward burst currents. Assuming that the membrane potential of the neighbors is similar to that of the impaled cell during current clamp, we can estimate g_c from the ratio of current difference between the active and silent phases to the voltage difference. Here, an estimate by eye of 10 pA/20 mV gives 0.5 nS, close to the actual value (6 connections of 100 pS each) present in the model. Another suggested way to synchronize islets is diffusion of K^+ and Ca^{2+} in the tight intercellular space. For example, K^+ released by an active cell would tend to depolarize neighboring cells. Stokes and Rinzel (1993) have shown that K^+ could contribute to synchronization. It is not likely to be the whole explanation, however, as K^+ diffusion is not strong enough for to account for the data of Eddlestone et al. (1984) showing that current injection in one cell can evoke an attenuated spike in a neighboring cell.

4. CONCLUSIONS

The bursting electrical activity of β-cells transduces plasma glucose levels into a mean $[Ca^{2+}]_i$ level, which partially determines insulin secretion. The multicell (islet) model, which only takes into account electrical activity and Ca^{2+} handling, suggests that glucose both recruits cells into activity and increases the individual cell output. The electrical coupling forces the cells to behave nearly synchronously, even though their intrinsic properties (their behavior when isolated) differ. The collective bursting behavior is determined by a nonlinear balance of tonically silent and active sub-populations. In this way, oscillations are achieved without a pacemaker. Heterogeneity broadens the response to glucose, while coupling sharpens it. It is not yet known whether gap-junctional coupling is indeed adequate to synchronize. Simulations suggest a way to measure coupling *in situ*.

ACKNOWLEDGMENTS

John Rinzel, Joel Keizer, and Cindy Stokes participated in many of the modeling studies and discussions from which these ideas were developed. The National Cancer Institute Biomedical Supercomputing Center and the National Institutes of Health Division of Computer Research and Technology Convex group provided computer time and technical assistance.

REFERENCES

[1] Beigelman, P. M., Ribalet, A., and Atwater, I., 1977, Electrical activity of mouse pancreatic beta-cells, *J. Physiol. (Paris)* 73:201.

[2] Chay, T. R., and Cook, D. L., 1988, Endogenous bursting patterns in excitable cells, *Math. Biosci.* 90:139.

[3] Chay, T. R., and Keizer, J., 1983, Minimal model for membrane oscillations in pancreatic β-cells, *Biophys. J.* 42:181.

[4] Cook, D., Porte, D., and Crill, W., 1981, Voltage dependence of rhythmic plateau potentials of pancreatic islet cells, *Am. J. Physiol.* 240:E290.

[5] Eddlestone, G. T., Gonçalves, A., Bangham, J. A., and Rojas, E., 1984, Electrical coupling between cells in islets of Langerhans in mouse, *J. Membr. Biol.* 77:1.

[6] Gembal, M., Gilon, P., and Henquin, J.-C., 1992, Evidence that glucose can control insulin secretion release independently from its action on ATP-sensitive K^+ channels in mouse B cells, *J. Clin. Invest.* 89:1288.

[7] Gylfe, E., Grapengieser, E., and Hellman, B., 1991, Propagation of cytoplasmic Ca^{2+} oscillations in clusters of pancreatic β-cells exposed to glucose, *Cell Calcium* 12:229.

[8] Keizer, J., and Smolen, P., 1991, Bursting electrical activity in pancreatic β cells cause by Ca^{2+}- and voltage-inactivated Ca^{2+} channels, *Proc. Natl. Acad. Sci. USA* 88:3897.

[9] Meda, P., Santos, R. M., and Atwater, I., 1986, Direct identification of electrophysiologically monitored cells within intact mouse islets of Langerhans, *Diabetes* 35:232.

[10] Meda, P., Bosco, D., Giordano, E., and Chanson, M., 1991, Junctional coupling modulation by secretagogues in two-cell pancreatic systems, *in:* "Biophysics of Gap Junction Channels," C. Peracchia, ed., CRC Press, Boca Raton.

[11] Perez-Armendariz, M., Roy, C., Spray, D. C., and Bennett, M. V L., 1991, Biophysical properties of gap junctions between freshly dispersed pairs of mouse pancreatic β-cells, *Biophys. J.* 59:76.

[12] Pipeleers, D., 1992, Heterogeneity in pancreatic β-cell population, *Diabetes* 41:777.

[13] Rinzel, J., 1987, A formal classification of bursting mechanisms in excitable systems, *in:* "Mathematical Topics in Population Biology, Morphogenesis, and Neurosciences," Teramoto, E., and Yamaguti, M., eds., Springer-Verlag, New York.

[14] Rojas, E., Stokes, C. L., Mears, D., and Atwater, I., 1995, Single micro-electrode voltage-clamp measurements of pancreatic β-cell membrane ionic currents *in situ*, *J. Membr. Biol.* 143:65.

[15] Santos, R. M., Rosario, L. M., Nadal, A., Garcia-Sancho, J., Soria, B., and Valdeolmillos, M., 1991, Widespread synchronous $[Ca^{2+}]_i$ oscillations due to bursting electrical activity in single pancreatic islets, *Pflügers Arch.* 418:417.

[16] Satin, L., and Smolen, P., Electrical bursting in β-cells of the pancreatic islets of Langerhans, *Endocrine J.* in press.

[17] Sheridan, R. L., Sorenson, R. L., Parsons, J. A., and Sheridan, J. D., 1987, Prolactin enhances cell-to-cell communication among β-cells in pancreatic islets, *Diabetes* 36:1098.

[18] Sherman, A., and Rinzel, J., 1991, Model for synchronization of pancreatic β-cells by gap junction coupling, *Biophys. J.* 59:547.

[19] Sherman, A., and Rinzel, J., 1992, Rhythmogenic effects of weak electrotonic coupling in neuronal models, *Proc. Natl. Acad. Sci. USA* 89:2471.

[20] Sherman, A., 1995, Theoretical aspects of synchronized bursting in β-cells, in: *Pacemaker Activity and Intercellular Communication*, J. D. Huizinga, ed., CRC Press, Boca Raton, FL, pages 323–337.

[21] Sherman, A., Xu L., and Stokes, C., Estimating and eliminating junctional current in coupled cell populations by leak subtraction. A computational study, Submitted to *J. Membr. Biol.*

[22] Smith, P. A., Ashcroft, F. M., and Rorsman, P., 1990, Simultaneous recordings of glucose dependent electrical activity and ATP-regulated K^+- currents in isolated mouse pancreatic β-cells, *FEBS Lett.* 261:187.

[23] Smolen, P., and Keizer, J., 1992, Slow voltage inactivation of Ca^{2+} currents and bursting mechanisms for the mouse pancreatic β-cell, *J. Membr. Biol.* 127:9.

[24] Smolen, P., Rinzel, J., and Sherman, A., 1993, Why pancreatic islets burst but single β-cells do not: The heterogeneity hypothesis, *Biophys. J.* 64:1668.

[25] Smolen, P., and Sherman, A., Phase-independent resetting in relaxation and burst oscillators, *J. Theo. Biol.* 169:339.

[26] Stokes, C., and Rinzel, J., 1993., Diffusion of extracellular K^+ can synchronize bursting oscillations in a model islet of Langerhans, *Biophys. J.* 65:597.

39

RECONSTRUCTING ISLET FUNCTION *IN VITRO*

Domenico Bosco and Paolo Meda

Department of Morphology
University of Geneva
C.M.U.
1211 Genève 4, Switzerland

INTRODUCTION

Throughout the day, insulin secretion and biosynthesis result from the activity of numerous β-cells which function in coordination. Until recently, it has been implicitly assumed that all these cells are alike, i.e. that they secrete synchronously and at the same rate under various conditions. However, several lines of evidence now show that the actual situation is more complex. Thus, in situ, individual β-cells show variable amounts of secretory granules and rough endoplasmic reticulum[1], different thresholds for glucose-induced electrical activity[2,3] and a variable ability to biosynthesize insulin[4]. Furthermore, the β-cells located at the periphery of the islets differ from those located in the center of the microorgan with regard to nucleus size[5,6], incorporation of [^{3}H]-thymidine[7], number of gap junctions[8], extent of dye coupling[9], electrical activity[10,11], and ability to secrete insulin[12]. In vitro studies have also revealed marked differences between individual β-cells with respect to insulin release[13–17], electrical activity[18] and Ca^{2+} changes during stimulation[19,20], as well as with respect to protein biosynthesis[4] and glucose-activated metabolic redox changes[21–23]. This wide heterogeneity, which is reviewed in the first part of this chapter, raises the question of how β-cells achieve the proper coordination which is necessary to ensure appropriate insulin biosynthesis and secretion under continously changing physiological conditions.

Such a coordination implies that β-cells communicate with each other to sense the state of activity of nearby cells and to coordinate accordingly their functioning. There are multiple mechanisms which could mediate these communications, including signaling by hormones, neuromediators, cytokines and other molecules (nutrients, ions, NO, …) that diffuse in the intercellular spaces of pancreatic islets. Furthermore, since insulin biosynthesis and secretion remain regulated events under in vitro conditions which perturb or even abolish native blood supply and innervation, as well as the flux of intercellular fluid which takes place in the intact pancreas, other mechanisms should also contribute to β-to-β-cell coordination. The findings that the functioning of islet cells is altered after their dispersion[24–26] and rapidly improves upon their reaggregation[25–29], suggest that these additional mecha-

Physiology and Pathophysiology of the Islets of Langerhans, edited by Soria.
Plenum Press, New York, 1997.

nisms depend on the proper establishment and maintenance of cell-to-cell contacts, presumably due to the involvement of specialized domains of the cell membrane. To elucidate these mechanisms, we have studied how individual β-cells change their functioning as a function of reaggregation to companion β-cells. These findings are reviewed in the second and third parts of this chapter.

FUNCTION OF SINGLE β-CELLS

The All/None Insulin Release Response

Hemolytic plaque assays have revealed that individual β-cells secrete insulin in a rather variable way after stimulation by glucose, non glucidic nutrient secretagogues and other non metabolizable stimuli[13–17,30]. Thus, irrespective of the secretagogue type and of the duration of stimulation, secreting β-cells consistently coexist with apparently similar β-cells that, as judged by the lack of formation of a hemolytic plaque, do not release detectable amounts of the hormone, if they secrete at all (Fig. 1). These non secreting cells were shown to exclude trypan blue, to display an electrophysiologically normal membrane and, at least in some cases, to be able of new protein biosynthesis[17,31], indicating that they were living and functional cells.

Most secreting and non secreting β-cells were also observed to maintain their rather different secretory behaviour during successive stimulations, and for various intervals of

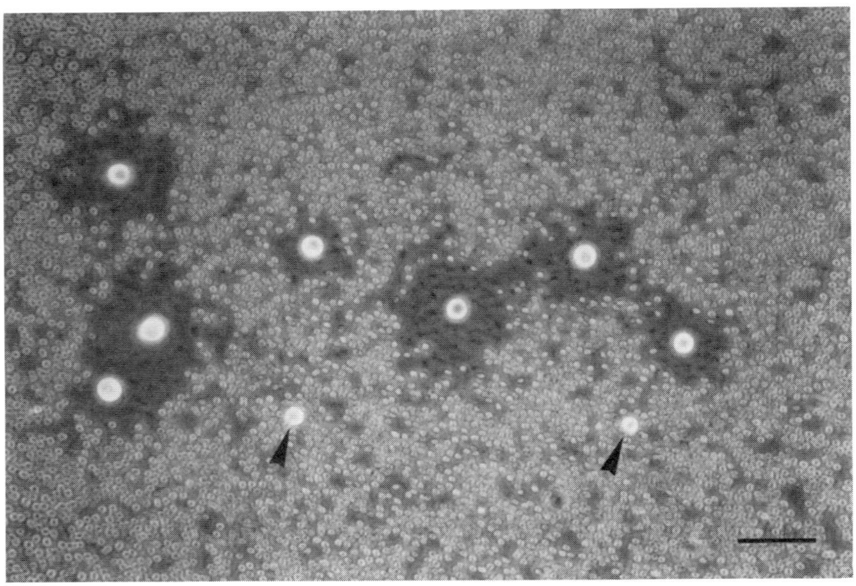

Figure 1. Heterogeneous insulin release from single β-cells. Examination of plaque assay chambers after a 30 min incubation in the presence of 16.7 mM glucose, revealed that individual β-cells, which appear brightly white after insulin immunostaining, release variable amounts of insulin, as judged by the variable size of the surrounding hemolytic plaque. In this field, two β-cells (arrowheads), apparently similar to the secreting ones, have not induced the formation of a hemolytic plaque, i.e. have failed to release detectable amounts of insulin. The bar represents 40 μm.

secretagogue challenge[16], suggesting that they likely represent functionally distinct, and quantitatively stable subpopulations of β-cells. Successive stimulations of the same β-cells by different secretagogues, further indicated that β-cells unresponsive to an acute glucose stimulation, were also usually unresponsive to other secretagogues[30]. Hence, there is presently no evidence for β-cell subpopulations, which may be specialized to respond to a given secretagogue.

Another level of secretory heterogeneity was detected by evaluating the proportion of cells forming a hemolytic plaque, a parameter which estimates the fraction of β-cells contributing to insulin output, and the individual areas of these plaques, which evaluate the amount of hormone released by each secreting cell. In the presence of 2.8 mM glucose, only a small fraction of β-cells was found able to form a hemolytic plaque (Fig. 2), usually of small size. Raising the concentration of D-glucose in the medium, significantly

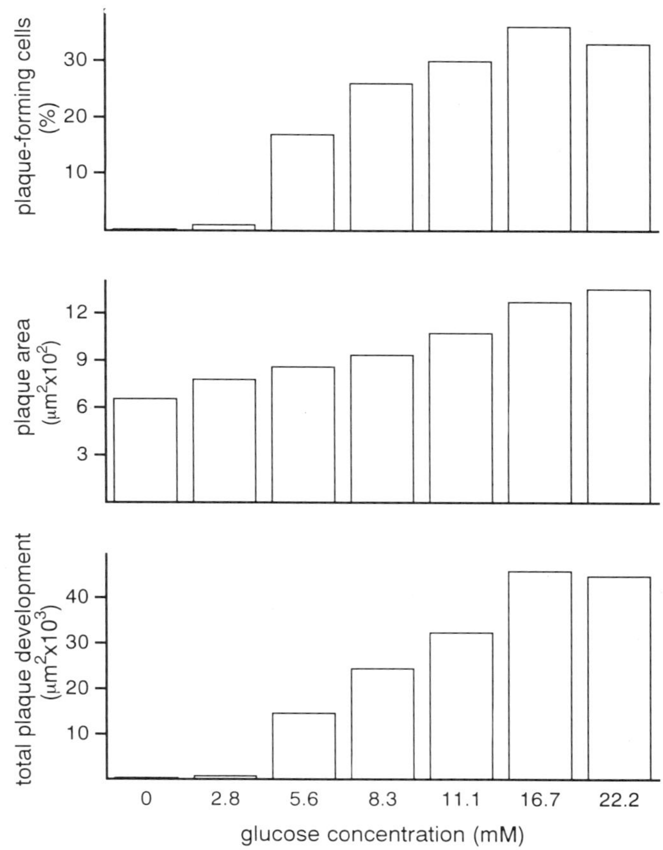

Figure 2. Glucose stimulation of single β-cells, as evaluated in the hemolytic plaque assay for insulin. The upper panel shows that the proportion of cells releasing detectable amounts of insulin increased as a function of glucose concentration, indicating a progressive recruitment of secreting cells with stimulation. The middle panel shows that the average area of hemolytic plaques also slightly enlarged with glucose stimulation, indicating an increase in the insulin output of individual β-cells. However, this increase was much smaller than that reflecting cell recruitment. The lower panel shows that, as a result of these changes, total insulin secretion of a single β-cell population increases with glucose stimulation in a sigmoidal fashion. In this typical experiment, the threshold level for glucose-induced insulin release was about 5.6 mM, and β-cells were maximally stimulated by glucose concentrations around 16.7 mM.

increased the proportion of secreting β-cells, up to a maximum of about 40% (a 10-fold increase as compared to basal value) in the presence of 16.7 mM glucose (Fig. 2).

Under these maximal stimulatory conditions, the areas of individual hemolytic plaques were again variable from one cell to another, and, on the average, only slightly elevated over those observed under basal conditions (Fig. 2).

Comparable observations were made with β-cells cultured 15–18 h in the presence of 2.8 mM glucose, and then exposed 30 min to a stimulatory concentration (16.7 mM) of the sugar. Under these conditions, overall insulin release was markedly decreased, due to a significant reduction in the proportion of cells that were recruited to secrete, but the amount of insulin which was released individually by these cells was essentially unaltered (Fig. 3).

These observations indicate first that secreting β-cells do not all release similar amounts of insulin, whatever the glucose concentration prevalent in the medium. Second, that the amount of insulin released by glucose sensitive cells, is not markedly influenced by the level of stimulation. Third, that the increased insulin secretion which is elicited by glucose is mostly due to an increased recruitment of secreting cells, which, as a population, release insulin at a rate similar to that observed under basal conditions. Fourth, that

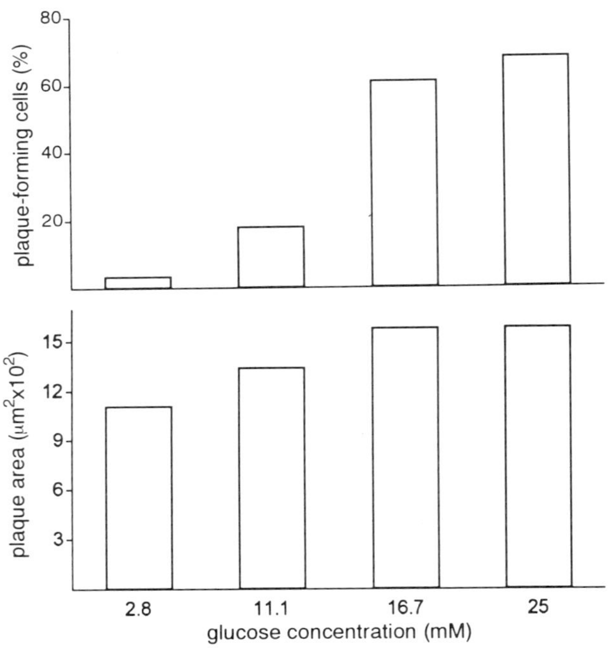

Figure 3. Glucose responsiveness of single β-cells cultured in the presence of various levels of the sugar. In this experiment, single β-cells were cultured 15–18 h in the presence of the various glucose concentrations indicated in the abscissa, and then stimulated 30 min by 16.7 mM glucose. The upper panel shows that the proportion of secreting cells was maximal in the population of β-cells which had been cultured in the presence of 16.7–25 mM glucose, much smaller in the population of β-cells which had been cultured in the presence of 11.1 mM glucose, and minimal in the population of β-cells which had been cultured in the presence of 2.8 mM glucose. The lower panel shows that, contrasting with these major changes, the average area of hemolytic plaques was about the same, whatever the glucose level used to culture the cells prior to the secretion test. Hence, whenever a β-cell is recruited to secrete, its secretory response appears rather constant, as judged by the amount of insulin released.

under conditions which seriously hinder glucose-induced insulin release, some β-cells still secrete the hormone in amounts comparable to those observed under conditions which optimalize secretion. Hence, β-cells appear to show a all/none type of secretory responsiveness.

One implication of these conclusions is that the total insulin output of a single β-cell population should take into account both the proportion of secreting cells and their average, individual rate of secretion. In the plaque assay, this can be done by calculating total plaque development, which is given by the product of the two primary data evaluated in the test. As shown in Fig. 2, this parameter revealed that glucose stimulation of single β-cells elicits a sigmoidal increase in insulin release, with a threshold level between 5 and 8 mM and a plateau at about 16.7 mM glucose. Hence, in spite of their marked individual heterogeneity, single β-cells show, as a population, a response pattern which is qualitatively similar to that observed in the intact pancreas.

What Determines the Heterogeneous Secretion of Individual β-Cells?

The reason why living, and apparently alike β-cells feature the marked secretory heterogeneity summarized above is still a matter of conjecture. Because normal secretory responsiveness requires that glucose is properly taken up and phosphorylated by β-cells, we have compared secreting and non secreting β-cells, as differentiated at the end of the plaque assay, for the presence of both GLUT2 and glucokinase. By immunofluorescence staining with specific antibodies, we have observed that these two proteins are virtually always expressed by single β-cells, whether these cells were able to induce the formation of a hemolytic plaque after an acute stimulation by D-glucose, or not[30]. Hence, the mere presence of either GLUT2 or glucokinase is not a sufficient determinant of the glucose responsiveness of individual β-cells.

In view of the critical importance of ionic events in the early steps of the stimulus-secretion coupling of β-cells, we further investigated whether secreting and non secreting β-cells have different electrophysiological characteristics. By combining the plaque assay with the recording of individual β-cells by either thin tip (high resistance) or patch-clamp electrodes (used in the attached, whole cell configuration), we have found that both secreting and non secreting β-cells are equipped with similar ions channels, including for voltage-dependent Na^+ currents, voltage-activated Ba^{2+} currents, voltage-dependent K^+ delayed-rectifier currents, voltage-dependent Ca^{2+}-activated K^+ currents, and voltage-independent and tolbutamide-sensitive K^+ currents[17]. In addition, both cell subpopulations showed a similar modulation of ions channels during both glucose and tolbutamide stimulation[17]. Hence, there is presently no evidence that electro-physiological differences determine the striking secretory heterogeneity of single β-cells.

After the suggestion that the heterogeneous secretory responsiveness of individual β-cells may be related to a variable metabolic handling of glucose[22], we have investigated β-cells showing markedly different changes in NAD(P)H autofluorescence after an acute glucose stimulation. In our assay, we first confirmed that the subpopulation of β-cells featuring a glucose-induced increase in the NAD(P)H signal secreted more insulin than the subpopulation showing no apparent redox shift[22], but also observed that both subpopulations comprised secreting and non secreting β-cells[32]. In these experiments, we were struck by the observations that the average size of β-cells differed in the two sorted-populations and that, when cells of comparable size were compared, no more difference in insulin output was found between the β-cells that appear to be metabolically active and those which seem to be metabolically quiescent[32]. Hence, the secretory heterogeneity of β-cells is related to a difference in size rather than to a marked, differential ability to activate metabolism in the presence of glucose.

In parallel experiments, we have found that very same β-cells respond to D-glucose and to non-glucidic nutrient secretagogues, and do so at the same extent, as judged both by a similar total insulin output and by a comparable number of cells contributing to it[30]. These findings strongly suggest that the factor(s) responsible for the responsiveness of individual β-cells are not tightly related to a specific metabolic event in the early steps of glucose transport and catabolism. Functional heterogeneity was also observed in the presence of non metabolized secretagogues[30], further indicating that the factors which rule the response of β-cells are likely to be somewhat distal in the sequence of steps which links stimulus to secretion in pancreatic β-cells. Eventually, the autoradiographic observations that individual β-cells are heterogeneous in terms of their ability to biosynthesise proteins, including insulin, and that glucose stimulates protein biosynthesis via a dose-dependent recruitment of β-cells which is similar to that observed for secretion[4], argues for the same factors controlling the secretory and biosynthetic ability of β-cells. To test this idea, we have combined the plaque assay for insulin with autoradiography, in order to monitor a number of β-cells for both insulin secretion and protein biosynthesis. We have observed that the β-cells which were biosynthetically active at the time of the test were preferentially recruited to secrete insulin during a short term stimulation by glucose, as compared to similar, but biosynthetically quiescent β-cells[31]. However, we have also found that a sizable proportion of biosynthetically active β-cells was not able to secrete insulin, and, conversely, that a number of biosynthetically quiescent β-cells could release detectable amounts of the hormone[31]. Hence, it is unlikely that a major metabolic perturbation accounts for the unresponsiveness of some β-cells to glucose.

FUNCTION OF β-CELLS IN CONTACT

The considerations summarized above, indicate that individual β-cells show a marked functional heterogeneity, whose cause(s) remain(s) uncertain. They also indicate that, in spite of this heterogeneity, single β-cells, as a population, have a response pattern which is qualitatively similar to that observed in the intact pancreas. However, as compared to the situation prevailing in the intact gland, the quantitative response of single cells to stimulation is severely reduced. This reduction is essentially due to a rather modest recruitment of single cells able to release and/or to biosynthesize insulin during secretagogue stimulation. Hence, some intraislet mechanism should ensure an enhanced recruitment of functioning β-cells under conditions requiring substantial insulin output or biosynthesis. Because such mechanism is apparently lost in single cells, we investigated whether it could be related to the establishment of cell-to-β-cell contacts.

As a first approach to this question, we have compared the glucose-induced insulin release of single β-cells to that of the smallest units in which cell-to-cell contact may be influential, i.e. pairs of β-cells. We have first observed that the response of both single cells and pairs increased as a function of the concentration of glucose prevalent in the medium (Fig. 4). We have also found that whereas in the presence of glucose concentrations less than 5.7 mM, i.e. below the average threshold level for stimulation, single β-cells and β-cell pairs behaved similarly, as judged by a comparable proportion of secreting units and a similar average size of hemolytic plaques (Fig. 4). However, this was no longer the case in the presence of 16.7 mM glucose. Under this maximally stimulatory condition, β-cell pairs secreted about twice more frequently than single β-cells and, as

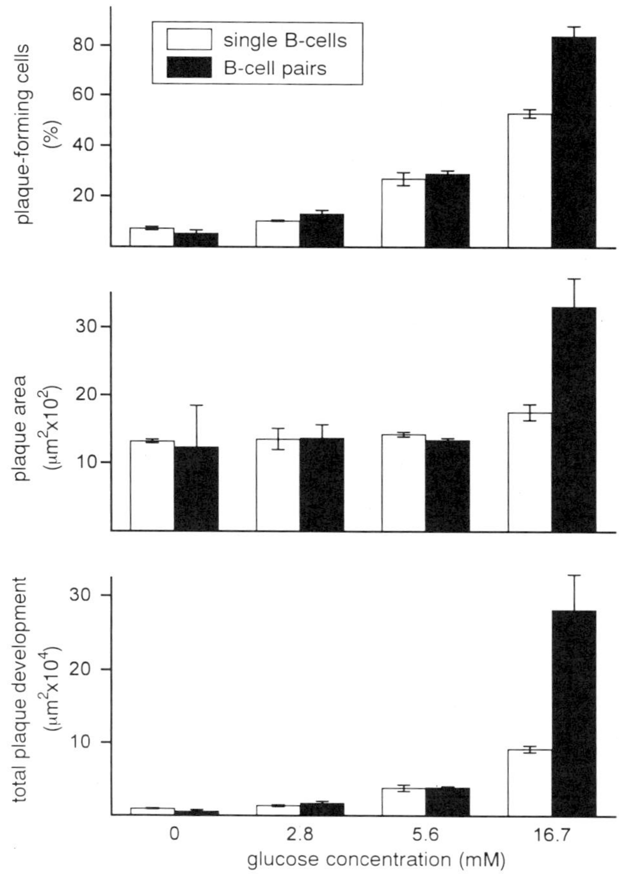

Figure 4. Effect of cell-to-cell contact on glucose-induced insulin release. The upper panel shows that the proportion of cells recruited to release insulin increased as a function of glucose concentration. Comparaison of single β-cells (open columns) and β-cell pairs (solid columns), revealed no difference in their recruitment for glucose concentrations in the 0–5.6 mM range. In contrast, when the secretion test was performed in the presence of 16.7 mM glucose, β-cell pairs were recruited for secretion significantly more than single β-cells. The middle panel shows that the average area of hemolytic plaques surrounding single β-cells (open columns) was almost constant for the glucose concentrations tested. β-cell pairs (solid columns) showed a similar pattern for glucose concentrations in the 0–5.6 mM range. In contrast, when the secretion test was performed in the presence of 16.7 mM glucose, β-cell pairs induced the formation of hemolytic plaques which were significantly larger than those surrounding single β-cells. The lower panel shows that, as a result of these changes, total insulin secretion of single (open columns) and paired β-cells (solid columns) was comparable in the presence of low levels of glucose. By contrast, maximally stimulatory levels of the sugar elicit 3–4 fold higher response from β-cell pairs than from single β-cells.

judged by the average size of the hemolytic plaques they induced, also released in average twice as much insulin (Fig.4).

Hence, whereas in pairs exposed to low glucose levels only one β-cell appears to contribute to secretion, in pairs exposed to high glucose levels, the two β-cells in contact do so in coordination. These results indicate first that, in the presence of a non stimulatory concentration of glucose, the mere contact between two β-cells is not sufficient to promote their functioning. They also suggest that a number of β-cells which are in an "off" functional state may be induced to secrete after contacting another β-cell. Eventually, they indicate that the mechanism which mediates the functional recruitment of previously quiescent cells is glucose-dependent.

To gain further insights into this mechanism, we investigated the time required to observe the four fold increase in secretory function that takes place, in the presence of high glucose, as single β-cells adhere to form pairs. To this end, we prelabeled single β-cells with inert fluorescent beads, which are conveniently stable cytoplasmic markers, and we cocultured these cells with similar but unlabeled β-cells. Using this approach, we established that β-cell pairs formed within 10 min already showed the full increase in secretory capacity that is observed in much older β-cell pairs. Hence, the mechanism which mediates the increased function of β-cells after establishment of cell contacts is activated.

In parallel experiments, we also observed that contact between insulin-producing cells upregulates their expression of the insulin gene[33].

IDENTIFYING THE CONTACT-DEPENDENT MECHANISM WHICH MODULATES β-CELL FUNCTIONING

The observations summarized above provide compelling evidence that a mechanism dependent on the physical contact of β-cells, ensures proper glucose responsiveness and upregulates secretagogue-induced insulin release, protein biosynthesis and the expression of the insulin gene. However, the reason why cell contact is required, if not obligatory, for proper β-cell functioning remains to be elucidated, as is the molecular mechanism underlying this requirement.

Conceivably, this mechanism may involve any of the events that take place as β-cells interact with one another, including changes in the polarity of cytoplasmic and membrane components, and in the surface molecules which ensure cell adhesion and comprise intercellular junctions. Surprisingly, the influence of several of these potential mechanisms has not yet been tested directly. However, the observation that, under stimulatory conditions, a sizable fraction of β-cell aggregates do not release insulin (as evaluated in the plaque assay) and do not synthesize proteins (as evaluated by autoradiography), indicates that the mere aggregation of β-cells is not alone sufficient to ensure an upregulation of β-cell function. Furthermore, since the phenotype of β-cells in functionally quiescent aggregates is alike that observed in active aggregates, it is unlikely that changes in the polarity of β-cell components and/or in the molecules and structures which ensure β-cell adhesion be a prime event in the contact-dependent regulation of insulin secretion and biosynthesis. An implication of this view is that another mechanism, activated by cell contact, should be prominent. Several lines of experimental evidence, including the rapid onset of secretion upregulation which takes place after reaggregation, suggest that such a control mechanism could be provided by junctional coupling, the form of cell-to-cell communication which is mediated by gap junctions.

Gap Junctional Coupling

Pancreatic β-cells are connected to each other by numerous and minute gap junctions made of a protein of the connexin family, called Cx43[34]. In a resting β-cell, there are 800–2000 gap junction channels that, altogether, occupy less than 1 μm^2 of the plasma membrane[35]. These channels allow for the β-to-β-cell exchange of current-carrying ions, low molecular weight probes, nucleotides and glycolytic intermediates[35–39]. Ionic and metabolic coupling is not observed between all β-cells[34], in agreement with the detection of gap junctions in only 30% of the β-to-β-cell interfaces, and at least metabolic coupling is spatially restricted to small groups of β-cells in both intact islets and monolayer cultures[37,38]. Hence, the 10–3,000 β-cells that comprise a pancreatic islet form an assembly of multiple communication territories rather than a single syncitium.

Several lines of evidence indicate a contribution of β-cell coupling to the control of insulin secretion. First, single β-cells (which cannot form gap junctions) show increased basal release of insulin, poor responsiveness to secretagogues, decreased protein biosynthesis, decreased basal expression of the insulin gene and loss of its normal, cAMP-dependent control[13,24,31,33,40]. Restoration of β-cell contacts is paralleled by a rapid secretory improvement, as judged by a decrease in the basal release of insulin and an increased responsiveness to secretagogues, as well as by a larger protein biosynthesis and expression of the insulin gene[13,24,31,33,40]. The finding that drugs blocking gap junctions prevent the increase in insulin secretion which normally takes place as single β-cells interact to form pairs[40], indicates that coupling may acutely control the recruitment of secreting β-cells as well as their individual level of activity.

Second, sustained stimulation of insulin release increases β-cell coupling in vivo and in vitro[35,41] due, at least in some cases, to increased expression of gap junctions and Cx43[34,35]. The almost immediate increase in coupling coefficient which is observed when islets are exposed to concentrations of glucose stimulating insulin release, further suggests that β-cell coupling may also be acutely regulated by changes in the conductance and/or permeability of existing gap junction channels[39].

Third, conditions that inhibit insulin release decrease or abolish β-cell coupling[41,42]. In vivo, however, this effect may be overcome whenever inhibition of β-cell secretion results in hyperglycemia[38,42], suggesting that the level of circulating glucose and the ability of β-cells to properly recognize the sugar stimulus independently control junctional coupling.

Fourth, the acute pharmacological blockade of gap junction channels markedly alters β-cell function, as indicated by increased basal insulin release and loss of stimulated insulin secretion[40,43]. These alterations appear specifically related to β-cell uncoupling since they could not be accounted for by consistent changes in the main second messengers that are known to control insulin secretion, they were rapidly and fully reversible after wash out of the uncoupling drugs and they were not observed with single β-cells[40,43]. Preliminary observations using antisense oligonucleotides, which are expected to be incorporated by β-cells and to hybridize to the endogenous mRNA coding for Cx43, further support this view. Indeed, these probes were found not to affect the glucose-induced insulin release of single β-cells but to markedly decrease that of β-cell aggregates.

Fifth, a number of tumoral and transformed insulin-producing cell lines (RIN, INS1, HIT, AtT20ins, CGT-5, CGT-6) which show abnormal glucose sensitivity, do not express connexins and gap junctions and are essentially uncoupled[44,45]. This coupling deficiency cannot be simply explained by an in vitro downregulation of gap junction channels since primary β-cells in monolayer culture continue to express Cx43, gap junctions and coupling[44,45]. It cannot be either ascribed solely to the proliferating ability of the cell lines, since the glucose-sensitive cells of a rat insulinoma, from which at least two of the communication-deficient clones (RIN and INS1) were derived, still express Cx43, gap junctions and coupling in vivo[45]. Hence, coupling defects appear to be a shared attribute of cell lines showing abnormal sensitivity to glucose, whatever the expression of several key factors (GLUT-2, glucokinase, hexokinase, ...) that rate-limit the entry and early metabolic response to the sugar. Preliminary observations on a few clones of INS cells that had retained junctional coupling, further support this coupling-glucose responsiveness relationship. Indeed, clones showing a junctional coupling analogous to that of primary β-cells, display a qualitatively normal dose-response curve to glucose, an enhanced glucose- and cAMP-induced insulin release and a marked increase in insulin content and in the expression of the insulin gene[45]. In addition, stable transfection of communication incompetent RIN and INS cells with the gene coding for Cx43, resulted in overexpression of Cx43, in restored junctional communication and in decreased levels of stored insulin and expression of the insulin gene[45]. Together, these observations provide compelling evidence for a prime role of coupling in the control of β-cell specific functions. What remains to be understood is why.

As compared to other forms of cell-to-cell communication, gap junctional coupling is unique in that it provides a direct mechanism to equilibrate ionic and molecular electrochemical gradients between nearby cells[46]. In such a system, the increase of cytoplasmic ions or molecules less than 900 Da into one cell is followed by their diffusion-driven passage into nearby cells. At steady state, this passage leads to the equilibration of electrochemical concentrations on the two sides of the channels. If the resulting concentration reaches a threshold level for activation of an effector mechanism, functioning will be modified not only in the cell in which the ionic and molecular change first occurred, but also in all other cells coupled to it. In this way, junctional coupling may ensure the functional recruitment of cells that could not be directly activated. Such a recruiting role of coupling has been experimentally verified in β-cell populations[13,29]. Furthermore, since individual β-cells secrete more insulin when they share gap junctions than when they are single[13,29], the coupling-induced equilibration should also optimize the concentration of factors critical for secretion. This view is consistent with the observation that the threshold level for activation of insulin secretion and biosynthesis is lowered under conditions promoting β-cell coupling[47]. Eventually, coupling would be expected to synchronize changes of factors exchanged through gap junctions. This expectation has also been verified for β-cells[48,49].

The identification of an intrinsic heterogeneity of β-cells provides a first clue to conceptualize why and how junctional coupling could modulate insulin secretion. What is not determined is the molecular mechanism underlying this modulation. A first possibility is that coupling may enhance the secretagogue-induced changes in free intracellular Ca^{2+}. The levels and oscillations of this cation, which plays a critical role in the control of insulin secretion, are differentially affected by the establishment of β-to-β-cell contacts[47,48]. Coupling may also regulate the electrophysiological characteristics of β-cells. It has been observed that resting membrane potentials and individual conductances become larger and more stable after establishment of cell-to-cell contacts, presumably because individual β-cells are equipped with so limited numbers of K^+ and Ca^{2+} channels that they cannot ensure stable ionic fluxes as channels fluctuate between the open and close state[50]. By mediating a non selective intercellular exchange of current-carrying ions, junctional coupling results in the functional sharing of ionic channels by several cells, thus ensuring that the number of opened channels be always sufficient[50]. Channel sharing could markedly promote the responsiveness of β-cells, since the activation of the distal, effector steps of their secretory machinery depends on proper control of membrane potentials and ionic fluxes. Third, coupling could ensure the spreading across large cell populations of signals controlling secretion. Secretagogue-induced Ca^{2+} waves, indicating a temporally and spatially coordinated change in the levels of this ion across multiple cells, have been observed throughout intact islets of Langerhans[49]. These waves, which may result from the intercellular passage of Ca^{2+} or IP_3 via gap junctions, could mediate the rapid recruitment of secreting cells at distance from the site of signaling. In other systems, cells devoid of specific receptors have been shown to be activated after establishment of junctional coupling with cells recognizing the cognate signal, probably as a result of a gap junction-mediated exchange of second messengers[51]. An analogous mechanism, resulting in the intercellular diffusion of Ca^{2+} [48,49] or cAMP[37], may similarly ensure the rapid recruitment of non secreting β-cells[13,29], some of which may be equipped with insufficient amounts of factors (GLUT2, glucokinase, ATP-sensitive K^+ channels, ...) which rate-limit insulin secretion. By sharing gap junctions with nearby cells equipped with these essential molecules, the defective cells may be adequately activated to secrete, eventhough, individually, they may be unable to directly recognize stimuli.

RELEVANCE FOR THE IN VIVO SITUATION

The relevance of these in vitro findings for the behaviour of β-cells in situ remains to be clarified. We have previously reported that the β-cells located in the center of the islets of Langerhans show more gap junction[8] and secrete insulin at a higher rate than the β-cells located at the periphery of the microorgans[12]. To assess whether centrally located β-cells also synthesize proteins more actively than peripheral β-cells, we in situ perfused the pancreas of glucose-infused rats with ^{3}H-leucine, for 10 min and in the presence of 16.7 mM glucose. Under these conditions, autoradiography showed that the incorporation of the labeled aminoacid into newly synthesized proteins was not homogeneous throughout the islets, and predominated over the β-cells which were located in the central part of the microorgans (Fig. 5).

These cells, which also appeared preferentially degranulated, as judged by faint insulin immunostaining (Fig. 5), featured a profile area significantly larger than that of β-cells which, in the very same islets, were poorly labeled by autoradiographic grains and showed intense insulin immunostaining. These differences were not observed in control rats infused with saline, nor when the ^{3}H-leucine perfusion was performed in the presence of 2.8 mM glucose. Hence, in vivo as well as in vitro, β-cells show a striking heterogeneity in size, and in their ability to release insulin and biosynthesize proteins. Furthermore,

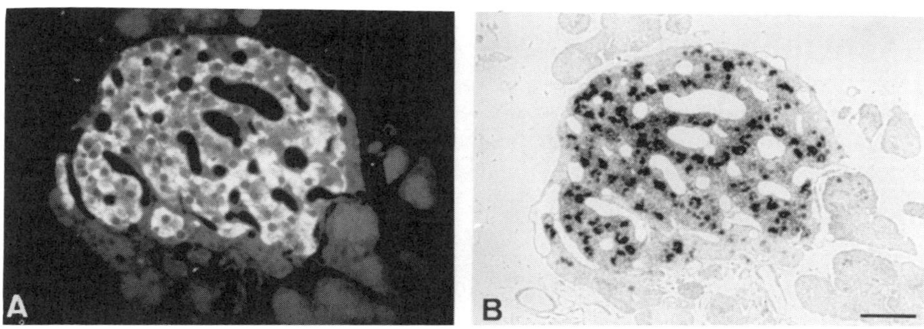

Figure 5. Heterogeneous protein biosynthesis of central and peripheral β-cells. **A:** Immunostaining of a rat islet after a 90 min in vivo stimulation by 20% glucose, revealed that the level of stored insulin was lower in the β-cells located in the center than in those located at the periphery of the microorgan, indicating that insulin had been mostly released by the former cell subpopulation; **B:** autoradiography of the very same islet, after a 10 min in situ perfusion of [^{3}H]-leucine, resulted in a higher labeling of the central, poorly granulated β-cells, indicating that these cells had also preferentially incorporated the labeled aminoacid into newly synthesized proteins.

both in vivo and in vitro, this heterogeneity is most easily revealed after glucose stimulation. The in vivo studies have also documented that the central part of the islets comprise β-cells which appear to be more sensitive and/or to function at a faster rate than the β-cells located at the islet periphery. Hence, the former cells may contribute predominantly to insulin homeostasis under most physiological conditions. The cause(s) of this regional intraislet heterogeneity remain(s) to be demonstrated. Differences in junctional coupling[9], as well as differential interactions (paracrine? hormonal? neural? ...) of central and peripheral β-cells with intraislet signaling molecules could both contribute to it.

The bar represents 40 m.

CONCLUSIONS AND PERSPECTIVES

Our work has identified multiple levels of functional heterogeneity between pancreatic β-cells, and has revealed that gap junctional communication plays a significant role in modulating this heterogeneity. Junctional communications and the secretory functioning of β-cells are tightly linked, and this link is implicated in the moment-to-moment regulation of insulin release as well as in the more long-term control of the expression of the insulin gene. Furthermore, defective coupling appears associated to loss of β-cell responsiveness to secretagogues. It is probable that junctional communication has become an obligatory feature in pancreas evolution, since it provides the most direct way to compensate intrinsic metabolic and effector differences of secretory cells. At this time, however, the molecular mechanism underlying the relationship between the control of β-cell coupling and of insulin secretion remains to be unravelled, and our understanding of whether such a relationship is causal remains, at best, quite limited. Experiments are underway to address these questions, using novel cell and molecular biology approaches which should permit to specifically interfere with the building and functioning of gap junction channels as well as with selected steps of the secretory machinery. These approaches can be combined with the testing of individual β-cells, as made possible by plaque assay, immunofluorescence and autoradiography. Future experiments will also test whether and how connexin and/or coupling defects participate in the early, and still obscure, pathogenesis of pancreatic dysfunctions in type II diabetes and in rodent models of this disease.

ACKNOWLEDGMENTS

We thank L. Burkhardt, A. Charollais, J.-P. Gerber and E. Sutter for excellent technical assistance. Supported by grants from the Swiss National Science Foundation (32-34090.92), the Juvenile Diabetes Foundation International (192467) and the Commission of the European Union (SC*1-CT92-0833).

REFERENCES

1. Orci, L., 1974, A portrait of the pancreatic B-cells. *Diabetologia* 10:163–187.
2. Mathews, E.K., and Dean, P.M., 1970, Electrical activity in islet cells, *In*: "Structure and Metabolism of Pancreatic Islets," S. Falkmer, B. Hellman and I.-B. Taljedal, eds., Cambridge University Press, Cambridge, pp. 305–313.
3. Beigelman, P., Ribalet, B., and Atwater, I., 1977, Electrical activity of mouse pancreatic beta-cells. II. Effects of glucose and arginine, *J. Physiol.* (Paris) 73:201–217.

4. Schuit, F.C., In't Veld, P.A., and Pipeleers, D.G., 1988, Glucose stimulates proinsulin biosynthesis by a dose-dependent recruitment of pancreatic beta cells, *Proc. Natl. Acad. Sci. USA* 85:3865–3869.
5. Hellman, B., and Hellerström, C., 1959, Size difference of the B-cell nuclei in the islet tissue of normal and alloxan-treated rats. *Acta Pathol. Microbiol. Scand.* 45:113–122.
6. Hellerström, C., Petersson, B., and Hellman, B., 1960, Some properties of the B-cells in the islets of Langerhans studied with regard to the position of the cells. *Acta Endocrinol.* 34:449–456.
7. Hellerström, C., Hellman, B., Brolin, S., and Larson, S., 1962, In vitro incorporation of thymidine-H3 in the pancreas of normal and obese-hyperglycemic mice. *Acta Pathol. Microbiol. Scand.* 54:1–8.
8. Meda, P., Denef, J.-F., Perrelet, A., and Orci, L., 1980, Nonrandom distribution of gap junctions between pancreatic B-cells. *Am. J. Physiol.* 238:C114–C119.
9. Michaels, R.L., and Sheridan, J.D., 1981, Dye coupling among immunocytochemically distinct cell types. *Science* 214:801–803.
10. Meda, P., Goncalves, A., Bangham, A., Orci, L., and Rojas, E., 1984, The topography of electrical synchrony among B-cells in the mouse islets of Langerhans. *Q. J. Exp. Physiol.* 69:719–735.
11. Perez-Armendariz, E., Atwater, I., and Rojas, E., 1985, Glucose-induced oscillatory changes in extracellular ionized potassium concentration in mouse islets of Langerhans. *Biophys. J.* 48:741–749.
12. Stefan, Y., Meda, P., Neufeld, M., and Orci, L., 1987, Stimulation of insulin secretion reveals heterogeneity of pancreatic B-cells in vivo. *J. Clin. Invest.* 80:175–183.
13. Salomon, D., and Meda, P., 1986, Heterogeneity and contact-dependent regulation of hormone secretion by individual B cells, *Exp. Cell Res.* 162:507–520.
14. Hiriart, M., and Matteson, D.R., 1988, Na channels and two types of Ca channels in rat pancreatic B cells identified with the reverse hemolytic plaque assay. *J. Gen. Physiol.* 91:617–639.
15. Lewis, C.E., Clark, A., Ashcroft, S.J.H., Cooper, G.J.S., and Morris, J.F., 1988, Calcitonin gene-related peptide and somatostatin inhibit insulin release from individual rat B cells. *Mol. Cell. Endocrinol.* 57:41–49.
16. Giordano, E., Bosco, D., Cirulli, V., and Meda, P., 1991, Repeated glucose stimulation reveals distinct and lasting secretion patterns of individual rat pancreatic B-cells. *J. Clin. Invest.* 87:2178–2185.
17. Soria, B., Chanson, M., Giordano, E., Bosco, D., and Meda, P., 1991, Ion channels of glucose-responsive and -unresponsive B-cells, *Diabetes* 40:1069–1078.
18. Misler, S., Falke, L.C., Gillis, K., and McDaniel, M.L., 1986, A metabolite-regulated potassium channel in rat pancreatic B-cells. *Proc. Natl. Acad. Sci. USA* 83:7119–7123.
19. Prentki, M., Glennon, M.C., Thomas, A.P., Morris, R.L, Matschinsky, F.M., and Corkey, B.E., 1988, Cell-specific pattern of oscillating free Ca^{2+} in carbamylcholine-stimulated insulinoma cells, *J. Biol. Chem.* 263: 11044–11047.
20. Longo, E.A., Tornheim, K., Oeeney, J.T., Varnum, B.A., Tillotson, D., Prentki, M., and Corkey, B.E., 1991, Oscillations in cytosolic free Ca^{2+}, oxygen consumption, and insulin secretion in glucose-stimulated rat pancreatic islets, *J. Biol. Chem.* 266:9314–9319.
21. Pipeleers, D., and Van de Winkel, M., 1989, Cellular endogenous fluorescence: a basis for preparing populations of functionally homogeneous cells, in: "Cell Structure and Function by Microspectrofluorometry," E. Kohen and J.G. Hirschberg, eds., Academic, San Diego, CA, pp. 391–404.
22. Kiekens, R., In't Veld, P., Mahler, T., Schuit, F., Van De Winkel, M., and Pipeleers, D., 1992, Differences in glucose recognition by individual rat pancreatic B cells are associated with intercellular differences in glucose-induced biosynthetic activity, *J. Clin. Invest.* 89:117–125.
23. Van Schravendijik, C.F.H., Kiekens, R., and Pipeleers, D.G., 1992, Pancreatic cell heterogeneity in glucose-induced insulin secretion, *J. Biol. Chem.* 267:21344–21348.
24. Lernmark, A., 1974, The preparation of, and studies on, free cell suspensions from mouse pancreatic islets, *Diabetologia* 10:431–438.
25. Pipeleers, D., Hooghe-Peters, E., Maes, E., Schuit, F., Van De Winkel, M., and Van Schravendijk, C., 1982a, Reconstructing the pancreatic islet and its glucose-induced insulin release, *Diabetologia* 23:191 (abstract).
26. Pipeleers, D., In't Veld, P., Maes, E., and Van de Winkel, M., 1982b, Glucose-induced insulin release depends on functional cooperation between islet cells, *Proc. Natl. Acad. Sci. USA* 79:7322–7325.
27. Halban, P.A., Wollheim, C.B., Blondel, B., Meda, P., Niersor, E.N., and Mintz, D.H., 1982, The possible importance of contact between pancreatic islet cells for the control of insulin release. *Endocrinology* 111:86–94.
28. Chertow, B.S., Baranetsky, N.G., Sivitz, W.I., Meda, P., Webb, M.D., and Shih, J.C., 1983, Cellular mechanisms of insulin release: effects of retinoids on rat islet cell-to-cell adhesion, reaggregation, and insulin release, *Diabetes* 32:568–574.
29. Bosco, D., Orci, L., and Meda, P., 1989, Homologous but not heterologous contact increases the functioning of individual secretory cells, *Exp. Cell Res.* 184:72–80.
30. Bosco, D., Meda, P., Thorens, B., and Malaisse, W.J., 1995, Heterogenous secretion of individual B-cells in response to D-glucose and to non-glucidic nutrient secretagogues, *Am. J. Physiol.* 268:C611–C618.

31. Bosco, D., and Meda, P., 1991, Actively synthetizing B-cells secrete preferentially during glucose stimulation, *Endocrinology* 129:3157–3166.
32. Giordano, E., Cirulli, V., Bosco, D., Rouiller, D., Halban, P., and Meda, P., 1993, B-cell size influences glucose-stimulated insulin secretion, *Am. J. Physiol.* 265:C358–C364.
33. Philippe, J., Giordano, E., Gjinovci, A., and Meda, P., 1992, cAMP prevents the glucocorticoid-mediated inhibition of insulin gene expression in rodent islet cells, *J. Clin. Invest.* 90:2228–2233.
34. Meda, P., Chanson, M., Pepper, M., Giordano, E., Bosco, D., Traub, O., Willecke, K., El Aoumari, A., Gros, D., Beyer, E., Orci, L., and Spray, D.C., 1991, In vivo modulation of connexin 43 gene expression and junctional coupling of pancreatic B-cells, *Exp. Cell Res.* 192:469–480.
35. Meda, P., Perrelet, A., and Orci, L., 1979, Increase of gap junctions between pancreatic B-cells during stimulation of insulin secretion, *J. Cell Biol.* 82:441–448.
36. Kohen, E., Kohen, C., Thorell, B., 1979, Mintz, D.H., and Rabinovitch, A., 1979, Intercellular communication in pancreatic islet monolayer cultures: a microfluorometric study, *Science* 204:862–865.
37. Meda, P., Amherdt, M., Perrelet, A., and Orci, L, 1981, Metabolic coupling between cultured pancreatic B-cells, *Exp. Cell Res.* 133:421–430.
38. Meda, P., Michaels, R.L., Halban, P.A., Orci, L., and Sheridan, J.D., 1983, In vivo modulation of gap junctions and dye coupling between B-cells of the intact pancreatic islet, *Diabetes* 32:858–868.
39. Eddlestone, G.T., Gonçalves, A., Bangham, J.A., and Rojas, E., 1984, Electrical coupling between cells in islets of Langerhans from mouse, *J. Membr. Biol.* 77:1–14.
40. Meda, P., Bosco, D., Chanson, M., Giordano, E., Vallar, L., Wollheim, C., and Orci, L., 1990, Rapid and reversible secretion changes during uncoupling of rat insulin-producing cells. *J. Clin. Invest.* 86:759–768.
41. Kohen, E., Kohen, C., and Rabinovitch, A., 1983, Cell-to-cell communication in rat pancreatic islet monolayer cultures is modulated by agents affecting islet cell secretory activity, *Diabetes* 32:95–98.
42. Appel, M.C., O'Neill, J.J., and Meda, P., 1988, Effects of glucose on islet gap junctional communication, *Diabetes* 37, suppl 1, 47A (abstract).
43. Bruzzone, R., and Meda, P., 1988, The gap junction: a channel for multiple functions? *Eur. J. Clin. Invest.* 18:444–453.
44. Ullrich, S., Vozzi, C., and Meda, P., 1993, Connexins of insulin-secreting cells: Quantification of mRNA by polymerase chain reaction, *Diabetologia* 36 (Suppl 1): A5 (abstract).
45. Vozzi, C., Ullrich, S., Bosco, D., Dupont, E., and Meda, P., 1994, Glucose-unresponsive insulin-producing cells show defects in gap junction coupling and improved secretion after Cx43 transfection. *Acta Anat.* 149:162 (abstract).
46. Loewenstein, W.R., 1981, Junctional intercellular communication. The cell-to-cell membrane channel, *Physiol. Rev.* 61:829–913.
47. Sorenson, R.L., and Parsons, J.A., 1985, Insulin secretion in mammosomatotropic tumor-bearing and pregnant rats. A role for lactogens, *Diabetes* 34:338–341.
48. Gylfe, E., Grapengiesser, E., and Hellman, B., 1991, Propagation of cytoplasmic Ca^{2+} oscillations in clusters of pancreatic β-cells exposed to glucose, *Cell Calcium* 12:229–240.
49. Santos, R.M., Rosario, L.M., Nadal, A., Garcia-Sancho, J., Soria, B., and Valdeomillos, M., 1991, Widespread synchronous $[Ca^{2+}]_i$ oscillations due to bursting electrical activity in single pancreatic islets, *Pfluegers Arch.* 418:417–422.
50. Atwater, I., Rosario, L., and Rojas, E., 1983, Properties of the Ca^{2+}-activated K^+ channel in pancreatic B-cells, *Cell Calcium* 4:451–461.
51. Lawrence, T.S., Beers, W.H., and Gilula, N.B., 1978, Transmission of hormonal stimulation by cell-to-cell communication, *Nature* 272:501–506.

Part VI. IDDM (INSULIN DEPENDENT DIABETES MELLITUS): WHAT WENT WRONG? MECHANISMS OF β-CELL DESTRUCTION AND DEFENSE

40

NEW ASPECTS TO THE FUNCTIONING AND REGENERATION OF PANCREATIC β-CELLS

Cyclic ADP-Ribose and *Reg* Gene

Hiroshi Okamoto

Department of Biochemistry
Tohoku University School of Medicine
Sendai 980-77, Japan

INTRODUCTION

In this paper, some of our recent experiments concerning a novel second messenger in β-cells, cyclic ADP-ribose (cADPR), and *Reg* gene which is involved in β-cell regeneration will be discussed.

By way of introduction, a brief description should be given of the historical background of this work and, especially, the mechanism of action of diabetogenic agents on pancreatic β-cells. We have proposed a unifying model for the action of alloxan and streptozotocin on pancreatic β-cells (Okamoto, 1981; Okamoto, 1985; Okamoto, 1990). As shown in Figure 1, central to the model are breaks in the nuclear DNA of β-cells, resulting from either an accumulation of oxygen radicals or from alkylation of DNA. These breaks induce DNA repair involving the activation of poly (ADP-ribose) synthetase, which uses cellular NAD^+ as a substrate. As a result, intracellular levels of NAD^+ fall dramatically. The fall in cellular NAD^+ inhibits cellular activities including insulin secretion and synthesis, and thus the β-cell ultimately dies (Yamamoto et al., 1981; Uchigata et al., 1982). If alloxan- and streptozotocin-induced β-cell damage is provoked by the mechanism shown in Figure 1, then, theoretically, it can be prevented by the inhibition of serial reactions originating from the DNA strand breaks. One possibility would be by scavenging the radicals with such radical scavengers as superoxide dismutase and desferrioxamine. Another would be by inhibiting the poly (ADP-ribose) synthetase with specific inhibitors such as nicotinamide and 3-aminobenzamide (Yamamoto et al., 1981; Uchigata et al., 1982).

The destruction of β-cells may be mediated by infiltrating lymphocytes. The ability of T-cells to adoptively transfer diabetes in diabetes-prone BB rats and in the NOD mouse indicates that T-cells participate in β-cell destruction (Like et al., 1985; Wicker et

Physiology and Pathophysiology of the Islets of Langerhans, edited by Soria.
Plenum Press, New York, 1997.

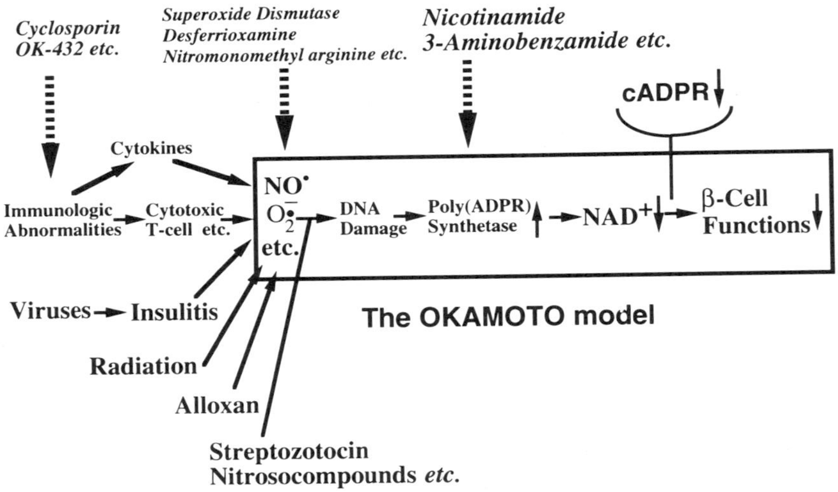

Figure 1. The OKAMOTO model for β-cell damage and its prevention in toxin- or virus-induced and immune diabetes.

al., 1986). Cytokines, released by infiltrating lymphocytes, have also been implicated as possible mediators of β-cell destruction. Treatment of isolated islets with interleukin-1β (IL-1β) resulted in a concentration- and time-dependent inhibition of glucose-stimulated insulin secretion that was followed by islet destruction after prolonged exposures of this cytokine (Bendtzen et al., 1986; Comens et al., 1987). The mechanisms of cytokine action on β-cells are unknown; however, the free-radical nitric oxide, resulting from cytokine-induced expression of nitric oxide synthase, has been implicated as the cellular effector molecule that mediates the inhibitory and cytotoxic effects of IL-1β on islets (Corbett and McDaniel, 1992). Nitric oxide, induced by IL-1β, causes DNA damage (Delaney et al., 1993), poly (ADP-ribose) synthetase activation, and NAD^+ depletion (Kallmann et al., 1992; Radons et al., 1994).

Thus, as shown in Figure 1, interest in the model for the mechanism of action of alloxan and streptozotocin has been heightened by its possible extension to the effects of viruses and inflammation, especially immune-mediated variants. It is thus reasonable to assume that, although insulin-dependent diabetes can be caused by many different agents such as immunologic abnormalities, inflammatory tissue damage, and β-cytotoxic chemical substances such as alloxan and streptozotocin, the final pathway for the toxic agents is the same. This pathway involves DNA damage, poly (ADP-ribose) synthetase activation, and NAD^+ depletion. The fall in cellular NAD^+ inhibits cellular activities. Therefore, insulin-dependent (Type I) diabetes is theoretically preventable by suppressing immune reactions, by scavenging free radicals, and by inhibiting the poly (ADP-ribose) synthetase activity (Okamoto, 1990). In fact, it has been reported that diabetes in the NOD mouse can be prevented by treatment with immunesuppressive agents (Mori et al., 1986), an immunomodulator (OK-432) (Okamoto, Sr., 1976; Toyota et al., 1986), radical scavengers (Nomikos et al., 1986), and poly (ADP-ribose) synthetase inhibitors (Yamada et al., 1982; Nomikos et al., 1986). Furthermore, Vague et al. reported that nicotinamide can extend the remission phase in human insulin dependent (Type I) diabetes (Vague et al., 1987).

A NOVEL SECOND MESSENGER IN β-CELLS, CYCLIC ADP-RIBOSE

As described above, maintenance of the cellular NAD^+ level is thought to be essential for the secretion and synthesis of insulin by β-cells. The question now arises as to why the maintenance of the NAD^+ level is necessary for these functions.

More recently, we found that a novel metabolite of NAD^+, cADPR, is a novel second messenger for intracellular Ca^{2+} mobilization in glucose-stimulated islets (Okamoto et al., 1992; Takasawa et al., 1993a). cADPR is a cyclic compound that is synthesized from NAD^+ by ADP-ribosyl cyclase (Clapper et al., 1987; Lee et al., 1989). We used rat islet microsomes as a cell-free system to study Ca^{2+} release and found that cADPR induced Ca^{2+} release from islet microsomes but IP_3 did not. The release of Ca^{2+} after additions of cADPR showed a steep dose-response relation with a clear effect at a concentration of 0.09 μM and a near maximum release at 0.5 μM. We then examined the effect of cADPR on insulin secretion using digitonin-permeabilized islets. As shown in Figure 2, both

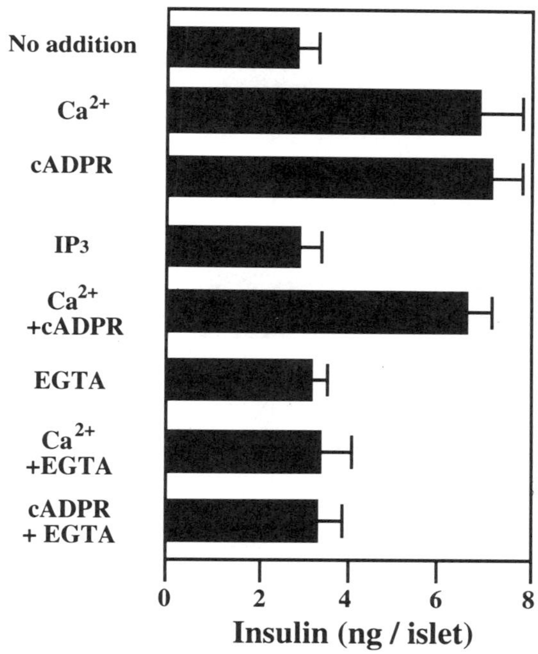

Figure 2. Effect of cADPR on insulin secretion from digitonin-permeabilized islets. Permeabilized islets were treated with cADPR (1 μM), IP_3 (1μM), Ca^{2+} (0.2 μM), and cADPR (1 μM) in the presence of Ca^{2+} (0.2 μM), and with cADPR (1 μM) in the presence of EGTA (10 mM). Values represent mean ± SEM of n = 5–14 measurements. Results of two-tailed Student's *t* test comparing the response to each addition versus the control (no addition) are shown. **Methods.** Freshly isolated islets were incubated in a modified Hepes-Krebs buffer (25 mM Hepes, 115 mM NaCl, 24 mM $NaHCO_3$, 5 mM KCl, 1 mM $MgCl_2$, 1 mM EGTA, 0.1% bovine serum albumin, pH 6.8) at 37°C with digitonin (20 μg/ml) for 20 min. Thirty islets were randomly selected, washed three times in Tris buffer (50 mM Tris, 100 mM KCl, 5 mM $MgCl_2$, 0.1% bovine serum albumin, pH 6.8), and incubated at 24°C for 15 min in 100 μl of Tris-Pipes buffer (55 mM Tris, 11 mM KCl, 5 mM $MgCl_2$, 1.1 mM EGTA, 1 mM ATP, 10 mM phosphocreatine, creatine kinase (10 units/ml), 0.1% bovine serum albumin, pH 7.5). Islets were treated with O_2:CO_2 (19:1). At the end of the incubation period, the medium was withdrawn and a radioimmunoassay kit (Novo Nordisk Biolabs, Baysvaerd, Denmark) was used to quantify the released insulin with rat insulin as the standard.

cADPR and Ca^{2+} induced insulin secretion, but IP_3 did not. The combined addition of cADPR and Ca^{2+} did not induce significantly more insulin secretion than the addition of cADPR or Ca^{2+} alone. The cADPR-induced insulin secretion was inhibited by the addition of EGTA. The dose-response curve between cADPR and insulin secretion from permeabilized islets was well fitted to that of Ca^{2+} release from islet microsomes. These results suggest that the cADPR-induced insulin secretion was mediated by Ca^{2+} mobilization from islet microsomes (Takasawa et al., 1993a).

When the extract from islets incubated with 2.8 mM or 20 mM glucose was added to a cell-free system of islet microsomes, a prominent Ca^{2+} release was found with the extract from islets treated with 20 mM glucose, but not with extracts from islets treated with 2.8 mM glucose. cADPR and 20 mM glucose-treated islet extract showed cross-desensitization in Ca^{2+} release from islet microsomes, suggesting that the active component generated in the 20 mM glucose-treated islet extract is cADPR (Takasawa et al., 1993a). In fact, we incu-

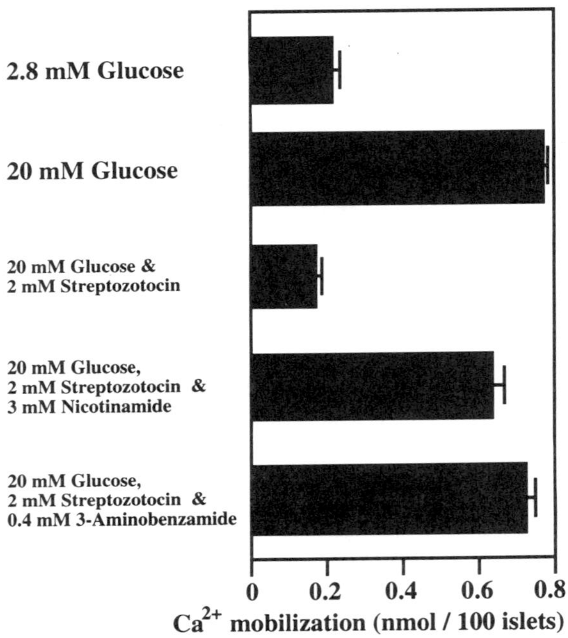

Figure 3. Effects of streptozotocin, nicotinamide, and 3-aminobenzamide on the Ca^{2+} mobilizing activity in islet extracts. Values are mean ± SEM. **Methods.** Five hundred islets were incubated at 37°C for 15 min in 100 µl of Krebs-Ringer's bicarbonate medium containing 2.8 mM glucose in the presence or absence of a poly (ADP-ribose) synthetase inhibitor (3 mM nicotinamide or 0.4 mM 3-aminobenzamide), then incubated for 20 min with or without the addition of 2 mM streptozotocin. After preincubation, islets were further incubated for 40 min with an additional 100 µl of medium containing 37.2 mM glucose. The final concentration of glucose was 20 mM. The islets were washed three times with cold acetate intracellular medium (AcIM) composed of 250 mM potassium acetate, 250 mM *N*-methyl-glucamine, 1 mM $MgCl_2$, and 20 mM Hepes (pH 7.2) supplemented with 0.5 mM ATP, 4 mM phosphocreatine, creatine phosphokinase (2 units/ml), 2.5 mM benzamidine, and 0.5 mM phenylmethylsulfonyl fluoride, and homogenized in 50 µl of AcIM. The homogenates were centrifuged at 4,100 *g* for 15 min, and the supernatant was used as islet extract. Calcium mobilization from microsomes was monitored in 3 ml of intracellular medium (GluIM) composed of 250 mM potassium gluconate, 250 mM *N*-methyl-glucamine, 1 mM $MgCl_2$, 20 mM Hepes (pH 7.2) containing 1 mM ATP, 4 mM phosphocreatine, creatine kinase (2 units/ml), 2.5 mM benzamidine, 0.5 mM phenylmethylsulfonyl fluoride, and 3 µM fluo 3, with the addition of 150 µl of microsome fraction. Fluorescence was measured at 490 nm excitation and 535 nm emission at 37°C with a circulating water bath. No changes in fluorescence were observed when islet extracts were added to the GluIM-fluo 3 system without microsomes.

bated islets with 20 mM glucose for 3 to 40 min, prepared the islet extract and measured its Ca^{2+} mobilizing activity, and found that the Ca^{2+} mobilizing activity in 20 mM glucose-treated islets attained a near maximal level by 3 min. As described in INTRODUCTION, β-cytotoxic agents deplete intracellular NAD^+ and inhibit cellular functions such as insulin secretion, and poly (ADP-ribose) synthetase inhibitors prevent the NAD^+ depletion and the β-cytotoxin-induced reduction of cellular functions (Okamoto, 1990). We incubated rat pancreatic islets with streptozotocin, prepared the islet extract, and measured its Ca^{2+} mobilizing activity (Figure 3). Streptozotocin greatly reduced the Ca^{2+} mobilizing activity in the islet extract, and nicotinamide and 3-aminobenzamide reversed this reduction. These results also indicate that cADPR acts a second messenger in glucose-stimulated islets for insulin secretion, as cADPR is synthesized from NAD^+ (Takasawa et al., 1993a).

From these results, the model presented as Figure 1 can be now understood more clearly; β-cytotoxins such as streptozotocin and alloxan cause DNA strand breaks which activate nuclear poly (ADP-ribose) synthetase, forming poly (ADP-ribose) and leading to NAD^+ depletion (Yamamoto et al., 1981; Uchigata et al., 1982; Okamoto, 1985; Okamoto, 1990). The NAD^+ depletion results in the inhibition of the cADPR-mediated Ca^{2+} mobilization. Poly (ADP-ribose) synthetase inhibitors such as nicotinamide and 3-aminobenzamide prevent the NAD^+ depletion and therefore the glucose-induced insulin secreting machinery continues to function (Takasawa et al., 1993b).

ADP-RIBOSYL CYCLASE / cADPR HYDROLASE

cADPR is synthesized from NAD^+ by ADP-ribosyl cyclase. We purified ADP-ribosyl cyclase from the soluble fraction of *Aplysia kurodai* ovotestes by sequential column chromatography. The enzyme has an apparent molecular mass of 30 kilo-dalton. The *Aplysia* enzyme catalyzes the formation of cADPR from NAD^+ (Okamoto et al., 1992, 1993; Takasawa et al., 1993a). We isolated a cDNA of the *Aplysia* ADP-ribosyl cyclase from an *Aplysia* ovotestes cDNA library, and determined the primary structure of the enzyme (Okamoto et al., 1993). The amino acid sequence of *Aplysia* cyclase shows a significant homology (31% identity) with that of a human lymphocyte surface antigen, CD38. Especially, the ten cysteine residues in both proteins are conserved, suggesting that *Aplysia* cyclase and human lymphocyte antigen CD38 may have some similar overall conformation (States et al., 1992: Okamoto et al., 1993; Koguma et al., 1994).

Then, we isolated a CD38 cDNA from a human insulinoma and constructed an expression vector under the control of an SV40 promoter. The expression vector was introduced into COS-7 cells. CD38 was mainly expressed in the plasma membrane fraction of the transfected COS-7 cells. We incubated ^{32}P-NAD^+ with the plasma membrane fraction for 20 min and analyzed the reaction product by HPLC. Some amount of cADPR was formed during the first 10 min, and, thereafter, the cADPR level decreased. In the overall reaction, a decrease in NAD^+ and the concomitant stoichiometric formation of ADP-ribose were observed. These results suggest that CD38 has both ADP-ribosyl cyclase activity and cyclic ADP-ribose hydrolase activity to produce ADP-ribose. To confirm this, we prepared ^{32}P-labeled cADPR and incubated it with the membrane fraction. cADPR was stoichiometrically converted to ADP-ribose. Both the ADP-ribosyl cyclase and the cADPR hydrolase activities were inhibited by the addition of an anti-CD38 antibody. These results indicate that CD38 has both the cyclase and the hydrolase activities (Takasawa et al., 1993b, 1993c).

We then examined the effect of ATP on cADPR hydrolysis using cADPR as a substrate. As shown in Figure 4, ATP inhibited the cADPR hydrolysis. Next, we examined the

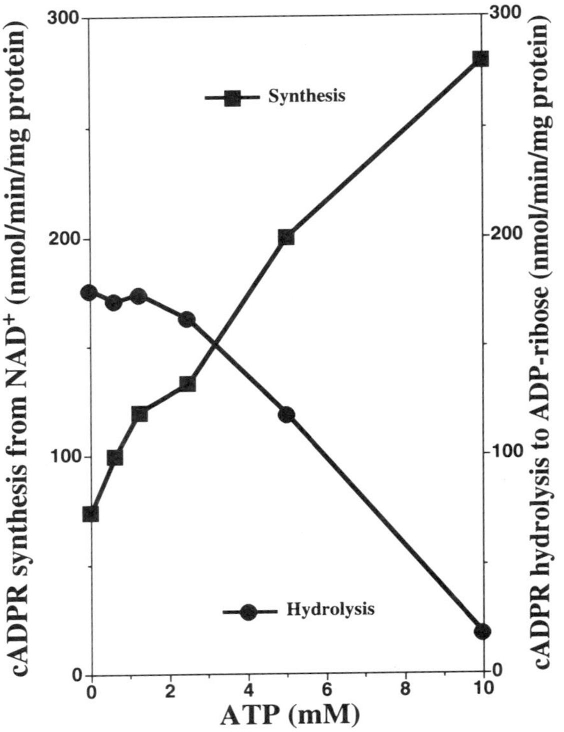

Figure 4. Effects of ATP on synthesis and hydrolysis of cADPR. cADPR synthesis from NAD^+ (■) and cADPR hydrolysis to ADPR (●) by the plasma membrane fraction of COS-7 cells into which the CD38 expression vector had been introduced. ATP was added to the assay for cADPR synthesis or hydrolysis. **Methods.** The plasma membrane fraction (10 μg protein) into which the CD38 expression vector or control vector (pSV2 vector) had been introduced was incubated at 37°C in 0.1 ml of phosphate buffered saline (137 mM NaCl, 2.7 mMKCl, 8.1 mM Na_2HPO_4, 1.5 mM KH_2PO_4, pH 7.4) with 0.2 mM NAD^+ containing 5 μCi of [^{32}P] NAD^+ (NEN) or 0.2 mM cADPR containing 5 mCi of [^{32}P] cADPR, prepared enzymatically from [^{32}P] NAD^+ with *Aplysia kurodai* ADP-ribosyl cyclase (Takasawa et al., 1993a). Reaction products were analyzed by HPLC (Okamoto et al., 1992, 1993; Takasawa et al., 1993a).

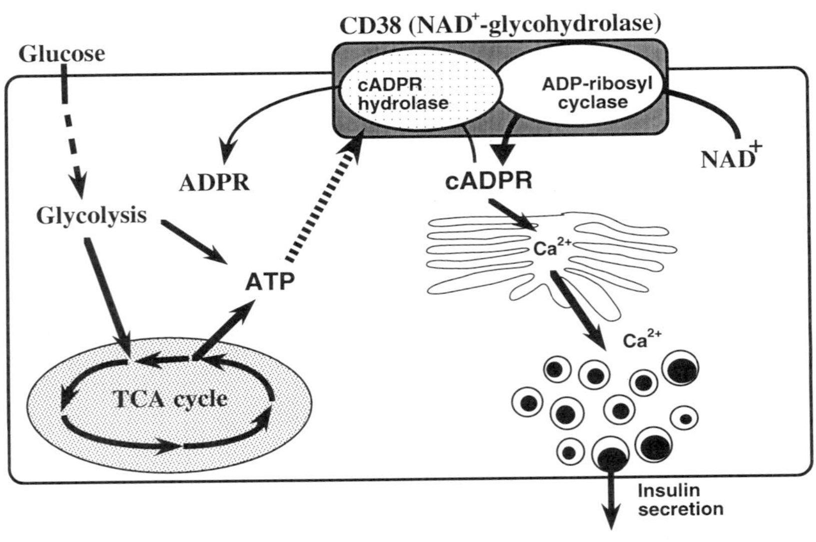

Figure 5. Diagram showing the role of CD38 in the regulation of the cADPR concentration in glucose-stimulated pancreatic β-cells. Glucose is metabolized to form ATP (Ashcroft et al., 1973; Matschinsky et al., 1976; Sener et al., 1978; Kawazu et al., 1980). ATP inhibits the hydrolysis of cADPR, which is synthesized from NAD^+ by the cyclase, and then the concentration of cADPR is elevated. cADPR mobilizes Ca^{2+} from the β-cell endoplasmic reticulum resulting in insulin secretion.

effect of ATP on the formation of cADPR using NAD^+ as a substrate. As shown in Figure 4, ATP stimulated the cADPR formation at concentrations of 2–10 mM. Based on these results, we concluded that CD38 has both cyclase and hydrolase activities, and that ATP can stimulate the formation of cADPR by inhibiting the hydrolase activity. And in the overall reaction, CD38 can exhibit the NADase activity (Takasawa et al., 1993c).

As described above, cADPR is a mediator of Ca^{2+} release from islet microsomes and is generated in islets by glucose stimulation, serving as a second messenger for Ca^{2+} mobilization for insulin secretion (Okamoto et al., 1992; Takasawa et al., 1993a). Thus, Figure 5 is our model for the induction of cADPR by glucose in the process of insulin secretion. Glucose stimuli induce the cADPR formation from NAD^+ by inhibiting the cADPR hydrolase activity of CD38 by ATP, which is generated in the process of glucose metabolism in β-cells.

β-CELL REGENERATION AND *Reg* GENE

From a practical point of view, strategies for influencing the replication of islet β-cells and the growth of the β-cell mass in order to ameliorate not only Type I diabetes but also Type II diabetes may be more important. We will now proceed to our experiments concerning β-cell regeneration and *Reg* gene. In 1984, we demonstrated that poly (ADP-ribose) synthetase inhibitors induce the regeneration of pancreatic β-cells, thereby ameliorating surgical diabetes (Yonemura et al., 1984). Male Wistar rats were 90% depancreatized. Also, beginning seven days before the partial pancreatectomy and continuing postoperatively, nicotinamide (0.5 g/kg body weight) or 3-aminobenzamide (0.05 g/kg body weight) was injected intraperitoneally every day. In 90% depancreatized rats, active DNA replication was observed in the islet β-cells of the remaining pancreas for 15 days. The regenerative process in the β-cells, however, could not continue further and the β-cells degenerated. In rats that were 90% depancreatized and treated with a poly (ADP-ribose) synthetase inhibitor, the replicative DNA synthesis increased and the β-cells continued to regenerate (Yonemura et al., 1988). The islets in the remaining pancreases of rats which had received the poly (ADP-ribose) synthetase inhibitors for 3 months were extremely large, and almost the entire area of the enlarged islet was densely stained for insulin. These results indicate that poly (ADP-ribose) synthetase inhibitors induced pancreatic β-cell regeneration, thereby ameliorating diabetes caused by partial pancreatectomy.

We isolated regenerating islets and constructed a cDNA library. In screening the regenerating islet-derived cDNA library, we came across a novel gene expressed in regenerating islets. The cDNA had one large open reading frame which encoded a 165-amino acid protein. The deduced protein has a putative signal sequence of 21 amino acids. We named the novel gene *Reg*, i.e., regenerating gene, with the implication that the gene may be involved in islet regeneration (Terazono et al., 1988).

We have constructed an expression vector in which a cDNA sequence encoded rat Reg protein was placed under the control of the PHO 5 promoter. The construct was transfected into a yeast recipient, *Saccharomyces cerevisiae* strain AH22. The yeast recipient produced a rat Reg protein of 16,000 daltons without the signal sequence and the protein was secreted into the culture medium. We purified the 16,000-dalton protein and prepared an antibody against it (Itoh et al., 1990; Terazono et al., 1990). We examined the localization of the Reg protein in normal and regenerating rat islets using immunocytochemical techniques. A normal islet was densely stained with insulin. However, in a thin serial section, the normal islet was not stained with the Reg protein. Two weeks–3 months after the

90% pancreatectomy and nicotinamide treatment, a regenerating islets was stained with Reg protein. The immunostaining for the Reg protein exhibited a distribution pattern almost identical to that of insulin-positive cells in a thin serial section of the regenerating islet. One year after the 90% pancreatectomy and nicotinamide treatment, the islet was scarcely stained with Reg protein, but islet cells showed an immunoreactivity for insulin comparable to that of normal islet cells. These results suggest that Reg protein is synthesized in regenerating β-cells, and that the expression of *Reg* is closely associated with β-cell regeneration (Terazono et al., 1990).

More recently, we examined the effect of recombinant rat Reg protein on pancreatic β-cell replication using both 90% depancreatized rats and isolated islets (Watanabe et al., 1994). We examined the effect of Reg protein on ^{3}H-thymidine incorporation into β-cells using isolated rat islets. As shown in Figure 6, Reg protein stimulated ^{3}H-thymidine incorporation in a dose dependent manner; there was a 2.8-fold increase in the presence of 180 nM Reg protein. Almost all the autoradiographically labeled cells were insulin positive and the grains were localized in the nuclei of β-cells. There was a 2.4-fold increase in the

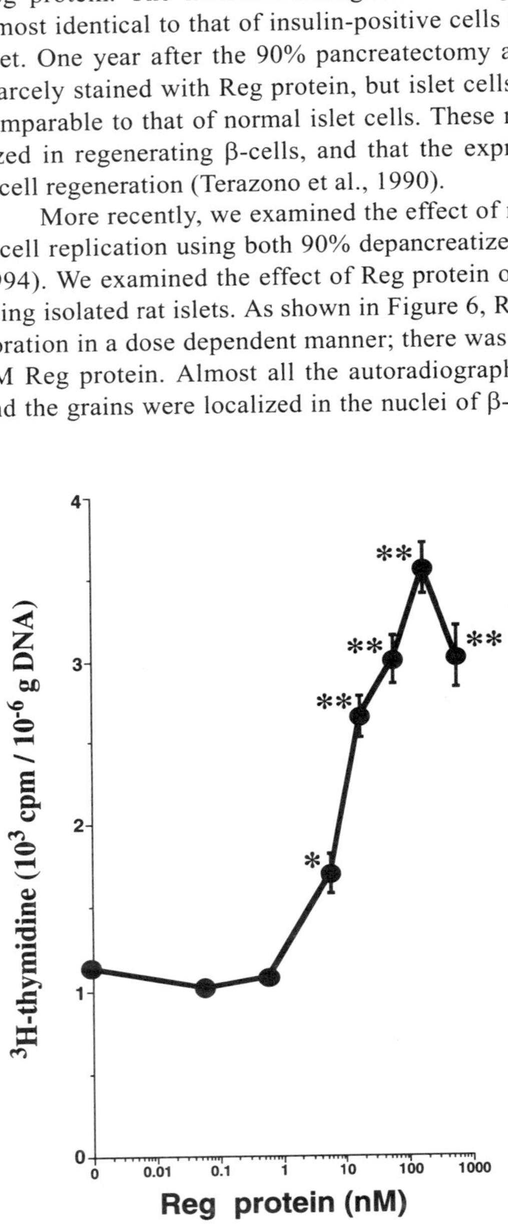

Figure 6. Reg protein stimulates ^{3}H-thymidine incorporation into islet DNA. Recombinant rat Reg protein was dissolved in 50 mM acetic acid as solvent and the final concentration of the acetic acid in the culture was 0.55 mM. Acetic acid alone at the same final concentration did not affect ^{3}H-thymidine incorporation. Data are expressed as radioactivity of ^{3}H-thymidine incorporation / μg of islet DNA. Values represent mean ± SEM of n = 4. Asterisks indicate difference from control without Reg protein (*$P < 0.05$, **$P < 0.001$ in ANOVA). **Methods.** Pancreatic islets were isolated from male Wistar rats (body weight 200–250 g) using density separation on a dextran gradient and cultured free floating in RPMI 1640 supplemented with 10% fetal calf serum, 100 μg/ml penicillin G and 100 μg/ml streptomycin for 48 hours to allow recovery from the isolation procedure. After this initial period, islets were transferred to 24-well culture dishes in groups of 50 islets. The islets were cultured in RPMI 1640 medium containing 2.7 mM D-glucose supplemented with 2% fetal calf serum, 100 μg/ml penicillin G and 100 μg/ml streptomycin in the presence of increasing concentrations of Reg protein for 72 hours. During the last 24 hours, the islets were cultured in the above medium to which 10 μCi/ml of [*methyl*-^{3}H] thymidine (Amersham) had been added. To estimate the amount of ^{3}H-thymidine incorporated into newly synthesized DNA, the islets were washed after the culture period, and sonicated in 10 mM Tris-HCl and 5 mM EDTA. DNA was precipitated by the addition of 7% ice cold trichloroacetic acid and trapped by filtration on a glass fiber disc (Whatman GF/C). The discs were dried and radioactivity was counted after the addition of scintillation fluid (Packard Ultima Gold F). The DNA content of the islets was measured by a flurometric DNA assay using Hoechst 33258. To estimate labeling indices for insulin positive cells, the ^{3}H-thymidine-labeled islets were fixed in 4% paraformaldehyde for 20 min and embedded in OCT compound. 10 μm sections were cut with a cryostat and immunostained with anti-porcine insulin guinea pig antiserum (DAKO, 1:500) and Vectastain ABC-GO kit (Vector, Burlingame, CA). Autoradiography of the immunostained sections was performed using Konica NR-M2 emulsion.

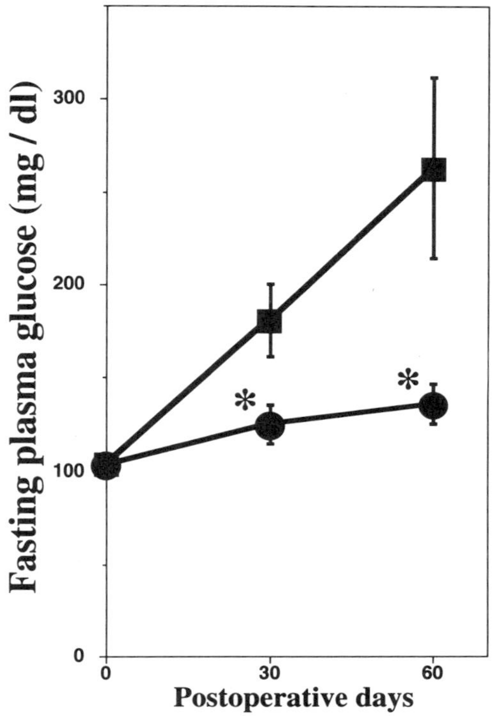

Figure 7. The 90% depancreatized rats that received daily intraperitoneal injections of 1 mg/kg body weight recombinant Reg protein showed an amelioration of the diabetes. Values represent mean ± SEM of samples from control rats (n=17) (B); and samples from Reg protein-treated rats (n=20) (J). Results of Student's *t* test comparing values of Reg protein-treated rats as compared to the control rats. $^*P < 0.05$ versus control rats. **Methods.** Thirty-seven male Wistar rats (200–220 g of weight) were 90% depancreatized (Yonemura et al., 1984, 1988; Terazono et al., 1988) and maintained on standard rat chow. Recombinant rat Reg protein, produced in *Saccharomyces cerevisiae*, purified (Itoh et al., 1990) and dissolved at a concentration of 1 mg/ ml in 50 mM acetic acid, was injected intraperitoneally at a dose of 1 mg/kg body weight into twenty rats every day. Seventeen control rats were injected intraperitoneally with 50 mM of acetic acid without Reg protein after the 90% pancreatectomy. In both groups the injections were continued until the 60th postoper ative day. Rats were fasted overnight before blood sampling and the plasma glucose level was measured by the glucose-oxidase method using Glucose Auto & Stat GA-1110 (Kyoto Daiichi Instrument Inc., Kyoto, Japan). The statistical significance of differences between rats injected with Reg protein (n=20) and those injected with acetic acid (n=17) was analyzed using Student's *t* test.

labeling index of β-cells (0.19 ± 0.02 vs. 0.08 ± 0.02, $p < 0.05$) when islets were incubated with 60 nM Reg protein. These results clearly indicate that Reg protein itself stimulates β-cell replication in the pancreatic islets of *Langerhans*.

We next injected 90% depancreatized rats intraperitoneally with recombinant rat Reg protein (1 mg/kg/day). On the 30th and 60th postoperative day, the fasting plasma glucose level of the rats receiving Reg protein was significantly lower than those of 90% depancreatized control rats (Figure 7), and the rats treated with Reg protein also showed increased body weight. These results indicate that the administration of Reg protein ameliorates surgically induced diabetes. We examined morphologically the remaining pancreas which had been stained for insulin. Normal islets of untreated, non-depancreatized rats are oval in shape and the diameters range from 100 μm to 200 μm. After 2 months, almost all the islets of 90% depancreatized control rats were destroyed, and the insulin positive cells were markedly decreased in number; fibrotic degeneration and degranulation were frequently encountered. In contrast, the islets of the remaining pancreas in Reg protein-treated rats were enlarged and the enlarged islets were densely and almost entirely stained for insulin. These results indicate that Reg protein stimulates the regeneration and/or growth of pancreatic β-cells, thereby ameliorating the diabetes (Watanabe et al., 1994).

The present study demonstrated that Reg protein can ameliorate diabetes in partially depancreatized rats. Morphologic and immunocytochemical examination of the remaining pancreas of Reg protein-treated rats showed a marked increase in the β-cell population. Therefore, it is reasonable to assume that Reg protein induces pancreatic β-cell regeneration, thereby improving diabetes caused by partial pancreatectomy. The present study also demonstrated that Reg protein directly stimulated islet β-cell replication *in vitro*. These results strongly suggest that Reg protein is a growth factor for pancreatic β-cells. This concept is reconcilable with the previous observations that the *Reg* gene was expressed in rat regenerating islets and in mouse hyperplastic islets (Terazono et al., 1988; Unno et al., 1993).

A low capacity for β-cell regeneration has been suggested as a predisposing factor for the development of human diabetes. We have already isolated human *REG* cDNA and gene (Terazono et al., 1988; Watanabe et al., 1990; Moriizumi et al., 1994), expressed the cDNA in yeast, and purified the human protein (Itoh et al., 1990). It is therefore possible that this protein could be used as a new treatment for human diabetes to stimulate the regeneration of pancreatic β cells.

REFERENCES

Ashcroft, S. J. H., Weerasinghe, L. C. C. and Randle, P. J., 1973, Interrelationship of islet metabolism, adenosine triphosphate content and insulin release, *Biochem. J.* 132: 223–231.

Bendtzen, K., Mandrup-Poulsen, T., Nerup, J., Nielsen, J. H., Dinarello, C. A. and Svenson, M., 1986, Cytotoxicity of human pI 7 interleukin-1 for pancreatic islets of Langerhans, *Science* 232: 1545–1547.

Clapper, D. L., Walseth, T. F., dargie, P. J. and Lee, H. C., 1987, Pyridine nucleotide metabolites stimulate calcium release from sea urchin egg microsomes desensitized to inositol trisphosphate, *J. Biol. Chem.* 262: 9561–9568.

Comens, P. G., Wolf, B. A., Unanue, E. R., Lacy, P. E. and McDaniel, M. L., 1987, Interleukin 1 is potent modulator of insulin secretion from isolated rat islets of Langerhans, *Diabetes* 36: 963–970.

Corbett, J. A. and McDaniel, M. L., 1992, Dose nitric oxide mediate autoimmune destruction of β-cells? — possible therapeutic interventions in IDDM, *Diabetes* 41: 897–903.

Delaney, C. A., Green, M. H., Lowe, J. E. and Green, I. C., 1993, Endogenous nitric oxide induced by interleukin-1β in rat islets of Langerhans and HIT-T15 cells causes significant DNA damage as measured by the 'comet' assay, *FEBS Lett.* 333: 291–295.

Itoh, T., Tsuzuki, H., Katoh, T., Teraoka, H., Matsumoto, K., Yoshida, N., Terazono, K., Watanabe, T., Yonekura, H., Yamamoto, H. and Okamoto, H., 1990, Isolation and characterization of human *reg* protein produced in *Saccharomyces cerevisiae*, *FEBS Lett.*, 272: 85–88.

Kawazu, S., Sener, A., Couturier, E. and Malaisse, W. J., 1980, Metabolic, cationic and secretory effects of hypoglycemic sulfonylureas in pancreatic islets, *Naunyn-Schmiedeberg's Arch. Pharmacol.* 312: 277–283.

Kallmann, B., Burkart, V., Kröncke, K. -D., Kolb-Bachofen, V. and Kolb, H., 1992, Toxicity of chemically generated nitric oxide towards pancreatic islet cells can be prevented by nicotinamide, *Life Sci.* 51: 671–678.

Koguma, T., Takasawa, S., Tohgo, A., Karasawa, T., Furuya, Y., Yonekura, H. and Okamoto, H., 1994, Cloning and characterization of cDNA encoding rat ADP-ribosyl cyclase / cyclic ADP-ribose hydrolase (homologue to human CD38) from islets of Langerhans, *Biochim. Biophys. Acta* 1223: 160–162.

Lee, H. C., Walseth, T. F., Bratt, G. T., Hayes, R. N. and Clapper, D. L., 1989, Structural determination of a cyclic metabolite of NAD^+ with intracellular Ca^{2+}-mobilizing activity, *J. Biol. Chem.* 264: 1608–1615.

Like, A. A., Weringer, E. J., Holdash, A., McGill, P., Atkinson, D. and Rossini, A. A., 1985, Adoptive transfer of autoimmune diabetes mellitus in biobreeding/Worrcester (BB/W) inbred and hybrid rats, *J. Immunol.* 134: 1583–1587.

Matschinsky, F. M., Pagliara, A. S., Stillings, S. N. and Hover, B. A., 1976, Glucose and ATP levels in pancreatic islet tissue of normal and diabetic rats, *J. Clin. Invest.* 58: 1193–1200.

Mori, Y., Suko, M., Okudaira, H., Matsuda, I., Tsuruoka, A., Sasaki, A., Yokoyama, H., Tanase, T., Shida, T., Nishimura, M., Terada, E. and Ikeda, Y., 1986, Preventive effects of cyclosporin on diabetes in NOD mice, *Diabetologia* 29: 244–247.

Moriizumi, S., Watanabe, T., Unno, M., Nakagawara, K., Suzuki, Y., Miyashita, H., Yonekura, H. and Okamoto, H., 1994, Isolation, structural determination and expression of a novel *reg* gene, human *reg* Iβ, *Biochim. Biophys. Acta* 1217: 199–202.

Nomikos, I. N., Prowse, S. J., Carotenuto, P. and Lafferty, K. J., 1986, Combined treatment with nicotinamide and desferrioxamine prevents islet allograft destruction in NOD mice, *Diabetes* 35: 1302–1304.

Okamoto, H., 1981, Regulation of proinsulin synthesis in pancreatic islets and a new aspect to insulin-dependent diabetes, *Mol. Cell. Biochem.* 37: 43–61.

Okamoto, H., 1985, Molecular basis of experimental diabetes: degeneration, oncogenesis, and regeneration of pancreatic B-cells of islets of Langerhans, *BioEssays* 2: 15–21.

Okamoto, H., 1990, The molecular basis of experimental diabetes, in "Molecular biology of the islets of Langerhans", pp. 209–231, H. Okamoto ed., Cambridge University Press, Cambridge.

Okamoto, H., Takasawa, S., Nata, K. and Yonekura, H., 1992, Cyclic ADP-ribose, a novel second messenger for intracellular Ca^{++} mobilization in pancreatic islets, in "The first conference of the international union of biochemistry and molecular biology: Biochemistry of diseases, June 1–6, 1992, Nagoya, Japan, Abstract" p. 218, Bridge Ltd., Nagoya.

Okamoto, H., Takasawa, S., Nata, K., Sugimoto, T., Noguchi, N., Takeyama, J. and Yonekura, H., 1993, ADP-ribosyl cyclase that synthesizes cyclic ADP-ribose, a second messenger for Ca^{2+} mobilization in β-cells, *Diabetes*, 42: 76A.

Okamoto, H. Sr., 1976, Antitumor activity of streptolysin S-forming streptococci. *In*: "Mechanisms in Bacterial Toxinology," A. W. Bernheimer, ed., John Wiley & Sons, New York, pp. 237–257.

Radons, J., Heller, B., Bürkle, A., Hartmann, B., Rodriguez, M. L., Kröncke, K. D., Burkart, V. and Kolb, H., 1994, Nitric oxide toxicity in islet cells involves poly (ADP-ribose) polymerase activation and concomitant NAD^+ depletion, *Biochem. Biophys. Res. Commun.* 199: 1270–1277.

Sener, A., Hutton, J. C., Kawazu, S., Boschero, A. C., Somers, G., Devis, G., Herchuelz, A. and Malaisse, W. J., 1978, The stimulus-secretion coupling of glucose-induced insulin release — metabolic and functional effects of NH_4^+ in rat islets, *J. Clin. Invest.* 62: 868–878.

States, D. J., Walseth, T. F. and Lee, H. C., 1992, Similarities in amino acid sequences of Aplysia ADP-ribosyl cyclase and human lymphocyte antigen CD38, *Trends Biochem. Sci.* 17: 495.

Takasawa, S., Nata, K., Yonekura, H. and Okamoto, H., 1993a, Cyclic ADP-ribose in insulin secretion from pancreatic β cells, *Science*, 259: 370–373.

Takasawa, S., Nata, K., Yonekura, H. and Okamoto, H., 1993b, Cyclic ADP-ribose in β cells, *Science*, 262: 585.

Takasawa, S., Tohgo, A., Noguchi, N., Koguma, T., Nata, K., Sugimoto, T., Yonekura, H. and Okamoto, H., 1993c, Synthesis and hydrolysis of cyclic ADP-ribose by human leukocyte antigen CD38 and inhibition of the hydrolysis by ATP, *J. Biol. Chem.*, 268: 26052–26054.

Terazono, K., Yamamoto, H., Takasawa, S., Shiga, K., Yonemura, Y., Tochino, Y. and Okamoto, H., 1988, A novel gene activated in regenerating islets, *J. Biol. Chem.*, 263, 2111–2114.

Terazono, K., Uchiyama, Y., Ide, M., Watanabe, T., Yonekura, H., Yamamoto, H. and Okamoto, H., 1990, Expression of reg protein in rat regenerating islets and its co-localization with insulin in the beta cell secretory granules, *Diabetologia*, 33: 250–252.

Toyota, T., Satoh, J., Oya, K., Shintani, S. and Okano, T., 1986, Streptococcal preparation (OK-432) inhibits development of type I diabetes in NOD mice, *Diabetes* 35: 496–499.

Uchigata, Y., Yamamoto, H., Kawamura, A. and Okamoto, H., 1982, Protection by superoxide dismutase, catalase, and poly (ADP-ribose) synthetase inhibitors against alloxan- and streptozotocin-induced islet DNA strand breaks and against the inhibition of proinsulin synthesis, *J. Biol. Chem.*, 257: 6084–6088.

Unno, M., Yonekura, H., Nakagawara, K., Watanabe, T., Miyashita, H., Moriizumi, S., Okamoto, H., Itoh, T. and Teraoka, H., 1993, Structure, chromosomal localization, and expression of mouse *reg* genes, *reg* I and *reg* II — a novel type of *reg* gene, *reg* II, exists in the mouse genome, *J. Biol. Chem.*, 268: 15974–15982.

Vague, Ph., Vialettes, B., Lassmann-Vague, V. and Vallo, J. J., 1987, Nicotinamide may extend remission phase in insulin-dependent diabetes, *Lancet* i: 619–620.

Watanabe, T., Yonekura, H., Terazono, K., Yamamoto, H. and Okamoto, H., 1990, Complete nucleotide sequence of human *reg* gene and its expression in normal and tumoral tissues — the *reg* protein, pancreatic stone protein, and pancreatic thread protein are one and the same product of the gene, *J. Biol. Chem.*, 265: 7432–7439.

Watanabe, T., Yonemura, Y., Yonekura, H., Suzuki, Y., Miyashita, H., Sugiyama, K., Moriizumi, S., Unno, M., Tanaka, O., Kondo, H., Bone, A. J., Takasawa, S. and Okamoto, H., 1994, Pancreatic beta-cell replication and amelioration of surgical diabetes by Reg protein, *Proc. Natl. Acad. Sci. USA*, 91: 3589–3592.

Wicker, L. S., Miller, B. J. and Mullen, Y., 1986, Transfer of autoimmune diabetes mellitus with splenocytes from nonobese diabetic (NOD) mice, *Diabetes* 35: 855–860.

Yamada, K., Nonaka, K., Hanafusa, T., Miyazaki, A., Toyoshima, H. and Tarui, S., 1982, Preventive and therapeutic effects of large-dose nicotinamide injections on diabetes associated with insulitis — an observation in nonobese diabetic (NOD) mice, *Diabetes* 31: 749–753.

Yamamoto, H., Uchigata, Y. and Okamoto, H., 1981, Streptozotocin and alloxan induce DNA strand breaks and poly (ADP-ribose) synthetase in pancreatic islets, *Nature*, 294: 286–286.

Yonemura, Y., Takashima, T., Matsuda, Y., Miwa, K., Sugiyama, K., Miyazaki, I, Yamamoto, H. and Okamoto, H., 1984, Amelioration of diabetes mellitus in partially depancreatized rats by poly (ADP-ribose) synthetase inhibitors — Evidence of islet B-cell regeneration, *Diabetes*, 33: 401–404.

Yonemura, Y., Takashima, T., Matsuda, Y., Miwa, K., Sugiyama, K., Miyazaki, I., Yamamoto, H. and Okamoto, H., 1988, Induction of islets B-cell regeneration in partially pancreatectomized rats by poly (ADP-ribose) synthetase inhibitors, *Int. J. Pancreatol.*, 3: 73–82.

41

A ROLE FOR NITRIC OXIDE AND OTHER INFLAMMATORY MEDIATORS IN CYTOKINE-INDUCED PANCREATIC β-CELL DYSFUNCTION AND DESTRUCTION

Michael L. McDaniel,[1] John A. Corbett,[1] Guim Kwon,[1] and Jeanette R. Hill[1]

Department of Pathology
Washington University School of Medicine
Saint Louis, Missouri 63110-8118

INTRODUCTION

Insulin-dependent diabetes mellitus is an autoimmune disease characterized by the selective destruction of the pancreatic β-cell. The autoimmune response that is ultimately responsible for the destruction of the β-cell consists of a number of complex components. Cytokines released during this inflammatory reaction have been implicated as effector molecules which mediate β-cell destruction[1–3]. Our studies have focused primarily in attempting to define the role of cytokines released by both T-lymphocytes and activated macrophages to produce deleterious effects directly on the β-cell during the initial inflammatory response associated with autoimmune diabetes. Our studies have described the ability of the cytokine, interleukin-1 (IL-1), to both inhibit insulin secretion from the β-cell and also to produce cytotoxic effects via the formation of the free radical nitric oxide (NO). Our more recent studies have revealed that the ability of cytokines such as IL-1 to produce nitric oxide by islets is also directly linked to the production of the proinflammatory prostaglandins and thromboxanes that may play an important role in the initial inflammatory response that is the hallmark of autoimmune diabetes.

RESULTS AND DISCUSSION

Effects of IL-1 on β-Cell Function

Our previous studies in 1990 demonstrated that the continuous exposure of rat islets to IL-1 for 18 h potently inhibited glucose-stimulated insulin secretion and the degree of inhibition depended on the concentration of IL-1[4]. Maximum inhibition (95%) was observed

Physiology and Pathophysiology of the Islets of Langerhans, edited by Soria.
Plenum Press, New York, 1997.

with an IL-1 concentration of 5 U/ml. The time dependency of IL-1's effects indicated that exposure of islets to 5 U/ml IL-1 for periods up to 5 h had essentially no effect on glucose-stimulated insulin secretion, whereas exposure of islets for periods > 5 h resulted in potent inhibition of glucose-stimulated insulin secretion with complete inhibition observed at 15–18 h. The appearance of the initial lag period of 5 h before IL-1 exerted its potent inhibitory effects on insulin secretion suggested a requirement for new protein synthesis for IL-1 to exert its inhibitory effects. This turned out to be the case since the inhibitory effects of IL-1 on insulin secretion from islets could be divided into a transcriptional phase occurring within the first h of exposure to IL-1, and a translational phase occurring after the first h of exposure to IL-1. A summary of IL-1's effects as described in our early studies on β-cell dysfunction include the following: 1) a time-dependent inhibition of glucose-stimulated insulin secretion that requires > than 5 h to develop, 2) inhibition of insulin secretion requires both gene transcription and mRNA translation suggesting a requirement for new protein synthesis, 3) inhibition of β-cell function is also associated with significantly impaired glucose oxidation by islet-cell mitochondria and 4) destruction of islets occurs after prolonged exposure to IL-1. These observations and others raised the question in our laboratory as to whether the free radical NO may mediate IL-1's inhibitory effects on the pancreatic β-cell.

Nitric Oxide Synthase (NOS)

The enzyme nitric oxide synthase (NOS) catalyzes the mixed functional oxidation of L-arginine to nitric oxide and L-citrulline. At least three isoforms of NOS have been described[5]. These isoforms include endothelial (eNOS) and neuronal (nNOS) that are constitutively expressed and an inducible NOS or iNOS. The constitutive isoforms are Ca^{2+} and calmodulin-dependent and found in many tissues including endothelial cells, brain, and also the pancreatic β-cell[6]. The other isoform referred to as iNOS is induced by cytokines and lipopolysacchride. iNOS is Ca^{2+}-independent, and was originally isolated from activated macrophages[7]. Our studies have focused primarily on the cytokine-inducible isoform of NOS that results in the overproduction of NO for extended periods of time.

Role for NO in IL-1-Induced Inhibition of Insulin Secretion

Our laboratory and others demonstrated that IL-1-induced inhibition of insulin secretion depended on the metabolism of L-arginine to NO[8–10]. N^G-monomethyl-arginine (NMMA), a competitive inhibitor of the enzyme NOS, completely prevents IL-1 induced inhibition of insulin secretion as well as nitrite, a stable oxidation product of NO, by islets. The cellular mechanisms responsible for the ability of NO to inhibit β-cell function as well as exert its cytotoxic effects are believed to be mediated by inactivation of enzymes that contain iron-sulfur centers or clusters. Our studies demonstrated that IL-1 induces NO formation in islets as evidenced by an electron paramagnetic resonance feature at g=2.04 which is identical to previously reported iron-nitrosyl complexes as illustrated schematically in Figure 1[10].

Inhibition of NOS by NMMA completely prevents the formation of this EPR signal in islets. We have also used this EPR technique to confirm that we are characterizing the cytokine-inducible isoform of iNOS. IL-1 was shown to induce the formation of a g=2.04 iron-nitrosyl feature in islets which is prevented by cycloheximide, demonstrating the requirement of new protein synthesis for IL-1-induced NO formation[11]. These results indicated that NO mediates its inhibitory effects on the β-cell by destruction of iron-sulfur

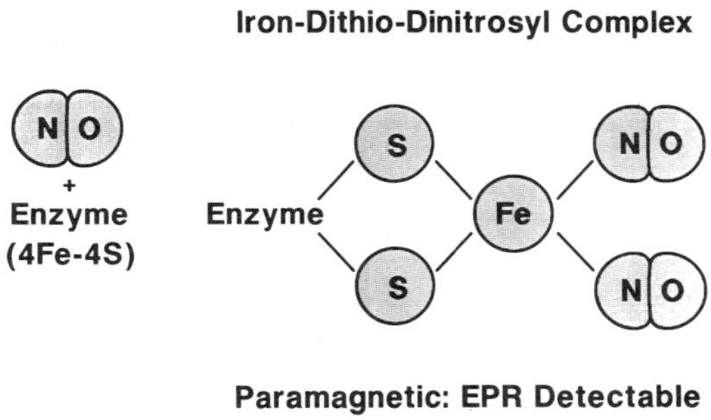

Figure 1. Iron-dithio-dinitrosyl complex.

centers of enzymes primarily localized to the islet-cell mitochondria. We and others have further demonstrated that treatment of rat islets with IL-1 for 18 h results in significant inhibition of mitochondrial aconitase activity and this inhibition of aconitase is completely prevented by NMMA[9,12].

β-Cell as a Source of NO Production

As indicated in Figure 2, the islet of Langerhans represents a heterogeneous cell population consisting of both endocrine and non-endocrine cells. Approximately 65% of the cells of an islet are β-cells that both synthesize and secrete insulin and are located in the core of the islet. Scattered around the periphery of the islet are also glucagon secreting α-cells and somatostatin secreting δ-cells. The islet also contains non-endocrine cells including fibroblasts, endothelial, dendritic and some resident macrophages. We were particularly interested in the cellular source of IL-1-induced NO production and whether the β-cell which is selectively destroyed in autoimmune diabetes could express iNOS and if the overproduction of NO would exert a deleterious effect directly on the β-cell.

To address this question, islets were dispersed into individual islet cells and a β-cell population > 95% purity and an α-cell population of ~85% purity was obtained by fluorescence-activated cell sorting (FACS). Using antiserum specific for mouse macrophage iNOS, we immunoprecipitated a 130 kDa protein (iNOS) from purified β-cells treated

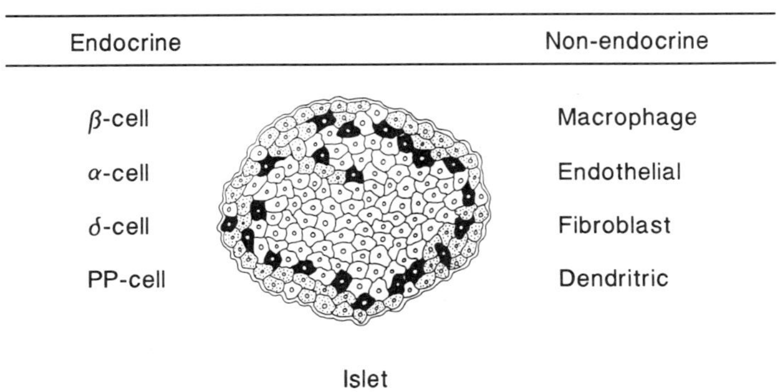

Figure 2. Cellular source of IL-1-induced NO production by islets.

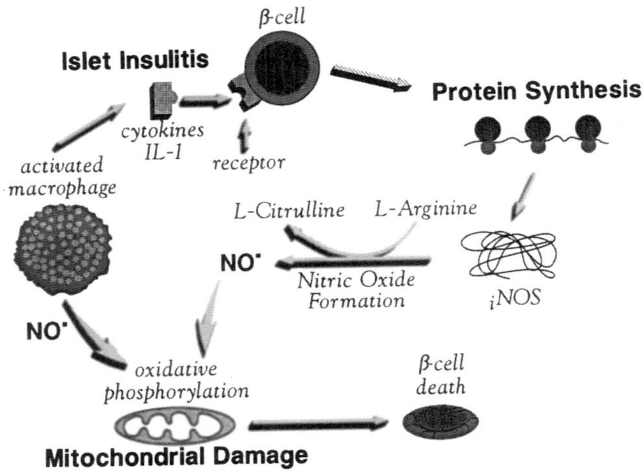

Figure 3. Model of IL-1's effects on β-cell dysfunction and destruction.

with IL-1. The expression of iNOS was inhibited by actinomycin D, an inhibitor of gene transcription, and not observed in purified α-cells exposed to IL-1[13]. These studies provided the initial evidence that the cytokine IL-1 has the ability to induce iNOS expression in the β-cell which is selectively destroyed in autoimmune diabetes[12].

Figure 3 illustrates a proposed model to explain the ability of the cytokine IL-1 to both potently inhibit insulin secretion and produce cytotoxic effects by the overproduction of the free radical nitric oxide.

In this model, IL-1 binds to a β-cell specific receptor, a type 1 IL-1 receptor, that then initiates a series of signal transduction events that include activation of a post-receptor tyrosine kinase activity[14] and a role for the early transcription factors c-fos, c-jun and NFKB that ultimately culminates in the expression of iNOS. The overproduction of NO by iNOS damages the β-cell mitochondria by inactivating iron-sulfur containing enzymes and also inhibits DNA synthesis that is believed to ultimately contribute to β-cell death. Activated macrophages present during this initial insulitis or inflammation also play an important role in this cascade by directly producing NO and also, more importantly, by releasing the cytokine IL-1 which following brief exposures to IL-1 is sufficient to initiate this signal transduction cascade that results in the overproduction of NO[4,14]. Our studies suggest that activation of resident macrophages stimulate the release of IL-1 which then results in the overproduction of NO by the islet β-cell. The production of NO by activation of resident macrophages in the islet exerts minor effects on β-cell function.

Cytokines Coexpress Both NOS and Cyclooxygenase (COX)

Autoimmune diabetes is characterized by the selective destruction of the β-cell and also by an initial insulitis or inflammation. Cytokines released during this inflammatory reaction have been implicated as effector molecules which mediate β-cell destruction. Our recent studies indicate that the cytokine IL-1 induces the coexpression of both iNOS and also cyclooxygenase (COX), the rate limiting enzyme responsible for the production of the proinflammatory prostaglandins and thromboxanes[15]. Figure 4 reviews the cyclooxygenase pathway for arachidonic acid metabolism by islets to produce the

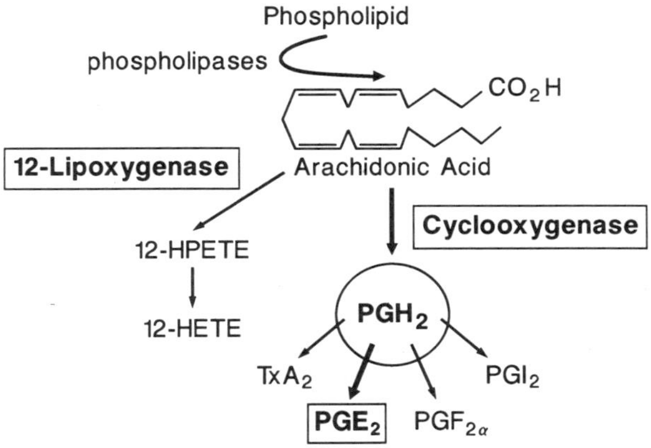

Figure 4. Arachidonic acid metabolism in pancreatic islets.

prostaglandins and the thromboxane, TxA_2. In rat pancreatic islets, the most abundant prostaglandin is PGE_2[16].

Similar to NOS, two isoforms of COX have been characterized. One isoform (COX-1) is constitutively expressed and the expression of the other isoform (COX-2) is stimulated by cytokines and mitogens. Of particular importance is that both isoforms of COX contain an iron-heme prosthetic group at their active site. This is illustrated in Figure 5.

As illustrated on the left of Figure 5, the ability of NO to avidly combine with enzymes that contain iron-sulfur centers or clusters is believed to be the cellular mechanism responsible for the ability of NO to cause mitochondrial damage. In contrast, as shown on the right of Figure 5, the ability of NO to interact with enzymes that contain an iron-heme center that results in the formation of a NO iron-heme complex is believed to mediate the ability of NO to activate enzymes such as guanyl cyclase. Our interest in cyclooxygenase was two-fold. We wanted to determine if the cytokine IL-1 would coex-

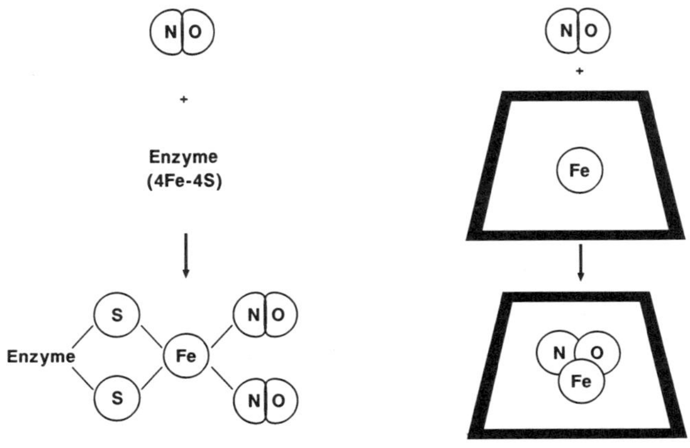

Figure 5. NO formation of iron-dinitrosyl versus iron-heme complexes.

press both iNOS and COX-2 in islets and also determine if by a completely separate mechanism whether NO possibly interacting with the heme prosthetic group of COX or other mechanisms would stimulate the production of PGE_2.

In this approach, exposure of rat islets to 5U/ml IL-1 induces a similar time-dependent production of both nitrite and PGE_2[15]. Furthermore, IL-1-induced nitrite and PGE_2 production is inhibited by the NOS inhibitor, NMMA. Using metabolically labeled islets it was shown by immunoprecipitation that IL-1 exposure to islets results in the coexpression of iNOS and COX-2 and that NMMA has no effects on the expression of either iNOS or COX-2. In addition, treatment of islets for 10 min with 50 μM arachidonic acid results in a 10-fold increase in PGE_2 production by islets cultured with IL-1 before arachidonic acid stimulation that is inhibited 70% by the NOS inhibitor NMMA. Arachidonic acid also induces PGE_2 production by both control islets and islets treated with IL-1 and actinomycin D which is inhibited by NMMA suggesting that NO also stimulates the activity of COX-1 in islets. Overall, these results indicate that IL-1 induces the coexpression of both iNOS and COX-2 by islets and that NO produced by iNOS further stimulates the activities of both COX-1 and COX-2 resulting in the overproduction of the proinflammatory mediator, PGE_2.

CONCLUSION

As shown in Figure 6, autoimmune diabetes is characterized by the destruction of the pancreatic β-cell which is believed to be mediated, in part, by the expression of iNOS by the β-cell resulting in the overproduction of the free radical, NO. Autoimmune diabetes is also characterized by an islet inflammation or insulitis involving the proinflammatory prostaglandins. Our working model is that coexpression of both iNOS and COX-2 by cytokines and the overproduction of NO by iNOS and prostaglandins by COX-2 results in the overproduction of these proinflammatory mediators. The ability of NO to directly activate both constitutive (COX-1) and inducible (COX-2) by a separate mechanism further augments the production of these mediators. The overproduction of these proinflammatory mediators by these cellular mechanisms could play an important role in initiating and maintaining islet inflammation which is the hallmark of autoimmune mediated diabetes.

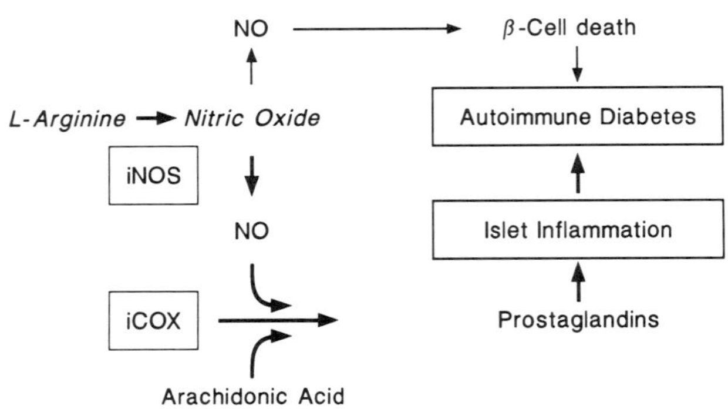

Figure 6. Overall proposed model suggesting a role for NO in islet inflammation.

REFERENCES

1. J.A. Corbett, and M.L. McDaniel, Perspectives in Diabetes: Does nitric oxide mediate autoimmune destruction of β-cells? Possible therapeutic interventions in IDDM, *Diabetes* 41:897 (1992).
2. T. Mandrup-Poulsen, S. Helqvist, L.D. Wogensen, J. Molvig, F. Pociot, J. Johannesen, and J. Nerup, Cytokines and free radicals as effector molecules in the destruction of pancreatic beta cells, *Curr. Top. Microbiol. Immunol.* 164:169 (1990).
3. A. Rabinovitch, Roles of cytokines in IDDM pathogenesis and islet β-cell destruction, *Diabetes Rev.* 1: 215 (1993).
4. J.H. Hughes, J.R. Colca, R.A. Easom, J. Turk, and M.L. McDaniel, Interleukin-l inhibits insulin secretion from isolated rat pancreatic islets by a process that requires gene transcription and mRNA translation, *J Clin Invest* 86:856 (1990).
5. U. Forstermann, H.H.H.W. Schmidt, J.S. Pollock, H. Sheng, J.A. Mitchell, T.D. Warner, M. Nakane, and F. Murad, Isoforms of nitric oxide synthase, *Biochem. Pharmacol.* 42:1849 (1991).
6. J.A. Corbett, J.L. Wang, T.P. Misko, W. Zhao, W. Hickey, and M.L. McDaniel, Nitric oxide mediates IL-lβ-induced islet dysfunction and destruction: Prevention by dexamethasone, *Autoimmunity* 15:145 (1993).
7. C. Nathan, Nitric oxide as a secretory product of mammalian cells, *FASEB J.* 6:3051 (1992).
8. C. Southern, D. Schulster, and I.C. Green, Inhibition of insulin secretion by interleukin-1β and tumor necrosis factor α via an L-arginine-dependent nitric oxide generation mechanism, *FEBS Lett.* 276:42 (1990).
9. N. Welsh, D.L. Eizirik, K. Bendtzen, and S. Sandler, Interleukin-1β induced nitric oxide production in isolated rat pancreatic islets requires gene transcription and may lead to inhibition of Krebs cycle enzyme aconitase, *Endocrinol.* 129:3167 (1991).
10. J.A. Corbett, J.R. Lancaster, M.A. Sweetland, and M.L. McDaniel ML, Interleukin 1 induced inhibition of glucose stimulated insulin secretion and the formation of EPR-detectable iron-nitrosyl complexes in islets of Langerhans, *J. Biol .Chem.* 266:21351 (1991).
11. J.A. Corbett, J.L. Wang, J.H. Hughes, B.A. Wolf, M. Sweetland, J.R. Lancaster, and M.L. McDaniel, Nitric oxide and cGMP formation induced by interleukin-lβ in islets of Langerhans: Evidence for an effector role of nitric oxide in islet dysfunction, *Biochem. J.* 287:229 (1992).
12. J.A. Corbett JA, J.L. Wang, M.A. Sweetland, J.R. Lancaster, and M.L. McDaniel, IL-lβ induces the formation of nitric oxide by β-cells purified from rodent islets of Langerhans: Evidence for the β-cell as a source and site of action of nitric oxide, *J. Clin. Invest*. 90:2384 (1992).
13. J.A. Corbett, G. Kwon, T.P. Misko, C.P. Rodi, and M.L. McDaniel, Tyrosine kinase involvement in IL-1β expression of iNOS by β-cells purified from islets of Langerhans, *Am. J. Physiol.* 267:(Cell Physiol. 36) C48 (1994).
14. J.A. Corbett, M.A. Sweetland, J.R. Lancaster, and M.L. McDaniel, A 1 hour pulse with IL-lβ induces the formation of nitric oxide and inhibits insulin secretion by rat islets of Langerhans: Evidence for a tyrosine kinase signaling mechanism, *FASEB J.* 7:369 (1993).
15. J.A. Corbett, G. Kwon, J. Turk, and M.L. McDaniel, IL-1β induces the coexpression of both nitric oxide synthase and cyclooxygenase by islets of Langerhans: Activation of cyclooxygenase by nitric oxide, *Biochemistry* 32:13767 (1993).
16. J. Turk, B.A. Wolf, and M.L. McDaniel, The role of phospholipid-derived mediators including arachidonic acid, its metabolites, inositoltrisphosphate and intracellular Ca^{2+} in glucose-induced insulin release by islets, *Progress in Lipid Research,* 26:125 (1987).

42

THE REG GENE AND ISLET CELL REPAIR AND RENEWAL IN TYPE 1 DIABETES

Adrian J. Bone,[1] Susan H. Banister,[2] and Shaoli Zhang[2]

[1]Department of Pharmacy
University of Brighton
Moulsecoomb
Brighton, BN2 4GJ, United Kingdom
[2]University Medicine
Southampton General Hospital
Tremona Road
Southampton, SO9 4XY, United Kingdom

INTRODUCTION

The characteristic inability to maintain glucose homeostasis in diabetes mellitus reflects an absolute or partial insulin deficiency. This lack of insulin is due to an overall reduction in the mass of properly functioning β-cells. Such a reduction occurs as a result of a combination of an increased rate of cell destruction and a decreased rate of cell repair and renewal. Whilst considerable attention has been focussed on the elucidation of factors resulting in β-cell loss, much less information is available regarding possible common genetic control mechanisms implicating alterations in islet cell repair and/or adaptive β-cell regeneration as causative factors in diabetes. The difficulties in performing studies of β-cell repair and renewal in diabetes in man are obvious. Thus, it has been earlier investigations performed in models of diabetes which have provided some insight into the defence and repair/regeneration mechanisms activated in the islet cells following injury and onset of disease(11). The hypothesis that pancreatic β-cells possess defence mechanisms against cell injury gained support from observations that islets are able to survive and even recover functional activity after exposure to cytotoxic attack or disturbed metabolism (21,17). However, the magnitude and subsequent effectiveness of the islet cell defence and repair mechanisms is dependent upon the nature and extent of the cytotoxic insult (5). Thus, exposure of rodent islets to alkylating agents (6), IL-1β(8) or heat shock (25) induces a sustained but reversible inhibition of β-cell function. On the other hand, treatment of mouse islets with streptozotocin (SZ) impairs mitochondrial gene expression leading to a persistent decrease in glucose stimulated insulin secretion (20). The existence of islet cell defence and repair

Physiology and Pathophysiology of the Islets of Langerhans, edited by Soria.
Plenum Press, New York, 1997.

mechanisms has also been demonstrated in vivo in studies performed in spontaneously diabetic animal models. Thus, infiltrated islets isolated from prediabetic NOD mice showed a reduction in the inflammatory lesion and a recovery of insulin release and glucose oxidation following a period of tissue culture(21). It would appear, therefore, that removal of islets from the diabetogenic environment is followed by induction of repair mechanisms leading to a restoration of normal β-cell function.

The precise nature of the defence/repair mechanisms activated in islet cells remains unclear but cytotoxic insult is known to evoke a stress response in mammalian cells. This response is characterised by a rapid increase in the synthesis of specific stress or heat shock proteins (HSP) which are thought to be essential for subsequent cell survival(26). There is evidence both in vitro and in vivo for a possible regulatory role of HSP's in the pathogenesis of IDDM. Pancreatic islet content of HSP 70 is reported to be increased following exposure of isolated islets to IL-1β (9). Moreover, the observed induction of HSP 70 expression appeared to coincide with a recovery of β-cell function after subsequent withdrawal of IL-1β (8). Furthermore, liposomal delivery of HSP 70 into rat islets protected against IL-1β induced impairment of pancreatic β-cell function (15). Recent in vivo studies demonstrated the presence of HSP 60 in pancreatic islets in both control and prediabetic NOD mice (2). There was, however, an insulitis-dependent redistribution of HSP 60 in prediabetic animals leading to increased cytoplasmic levels and subsequent induction of HSP 60 autoantibodies (1). Thus it has been suggested that cell mediated immunity initiates redistribution of HSP 60 which acts as a defence mechanism to help in the stabilisation or disposal of denatured proteins (7).

In a recent review, Eizirik and co-workers suggested that the natural repair mechanisms of the β-cell could be enhanced by agents such as nicotinamide (7), an inhibitor of poly(ADP-ribose)synthetase. High concentrations of nicotinamide can block the cytotoxic effects of nitric oxide and IL-1β on islet cells in vitro (3,13). Administration of nicotinamide in vivo has been shown to ameliorate surgically and chemically induced diabetes (29,18) and prevent the development of disease in NOD mice (27).

A novel gene (designated REG) has been identified in a cDNA library constructed from islets isolated from the pancreatic tissue of rats subjected to a 90% pancreatectomy and subsequently treated with nicotinamide (23). The authors suggested that expression of the REG gene was restricted to regenerating islet tissue and was associated with replication, growth or maturation of pancreatic β-cells (23). However, it has recently become apparent that a family of proteins including the REG protein, pancreatic stone protein (PSP) and pancreatic thread protein (PTP) are derived from a single REG gene (24). Moreover, REG protein PSP and PTP are considered to be just different names for a single protein which exists in several molecular forms and is expressed in both exocrine and endocrine pancreatic tissues (28). Further analysis of the REG gene products revealed a high degree of homology with a consensus motif almost invariably present in calcium dependent (C-type) animal lectins (4). Lectins are a family of proteins with diverse properties including growth promotion, tissue recognition and immunomodulation. More specifically, lectins have been reported to suppress autoimmune experimental diabetes (14). Against this background, we have previously demonstrated increased expression of the REG gene in isolated islets exposed to IL-1β, with the rise in REG mRNA levels being accompanied by raised islet specific production of HSP 65 (19). Furthermore, a very recent study has demonstrated the presence of REG gene encoded products in islets of BB rats during temporary, insulin-induced remission of diabetes (12). In the present study, we have examined the association between expression of the REG gene and the development of diabetes in the spontaneously diabetic BB/S rat.

MATERIALS AND METHODS

Groups of age-matched Diabetes Prone (DP) and Diabetes Resistant (DR) BB/S rats were given a series of repeat pancreatic biopsies from 30–90 days of age (prediabetic period). Each individual animal receiving a total of 4 biopsies with a three week interval between procedures.

Pancreatic tissue samples were divided in half and immediately snap frozen in liquid nitrogen. One portion of tissue was reserved for analysis of total pancreatic RNA and the other retained for histological evaluation of insulitis.

The RNA was prepared by homogenisation in guanidinium isothiocyanate followed by ultracentrifugation on a caesium chloride gradient. Northern and Dot Blot analyses were performed by sequential hybridisation using REG (Pst1–Dra1 fragment) and rat pre-proinsulin (Pst1 insert of pBR322) cDNA probes, the kind gifts of Professor H. Okamoto and Dr W. Kastern respectively.

RESULTS AND DISCUSSION

Northern blot analysis of fractionated RNA revealed Reg mRNA as an approximate 0.9 Kb nucleotide band present in all pancreatic biopsy samples from both DP and DR BB/S rats. However, there appeared to be increased expression of Reg mRNA in tissue samples from DP compared to DR BB/S rats at 70 and 90 days of age (Fig. 1). This observation was confirmed by semiquantitative dot blot analysis of unfractionated RNA samples from all study animals. The pancreatic Reg mRNA levels in DP and DR BB/S rats during the prediabetic period (30–90 days of age) are given in Table 1 and illustrated in Figure 2. Thus, DR BB/S rats showed a steady decline in Reg mRNA levels from high values at 30 days (1.14 ± 0.42 mean density ratio Reg/β-actin) to a 50% reduction in levels at 90 days (0.57 ± 0.42 Reg/β-actin). The DP BB/S rats on the other hand, showed a similar decline in Reg gene expression from 30 to 70 days of age but at age 90 days Reg mRNA levels increased to values approaching those seen at 30 days (0.88 ± 0.49 Reg/β-actin; $P < 0.05$ vs DR BB/S rat values at 90 days).

Following removal of the labelled Reg probe by stringent washing at 80°C, the membrane-bound unfractionated RNA samples were rehybridised with a radiolabelled cDNA probe for rat pre-proinsulin (PPI). The mean values of PPI mRNA levels in DP and DR BB/S rats at ages 30, 50, 70 and 90 days are shown in Table 2. There were no significant changes in PPI mRNA levels with increasing age in either the DP or DR study animals.

Thus in the present study, the changes in Reg gene expression observed in the spontaneously diabetic BB/S rat during the prediabetic period appear to occur whilst the mass of properly functioning β-cells is being maintained. This would suggest therefore, that the previously reported relationship between expression of the Reg gene and experimentally

Table 1. Changes in rat REG mRNA levels in DP and DR BB/S rats aged between 30–90 days. REG mRNA expression is related to β-actin mRNA levels and calculated as a ratio of the densities of REG/β-actin

	30/40 days	50/60 days	70/80 days	90/100 days
DP BB/S rats (n=23)	1.01 (± 0.37)	0.92 (± 0.53)	0.64 (± 0.63)	0.88* (± 0.49)
DR BB/S rats (n=23)	1.14 (± 0.42)	0.99 (± 0.58)	0.64 (± 0.41)	0.57* (± 0.42)

*$p<0.05$, t test; DP vs DR rats.

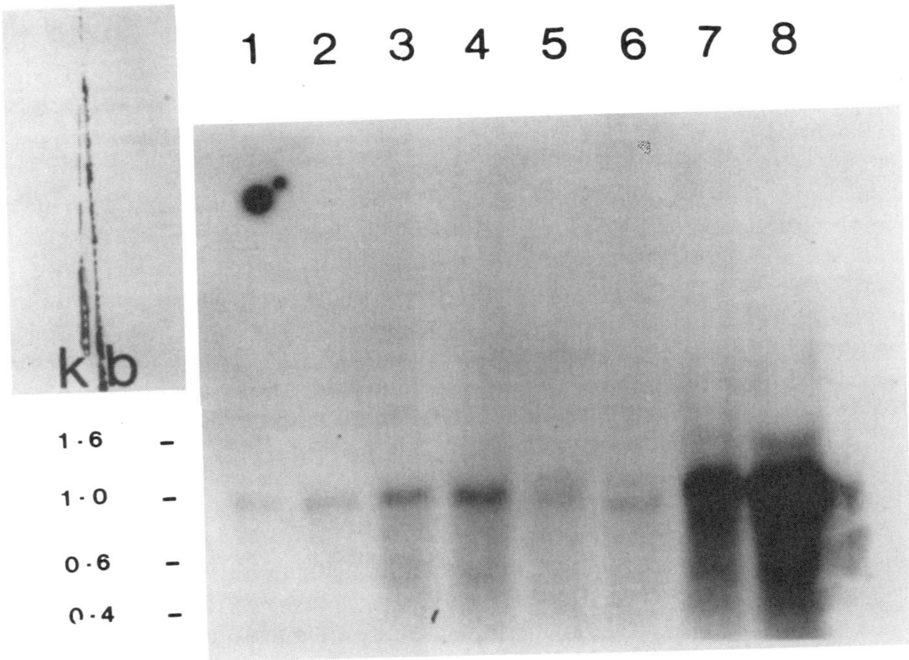

Figure 1. Northern blot analysis of fractionated total RNA isolated from pancreatic biopsies after hybridisation with a rat Reg cDNA probe. Lanes 1,2 and 5,6 have been loaded with two concentrations (1 and 5 µg) of RNA isolated from a DR rat biopsied at 70 and 90 days of age. Lanes 3,4 and 7,8 are loaded with similar amounts of RNA isolated from a DP rat biopsied at the same ages.

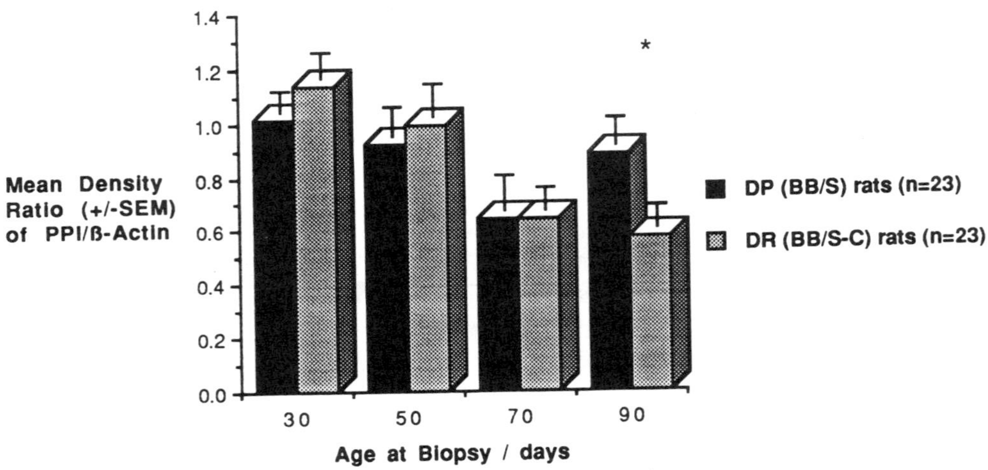

Figure 2. Changes in pancreatic Reg mRNA levels in DP and DR BB/S rats aged between 30–90 days. Reg mRNA expression assessed in pancreatic biopsy samples is related to β-actin mRNA levels and calculated as a ratio of the densities of Reg/β-actin. *Significant difference in Reg mRNA levels between DP and DR BB/S rats at 90 days of age, $P < 0.05$.

Table 2. Changes in rat pre-proinsulin (PPI) mRNA levels in DP and DR BB/S rats aged between 30–90 days. PPI mRNA expression is related to β-actin mRNA levels and calculated as a ratio of the densities of PPI/β-actin

	Age at biopsy			
	30 days	50 days	70 days	90 days
DP BB/S rats (n=23)	0.85 ± 0.44	0.83 ± 0.48	0.80 ± 0.53	0.79 ± 0.42
DR BB/S rats (n=23)	0.87 ± 0.43	0.82 ± 0.53	0.85 ± 0.47	0.88 ± 0.46

induced islet cell proliferation (16,10) is unlikely to be solely a response of cells to the stress of acute changes in glucose concentrations. Earlier studies have reported a decrease in islet cell replication with increasing age in the rat (22). The present observation of a steady decline in Reg mRNA levels in DR BB/S rats between 30 and 90 days of age lends further support for an association between Reg gene expression and islet cell proliferative activity.

In the DP BB/S rats studied, there was a significant increase in Reg mRNA levels at 90 days of age compared to values in DR rats of the same age. This observation indicated an enhancement of Reg gene transcription in DP BB/S rats at or around the time of development of overt diabetes since the current mean age at onset of diabetes for the Southampton colony of BB/S rats is approximately 96 days. Indeed, a histological evaluation of the pancreatic biopsies performed in parallel revealed an early insulitis present in the DP study animals at 90 days of age (S. H. Banister, PhD Thesis — University of Southampton, 1993). Cell mediated immunity is reported to evoke a stress response in mammalian cells characterised by an increase in the synthesis of stress or heat shock proteins (HSP) which involves enhanced gene transcription and translation (26). In this respect, pancreatic islet cell content of HSP 70 is reported to be increased following exposure of isolated islets to IL-1β in tissue culture (9). Furthermore, the observed induction of HSP 70 expression appeared to coincide with a restoration of β-cell function after subsequent culture in the absence of IL-1β (8). In an earlier preliminary study, we have reported an increase in pancreatic islet Reg gene expression following exposure of rat islets to IL-1β (19). Moreover, the rise in Reg mRNA levels appeared to correlate with an increased production of HSP 65. Our evidence therefore suggests an analogous situation to the insulitis driven redistribution of HSP 60 (1) which may serve to stabilise or remove denatured proteins from the β-cells of prediabetic NOD mice (7).

CONCLUSIONS

Thus, the present study and previous in vitro findings suggest a close association between REG gene expression and an activation of possible islet cell adaptive defence and repair/regeneration responses to cell mediated immune attack. These studies do not however indicate the extent to which the REG gene encoded proteins are capable of exerting direct growth promoting or protective effects on pancreatic islet cells. We should like to suggest that the REG proteins are stress proteins produced by both endocine and exocrine pancreatic cells in response to cell injury and that they are capable of modulating islet cell homeostasis. This hypothesis is currently under investigation in studies of the direct effects of recombinant REG protein both in depancreatectomised animals and in isolated rat islets.

ACKNOWLEDGMENTS

The financial support of the Wellcome Trust and the Glaxo Research Institute is kindly acknowledged. We are greatly indebted to Mrs Jasmine Barley and her staff for maintenance of the BB/S rat colony and to Professor Hiroshi Okamoto for generous collaborative support.

REFERENCES

1. Brudzynski K: Insulitis-caused redistribution of heat shock protein HSP60 inside β-cells correlates with induction of HSP60 autoantibodies. Diabetes 42: 908–13, 1993
2. Brudzynski K, Martinez V, Gupta RS: Immunocytochemical localization of heat shock protein 60-related protein in β-cell secretory granules and its altered distribution in nonobese diabetic mice. Diabetologia 35: 316–24, 1992
3. Buscema M, Vinci C, Gatta C, Rabuazzo MA, Vignen, Purrello F: Nicotinamide partially reverses the interleukin-1β inhibition of glucose-induced insulin release in pancreatic islets. Metabolism 41: 296–300, 1992
4. Drickamer K: Two distinct classes of carbohydrate-recognition domains in animal lectins. J. Biol. Chem. 263: 9557–9560, 1988
5. Eizirik DL, Sandler S: Function and metabolism of pancreatic β-cells maintained in culture following experimentally induced damage. Pharmacol Toxicol 65: 114–18, 1989
6. Eizirik DL, Sandler S, Ahnström G, Welsh M: Exposure of pancreatic islets to different alkylating agents decreases mitochondrial DNA content, but only streptozotocin induces long-lasting functional impairment of β-cells. Biochem Pharmacol 42: 2275–82, 1991
7. Eizirik DL, Sandler S, Palmer JP: Repair of pancreatic β-cells — a relevant phenomenon in early IDDM? Diabetes 42: 1383–91, 1993
8. Eizirik DL, Strandell E, Bendtzen K, Sandler S: Functional characteristics of rat pancreatic islets maintained in tissue culture following exposure to interleukin-1. Diabetes 37: 916–19, 1988
9. Eizirik DL, Welsh M, Strandell E, Welsh N, Sandler S: Interleukin-1β depletes insulin messenger ribonucleic acid and increases the heat shock protein HSP70 in mouse pancreatic islets without impairing the glucose metabolism. Endocrinology 127: 2290–97, 1990
10. Francis PJ, Southgate JL, Wilkin TJ & Bone AJ: Expression of an islet regenerating reg gene in isolated rat islets: effects of nutrient and non-nutrient growth factors. Diabetologia 35: 238–42, 1992
11. Hellerström C, Swenne I: Growth pattern of pancreatic islets in mammals. In The Diabetic Pancreas. 2nd ed. Volk BW, Arquilla ER, Eds. New York, Plenum, 1985, p. 53–70
12. Ishii C, Kawazu S, Tomono S, Ohno T, Shimizu M, Kato N, Fukuda M, Ito Y, Kurihara S, Murata K & Komeda K: Appearance of a regenerating (reg) gene protein in pancreatic islets of remission BB/Wor/Tky rats. Endocrine Journal 40 (2): 269–273, 1993
13. Kallmann B, Burkark V, Kröncke K-D, Kolb-Bachofen V, Kolb H: Toxicity of chemically generated nitric oxide towards pancreatic islet cells can be prevented by nicotinamide. Life Sci 51: 671–78, 1992
14. Kolb H, Oschilewski M, Schwab E, Greulich B, Roos P & Kiesel U: Suppression of low-does streptozotocin-induced diabetes by immunomodulatory lectins. Diab Res 3: 183–86, 1986
15. Margulis BA, Sandler S, Eizirik DL, Welsh M: Liposomal delivery of purified heat shock protein HSP70 into rat pancreatic islets as protection against interleukin-1β–induced impaired β-cell function. Diabetes 40: 1418–22, 1991
16. Miyaura C, Ling C, Appel M: Expression of reg/PSP, a pancreatic exocrine gene: relationship to changes in islet β-cell mass. Mol.Endocrinol. 5:226–234, 1991
17. Pipeleers D, Van de Winkel M: Pancreatic B cells possess defense mechanisms against cell-specific toxicity. Proc Natl Acad Sci USA 83: 5267–71. 1986
18. Schein PS, Cooney DA, Vernon ML: The use of nicotinamide to modify the toxicity of streptozotocian diabetes without loss of antitumor activity. Cancer Res 27: 2324–32, 1967
19. Southgate J, Francis PJ, Wilkin TJ, Bone AJ: Islet cell defence and repair mechanisms in type 1 diabetes: role for the reg gene? Diabetologia 34: (Suppl. 2)A96, 1991
20. Strandell E, Eizirik DL, Sandler S: Functional characteristics of cultured mouse pancreatic islets following exposure to different streptozotocin concentrations. Mol Cell Endocrinol 59: 83–91, 1988

21. Strandell E, Eizirik DL, Sandler S: Reversal of β-cell suppression in vitro in pancreatic islets isolated from nonobese diabetic mice during the phase preceding insulin-dependent diabetes mellitus. J Clin Invest 85: 1944–50,1990
22. Swenne I: Effects of aging on the regenerative capacity of the pancreatic β-cell of the rat. Diabetes 32: 14–19, 1983
23. Terazono K, Yamamoto H, Takasawa S, Shiga K, Yonemura Y, Tochino Y, Okamoto H: A novel gene activated in regenerating islets. J Biol. Chem. 263: 2111–2114, 1988
24. Watanabe T, Yonekura H, Terazono K, Yamamoto H, Okamoto H: Complete nucleotide sequence of human reg gene and its expression in normal and tumoral tissues. The reg protein, pancreatic stone protein and pancreatic thread protein are one and the same product of the gene. J Biol. Chem. 265:7432–7439, 1990
25. Welsh M, Eizirik DL, Strandell E: Heat shock treatment of mouse pancreatic islets results in a partial loss of islet cells but no remaining functional impairment among the surviving β-cells. J Mol Endocrinol 1: 27–31, 1988
26. Welch WJ: Mammalian stress response: cell physiology, structure/function of stress proteins, and implications for medicine and disease. Physiol Rev 72: 1063–81, 1992
27. Yamada K, Novaka K, Hanafusa T, Miyazaki T, Toyoshima H, Tarui S: Preventive and therapeutic effects of large-dose nicotinamide injections on diabetes associated with insulitis: an observation in nonobese diabetic (NOD) mice. Diabetes 31: 749–53, 1992
28. Yonekura H, Unno M, Watanabe T, Moriizumi S, Suzuki Y, Miyashita H, Yonemura Y, Sugiyama S & Okamoto H : Structure and expression of reg gene family in Frontiers of insulin secretion and pancreatic β-cell research (Flatt PR & Lenzen S, eds.), Smith Gordon, London, 1994, pp. 581–588
29. Yonemura Y, Takashima T, Miwa K, Miyazaki I, Yamamoto H, Okamoto H: Amelioration of diabetes melitus in partially depancreatized rats by poly synthetase inhibitors: evidence of islet β-cell regeneration. Diabetes 33: 401–4, 1984

43

DNA-DAMAGE AND NAD$^+$-DEPLETION ARE INITIAL EVENTS IN OXYGEN RADICAL INDUCED ISLET CELL DEATH

B. Heller,[1] A. Bürkle,[2] J. Radons,[1] E. Fengler,[1] M. Müller,[2] V. Burkart,[1] and H. Kolb[1]

[1]Diabetes-Forschungsinstitut
Heinrich-Heine Universität Düsseldorf
Auf'm Hennekamp 65, D-40225 Düsseldorf, Germany
[2]Deutsches Krebsforschungszentrum
Im Neuenheimer Feld 242, D-69120 Heidelberg, Germany

INTRODUCTION

Previous studies in vitro and in animal models indicate that reactive oxygen intermediates (ROI) contribute to the destruction of pancreatic islet cells in the pathogenesis of insulin dependent diabetes (Mendola et al., 1989; Rabinovitch et al., 1992). During islet inflammation endothelial cells and infiltrating macrophages are thought to release cytotoxic amounts ROI (Zweier et al., 1988; Brenner et al., 1993). In addition it was shown, that islet cells are highly susceptible to ROI since they possess only low levels of oxygen radical defense systems (Grankvist et al., 1981; Malaisse et al., 1982). We recently have described an in vitro model of oxygen-radical induced islet cell death where ROI are generated by xanthine oxidase in the presence of hypoxanthine (Burkart et al., 1992). In the present study we investigated the initial events of ROI-induced pancreatic islet cell destruction. We observed that DNA strand breaks and the activation of poly(ADP-ribose) polymerase in islet cell nuclei are prominent early consequences of ROI action. The subsequent islet cell death occured several hours after ROI treatment, which appeared to result from depletion of cellular NAD$^+$ pools. Inhibition of poly(ADP-ribose) polymerase by nicotinamide resulted in the preservation of the NAD$^+$ pool and in islet cell survival.

MATERIALS AND METHODS

Islet Cell Preparation

Pancreatic islet cells were prepared from Wistar rats (provided from our own breeding colony) as described previously (Appels et al., 1989). Briefly, after ductal injection of

Physiology and Pathophysiology of the Islets of Langerhans, edited by Soria.
Plenum Press, New York, 1997.

a collagenase solution and digestion for 40 minutes at 37°C the pancreatic tissue was dispersed and the islets were enriched on a Ficoll density gradient (Ficoll 400, Pharmacia GmbH, Freiburg, Germany) with subsequent handpicking. Single islet cells were prepared by dissociation of the islets in the presence of trypsin (Boeringer Mannheim, Mannheim, Germany). For the in vitro assays islet cells were incubated (37°C, 5% CO_2) in culture medium RPMI 1640 (GIBCO EUROPE, Heidelberg, Germany) with 10% fetal calf serum (Radons et al., 1994).

Generation of Reactive Oxygen Intermediates (ROI)

Islet cells were exposed to reactive oxygen intermediates (ROI) generated during the oxidation of hypoxanthine (HX, 0.1 mM, Sigma, Deisenhofen, Germany) by the enzyme xanthine oxidase (XO; EC 1.1.3.22, 25 mU/ml, Sigma, Germany) (Burkart et al., 1992). For time course experiments, the reaction was terminated by washing the samples with ice-cold medium. Inhibitors were added 30 min prior to ROI treatment.

Islet Cell Death

Islet cell death was analysed by the Trypan blue exclusion assay. At least 200 cells were evaluated microscopically, and islet cell lysis was expressed as percent of Trypan blue-positive cells (Kallmann et al., 1992).

Detection of DNA Damage

DNA strand breaks in individual islet cells were determined using a modified situ nick translation method as previously described (Fehsel et al., 1991). Results are expressed as the percentage of cells with stained nuclei.

Activity of Poly(ADP-Ribose) Polymerase (PARP)

The activity of the chromatin associated enzyme poly(ADP-ribose) polymerase (EC 2.4.2.30) in living cells was assessed by immunofluorescence detection of its product, poly (ADP-ribose) (Bürkle et al., 1993; Heller et al., 1994). Immunofluorescence was evaluated by determining the percentage of cells with positive nuclei.

NAD^+ Determination

The intracellular NAD^+ content of islet cells was measured by an enzymatic cycling method using alcohol dehydrogenase from *S. cerevisiae* (Boehringer Mannheim, Mannheim, Germany), as previously described (Hinz et al., 1973; Nisselbaum and Green, 1969) with modifications according to Heller et al., 1994.

RESULTS

ROI-Induced DNA-Damage and PARP Activation

In order to investigate the appearence of ROI-induced DNA strand breaks and a possible PARP activation, pancreatic islet cells were exposed to 25 mU/ml XO and 0.1 mM

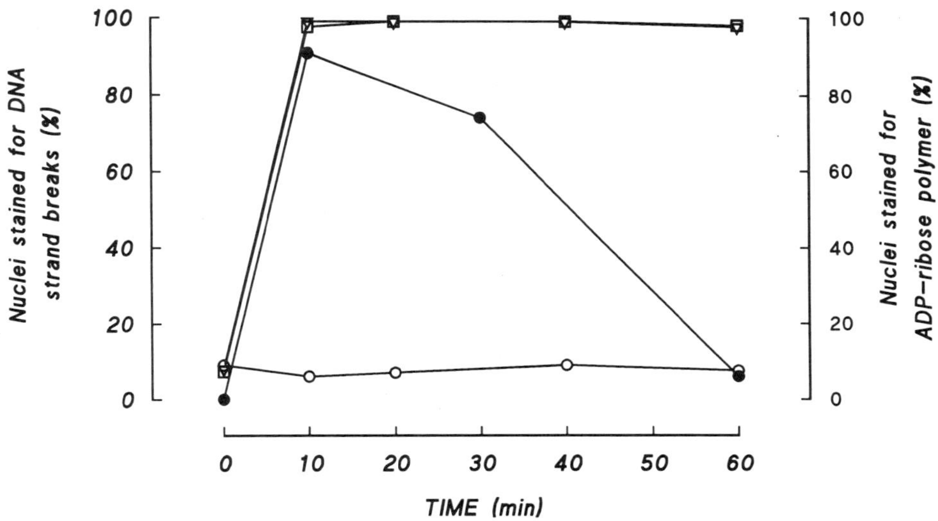

Figure 1. Effect of ROI treatment on the induction of DNA strand breaks and the formation of ADP-ribose polymer. Islet cells remained untreated (○) or were exposed to 25 mU/ml XO and 0.1 mM HX in the absence (▽) or presence of 10 mM NA (□) followed by analysis of DNA strand breaks by in situ nick translation. In parallel the formation of ADP-ribose polymer (●) was determined by indirect immunofluorescence in ROI exposed islet cells. Modified after Heller et al., 1994.

HX. As shown in Fig. 1, DNA strand breaks were observed within 5 minutes. In the presence of 10 mM nicotinamide (NA), an ADP-ribosylation inhibitor and weak oxygen radical scavenger, islet cells were not protected from ROI-induced DNA strand breaks. At all time points control cells showed less than 10% of nuclei with DNA strand breaks.

PARP activity was monitored by the appearence of immunofluorescence signals caused by nuclear poly(ADP-ribose) polymer. In this experiment the peak of polymer immunostaining was at 10 minutes. Background staining of islet cell nuclei ranged between 0 and 10%.

ROI-Induced Depletion of Intracellular NAD$^+$

Since poly(ADP-ribosyl)ation can consume large amounts of NAD$^+$, we determined the NAD$^+$ levels of islet cells after exposure to ROI. As shown in Table 1, ROI treated islet cells showed a rapid loss of intracellular NAD$^+$ and subsequent recovery was not

Table 1. Effect of NA (10 mM) and 3-AB (10 mM) on the NAD$^+$ content of pancreatic islet cells after exposure to ROI (25 mU/ml XO and 0.1 mM HX). Data are means of 4–8 experiments ± SD

Time	Control			XO/HX treated		
(min)	—	+ NA	+ 3-AB	—	+ NA	+ 3-AB
0	0.27 ± 0.01			0.27 ± 0.01		
30	0.28 ± 0.01	0.36 ± 0.05	0.32 ± 0.01	0.03 ± 0.01	0.17 ± 0.02	0.11 ± 0.02
60	0.29 ± 0.03	0.41 ± 0.08	0.33 ± 0.06	0.02 ± 0.01	0.16 ± 0.03	0.10 ± 0.02
120	0.32 ± 0.05	0.49 ± 0.11	0.38 ± 0.06	0.03 ± 0.02	0.18 ± 0.02	0.14 ± 0.34

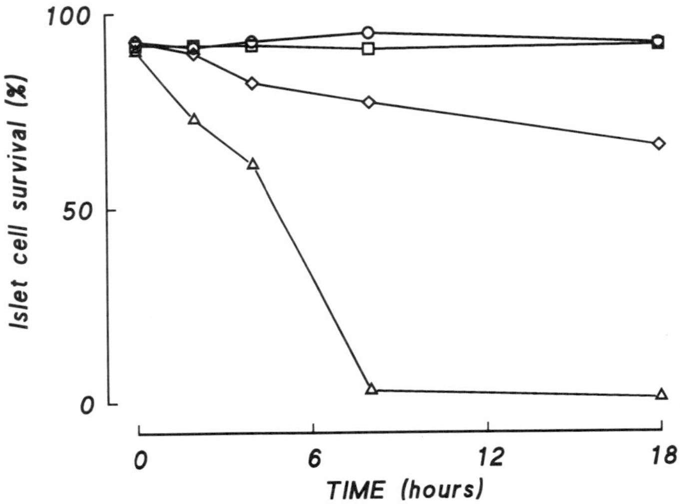

Figure 2. Improved islet cell survival by the PARP inhibitor NA after exposure to ROI. Islet cells remained untreated (○) or were exposed to 25 mU/ml XO and 0.1 mM HX in the absence (△) or presence of NA (◇, 10 mM). Controls (□) were incubated with NA alone. After several time intervals the percentage of surviving islet cells was determined by Trypan blue exclusion assay. Data show means of 2–3 experiments performed in triplicates. Modified after Heller et al., 1994.

observed. In the presence of NA or 3-aminobenzamide (3-AB) the NAD^+ depletion was diminished. Modified after Heller et al., 1994.

Effect of Nicotinamide on Islet Cell Survival

In order to study the effect of nicotinamide on islet cell survival, islets cells were incubated with 10 and 20 mM NA. As shown in Fig. 2, NA supported islet cell survival after ROI treatment. There was only a slight decrease in islet cell survival between 8 and 18 hours in the presence of NA while ROI-induced cell lysis was maximal already after 8 hours.

DISCUSSION

Reactive oxygen intermediates are highly toxic to pancreatic islet cells (Burkart et al., 1992). The concentrations of XO used here were comparable to levels detected in rat pancreatic islets (Parks and Granger, 1986). When XO is added to islet cell culture, HX is oxidated and mainly hydroxyl radicals are released (Sakurai and Ogiso, 1989). Former studies revealed that ROI are released in the first 45–60 minutes, whereas islet cell death occurs after several hours (Burkart et al., 1992). Thus, plasma membrane disintegration is not a direct consequence of ROI action, such as through lipid peroxidation. The present study focusses on the lytic action of ROI on pancreatic islet cells. In earlier studies we reported that NO, another important effector molecule, also induced DNA strand breaks (Fehsel et al., 1993). In many instances, an early consequence of DNA damage is the activation of the PARP, a chromatin-associated enzyme that is involved in the DNA repair (Molinete et al., 1993; Skidmore et al., 1979). Using the indirect immunofluorescence to detect endogenous poly(ADP-ribose) polymer, we have studied poly(ADP-ribose) polymerase activation in intact single islet cells in response to ROI treatment. The data show that in nearly all islet cell nuclei ADP-ribose polymers were formed and there was a strong correlation between the appearence of DNA strand breaks and PARP activation. A direct consequence of the PARP activation is the consumption of intracellular NAD^+ during the formation of ADP-ribose polymer (Yamamoto et al., 1981; Kallmann et al., 1992).Our data show a severe loss of NAD^+ within 30 minutes after exposure to ROI. These kinetics correlate with the formation of poly(ADP-ribose). The latter disappearance of the polymer most likely is a result of the loss of intracellular NAD^+ and the sustained activity of the polymer-degrading enzyme poly(ADP-ribose) glycohydrolase. Earlier studies indicated that the inhibition of PARP improves the survival of pancreatic islet cells treated with streptozotocin or alloxan (Uchigata et al., 1983). Furthermore treatment of NOD mice with nicotinamide prevented the immune destruction of islet cells (Yamada et al., 1982). The ADP-ribosylation inhibitors NA or 3-AB prevented the decrease of intracellular NAD^+ in ROI treated islet cells below a critical level required for cell survival. Our data show that there is no complete recovery of the NAD^+ pools in the presence of NA or 3-AB. This phenomenon has been described previously in lymphocytes despite nearly 100% inhibition of PARP activity (Carson et al., 1986). Some possible explanations may be the direct oxidative damage of NAD^+ by ROI, the hydrolysis of NAD^+ by other enzymatic activities induced by ROI (Richter and Schlegel, 1993) or a decreased biosynthesis of NAD^+ in ROI-damaged cells. However, the preservation of the NAD^+ pool above a critical level by PARP inhibition, as seen here, was sufficient to support islet cell survival.

In conclusion, the present study demonstrates at the level of single cells that ROI induces DNA damage, followed by PARP activation, the depletion of cellular NAD^+ pools and subsequent cell death. The inhibition of PARP by NA or 3-AB preserves NAD^+ pools and supports islet cell survival.

ACKNOWLEDGMENTS

We thank Dr. M. Miwa (University of Tsukuba, Tsukuba, Japan) for the kind gift of 10H hybridoma cells. This work was supported by the Deutsche Forschungsgemeinschaft, the Bundesminister für Gesundheit, the Minister für Wissenschaft und Forschung des Landes Nordrhein-Westfalen and the Werner & Gertrud Müller-Stiftung.

REFERENCES

Appels, B., Burkart, V., Kantwerk-Funke, G., Kolb-Bachofen, V., and Kolb, H., 1989, Spontaneous cytotoxicity of macrophages against pancreatic islet cells, *J. Immunol.* 142:3803–3808.

Brenner, H. H., Burkart, V., Rothe, H., and Kolb, H., 1993, Oxygen radical production is increased in macrophages from diabetes prone BB rats, *Autoimmunity* 15:93–98.

Burkart, V., Koike, T., Brenner, H. H., and Kolb, H., 1992, Oxygen radicals generated by the enzyme xanthine oxidase lyse rat pancreatic islet cells in vitro, *Diabetologia* 35:1028–1034.

Bürkle, A., Chen, G., Küpper, J. H., Grube, K., and Zeller, W. J., 1993, Increased poly(ADP-ribosyl)ation in intact cells by cisplatin treatment, *Carcinogenesis* 14:559–561.

Carson, D. A., Seto, S., and Wasson, D. B., 1986, Lymphocyte dysfunction after DNA damage by toxic oxygen species. A model of immunodeficiency, *J. Exp. Med.* 163:746–751.

Fehsel, K., Kolb-Bachofen, V., and Kolb, H., 1991, Analysis of TNFα-induced DNA strand breaks at the single cell level, *Am. J. Pathol.* 139:251–254.

Fehsel, K., Jalowy, A., Sun, Q., Burkart, V., Hartmann, B., and Kolb, H., 1993, Islet cell DNA is a target of inflammatory attack by nitric oxide, *Diabetes* 42:496–500.

Grankvist, K., Marklund, S. L. and Talledal, I. B., 1981, CuZn-superoxide dismutase, Mn-superoxide dismutase, catalase and glutathione peroxidase in pancreatic islets or other tissues in the mouse, *Biochem. J.* 199:393–398.

Heller, B., Bürkle, A., Radons, J., Fengler, E., Jalowy, A., Müller, M., Burkart, V., and Kolb, H., 1994, Analysis of oxygen radical toxicity in pancreatic islets at the single cell level, *Biol. Chem. Hoppe-Seyler* 375:597–602.

Hinz, M., Katsilambros, N., Maier, V., Schatz, H., and Pfeiffer, E. F., 1973, Significance of streptozotocin induced nicotinamide-adenine-dinucleotide (NAD^+) degradation in mouse pancreatic islets, *FEBS Letters* 30:225–228.

Kallmann, B., Burkart, V., Kröncke, K.-D., Kolb-Bachofen, V., and Kolb, H., 1992, Toxicity of chemically generated nitric oxide towards pancreatic islet cells can be prevented by nicotinamide. *Life Sci.* 51:671–678.

Malaisse, W. J., Malaisse-Lagae, F., Sener, A., and Pipeleers, D. G., 1982, Determinants of the selective toxicity of alloxan to the pancreatic B cell, *Proc. Natl. Acad. Sci. USA* 79:927–930.

Mendola, J., Wright, J. R., and Lacy, P. E., 1989, Oxygen free radical scavengers and immune destruction of murine islets in allograft rejection and multiple low-dose streptozotocin-induced insulitis, *Diabetes* 38:379–385.

Molinete, M., Verneulen, W., Bürkle, A., Ménissier-de Murcia, J., Küpper, J. H., Hoeijmakers, J. H. J., and de Murcia, G., 1993, Overproduction of the poly(ADP-ribose)polymerase DNA-binding domain blocks alkylation-induced DNA repair synthesis in mammalian cells, *EMBO J.* 12:2109–2117.

Nisselbaum, J. S., and Green, S., 1969, A simple ultramicro method for determination of pyridine nucleotides in tissues, *Analytical Biochemistry* 27:212–217.

Parks, D. A., and Granger, D. N., 1986, Xanthine oxidase: biochemistry, distribution and physiology, *Acta Phys. Scand.* (Suppl. 548):87–99.

Rabinovitch, A., Suarez, W. L., Thomas, P. D., Strynadka, K., and Simpson, I., 1992, Cytotoxic effects of cytokines on rat islets: evidence for involvement of free radicals and lipid peroxidation, *Diabetologia* 35:409–413.

Radons, J., Heller, B., Bürkle, A., Hartmann, B., Rodriguez, M.-L., Kröncke, K.-D., Burkart, V., and Kolb, H., 1994, Nitric oxide toxicity in islet cells involves poly(ADP-ribose) polymerase activation and concomitant NAD depletion, *Biochem. Biophys. Res. Comm.* 199:1270–1277.

Richter, C., and Schlegel, J., 1993, Mitochondrial calcium release induced by prooxidants, *Toxicol. Lett.* 67:119–127.

Sakurai, K. and Ogiso, T., 1989, Studies on the biological damage by active oxygen. III. Generation of hydroxyl radical and inhibition of insulin release in hypoxanthine-xanthine oxidase system in the presence of pancreatic islet cells. *Yakugaku Zasshi* 109:102–106.

Skidmore, C. J., Davies, M. I., Goodwin, P. M., Halldorsson, H., Lewis, P. J., Shall, S., and Zia'ee, A.-A., 1979, The involvement of poly(ADP-ribose) polymerase in the degradation of NAD+ caused by gamma irradiation and N-methyl-N-nitrosourea, *Eur. J. Biochem.* 101:135–142.

Uchigata, Y., Yamamoto, H., Nagai, H., and Okamoto, H., 1983, Effect of poly(ADP-ribose) synthetase inhibitor administration to rats before and after injection of alloxan and streptozotocin on islet proinsulin synthesis, *Diabetes* 32:316–318.

Yamada, K., Nonaka, K., Hanafusa, T., Miyazaki, A., Toyoshima, H., and Tarui, S., 1982, Preventive and therapeutic aspects of large dose nicotinamide injections on diabetes associated with insulitis: an observation in non-obese diabetic (NOD) mice, *Diabetes* 31:749–753.

Yamamoto, H., Uchigata, Y., and Okamoto, H., 1981, Streptozotocin and alloxan induce DNA strand breaks and poly(ADP-ribose) synthetase in pancreatic islets, *Nature* 294:284–286.

Zweier, J. I., Kuppusamy, P., Lutty, G. A., 1988, Measurement of endothelial cell free radical generation: evidence for a central mechanism of free radical injury in postischaemic tissues, *Proc. Natl. Acad. Sci.* 85:4046–4050.

44

NITRIC OXIDE RATHER THAN SUPEROXIDE OR PEROXYNITRITE INHIBITS INSULIN SECRETION AND CAUSES DNA DAMAGE IN HIT-T15 CELLS

C. A. Delaney, J. M. Cunningham, M. H. L. Green, and I. C. Green

[1]Biochemistry Group, School of Biological Sciences
University of Sussex
Falmer, Brighton, BN1 9QG
[2]MRC Cell Mutation Unit
University of Sussex
Brighton, BN1 9RR, United Kingdom

INTRODUCTION

We have previously demonstrated that treatment of rat islets of Langerhans with the nitric oxide donors 3-morpholinosydnonimine (SIN-1) and S-nitrosoglutathione (GSNO) inhibits insulin secretion and increases cyclic GMP, thus mimicking the effects of the cytokine interleukin-1β [1] and [2]. We have recently found that nitric oxide, derived exogenously from nitric oxide donors or endogenously by IL-1β induction of nitric oxide synthase, causes DNA damage in islets of Langerhans and in HIT-T15 cells when measured by the 'comet' assay [3].

SIN-1 releases superoxide ions as well as nitric oxide [4] as does purified neuronal nitric oxide synthase [5]. The combination of superoxide and nitric oxide can form peroxynitrite and this may decompose to form the highly toxic hydroxyl radical [6]. A similiar series of events may follow the induction of nitric oxide synthase. Evidence has recently been presented that peroxynitrite is responsible for the neurotoxicity of nitric oxide, and paradoxically nitric oxide in the form of the nitronium ion (NO^+) has been suggested to be neuroprotective [7].

This study examines the effects of short term incubation with the nitric oxide donors GSNO and SIN-1 on inhibition of insulin secretion and production of DNA strand breaks in HIT-T15 cells, and whether nitric oxide itself is the damaging species. We used superoxide dismutase (SOD) to test whether the deleterious effects on insulin secretion and DNA damage induced by SIN-1 might arise from superoxide or from the combination of nitric oxide and superoxide to form peroxynitrite ($ONOO^-$).

Physiology and Pathophysiology of the Islets of Langerhans, edited by Soria.
Plenum Press, New York, 1997.

METHODS

The transformed clonal beta cell line HIT-T15 (passage no 69–75) was used. Insulin secretion studies were carried out as decribed previously [2]. Nitric oxide formation was assessed by assay of the oxidative products nitrite and nitrate [8] after incubating HIT-T15 cells with the nitric oxide donors ± superoxide dismutase in Gey and Gey buffer for 30 mins. To ascertain the proportion of nitrate relative to nitrite produced by cells, nitrate in the incubation medium was reduced using cadmium powder and ammonium chloride/ borax buffer prior to analysis for nitrite [9]

DNA damage was determined by a novel single cell gel electrophoresis method, the 'comet' assay [10] and [3]. Briefly, single cells were embedded in agar on a frosted microscope slide and treated with SIN-1 (0.1 mM), GSNO (0.3 mM) or SOD (200 U/ml) on the slide for 30 min. The cells were lysed, placed in alkali, and an electric current applied. DNA containing strand breaks unwinds and the fragments stream towards the anode in a comet tail during electrophoresis. DNA was stained with ethidium bromide, viewed under a fluorescent microscope and quantified by an image analysis system which compares the length of intact nuclei versus damaged nuclei with a comet tail.

RESULTS AND DISCUSSION

The inhibitory effect of SIN-1 on 20mM glucose-induced insulin secretion was not altered by the co-treatment with SOD (Fig. 1).

The nitric oxide donors SIN-1 and GSNO cause DNA damage in HIT-T15 cells as measured by an increase in the number of nuclei with comet tails (right hand shift towards increased nuclear/comet diameter) (Fig. 2).

The removal of superoxide with exogenous superoxide dismutase, which should substantially reduce peroxynitrite formation from SIN-1, did not prevent the DNA damaging effects of SIN-1 or GSNO. Cells treated with SOD alone behaved as controls (Fig. 3).

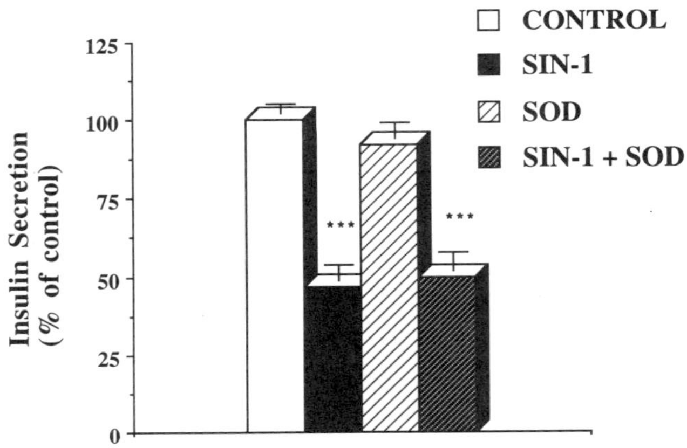

Figure 1. The effect of SIN-1 (100 μM) and superoxide dimutase (200 U/ml) on 20 mM glucose-induced insulin secretion in HIT-T15 cells in 30 mins. Data are standardised as a % of control, n = 28–30, $^{**}p < 0.001$ versus control. Mean control value was 18 fmol insulin secreted/μg cell protein.

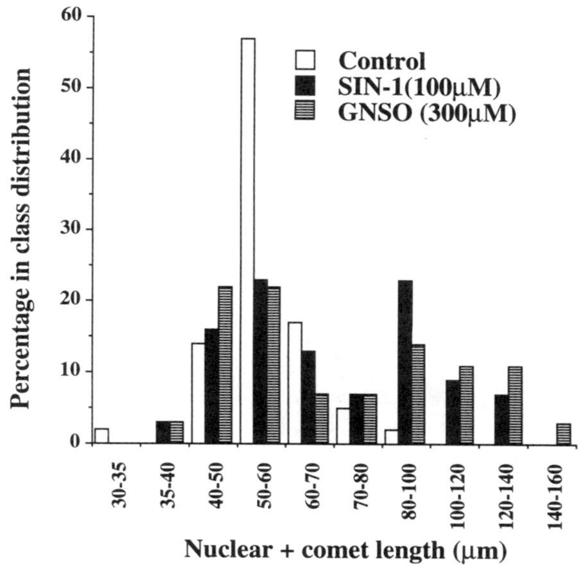

Figure 2. Percentage distribution of mean comet lengths in HIT-T15 cells exposed to SIN-1 (100 µM) and GSNO (300 µM). There is a right hand shift towards increased nuclear/ comet diameter indicative of increased DNA damage. Data from 3 separate experiments.

The rate of generation of nitric oxide from the compounds used in this study was assessed by measuring nitrite and nitrate, which are formed in aqueous solution following oxidation of nitric oxide. As shown in Fig. 4, SIN-1 generated nitrite in the incubation medium, and as expected, a large proportion of nitrite appeared to be oxidised further to nitrate. The smaller amount of nitrate formed in the presence of superoxide dismutase may

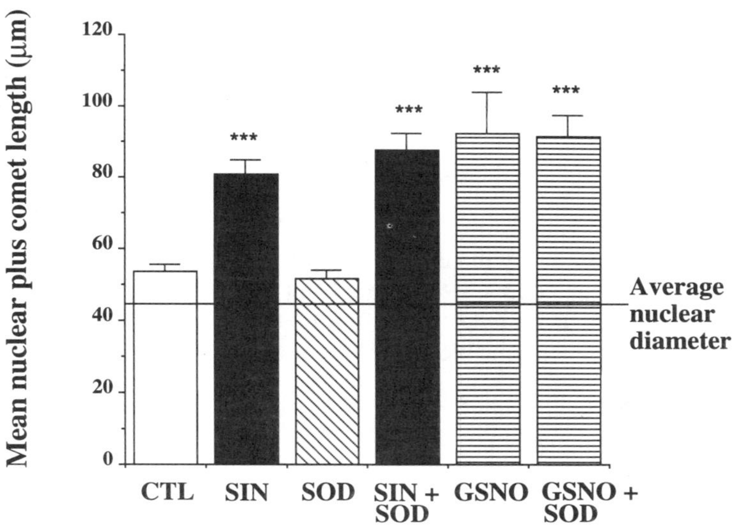

Figure 3. Single cells obtained after trypsinising HIT-T15 cells were embedded in agar on frosted slides and left for 1 h prior to treatment. HIT-T15 cells were exposed to SIN-1 (100 µM), GSNO (300 µM) or SOD (200 U/ml) and DNA damage assessed. Results are overall (head + tail) mean comet length ± SEM. Data from 2–3 separate experiments. ***$p < 0.001$.

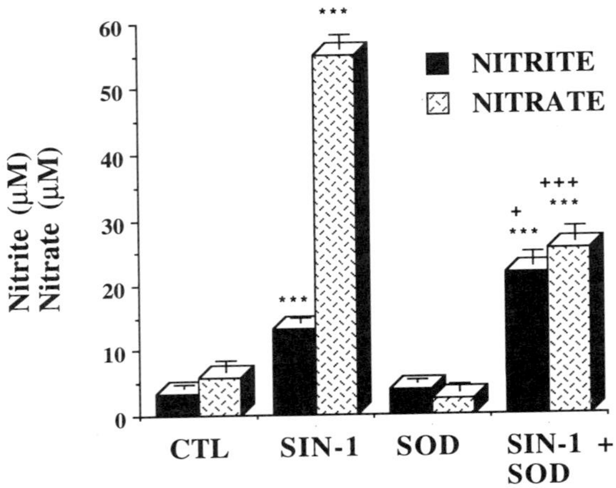

Figure 4. Nitite and nitrate were determined following incubation of the cells in physiological buffer containing SIN-1 (100 μM) and SOD (200 U/ml). ***$p < 0.001$ vs. control, $^{+}p < 0.05$ and $^{+++}p < 0.001$ vs values obtained with SIN-1 alone.

reflect reduced formation of peroxynitrite and suggests that the failure of superoxide dismutase to alter induction of strand breaks by SIN-1 cannot be because this enzyme is inactive in the system. We have also found that in rat islets, superoxide dismutase can increase cyclic GMP and decrease cyclic AMP even though it may not be penetrating the cell [2]. The generation of nitric oxide from SIN-1 in cell-free medium appears to be enhanced in the presence of superoxide dismutase by blocking the nitric oxide scavenging effect of superoxide [11].

CONCLUSIONS

Our results demonstrate that in HIT-T15 cells, 30 min exposure to SIN-1 and GSNO results in significant inhibition of glucose-induced insulin secretion and induction of DNA damage. These effects were not reduced by exogenous superoxide dismutase, suggesting that in this instance, peroxynitrite is not the active damaging species.

ACKNOWLEDGMENTS

Work supported in part by the British Diabetic Association, Medical Research Council, Science and Engineering Research Council and Commission of the European Communities. We wish to thank R. Knowles (Wellcome) for GSNO, Cassella AG for SIN-1, Rohit Kulkarni (Hammersmith Hospital) for HIT cells and our other colleagues for help and discussion.

REFERENCES

1. Green, I.C., C.A. Delaney, J.M. Cunningham, V. Karmiris, and C. Southern. Diabetologia, 1993. **36**: 9–16.
2. Cunningham, J.M., J.G. Mabley, C.A. Delaney, and I.C. Green. Mol. Cell. Endocrinol., 1994. **102**: 23–29.
3. Delaney, C.A., M.H.L. Green, J.E. Lowe, and I.C. Green. FEBS Lett, 1993. **333**: 291–295.
4. Feelisch, M., J. Ostrowski, and E. Noack. J. Cardiovasc. Pharmacol., 1989. **14 (suppl. 11)**: S13–S22.
5. Pou, S., W.S. Pou, D.S. Bredt, S.H. Snyder, and G.M. Rosen. J. Biol. Chem., 1992. **267 (34)**: 24173–24176.

6. Beckman, J.S., T.W. Beckman, J. Chen, P.A. Marshall, and B.A. Freeman. Proc. Natl. Acad. Sci. USA, 1990. **87**: 1620–1624.
7. Lipton, S.A., Y.B. Choi, Z.H. Pan, S.Z. Lei, H.S.V. Chen, N.J. Sucher, J. Loscalzo, D.J. Singel, and J.S. Stamler. Nature, 1993. **364**: 626–632.
8. Green, L., D. Wagner, J. Glogowski, P.L. Skipper, J.S. Wishnok, and S.R. Tannenbaum. Anal. Biochem., 1982. **126**: 131–138.
9. Davison., W. and C. Woof. Analyst, 1979. **104**: 385–390.
10. Green, M.H.L., J.E. Lowe, S.A. Harcourt, P. Akinluyi, T. Rowe, J. Cole, A.V. Anstey, and C.F. Arlett. Mutat. Res., 1992. **273**: 137–144.
11. Hogg, N., V.M. Darley-Usmar, M.T. Wilson, and S. Moncada. Biochem. J., 1992. **281**: 419–424.

45

ACTIVATION OF PERITONEAL MACROPHAGES DURING THE PREDIABETIC PHASE IN LOW-DOSE STREPTOZOTOCIN-TREATED MICE

Josefa Andrade, Manuel Conde, Francisco Sobrino, and Francisco J. Bedoya

Laboratorio de Sistemas Inmunológicos
Departamento de Bioquímica Médica y Biología Molecular
University of Sevilla
Spain

INTRODUCTION

It has been shown recently that islet cell lysis induced by *C. parvum*-activated macrophages is mediated by NO since cell destruction can be counteracted by NO synthase inhibitors [1]. However, evidence concerning the activation state of macrophages and the effector molecules that mediate islet destruction in experimental immune diabetes is lacking.

MATERIALS AND METHODS

Streptozotocin (STZ) administration. STZ was dissolved in cold citrate buffer, pH 4.5, and injected within 3 min i.p. at a dose of 40 mg/kg on 5 consecutive days to CD-1 mice.

Harvest of macrophages. Macrophages were harvested by peritoneal lavage. The viability of the collected cells was estimated from their ability to exclude trypan blue and was always higher than 95%.

Cell culture. Peritoneal cells were resuspended in culture medium consisting of either RPMI 1640 or EMEM without arginine, 10% FCS and antibiotics and plated (8×10^5 cells in 250 μL) in flat bottom, 96-well culture plates and incubated for 48 h at 37°C.

Assay of superoxide anion production. Macrophages (10^6 cells/mL) were incubated at 37°C in Krebs Ringer bicarbonate buffer containing 10 mM glucose and 80 μM cytochrome c. After 5 min, 100 nM PMA was added and superoxide dismutase-inhibitable decrease in absorbance at 550 nm was recorded continuously.

Physiology and Pathophysiology of the Islets of Langerhans, edited by Soria.
Plenum Press, New York, 1997.

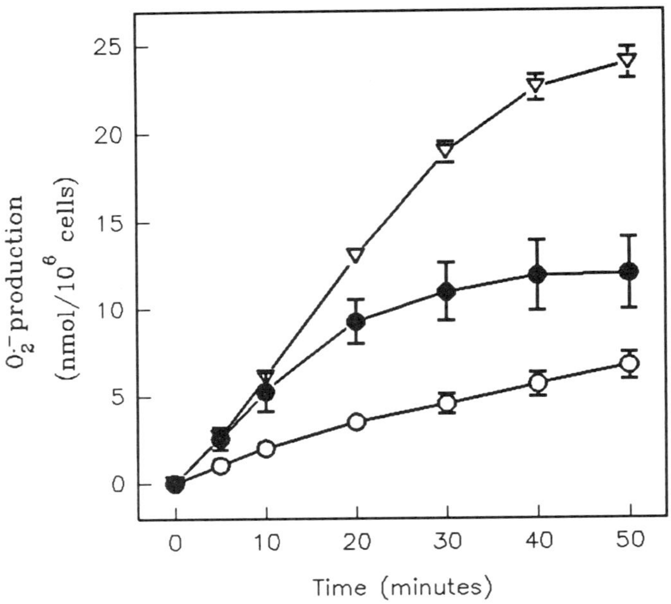

Figure 1. Evolution of superoxide anion production by peritoneal macrophages from mice treated with low-dose STZ. Superoxide anion production was measured at day 6 (●—●) and at day 12 (▽—▽). Control mice (○—○) received buffer alone. Values are means ± SEM for three experiments performed in triplicate.

Lactate determination. Lactate accumulation in medium was measured using a standard spectrophotometric assay [2].

Nitrite determination. The accumulation of NO_2^- in culture supernatants was measured with the Griess reagent [3]. Briefly, 100–150 μL of supernatant was mixed with 500 μL of Griess reagent. Absorbance was measured at 550 nm.

RESULTS

Fig. 1 shows that the treatment with low-dose STZ induced an increase in the PMA-induced O_2^- production by peritoneal macrophages.

On day 6 after beginning of the treatment with STZ, O_2^- production was increased 79% over control. This increase was more evident when the time elapsed was 12 days (259% over control).

Table 1 shows that NO_2^- production is significantly increased in macrophages from the 12-day group. Lactate production by macrophages was also significantly higher than macrophages from control mice.

DISCUSSION

The administration of multiple low doses of STZ to CD-1 mice results in a progressive destruction of pancreatic β-cell [4]. Macrophages have been reported to be the cells

Table 1. Nitrite production and lactate output in macrophages from control and STZ injected CD-1 mice

	NO_2^- (nmoles/well)	Lactate (μmoles/well)
Controls	1.86 ± 0.15	0.32 ± 0.05
STZ-treated	9.29 ± 2.32*	0.90 ± 0.12*

Macrophages (10^5 cells per well) were collected from citrate injected mice and from mice 12 days after the first STZ injection and cultured in RPMI 1640 for 48 hours. Values are the means ± SEM from 5 replicates and are representative of 4 separate experiments. *$p < 0.002$.

that initiate the immune attack against the pancreatic β-cell in this experimental model [5]. We have found that peritoneal macrophages from STZ- treated mice display an enhanced production of O_2^- in response to PMA (Fig. 1). This increase in O_2^- generation by macrophages is a consequence of their activation and may affect pancreatic β-cell since superoxide dismutase activity is low in these cells [6].

Table 1 shows that peritoneal macrophages collected 12 days after beggining of the STZ treatment produced significantly higher amounts of lactate than macrophages from control mice. Similar findings have been reported in *E. coli-* and in *C. parvum*-activated macrophages and indicate that these cells metabolize glucose at high rate to supply energy for the activation processes [2].

NO production (measured as nitrite accumulation in the culture medium) is also increased after STZ treatment at saturating concentrations of arginine (Table 1). These results show that NO is released by macrophages at a time when macrophage infiltration of the islet is in progress. It is thus possible that the generation of NO by activated macrophages is critical for the destruction of the β-cell in this model of immune mediated diabetes as is the case in *C. parvum*-activated macrophages [1].

CONCLUSIONS

The experimental evidence presented in this report indicates that peritoneal macrophages are metabolically active during the prediabetic phase and produce effector molecules such as O_2^- and NO which could participate in the destruction of pancreatic islets in this experimental model of type I diabetes.

ACKNOWLEDGMENTS

This study was supported by the DGICYT (grant no. PM90-0154).

REFERENCES

1. Kröncke, K.-D., Rodríguez, M.-L., Kolb, H. and Kolb-Bachofen, V. (1993) Diabetologia 36:1329–1331.
2. Bustos, R. and Sobrino, F. (1992) Biochem J. 282:299–303.
3. Green, L.C., Wagner, D.A., Glogowski, J., Skipper, P.L., Wishnok, J.S. and Tannenbaum, S.R. (1982) Analyt. Biochem. 126:131–138.
4. Like, A.A. and Rossini, A.A. (1976) Science 193:415–417.
5. Kolb-Bachofen, V., Epstein, S., Kiesel, V. and Kolb, H. (1988) Diabetes 37:21–27.
6. Malaisse, W.J., Malaisse-Lagae, F., Sener, A. and Pipeleers, D.G. (1982) Proc. Natl. Acad. Sci. USA 79: 927–930.

IMMUNOLOGICAL REACTIVITY OF DIABETES-PRONE BB/OK RATS TO SYNGENEIC ANTIGENS

Effect on β-Cell Destruction and Diabetes Onset

Dieter Schröder, Siegfried Schmidt, Ingrid Klöting, Anke Honig, Silke Lucke, Bernd Hehmke, and Michael Schlosser

Institute of Diabetes "Gerhardt Katsch"
Ernst-Moritz-Arndt-University
D-17495 Karlsburg, Greifswald, Germany

INTRODUCTION

The spontaneously diabetic BB rat represents an accepted and widely studied animal model for insulin-dependent diabetes (Nakhooda et al., 1977). In BB rats cellular immune processes (Koevary et al., 1983; Logothetopoulos et al., 1984) as well as humoral immunological phenomena (Dyrberg et al., 1984; Martin and Logothetopoulos, 1984) are involved in or are associated with β-cell destruction and the development of diabetes. Not only the endocrine pancreas is affected by immune-mediated cytolytic reactions but also alterations of the exocrine pancreas were morphologically evidenced (Hanenberg et al., 1989). Humoral-mediated cytotoxicity to islet cells, pancreatic exocrine cells and spleen lymphocytes were detected in serum of diabetes-prone BB/OK rats (Schröder et al., 1991).

At the age of 20–50 days 90–100% of the BB/OK rats exhibit complement-dependent antibody-mediated cytotoxicity (C′AMC) to islet cells as well as to pancreatic exocrine cells (Hehmke et al., 1990; Schröder et al., 1991) but only 50–60% of the animals become diabetic. However, this does not exclude that C′AMC is involved in β-cell alteration in vivo. It might be that in young BB/OK rats only weak lesions of islet cells or adjacent non-endocrine tissue are caused by C′AMC but liberated antigenic components subsequently initiate inflammatory processes thus being of importance for the extent of β-cell destruction. In the course of testing this hypothesis an increase of anti-islet C′AMC upon stimulation with syngeneic islet tissue was recently observed in prediabetic BB/OK rats (Schröder et al., 1993). Therefore this study was aimed to compare the immunological reactivity of diabetes-prone BB/OK rats in response to intrasplenic in vivo application of syngeneic antigens, i.e. homogenates of Langerhans' islets, pancreatic exocrine cells and

Physiology and Pathophysiology of the Islets of Langerhans, edited by Soria.
Plenum Press, New York, 1997.

spleen lymphocytes by measuring the appearance of C′AMC to islet cells, exocrine cells and lymphocytes in vitro and to estimate the impact on the development of diabetes.

MATERIALS AND METHODS

Animals

Diabetes-prone Bio Breeding/Ottawa–Karlsburg (BB/OK) rats expressing the RT1u haplotype of the major histocompatibility complex (MHC) were used throughout the study.

Haplotype-identical (RT1u) diabetes-resistant WOK rats and LEW.1W/Max K rats served as control serum donors or were used for target tissue preparation, respectively.

Islet Isolation and Cell Preparation Procedures

Islets of Langerhans were isolated from the pancreata of 6-to 14-day-old BB/OK or LEW.1W/Max K rats by collagenase digestion followed by Dextran M 70 density gradient centrifugation (Hehmke et al., 1986).

Cell suspensions were prepared from islets of Langerhans and from pancreatic exocrine tissue of these rat strains by enzymatic treatment with dispase (Schröder et al., 1991).

Lymphocytes were prepared from rat spleens and enriched by gradient centrifugation (Hehmke et al., 1990).

Preparation of Antigen

Unfractionated homogenate prepared from islets of Langerhans, pancreatic exocrine tissue and spleen lymphocytes of 6-to 14-day-old BB/OK rats was used as syngeneic antigen. The tissue was resuspended in phosphate-buffered saline solution (PBS) pH 7.2 and homogenized as earlier described (Schröder et al., 1993).

Antigen Administration and Monitoring of the Animals

At the age of 30 to 35 days BB/OK rats were subjected to a single intrasplenic injection of homogenate of either approximately 500 BB/OK rat islets or 1.6×10^6 pancreatic exocrine cells or 3.0×10^6 spleen lymphocytes, respectively (Schröder et al., 1993). Buffer-treated animals served as controls.

In a follow-up study BB/OK rats were observed up to 200 days of age. The rats were screened twice weekly for glucosuria and diabetes was confirmed by plasma glucose determination. Serum was sampled at intervals and stored at –20°C until use.

Determination of Complement-Dependent Antibody-Mediated Cytotoxicity (C′AMC)

In dependence on the injected antigen preparation C′AMC to either islet cells, pancreatic exocrine cells or spleen lymphocytes was assayed in BB/OK rat serum.

C′AMC was determined by measuring ^{51}Cr-release from prelabelled islet cells, pancreatic exocrine cells or spleen lymphocytes prepared from LEW.1W Max K rats in a two-step or in a one-step ^{51}Cr-release assay, respectively (Schröder et al., 1991). BB/OK rat sera inducing a specific ^{51}Cr-release exceeding the mean + 2SD of that caused by WOK rat control sera against the corresponding target cells as indicated were defined as cytotoxic.

Morphological Studies

The appearance of insulitis was examined in hematoxylin/eosin stained sections obtained from Bouin-fixed and paraffin-embedded pancreatic tissue as described by Lucke et al., 1988.

Relative islet and β-cell volume density were evaluated by morpho-metric analysis of immunostained sections (Lucke et al., 1985).

Analytical Procedures

IgG-antibodies to glutamate decarboxylase (GAD) in BB/OK rat sera were determined by ELISA (Ziegler et al., 1994).

Insulin and glucagon extracted from pancreatic tissue by acid/ ethanol was measured radioimmunologically (Besch et al., 1987).

Statistics

Results are expressed as mean ± SEM and were checked for statistical significance by student's t test. Differences were considered significant at the level $p < 0.05$.

RESULTS AND DISCUSSION

The single intrasplenic application of homogenates of syngeneic islets of Langerhans, pancreatic exocrine cells or lymphocytes neither influenced glucose tolerance of BB/OK rats in the prediabetic period (data not shown) nor plasma glucose and age at onset of diabetes as well as the incidence of diabetes (Table 1).

The retrospective analysis of islet antigen-treated BB/OK rats revealed that animals developing diabetes exhibited an increase of C′AMC to islet cells within 7 days after islet homogenate application which was not found in rats remaining long-term normoglycaemic (Figure 1) or which were treated with PBS, respectively, (data not shown).

In contrast, the time course of the appearance of C′AMC to pancreatic exocrine cells in BB/OK rats was not influenced by the intrasplenic application of homogenate of syngeneic pancreatic exocrine cells (Figure 2, panel A). Diabetic and long-term normoglycaemic animals displayed a nearly identical time pattern of C′AMC (Figure 2, panel A).

Table 1. Effect of intrasplenic application of syngeneic antigens on diabetes-prone BB/OK rats. Characteristics of diabetic animals at onset of the disease

Treatment of the animals	Age at manifestation (days)	Plasma glucose at manifestation (mmol/l)	Incidence of diabetes (%)
Injection of islet homogenate	115 ± 30.8 n = 11	24.6 ± 2.2 n = 11	28.2 (11/39)
Injection of homogenate of pancreatic exocrine cells	132 ± 32.6 n = 10	26.3 ± 1.9 n = 10	22.7 (10/44)
Injection of homogenate of lymphocytes	135 ± 35.2 n = 16	20.7 ± 1.9 n = 16	39.0 (16/41)
Injection of phosphate-buffered saline (PBS) (control)	121.9 ± 28.4 n = 22	21.6 ± 1.1 n = 22	40.0 (22/55)

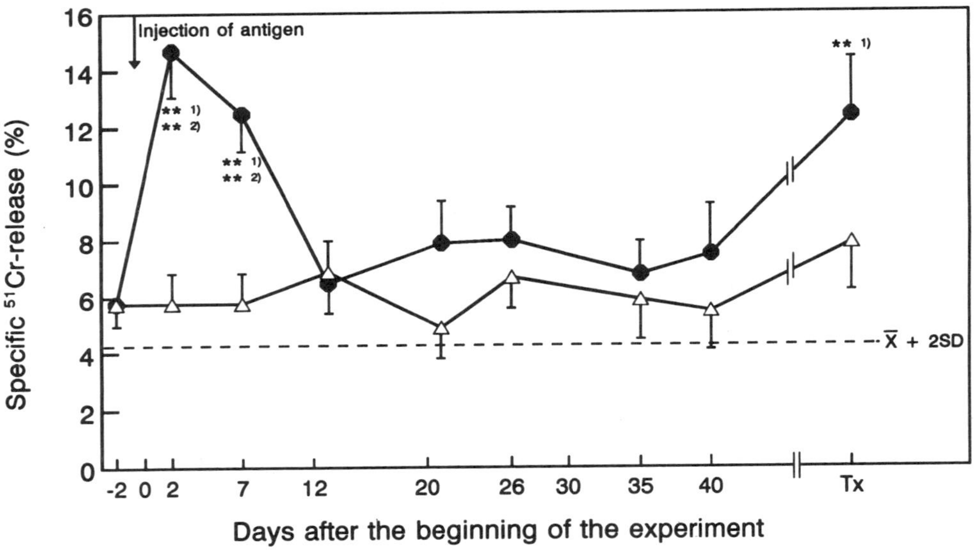

Figure 1. Comparison of C′AMC to islet cells in sera from BB/OK rats becoming diabetic (●—● n=11) or remaining normoglycaemic (Δ—Δ n=22) after syngeneic islet antigen injection as measured by ^{51}Cr-release. Tx marks day 81 in animals remaining normoglycaemic and the time of manifestation in diabetic rats. **1)** denotes significantly increased C′AMC compared to the initial value. **2)** indicates significant differences between diabetic and normoglycaemic animals. The dashed line (---) respresents the mean + 2SD of ^{51}Cr-release caused by WOK rat sera. Values are given as mean ± SEM. $^{**}p < 0.01$.

The administration of homogenate of syngeneic lymphocytes to diabetes-prone BB/OK rats also did not induce a differential time course of the appearance of humoral-mediated cytotoxicity to spleen lymphocytes in rats becoming diabetic or maintaining normoglycaemia (Figure 2, panel B).

Consequently, a differential immunological reactivity of diabetic and long-term normoglycaemic BB/OK rats as expressed by the pattern of C′AMC found upon syngeneic islet homogenate application (Figure 1) is not always produced after contact of the organism with destroyed own tissue and therefore does not reflect a generalized response on syngeneic antigens but seems to be related to the presence of islet antigen constituents.

By estimating the behaviour of anti-islet C′AMC in individual BB/OK rats 7 days after intrasplenic islet antigen administration it was found that 39.3% (13/33) of all islet homogenate-treated BB/OK rats exhibited C′AMC exceeding the mean + 1SD of the initial value of C′AMC of the animal group before islet antigen application (^{51}Cr-release of 9.4%). Among those BB/OK rats 61.5% (8/13) subsequently developed diabetes whereas 38.5% (5/13) remained long-term normoglycaemic. Thus, an increase of C′AMC to islet cells as detected in the investigated animal group upon challange with syngeneic islet antigen seems to define a subgroup of BB/OK rats with an increased risk of diabetes but does not allow to definitely predict an impending onset of the disease in the individual animal.

To further elucidate the immunological reactivity of diabetes-prone BB/OK rats the appearance of antibodies to glutamate decarboxylase (GAD) upon islet antigen administration was assayed. It might be expected that GAD as a constituent of the injected islet homogenate may influence the time course of the formation of GAD antibodies. However, islet homogenate and buffer-treated BB/OK rats exhibited a similar time course of the

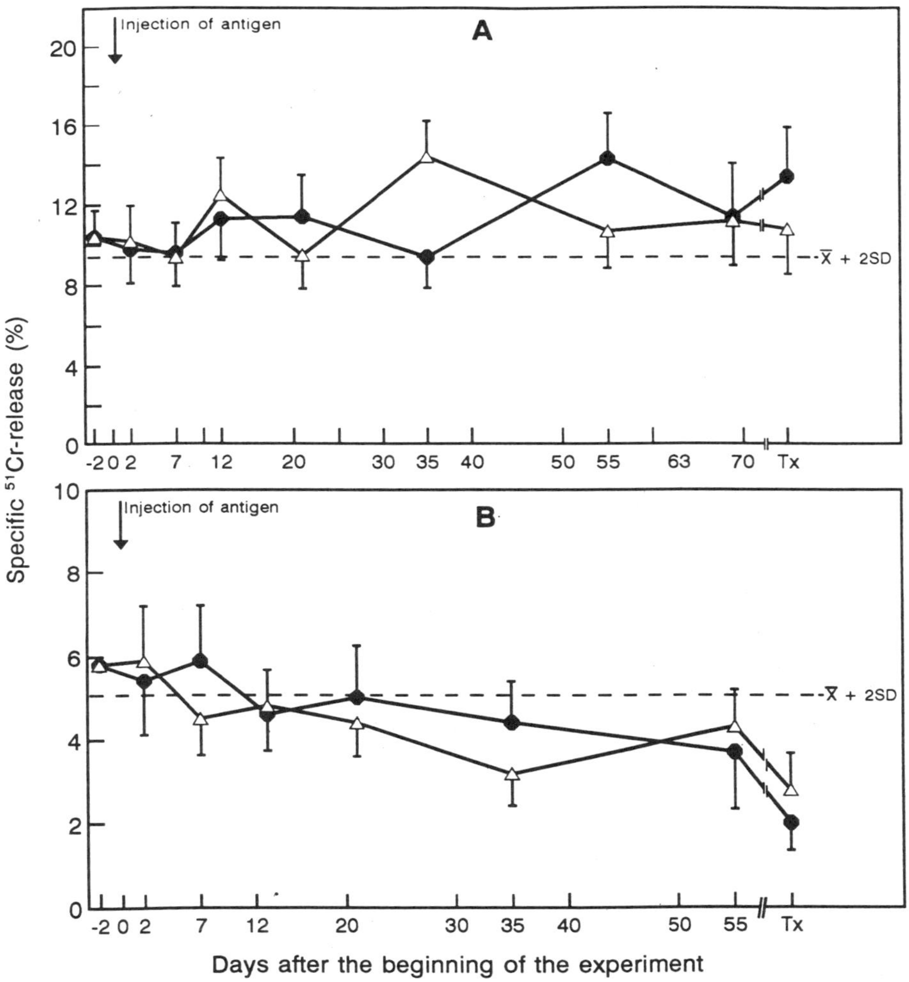

Figure 2. Comparison of C'AMC to pancreatic exocrine cells in sera from BB/OK rats becoming diabetic (●—● n=10) or remaining normoglycaemic (△—△ n=16) after intrasplenic administration of homogenate of syngeneic pancreatic exocrine cells (panel A) as well as comparison of humoral-mediated cytotoxicity to lymphocytes in sera from BB/OK rats becoming diabetic (●—● n=16) or remaining normoglycaemic (△—△ n=20) after injection of homogenate of syngeneic lymphocytes (panel B) as measured by ^{51}Cr-release. Tx marks day 81 in animals remaining normoglycaemic and the time of manifestation in diabetic rats. The dashed line (---) represents the mean + 2SD of ^{51}Cr-release caused by WOK rat sera. Values are given as mean ± SEM.

appearance of GAD antibodies (Figure 3, panel A and B). Independent on whether the animals were subjected to an administration of islet antigen (Figure 3, panel A) or buffer (Figure 3, panel B) GAD antibodies were detectable for the first time 20 to 26 days after the corresponding treatment when the rats were 50 to 55 days old. This parallels recent findings also proving the earliest appearance of GAD antibodies in untreated BB/OK rats at around 50 days of age (Schlosser et al., 1993). Islet antigen-treated BB/OK rats becoming diabetic or remaining long-term normoglycaemic displayed nearly identical time patterns of the appearance of GAD antibodies (Figure 3, panel A), thus giving no hints to a differential immunological reactivity of the animals with respect to the GAD antibody response.

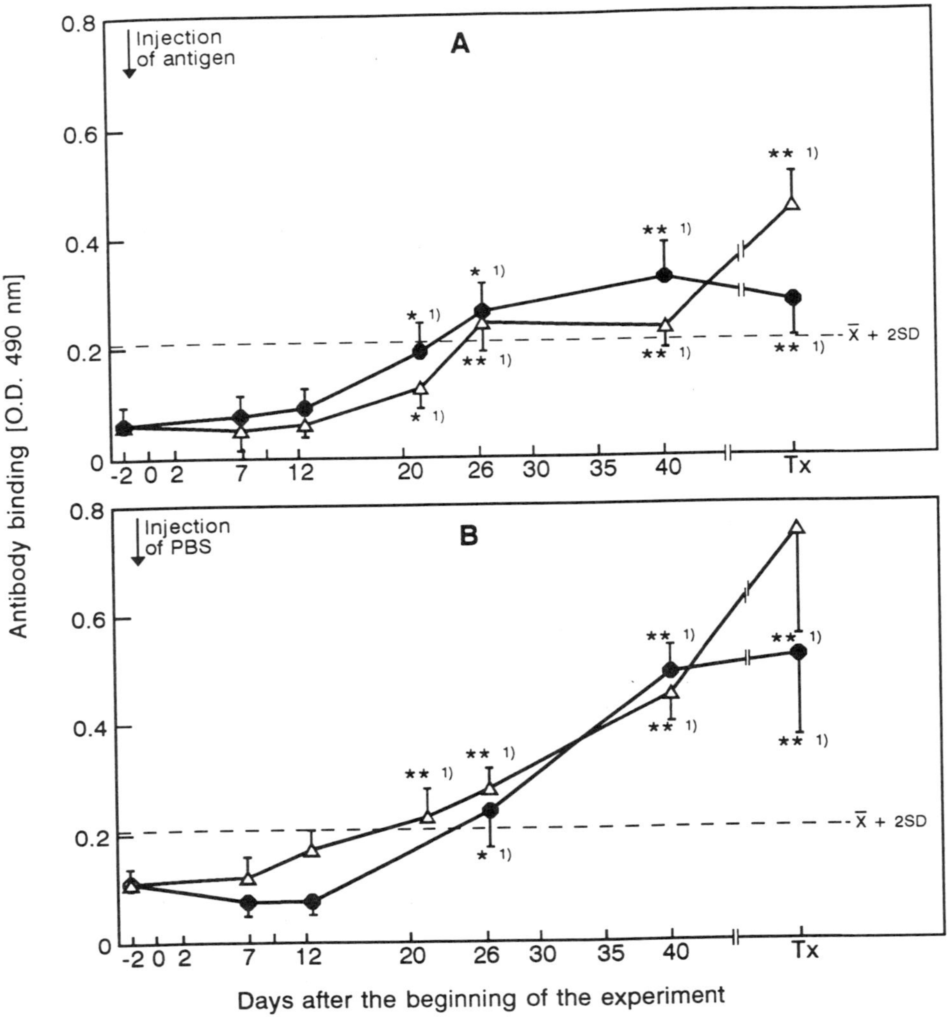

Figure 3. Time course of the appearance of antibodies to glutamate decarboxylase (GAD) as measured by ELISA in sera from BB/OK rats becoming diabetic (●—● n=10) or remaining normoglycaemic (Δ—Δ n=10) after intrasplenic administration of syngeneic islet antigen (panel A) or PBS (panel B). The cut off point for antibody positivity (mean + 2SD, O.D. 0.22) was determined by the investigation of sera from diabetes resistant LEW.1A rats and is indicated by the dashed line (---). Tx marks day 81 in normoglycaemic rats and the time of manifestation in diabetic animals. 1) denotes a significant difference to the initial value. Values are given as mean ± SEM. $*p < 0.05$; $**p < 0.01$.

The increase of C'AMC to islet cells upon islet antigen applica-tion in BB/OK rats becoming diabetic but the failure to accelerate diabetes onset or to affect the incidence of diabetes would suggest that anti-islet C'AMC is not decisively involved in the initiation of β-cell destruction in BB/OK rats. However, at the time of manifestation the pancreatic insulin content of diabetic BB/OK rats subjected to islet homogenate application was decreased compared to animals treated with pancreatic exocrine tissue or spleen lymphocytes as well as with buffer whereas the glucagon content was not affected (Table 2). This reduction of the pancreatic insulin content was accompanied by a slightly but not signifi-

Table 2. Effect of intrasplenic administration of syngeneic antigens on diabetes-prone BB/OK rats. Characteristics of the endocrine pancreas of diabetic animals at onset of the disease. Values are given as mean ± SEM

Treatment of the animals	Pancreatic insulin content (pmol/mg wet/wt)	Pancreatic glucagon content (pmol/mg wet/wt)	Relative islet volume density (%)	Relative β-cell volume density (%)	Insulitis (%)
Injection of islet homogenate	1.26 ± 0.23 n = 10	1.16 ± 0.26 n = 10	0.59 ± 0.10 n = 6	below the detection limit	80.6 ± 8.52 n = 7
Injection of homogenate of pancreatic exocrine cells	2.97 ± 0.54 n = 9	0.96 ± 0.15 n = 10	0.70 ± 0.23 n = 6	0.015 ± 0.009 n = 6	81.3 ± 6.13 n = 6
Injection of homogenate of lymphocytes	3.25 ± 0.71 n = 16	0.85 ± 0.11 n = 16	0.73 ± 0.22 n = 19	0.079 ± 0.03 n = 9	77.7 ± 9.99 n = 9
Injection of phosphate-buffered saline (PBS) (control)	3.34 ± 0.05 n = 21	0.91 ± 0.12 n = 21	0.95 ± 0.13 n = 14	0.037 ± 0.016 n = 15	79.4 ± 5.65 n = 14

(Pancreatic insulin content: islet homogenate vs. exocrine cells **; islet homogenate vs. lymphocytes **; islet homogenate vs. PBS *)

cantly reduced relative islet volume density and β-cells were morphologically nearly not detectable in these animals (Table 2). Thus, it seems that C′AMC to islet cells is able to influence the extent of β-cell alteration in an already initiated process leading to overt diabetes and to contribute to an additional loss of remaining β-cells. This suggestion is supported by previous findings demonstrating an increase of C′AMC to islet cells after transplantation of syngeneic islets into newly diagnosed diabetic BB/OK rats (Schröder et al., 1987) as well as into long-term diabetic BB/OK rats (Schröder et al., 1990) in those animals which rejected the islet graft.

CONCLUSIONS

Diabetic and long-term normoglycaemic BB/OK rats display a differential immunological reactivity to syngeneic islet antigens but not to syngeneic antigens in general as indicated by a selective increase of anti-islet C′AMC in a portion of animals developing diabetes. An increase of anti-islet C′AMC following syngeneic islet antigen application seems to define a subgroup of BB/OK rats at high risk of diabetes but does not allow to definitely predict an onset of the disease in the individual animal. C′AMC to islet cells is not decisively involved in the initiation of β-cell destruction and promotion of diabetes development but seems to affect the loss of remaining pancreatic insulin content in the course of an already on going β-cell destructive process leading to diabetes.

ACKNOWLEDGMENTS

The authors wish to thank Mrs. J. Stephan, Mrs. D. Schulz, Mrs. S. Sadewasser for skilful technical assistance and Mrs. M. Luedecke for typing of the manuscript. This study was supported by the Federal Initiative for the Development of Research in the new Federal States of Germany (KAI e.V., project No 018293/M) and the Deutsche Forschungsgemeinschaft grant Schr. 401/1-1.

REFERENCES

Besch, W., Woltanski, K.P., Keilacker, H., Diaz-Alonso, J.M., Schulz, B., Amend, P., Kohnert, K.D. and Ziegler, M., 1987, Measurement of insulin in human sera using a new RIA Kit. 1. Insulin determination in the absence of insulin antibodies — conventional assay and micro modification. Exp. Clin. Endocrinol., 90: 264–270.

Dyrberg, T., Poussier, P., Nakhooda, F., Marliss, E.B. and Lernmark, A., 1984, Islet cell surface and lymphocyte antibodies often precede the spontaneous diabetes in the BB rat. Diabetologia, 26: 159–165.

Hanenberg, H., Kolb-Bachofen, V., Kantwerk-Funke, G. and Kolb, H., 1989, Macrophage infiltration precedes and is a prerequisite for lymphocytic insulitis in pancreatic islets of prediabetic BB rats. Diabetologia, 32: 126–134.

Hehmke, B., Kohnert, K.D. and Odselius, R., 1986, The use of a new dextran gradient medium for rapid isolation of functionally intact neonatal rat pancreatic islets. Diabetes Res., 3: 13–16.

Hehmke, B., Schröder, D. and Klöting I., 1990, Early appearance of complement-dependent antibody-mediated cytotoxicity (C′AMC) to islet cells in serum of diabetes- prone BB/OK rats. Diabetes Res., 13: 183–186.

Koevary, St., Rossini, A., Stoller, W., Chick, W. and Williams, R.M., 1983, Passive transfer of diabetes in the BB/W rat. Science, 220: 727–728.

Logothetopoulos, J., Valiquette, N., Madura, F. and Cvet, D., 1984, The onset and progression of pancreatic insulitis in the overt spontaneously diabetic, young adult BB rat studied by pancreatic biopsy. Diabetes, 33: 33–36.

Lucke, S., Ziegler, B., Diaz-Alonso, J.M. and Hahn, H.J., 1985, Eignung spezifischer Färbemethoden für die Bestimmung des β-Zellvolumens im Pankreas mit normalem und reduziertem Insulingehalt. Acta histochem., 77: 106–116.

Lucke, S., Besch, W., Kauert, Ch. and Hahn, H.J., 1988. The endocrine pancreas of BB/OK rats before and at diagnosis of hyperglycaemia. Exp. Clin. Endocrinol., 91: 161–170.

Martin, D.R. and Logothetopoulos, J., 1984, Complement-fixing islet cell antibodies in the spontaneously diabetic BB rat. Diabetes, 33: 93–96.

Nakhooda, A.F., Like, A.A., Chappel, C.J., Murray, F.T. and Marliss, E.B., 1977, The spontaneously diabetic Wistar rat. Metabolic and morphological studies. Diabetes, 26: 100–112.

Schlosser, M., Ziegler, B., Hamann, J., Vieregge, P., Klöting, I. and Ziegler, M., 1993, Autoantibodies to glutamate decarboxylase have no predictive value for onset of diabetes in BB/OK rats. Diabetologia, 36: Suppl. 1, A 10 abstract 31.

Schröder, D., Hehmke, B., Klöting, I., Besch, W. and Hahn, H.J., 1987, Complement-dependent cytotoxicity to islet cells and lymphocytes in diabetes-prone BB/OK rats. Diabetologia, 30: 579 A.

Schröder, D., Wanka, H., Hehmke, B., Klöting, I., Köhler, E., Knospe, S. and Schmidt, S., 1990, Beta cell destruction of pancreatic islets transplanted into diabetic BB/OK rats may be reflected by increased antibody-mediated anti-islet cytotoxicity. Diabetes Res., 15: 27–32.

Schröder, D., Hehmke, B., Klöting, I. and Schmidt, S., 1991, Detection and time course of humoral-mediated cytotoxicity to different cell types in diabetes-prone BB/OK rats. Diabetes Res., 17: 81–91.

Schröder, D., Schmidt, S., Klöting, I. and Hehmke, B., 1993, Effect of syngeneic islet antigen administration on complement-dependent antibody-mediated cytotoxicity to islet cells and diabetes onset in diabetes-prone BB/OK rats. Autoimmunity, 14: 283–289.

Ziegler, M., Schlosser M., Hamann, J., Vieregge, P., Lühder, F., Klöting, I. and Ziegler, B., 1994, Autoantibodies to glutamate decarboxylase detected in diabetes-prone BB/OK rats do not distinguish onset of diabetes. Exp. Clin. Endocrinol., 102: 98–103.

47

EFFECTS OF OXIDANTS ON MEMBRANE POTENTIAL, K^+ AND Ca^{2+} CURRENTS OF MOUSE PANCREATIC B-CELLS

Peter Krippeit-Drews,[1] Stefan Britsch,[2] Florian Lang,[1] and Gisela Drews[1]

[1]Department of Physiology, Gmelinstr. 5
[2]Department of Gastroenterology, Otfried-Müller-Str. 10
University of Tübingen
D-72076 Tübingen, Germany

INTRODUCTION

K^+ATP channels play a key role in controlling membrane potential and insulin secretion in pancreatic B-cells (Ashcroft and Rorsman, 1989). Therefore, the regulation of these and of other channels involved in the control of the B-cell membrane potential is of great interest. Agents oxidizing SH-groups have been shown to influence K^+ channel activity and function in a variety of different cell types such as skeletal muscle cells (Weik and Neumcke, 1989), neurons (Ruppersberg *et al.*, 1991), lung adenocarcinoma cells (Kuo *et al.*, 1993) and liver cells (Hallbrucker *et al.*, 1993). Islam *et al.* (1993) have shown that the oxidizing agent 2,2′-dithio-bis(5-nitropyridine) (DTBNP) leads to closure of K^+ATP channels in pancreatic B-cells. They propose that this effect would increase insulin secretion. However, it has also been shown that SH-group oxidizing agents diminish insulin release (Ammon *et al.*, 1983), an effect which may be a result of the opening of K^+ channels. Our data demonstrate that H_2O_2 in contrast to DTBNP stimulates the K^+ATP current in mouse pancreatic B-cells and that thiol reagents also affect the current through voltage-dependent Ca^{2+} channels.

METHODS

Experiments were performed with islets and islet cells of fed female NMRI mice. The membrane potential of single B-cells was continuously recorded with high-resistance microelectrodes according to Meissner and Schmelz (1974). The bath medium contained (in mmol/l): 120 NaCl, 4.8 KCl, 2.5 $CaCl_2$, 1.2 $MgCl_2$, 24 $NaHCO_3$, gassed with O_2:CO_2 (95:5) to maintain a pH of 7.4 at 37°C.

Patch-clamp experiments were performed with islet cells, isolated and cultured as described by Plant (1988). Whole-cell recordings of the K^+_{ATP} current were performed without

Physiology and Pathophysiology of the Islets of Langerhans, edited by Soria.
Plenum Press, New York, 1997.

(fast whole-cell, FWC) or with nystatin (slow whole-cell, SWC) (Horn and Marty, 1988) in the pipette solution (150–250 mmol/l). The pipette solution also contained (in mmol/l): 140 KCl, 4 $MgCl_2$, 2 $CaCl_2$, 10 EGTA, 0.65 Na_2-ATP, 20 HEPES, pH 7.15 adjusted with KOH in the FWC mode or 10 KCl, 10 NaCl, 70 K_2SO_4, 4 $MgCl_2$, 2 $CaCl_2$, 10 EGTA, 20 HEPES, pH 7.15 adjusted with KOH in the SWC mode. Bath solution was composed of (in mmol/l): 140 NaCl, 5.6 KCl 1.2 $MgCl_2$, 2.6 $CaCl_2$, 0.5 glucose, 10 HEPES, pH 7.4 adjusted with NaOH. Currents were measured as described by Garrino et al. (1989). The holding potential was –70 mV.

B-cell Ca^{2+} channel currents were also recorded in the FWC and SWC mode. Cells were bathed in a solution containing (in mmol/l): 115 NaCl, 20 TEACl, 10 $CaCl_2$ or $BaCl_2$, 1.2 $MgCl_2$, 0.1 tolbutamide, 15 glucose, 10 HEPES, pH 7.4 adjusted with NaOH. For fast whole-cell experiments the pipette solution was composed of (in mmol/l): 50 CsCl, 70 N-methyl-D-glucamine, 58 HCl, 4 $MgCl_2$, 3 Na_2ATP, 10 EGTA, 2 $CaCl_2$, 10 HEPES, pH 7.15 adjusted with CsOH. For slow whole-cell experiments the pipette solution was (in mmol/l): 70 Cs_2SO_4, 10 NaCl, 10 KCl, 7 $MgCl_2$, 10 HEPES, pH 7.4 with NaOH. The nystatin concentration in the pipette was up to 250 μmol/l.

The patch-clamp experiments were carried out at 25°C.

Results are presented as means ± SEM or as representative recordings for n = number of experiments. Statistical significance was accepted for $P \leq 0.05$.

RESULTS AND DISCUSSION

Pancreatic B-cells exhibit a typical electrical activity in the presence of 15 mmol/l glucose (control conditions). This activity consists of slow waves of the membrane potential with superimposed Ca^{2+} action potentials on the plateau potential. Part A of Figure 1 illustrates a

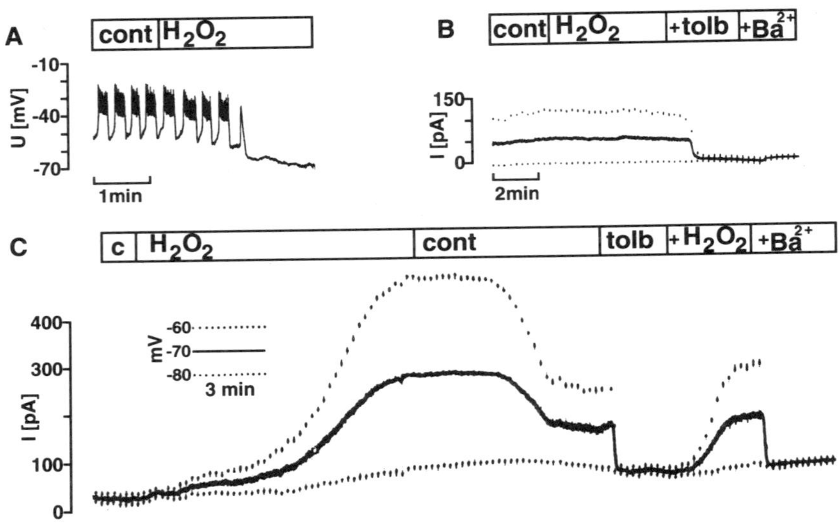

Figure 1. **A:** Effect of 1 mmol/l H_2O_2 on the membrane potential of mouse pancreatic B-cells recorded with an intracellular microelectrode in the presence of 15 mmol/l glucose. **B–C:** Effects of H_2O_2 (1 mmol/l), tolbutamide (100 μmol/l) and $BaCl_2$ (10 mmol/l) on K^+_{ATP} currents measured in the FWC mode (B) or SWC mode (C). Pulse protocol as shown in the inset in C. Holding potential –70 mV.

recording of the membrane potential, representative of six experiments with similar results. Under control conditions the fraction of the plateau phase was 46 ± 6%. Addition of H_2O_2 (1 mmol/l) led to a fast and marked hyperpolarization of the membrane potential by 18 ± 1 mV (Krippeit-Drews *et al.*, 1994a). This hyperpolarization abolished electrical activity which was not restored after wash-out of H_2O_2. The membrane potential remained hyperpolarized in the steady state. A lower concentration of H_2O_2 (0.1 mmol/l) was without effect.

Part C of Figure 1 illustrates an SWC K^+_{ATP} current recording measured with 250 µmol/l nystatin in the pipette. The current at the holding potential and during voltage steps to –80 mV and to –60 mV (pulse protocol in the inset) is low under control conditions and almost entirely a result of K^+_{ATP} channel activity. There was a difference of 33 ± 8 pA between the currents at –70 mV and –60 mV (n=11). This difference was always calculated as a means of quantifying effects on the current. After addition of 1 mmol/l H_2O_2 the outward current slowly increased to a difference of 169 ± 19 pA (n=8) (Krippeit-Drews *et al.*, 1994a). It is very likely that this outward current is responsible for the observed hyperpolarization. However, wash-out of H_2O_2 partly reversed the effect on the SWC current to a difference of 90 ± 22 pA (n=6). This remaining outward current was almost entirely K^+_{ATP} current, because it was blocked by tolbutamide (100 µmol/l) to only 7 ± 3 pA (n=6).

Part B of Figure 1 (1 representative recording of 4) shows that in the FWC mode 1 mmol/l H_2O_2 has no effect on the K^+_{ATP} current. Apparently, the effect of H_2O_2 requires an intracellular component which is lost by the cell dialysis in the FWC mode. In endothelial cells and in a macrophage-like cell line, H_2O_2 treatment leads to an exhaustion of intracellular ATP (Spragg *et al.*, 1985). If this holds true for B-cells, one can speculate that the increase in K^+_{ATP} current after wash-out of H_2O_2 versus control is due to the H_2O_2-induced ATP depletion. The remaining increase in K^+_{ATP} current may in turn explain why the membrane potential remains hyperpolarized, even after wash-out of H_2O_2.

A second addition of 1mmol/l H_2O_2, in the presence of 100 µmol/l tolbutamide (Figure 1, part C), led to an increase of an outwardly directed current to a mean difference of 62 ± 11 pA (n=6) between currents at –70 mV and –60 mV. This current is totally blocked by the subsequent addition of 10 mmol/l $BaCl_2$ (2 ± 1 pA, n=3), demonstrating that it is a K^+ current. Experiments in the SWC mode where different concentrations of tolbutamide have been added in the presence of H_2O_2 suggest that the sulfonylurea sensitivity has been reduced during the exposure to the oxidant (Krippeit-Drews *et al.*, 1994a).

Recently, Islam *et al.* (1993) have shown that oxidation of SH-groups with DTBNP leads to the closure of K^+_{ATP} channels. This observation, opposite to the effect of H_2O_2, is confirmed by our results (Fig. 2). Under control conditions, the FWC K^+_{ATP} current measured during a 10 mV depolarizing step from the holding potential of –70 mV was 109 ± 17 pA (n=6). It decreased to 31 ± 7 pA with 20 µmol/l DTBNP (n=4) and to 8 ± 5 pA with 100 µmol/l DTBNP (n=3) (Krippeit-Drews *et al.*, 1994b). The effect of DTBNP was at least partly reversed by the reducing agent DTE (dithioerythritol) (Fig. 2, Islam *et al.*, 1993). The effects of DTBNP have been observed in the FWC mode where the cell interior is dialyzed. This suggests that it acts on SH-groups located on the channel or on channel regulating proteins in the membrane.

DTBNP also strongly reduced the current through voltage-dependent Ca^{2+} channels (Fig. 3). In these experiments Ba^{2+} was used as charge carrier and the current elicited by depolarizing steps from the holding potential of –70 mV to 0 mV was monitored. On average, the inward current under control conditions was –94 ± 14 pA (n=6) in the FWC configuration. The current amplitude was reduced to –36 ± 5 pA (n=6) after addition of 20 µmol/l DTBNP and to –10 ± 3 pA when the DTBNP concentration was increased to 100 µmol/l (Krippeit-Drews *et al.*, 1994b).

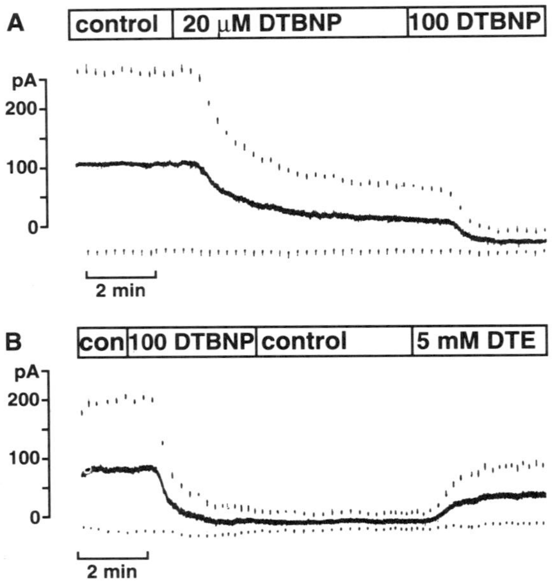

Figure 2. Effects of 20 μmol/l and 100 μmol/l DTBNP on FWC K^{+}_{ATP} currents (A) and of subsequent addition of 5 mmol/l DTE (B). Same pulse protocol as in Fig. 1.

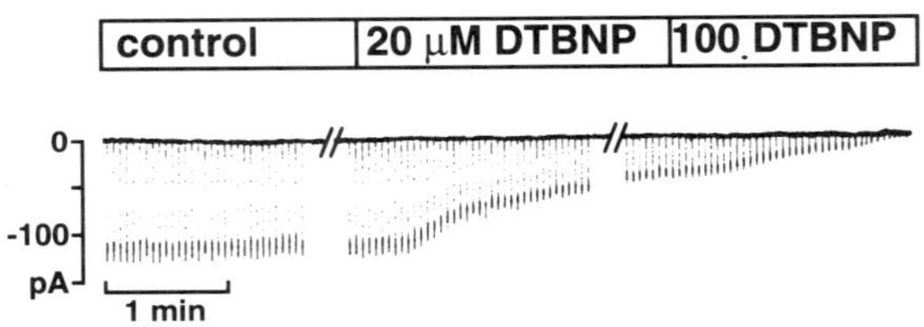

Figure 3. Effects of 20 μmol/l and 100 μmol/l DTBNP on FWC Ba^{2+} current through voltage-dependent Ca^{2+} channels. Currents were elicited every 3 s during 50 ms pulses from the holding potential of −70 mV to 0 mV.

In contrast, H_2O_2 neither affected the current through Ca^{2+} channels in the conventional nor in the perforated patch configuration (Krippeit-Drews *et al.*, 1994b).

In conclusion, SH-group oxidation by DTBNP inhibits K^{+}_{ATP} and Ca^{2+} channel currents in mouse pancreatic B-cells, suggesting that functional important SH-groups are located in the channels or in proteins influencing the activity of the channels. H_2O_2 influences B-cell function by a distinct mechanism, whereby the reduction of the cytoplasmic ATP concentration might be involved.

ACKNOWLEDGMENTS

This work was supported by grants of the Deutsche Forschungsgemeinschaft (Dr 225/1-2 and Kr 1386/1-1). We are grateful to Drs. M. Rack, H. Heinle, A. and G.L. Busch for helpful discussions. We thank Mrs. U. Hamacher, Mrs. V. Janle and Mrs. U. Emerich for skillful technical assistance.

REFERENCES

Ammon, H.P.T., Hägele, R., Youssif, N., Eujen, R., El-Amri, N., 1983, A possible role of intracellular and membrane thiols of rat pancreatic islets in calcium uptake and insulin release, *Endocrinology* 112:720.

Ashcroft , F.M., Rorsman, P., 1989, Electrophysiology of the pancreatic B-cell, *Prog. Biophys. Molec. Biol.* 54:87.

Garrino, M.G., Plant, T.D., Henquin, J.C., 1989, Effects of putative activators of K^+ channel in mouse pancreatic B-cells, *Br. J. Pharmacol.* 98:957.

Hallbrucker, C., Ritter, M., Lang, F., Gerok, W., Häussinger, D., 1993, Hydroperoxide metabolism in rat liver. K^+ channel activation, cell volume changes and eicosanoid formation, *Eur. J. Biochem.* 211: 449.

Horn, R., Marty, A., 1988, Muscarinic activation of ionic currents measured by a new whole-cell recording method, *J. Gen. Physiol.* 92:145.

Islam, M.S., Berggren, P.-O., Larsson, O., 1993, Sulhydryl oxidation induces rapid and reversible closure of the ATP-regulated K^+ channel in the pancreatic B-cell, *FEBS Lett.* 319:128.

Krippeit-Drews, P., Lang, F., Häussinger, D., Drews, G., 1994a, H_2O_2 induced hyperpolarization of pancreatic B-cell. *Pflügers Arch.* 426:552.

Krippeit-Drews, P., Britsch, S., Drews, G., 1994b, Effects of SH-group reagents on Ca^{2+} and K^+ channel currents of pancreatic B-cells, *Biochem. Biophys. Res. Commun.* 200:860.

Kuo, S.S., Saad, A.H., Koong, A.C., Hahn, G.M., Giaccia, A.J., 1993 Potassium-channel activation in response to low doses of γ-irradation involves reactive oxygen intermediates in nonexcitory cells, *Proc. Natl. Acad. Sci.* 90:908.

Meissner, H.P., Schmelz H., 1974, Membrane potential of Beta-cells in pancreatic islets, *Pflügers Arch.* 351:195.

Plant, T.D., 1988, Properties and calcium-dependent inactivation of calcium currents in cultured mouse pancreatic β-cells, *J. Physiol.* 404:731.

Spragg, R.G., Hinshaw, D.B., Hyslop, P.A., Schraufstätter, I.U., Cochrane, C.G., 1985, Alterations in adenosine triphosphate and energy charge in cultured endothelial and $P338D_1$ cells after oxidant injury, *J. Clin. Invest.* 76:1471.

Weik, R., Neumcke, B., 1989, ATP-sensitive potassium channels in adult mouse skeletal muscle: Characterization of the ATP-binding site. *J. Membrane Biol.* 110:217.

Part VII. PATHOPHYSIOLOGY OF THE NIDDM

48

IAPP AND INSULIN REGULATION IN HUMAN PANCREATIC ISLETS

A. Novials, R. Gasa, J. Fernandez-Alvarez, and R. Gomis*

Endocrinology and Diabetes Unit. Hospital Clínic
School of Medicine
Barcelona University

INTRODUCTION

One of the characteristic features of type 2 diabetes is the presence of extracellular deposition of amyloid in the islets of Langerhans (1). The storage of amyloid is characteristic of several animal species, i.e. humans, cats, and monkeys (2,3). The principal component of islet amyloid is a peptide designated as islet amyloid polypeptide (IAPP) or amylin, which is synthesized and stored in beta cells (4). In vivo and in vitro experiments in rats have shown that IAPP is coreleased with insulin in a regulated manner after different secretagogue stimulus (5).

The physiologic role of IAPP has not been defined but it has been suggested their participation in the process of glucose uptake by the skeletal muscle (6). This potential role of IAPP in the peripheral glucose metabolism suggests that the regulation of its synthesis and secretion in the beta cell might be relevant to understanding the pathogenesis of type 2 diabetes mellitus (7,8).

The aim of the present work was to analize the regulation of IAPP and insulin in isolated human pancreatic islets.

MATERIALS AND METHODS

Human Pancreatic Islet Isolation

A multicenter program on Islet Cell Trasplantation in Diabetes has been initiated in Spain with the support of *Fondo de Investigaciones Sanitarias*. The aim of this program is

* Correspondence should be adressed to R. Gomis. Endocrinology and Diabetes Unit. Hospital Clínic. Villarroel 170. Barcelona 08036, Spain.

to construct islet cell grafts of selected size and composition in order to test their potential in a clinical trial. Participating clinical centers collect the human donor organs and send them to the Experimental Diabetes Laboratory of Hospital Clínic in Barcelona where pancreatic islets are prepared, quality controlled and banked. Human cell aggregates are distributed to the associated laboratories to use them in approved research projects focusing on specific questions, and also to participating clinical centers to use them on clinical trials.

Human pancreatic islets were isolated following a modification of Ricordi's automatic technique. The pancreatic duct was cannulated and a solution of 2.5 mg of collagenase type P (Boehringer Mannheim, Germany) per ml of Hanks' Balanced salt solution was injected through the pancreatic duct at a rate of 2 ml per gram of tissue. After injection of the collagenase solution, the piece of pancreas was placed in a digestion chamber which contained five glass marbles to improve the efficiency of shaken. The chamber was connected to a close circuit where there was recircularization of the medium at 38°C and continously shaken. Afterwards, the samples were taken and tested every 3 minutes. These samples were stained with dithizone and then examined under stereomicroscope to select the endocrine from the exocrine tissue (see Fig. 1). When free islets were detected, less than 30 minutes in all cases, the digestion was stopped by quickly cooling the digestion chamber. The disintegrated pancreatic tissue was collected in precooled tubes containing 1% of newborn calf serum and washed several times by centrifugation. A 50 μl samples from this total digest were placed in reticulated Petri dishes, stained with dithizone and examined under an inverted microscope. A differential count by size of the islets was carried out using a calibrated grid. The equivalent number in relation to an standard islet of 150 μm diameter was calculated for each pancreas. In order to obtain purified material, islets were separated from exocrine tissue using a bovine-serum-albumin density gradient (9). Cell viability of the purified islets was assessed by ethidium bromide and acridine orange staining.

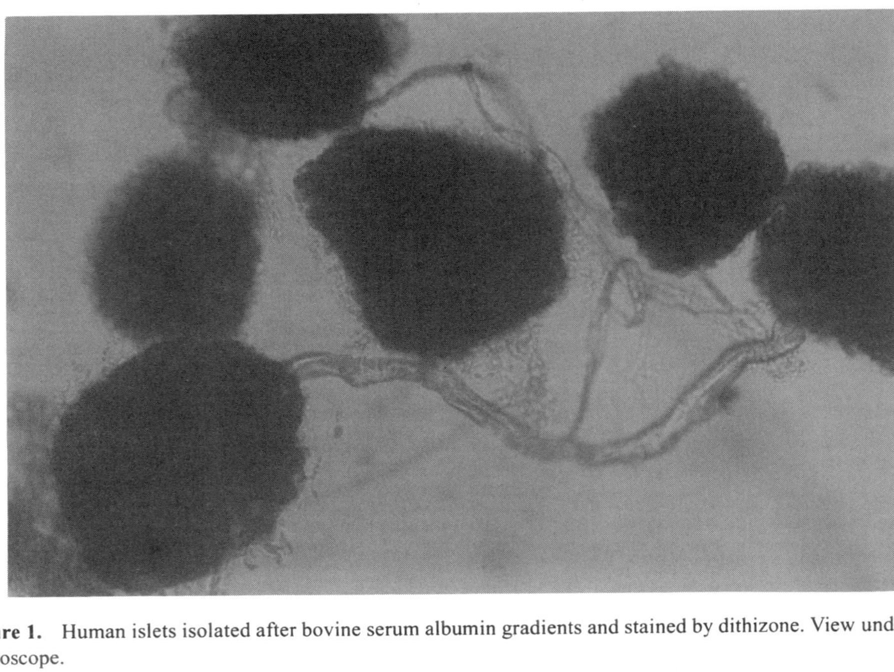

Figure 1. Human islets isolated after bovine serum albumin gradients and stained by dithizone. View under light microscope.

Islet Culture

Batches of 300 islets were placed in 10 ml of CMRL.1066 medium supplemented with 2.0 mM L-Glutamine, 10% heat-inactivated donor calf serum, penicillin (100 U/ml) and streptomycin (100 μg/ml) in Petri dishes. Final D-glucose concentration in the culture medium was 5.5 mM or 16.7 mM. All cultures were conducted at 37°C in a humidified atmosphere of 95% air–5% CO_2 for 1 or 7 days, and the medium was changed every 48 hours.

Insulin and IAPP Secretion

Batches of fresh and cultured islets were incubated in a shaking water bath for 90 min at 37°C in 1 ml of bicarbonate-buffered solution containing BSA 5mg per ml, 5.5 or 16.7 mM D-glucose plus 5 μM forskolin. At the end of incubation, supernatants were aliquoted and stored at −20°C until the radioimmunoassays for insulin (CIS Biointernational, Gif-Sur-Yvette, France) and IAPP (Peninsula, Belmont,CA) were performed.

Islet Insulin and IAPP Content

Fresh or cultured islets were disintegrated by the ultrasonic procedure in 0.5 ml acid-alcohol solution to analyze islet insulin and IAPP contents. The extracts were dried and reconstituted in 0.5 ml of the respective RIA buffer.

RNA Isolation and Northern Blot Analysis

Total RNA from islets was extracted by ultracentrifugation in cesium chloride gradient. The samples obtained per condition were loaded and electrophoresed on agarose-formaldehyde gel and transferred to a Z-probe nylon membrane. Filters were hybridized with ^{32}P-labeled probes. Complementary DNA probes a 1.7 kb BamHI fragment of human preproinsulin cDNA a 3.5-kb EcoRI/ Hind III fragment of human beta-actin cDNA (provided by G.Bell, Chicago, IL) and a 220-bp EcoRI/SmaI fragment of human IAPP cDNA (provided by J.C. Hutton, Cambridge,UK) were labeled with [^{32}P] CTP by random priming method and included at 1.2×10^6 cpm per ml. The autoradiograms were quantified by densitometry, and the area under the curve for each peak was calculated and normalized to the beta-actin control.

Statistical Analysis

All data were expressed as means ± SD. Statistical results were calculated with the use of the unpaired Student's t test.

RESULTS

A total of 41 glands reached to our laboratory in the course of 1990, 21 during 1991, 21 also during 1992 and 8 pancreases until july 1993. After digestion the average yield was 5800 islets per gram of processed tissue. The yield variability did not correlate with the age or the sex of the donor, the recorded time of cold ischemia, the donor center, the

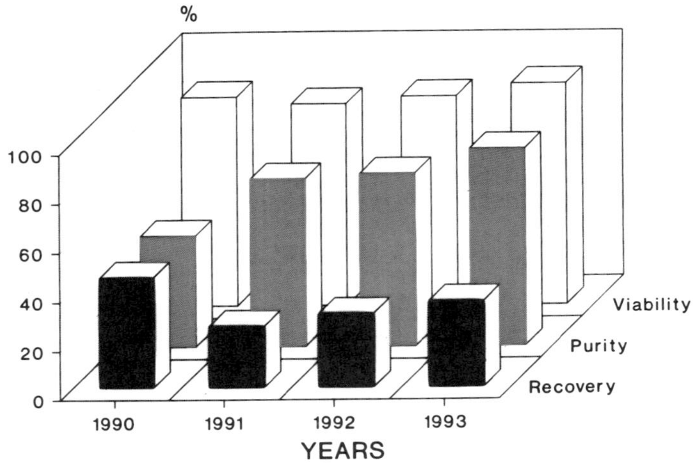

Figure 2. Human islets isolation. Percentage of viability, purity and recovery since the beginning of the Multicenter Program on Islet Cell Transplantation initiated in Spain.

amount of tissue available or the time required for digestion. As it is shown in Figure 2 the percentage of viability was maintained through the years. The recovery of islets diminished in relation to the first year, whereas the purity of the material improved because of modifications applied to the gradient's technique.

Figure 3 shows the IAPP and insulin secretory response of isolated human fresh islets to 0, 5.5 and 16.7 mM glucose and 5 μM forskolin. These results confirm that IAPP is cosecreted with insulin after a high glucose stimulus as it has been demontrated by other authors in animal models and cellular lines. However, while the insulin secretion was not affected by the previous culture, one or seven days at low or high glucose concentrations (Fig. 4), the islets were unable to enhance the IAPP secretion after culture at high glucose concentrations (Fig. 5). Table 1 summarizes the results of IAPP and insulin content of

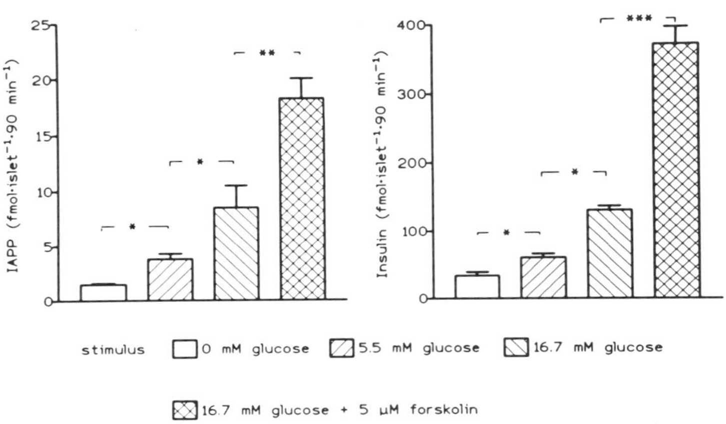

Figure 3. IAPP and Insulin secretory response of freshly isolated islets after different glucose stimulus. Data are means ± SE from 6 pancreases (2–4 experiments per pancreas). $^{*}P < 0.025$, $^{**}P < 0.005$, $^{***}P < 0.001$.

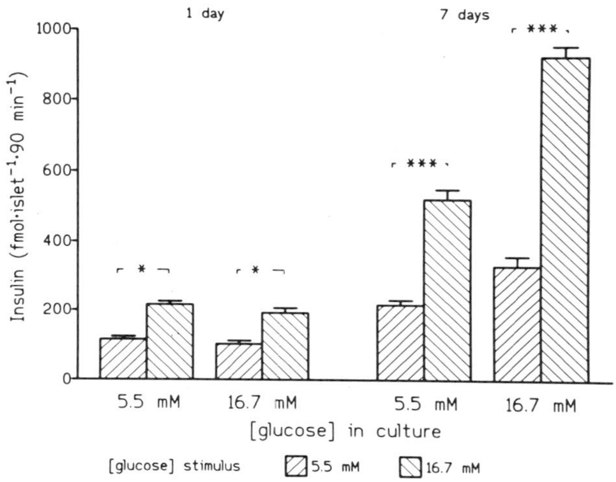

Figure 4. Insulin secretion from human islets cultured for 1 and 7 days at different glucose concentrations. Data are means ± SE from 4 pancreases (3–4 experiments per pancreas). $P < 0.01$, $***P < 0.001$.

fresh and cultured human islets. The most remarkable observation was the increase of IAPP content after seven days of culture at 16.7 mM glucose. In these conditions and compared with the seven days culture at 5.5 mM glucose the increase was more than 100% for IAPP and 50% for insulin.

The mRNA signals of IAPP, insulin and beta actin are shown in Figure 6. The IAPP and insulin signals increased after seven days culture in both low and high glucose concentrations. The densitometric analysis of signals normalized to the beta-actin control showed that the maximum mRNA expression for both transcripts was produced after the long exposure of islets to high glucose concentrations.

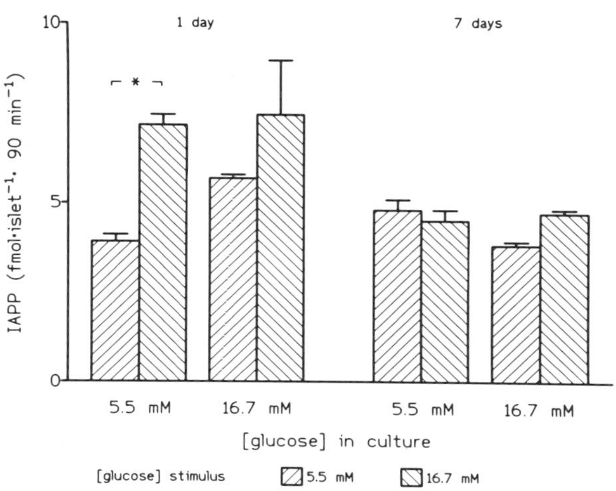

Figure 5. IAPP secretion from human islets cultured for 1 and 7 days at different glucose concentrations. Data are means ± SE from 4 pancreases (2–4 experiments per pancreas). $P < 0.01$.

Table 1. Human IAPP and insulin content of freshly and cultured islets

	Content		Fractional release	
	IAPP	Insulin	IAPP	Insulin
Freshly islets	166 ± 19	5600 ± 300	5.1%	2.3%
Cultured islets				
1 day				
5.5 mM	178 ± 10	5800 ± 300	4.0%	3.7%
16.7 mM	187 ± 24	5500 ± 300	4.0%	3.5%
7 days				
5.5 mM	209 ± 59*	10500 ± 300*	2.1%	4.9%
16.7 mM	462 ± 20	15600 ± 800	1.0%	5.9%

Data are taken from 2 pancreases (2–3 experiments per pancreas) and expressed as mean ± SEM (fmol of IAPP and insulin per islet). *$p < 0.05$.

DISCUSSION

IAPP, also called amylin, is the main peptide that has been isolated from amyloid deposits of type 2 diabetic pancreas. Controversy exists about the pathogenic role of IAPP in this metabolic disease.

The present work shows that the high glucose concentrations, mimicking chronic hyperglycemia are able to increase the expression of insulin mRNA, the hormone content and the secretion after an acute glucose stimulus in isolated human islets. However, while these conditions provoke a more relevant increase of IAPP mRNA and content, the islets are unable to increase their capacity to secrete IAPP after the same acute glucose stimulus, suggesting the existence of some regulatory differences between both peptides. Furthermore, the fractional release of insulin increases in relation to the duration of culture and the high glucose concentrations, meanwhile the IAPP fractional release diminishes despite its increase in islet content.

One emerging question after the observation of the present results is which signals derived from metabolism of glucose can modify the expresion of mRNA and protein contents of insulin and IAPP in islets. Preliminary results not shown in the paper, suggest a different way on the regulation of both peptides in human specimens related to the phos-

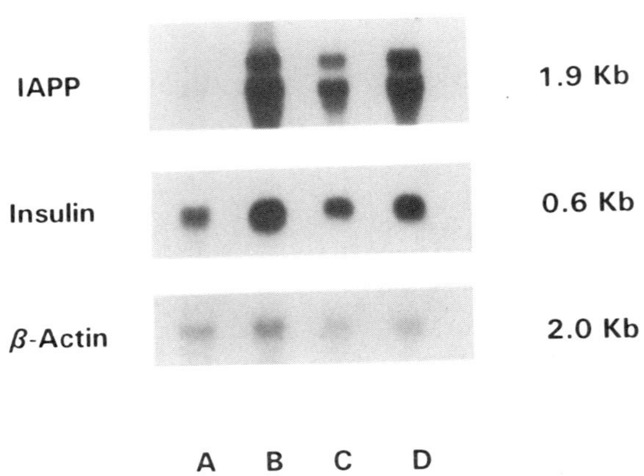

Figure 6. Northern blot analysis of IAPP, Insulin and Beta-Actin of islets cultured for 1 day at 5.5 and 16.7 mM glucose (A and B) and 7 days at same glucose concentrations (C and D).

phorylation and glycation of proteins, contrasting previous results obtained from rat or mice material.

The knowledge of the mechanisms that regulate gene expression, protein biosynthesis and secretory processes are relevant to investigate metabolic and molecular defects of islets in type 2 diabetes. The obtention of human islets from diseases related to the metabolism, i.e. obesity and type 2 diabetes mellitus might help this research project.

In summary, with the present results in mind, we conclude that glucose increases both IAPP mRNA and protein content in cultured human islets in the same way as for insulin, however, under the same conditions the secretory response to glucose of both peptides is dissociated (10). Additional investigations are needed to establish whether peptide processing or stimulus secretion coupling are regulated differently and to determine whether some alteration in these processes may result in IAPP deposition.

REFERENCES

1. Ehrlich JC, Ratner IM: Amyloidosis of the islets of Langerhans. Am J Pathol 38:49–59, 1961.
2. Westermark P, Wernstedt C, Wilander E, Haydn DW, O'Brien TD, Johnson KH: Amyloid fibrils in human insulinoma and islets of Langerhans of the diabetic cat are derived from a neuropeptide-like protein also present in normal islet cells. Proc Natl Acad Sci 84: 8628–8632, 1987.
3. Howard CF: Longitudinal studies on the development of diabetes in individual macaca nigra. Diabetologia 29: 301–306, 1986.
4. Cooper GJS, Willis AC, Clark A, Turner RC, Sim RB, Reid KBM: Purification and characterisation of a peptide from amyloid-rich pancreases of type 2 diabetic patients. Proc Nat Acad Sci 84: 8628–8632, 1987.
5. Fehmann HC, Weber V, Göke R, Göke B, Arnold R: Cosecretion of amylin and insulin from isolated rat pancreas FEBS Lett 262: 279–281, 1990.
6. Leighton B, Cooper GJS: Pancreatic amylin and calcitonin gene-related peptide cause resistance to insulin in skeletal muscle in vitro. Nature 335: 632–635, 1988.
7. Cooper GJS, Leighton B, Dimitradis GD, Parry-Billings M, Kowalchuk JM, Howland K, Rothbard JB, Willis AC, Reid KBM: Amylin found in amyloid deposits in human type 2 diabetes mellitus may be a hormone that regulates glycogen metabolism in skeletal muscle. Proc Natl Acad Sci 85: 7763–7766, 1988.
8. Porte D, Kahn SE: Hyperproinsulinaemia and amyloid in NIDDM: Clues to etiology of islet Beta cell dysfunction. Diabetes 38: 1333–1336, 1989.
9. Vives M, Sarri Y, Conget I, Somoza N, Alcalde L, Armengol P, Fernandez J, Lorenzo C, Martin M, Soldevila G, Fernandez-Usach E, Manalich M, Gomis R, Pujol-Borrell R: Human islet function after automatic isolation and bovine serum albumin gradient purification. Transplantation 53: 2443–2445, 1992.
10. Novials A, Sarri Y, Casamitjana R, Rivera F, Gomis R: Regulation of Islet Amyloid Polypeptide in Human Pancreatic Islets. Diabetes 42: 1514–1519, 1993.

49

HYPERPROINSULINAEMIA AND ISLET DYSFUCTION IN THE NIDDM-LIKE SYNDROME OF *Psammomys obesus*

Nurit Kaiser, Michal Gadot, Gil Leibowitz, Erol Cerasi, and David J. Gross

Departments of Endocrinology and Metabolism
Hebrew University-Hadassah Medical Center
Jerusalem 91120, Israel

INTRODUCTION

Patients with Type 2, non-insulin dependent diabetes (NIDDM) exhibit elevated plasma proinsulin to insulin ratios [1–9]. Recently, it has been shown that the plasma proinsulin-like fraction in these patients as well as in normal individuals is comprised of both proinsulin and partially cleaved proinsulin, primarily des 31,32 proinsulin [7,8]. It is assumed that the elevated ratio between proinsulin-related peptides and insulin reflects a β-cell abnormality, since the metabolic clearance rate of these peptides does not differ appreciably between normal individuals and patients with diabetes [10]. Reduction of the plasma glucose concentration in patients with NIDDM, irrespective of the means, was shown to improve insulin production and reduce the degree of hyperproinsulinaemia [3, 11–15]. These observations in man, as well as studies in animal models of diabetes [16–23] have led to the notion that hyperglycaemia *per se* might be implicated in the generation of a defective β-cell secretory response [24]. Alternatively, hyperglycaemia may play an important contributory role by amplifying a genetically determined β-cell defect, which may not be apparent until unmasked by a chronic increase in secretory demand.

In an attempt to investigate the relationship between chronic increase in insulin demand and the elevated ratio of proinsulin to insulin in the plasma of patients with NIDDM, we chose the *Psammomys obesus* as an experimental model [25,26]. This desert gerbil, trivially nicknamed "sand rat," is not known to develop diabetes in nature where it feeds on plants with low-calorie and high electrolyte content. However, when maintained in captivity and fed standard laboratory chow, it tends to develop obesity, hyperinsulinaemia and hyperglycaemia [25–27]. The hyperinsulinaemia usually precedes the onset of hyperglycaemia, and the high blood levels of immunoreactive insulin (IRI) suggest that insulin resistance contributes to the diabetic syndrome [28,29]. In the final stages of the disease, the animals become hypoinsulinaemic and ketotic and die unless treated with insulin [27]. The genetic background for diabetes tendency was recently demon-

Physiology and Pathophysiology of the Islets of Langerhans, edited by Soria.
Plenum Press, New York, 1997.

strated in the Hebrew University *Psammomys obesus* colony by the isolation of two lines which differ in their susceptibility to the diet-induced diabetes [30]. Thus, unlike other animal models utilized to study the relationship between hyperglycaemia and impaired islet cell function [16, 21,23,31], it offers the advantage of a genetically-determined, nutrition-evoked obesity and hyperglycaemia resembling some forms of NIDDM in man.

This study was aimed at evaluating the role of the endocrine pancreas in the development of the NIDDM-like syndrome in *Psammomys obesus*.

MATERIALS AND METHODS

Animals

Diabetic and non-diabetic hyperinsulinaemic *Psammomys obesus* of the Hebrew University colony [30] were used. Animals were weaned at 3 weeks and maintained on laboratory chow thereafter. Food and water were given *ad libitum*, unless stated otherwise. Blood glucose and body weight were monitored weekly. Animals were defined as diabetic when at least two consecutive blood glucose levels exceeded 11.1 mmol/l. All non-fasted *Psammomys* with blood glucose concentrations under 7.6 mmol/l were considered non-diabetic. Male Sprague-Dawley rats maintained on the same diet served as a control non-diabetic species in some of our studies. In experiments in which a fast was necessary, animals were deprived of food for 16–20 hours.

Islet Isolation

Psammomys anaesthetized with ketamine (Ketalar, Park-Davis, 0.5 ml of 50 mg/ml solution i.p.) were exsanguinated by cardiac puncture. Plasma samples were collected and frozen at –20°C prior to further analysis of glucose and insulin content. Fresh islets were prepared by collagenase digestion [32]. This method is being used routinely in our laboratory and described in detail elsewhere [33,34]. Islets free of exocrine tissue were obtained by repeated hand-picking under the stereo-microscope. We routinely obtain 200–400 islets per pancreas.

Extraction of Insulin-like Peptides

Each pancreas was homogenized in 6 ml of ice-cold 0.7 mmol/l HCl/ethanol (1:3 vol/vol) using a Kinematica Polytron (1 min, 27,000 rpm). The homogenates were stirred overnight at 4°C, followed by centrifugation at 10,000 rpm (Sorvall, RC-5B, SS-34 rotor) for 20 minutes, and insulin-like peptides precipitated with a modification of the Davoren method [23]. The precipitates were resolubilized in 1 mol/l acetic acid and insulin-related peptides determined by RIA, or resolved by HPLC. Freshly isolated islets were extracted by repeated freeze-thawing in 1 mol/l acetic acid, centrifuged in a microfuge for 10 min at maximal speed, and insulin-related peptides determined as described above.

HPLC Separation of Insulin-Like Peptides

Insulin-related peptides were resolved by reverse-phase HPLC using a modification of the conditions of Seino et al. [35]. Prior to the application to a C_{18} Synchropac column (Hewlett-Packard, Boeblingen, Germany), plasma samples were partially purified and concentrated using C_{18} Sep-Pak cartridges (Waters & Associates, Milford, MA), as described [36], whereas islet and pancreatic extract preparations were filtered through Iso-Disc N-34 nylon membranes (pore size 0.45 μm, Supelco, Bellefonte, PA). Elution rate was one ml/minute with 0.2% trifluoroacetic acid in water (solution A) and 0.2% trifluoroacetic acid in acetonitrile (solution B). Solution B was held at 30.5% for 25 minutes for elution of insulin and then increased linearly to 35.5% over an additional 55 minutes to elute proinsulin and proinsulin conversion intermediates. The fractions were either used for determination of insulin-like peptides by RIA, or measurement of radioactivity following pulse-chase experiments. For determination of insulin immunoreactivity, the samples were dried in a Speed-Vac apparatus (Savant Instruments, Inc., Farmingdale, NY) and reconstituted in 1 ml RIA buffer (PBS containing 0.1% BSA).

Secretion Studies in Static Incubations of Isolated Islets

Isolated islets were preincubated for 60 min in Krebs-Ringer bicarbonate buffer containing 20 mmol/l Hepes, 0.1% BSA (KRBH/BSA), and a basal concentration of glucose (3.3 mmol/l). For the secretion studies islets were placed in 24 well culture dishes, 1–2 islets per well, and incubated for 60 min in 1 ml KRBH/BSA with various concentrations of glucose. Secretion was calculated both per islet, and as percent of islet IRI content determined following extraction as outlined above.

Determination of Insulin-Like Immunoreactivity

Insulin-related peptides were quantitated by RIA using rat insulin as a standard (Novo-Nordisk, Bagsvaerd, Denmark) and iodinated porcine insulin (Diagnostic Products, Los Angeles, CA). Preliminary studies showed that the anti-insulin antibody used in our studies (Serono, Coinsins, Switzerland) gave parallel dilution curves for *Psammomys* and rat insulins.

RESULTS

In preliminary studies we identified insulin, proinsulin, and putative proinsulin conversion intermediates in the plasma and pancreas of *Psammomys obesus* by the use of HPLC analysis. A HPLC profile of immunoreactive insulin (IRI) extracted from the pancreas of non-fasted diabetic *Psammomys* is shown in Fig. 1.

The identification of the peaks is based on their temporal appearance following pulse-chase experiments and verification of size by gel filtration chromatography on a Superdex 75 HR column (not shown). HPLC analysis of plasma samples of diabetic and non-diabetic *Psammomys* revealed a marked increase in proinsulin and putative proinsulin conversion intermediates relative to insulin in the plasma of diabetic *Psammomys* (61.0 ± 14.4 and 7.3 ± 3.2%, in non-fasted diabetic and non-diabetic animals, respectively). Most diabetic animals exhibited a lower level of 'true' insulin relative to non-diabetic animals despite their higher plasma glucose levels (Table 1).

To test whether the observed high proportion of proinsulin and its conversion intermediates was related to their relative increase in the pancreas of the diabetic animals, pancreatic extracts were analyzed for content of total IRI and relative levels of proinsulin. A marked increase in the proportions of proinsulin and proinsulin conversion intermediates (not shown) in the pancreas of non-fasted diabetic *Psammomys* was associated with 90% reduction in the insulin stores of the pancreas (Fig. 2A and 2B).

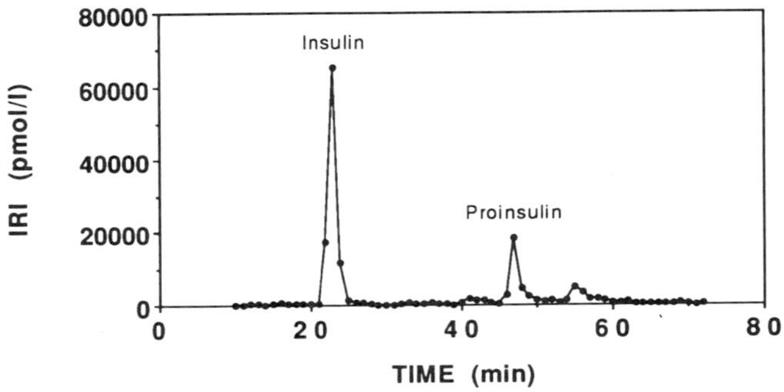

Figure 1. HPLC elution profile of a pancreatic extract from non-fasted hyperinsulinaemic, hyperglycaemic *Psammomys obesus*.

After a 16–20 hour fast the depletion of pancreatic insulin in the diabetic animals was partially corrected, and the proinsulin/insulin ratio normalized. In contrast, non-diabetic *Psammomys* showed only 50% reduction in pancreatic insulin stores under non-fasting conditions with no change in proinsulin/insulin ratio. No effect of fasting on pancreatic insulin content was observed in Sprague-Dawley rats which served as a control species (not shown).

In an attempt to further characterize the β-cell pathophysiology in the diabetic *Psammomys*, we investigated the glucose concentration dependency of insulin secretion from islets of diabetic and non-diabetic *Psammomys* and Sprague Dawley rats. Islets isolated from diabetic animals exhibited increased sensitivity to glucose (Fig. 3). They released as much insulin at 3.3 as at 16.7 mmol/l glucose (~25% of content), but lowered their insulin output to ~4% of content in the absence of extracellular glucose. Rat islets studied in parallel, exhibited a low secretion rate both at 0 and 3.3 mmol/l glucose (<0.5% of content) and increased their insulin secretion ~10-fold in response to 16.7 mmol/l glucose (Fig. 3). Islets of non-diabetic *Psammomys* elevated their insulin output ~6 fold (from 0.3 to 1.8% of islet content) when the level of glucose was increased from 3.3 to 16.7 mmol/l (Table 2). Insulin content per islet was significantly lower in islets from diabetic *Psammomys* as compared to non-diabetic ones, in agreement with the observed reduction in whole pancreatic IRI stores in these animals (compare Table 2 and Fig. 2).

DISCUSSION

The most prevalent form of NIDDM is characterized by obesity, insulin resistance, and insulin secretory dysfunction [37,38]. The relative roles of these metabolic abnormali-

Table 1. Plasma glucose and insulin levels in non-fasted *Psammomys*

Group	Glucose (mmol/l)	IRI (pmol/l)
Normoglycaemic, hyperinsulinaemic	5.6 ± 0.5	4600 ± 1220
Hyperglycaemic, hyperinsulinaemic	21.7 ± 2.1[a]	4120 ± 1110[b]

Results are mean ± SEM.
[a]P < 0.01 relative to the normoglycaemic group (by Mann–Whitney U test).
[b]No statistically significant difference from the normoglycaemic group.

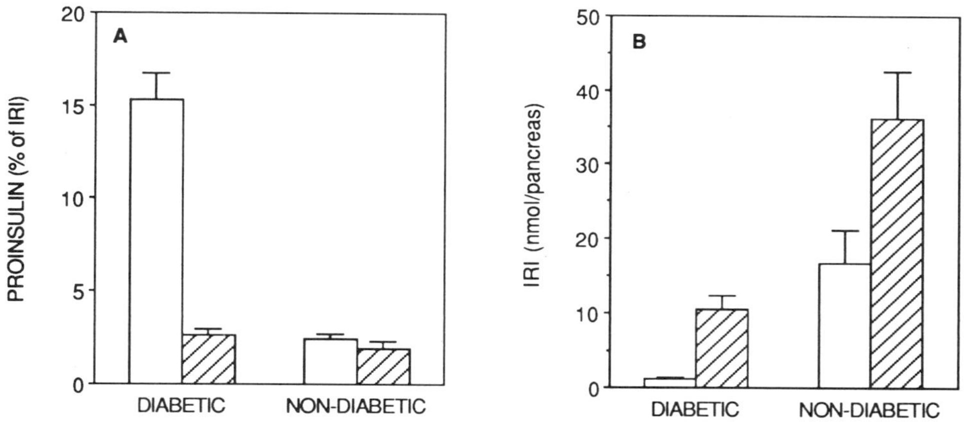

Figure 2. Percentage of proinsulin (**A**) and pancreatic content of total IRI (**B**) in diabetic and non-diabetic *Psammomys* in the non-fasting state (open bars) and after an overnight fast (cross-hatched bars). Results are shown as mean ± SEM of 4–10 animals per group.

ties is controversial, although it is well documented that many obese insulin resistant subjects never develop hyperglycaemia, suggesting that insulin resistance alone is not sufficient for progression to diabetes [39,40]. Likewise, the *Psammomys obesus,* when maintained in captivity and fed calorie rich laboratory chow, develops obesity and insulin resistance and may become diabetic [25–28,30]. The observation that not all obese hyperinsulinaemic *Psammomys* develop hyperglycaemia makes this animal an attractive model to study the role of the pancreas in the pathogenesis of NIDDM. An increased ratio of plasma proinsulin-related peptides to insulin was observed in individuals with NIDDM [1–9] and in the present study also in the plasma of hyperinsulinaemic, hyperglycaemic Psammomys. Unlike obese non-diabetic *Psammomys*, diabetic ones exhibited a very low pancreatic content of IRI, in agreement with a previous report in this animal [41]. Pancreatic depletion of IRI was associated with an increase in the relative content of proinsulin in non-fasted, diabetic *Psammomys*. However, an overnight fast was sufficient to correct the hyperglycaemia of these animals, partially restore the content of IRI and normalize the pancreatic proinsulin/insulin ratio. The relatively rapid recovery of insulin stores and normalization of proinsulin/insulin ratio in the pancreas after an overnight fast, makes it unlikely that hyperglycaemia *per se* (i.e. "toxic" effect of glucose) impairs the biosynthesis and/or processing of proinsulin. An alternative explanation compatible with our findings is that the relative

Table 2. Insulin secretion from islets of diabetic and non-diabetic *Psammomys*

Group	Glucose (mmol/l)	Secretion (pmol/islet/h)	Content (pmol/islet)	Secretion (% of content)
Diabetic				
	3.3	0.28 ± 0.04	1.13 ± 0.14	25.7 ± 3.6
	16.7	0.22 ± 0.03	0.92 ± 0.12	25.0 ± 2.6
Non-diabetic				
	3.3	0.08 ± 0.01	28.0 ± 2.5	0.3 ± 0.04
	16.7	0.49 ± 0.06	28.0 ± 1.9	1.8 ± 0.27

Results are mean ± SEM of 8–14 islet single replicates incubated for 1 h in KRBH/BSA buffer containing either 3.3 or 16.7 mmol/l glucose.

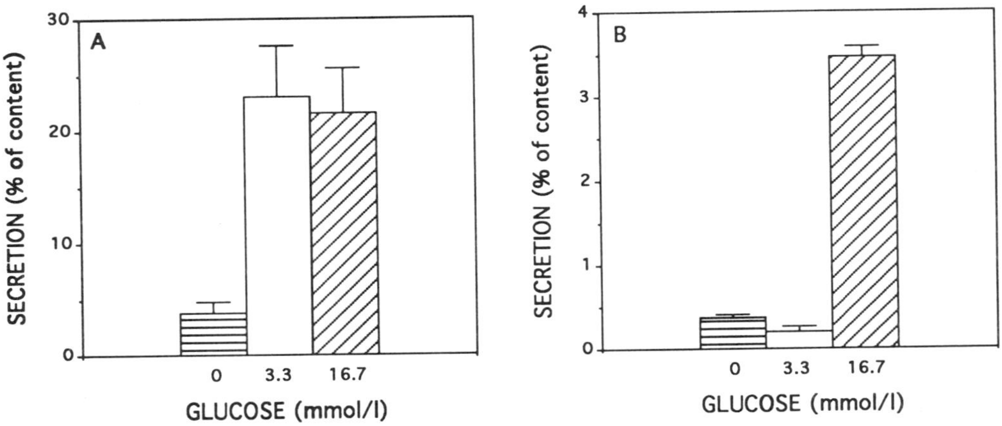

Figure 3. Insulin secretion from isolated islets of diabetic *Psammomys* (**A**) and Sprague-Dawley rats (**B**) in response to various concentrations of glucose. Results are shown as mean ± SEM of 3–4 islets per treatment.

hyperproinsulinaemia in the diabetic *Psammomys* may result from the inability of the pancreas to cope with the increase in secretory demand imposed by insulin resistance. This leads to depletion of pancreatic IRI content, and enrichment of the depleted pancreas with immature granules rich in proinsulin and related peptides. The reduction in the pancreatic insulin stores must be quite pronounced for hyperproinsulinaemia to appear, as indicated by the observation in non-diabetic *Psammomys*, in which a 50% reduction in insulin content in the non-fasting state did not affect either plasma or pancreatic proinsulin/insulin ratios. The observation that islets derived from diabetic *Psammomys* exhibited a reduced IRI content suggests that reduced pancreatic content observed in non-fasted animals is not a result of the mere reduction in the number of islets per pancreas, but that the islets themselves have a reduced insulin content.

The functional integrity of the diabetic pancreas was assessed in islets isolated from diabetic *Psammomys* by the insulin response to an acute glucose stimulus. Interestingly, these islets exhibited increased sensitivity to low concentrations of glucose, reminiscent of the leftward shift in the glucose dose-response curve observed in glucose intolerant subjects during progression to overt NIDDM and in a rat model of hyperglycaemia [42,43].

What could be the underlying defect(s) accounting for the pancreatic dysfunction displayed by the diabetic *Psammomys*? Possible changes compatible with reduced pancreatic insulin stores and the elevated ratio of precursor to mature insulin in both the pancreas and the plasma are: 1. increased rate of insulin output under basal conditions, 2. increased rate of insulin degradation in the β-cell (crinophagy), and 3. reduction in the maximal rate of proinsulin synthesis and/or processing. The secretory dysfunction observed in our preliminary studies on glucose responsiveness of the diabetic islets may result from defects in 1. the β-cell glucose sensing component(s), and/or 2. the stimulus-secretion coupling. In addition, under low ambient glucose the β-cells may secrete insulin in response to endogenous glucose derived from glycogenolysis of the glycogen loaded diabetic islets [41].

Further studies on processes affecting the storage capacity of insulin in the pancreas of diabetic and non-diabetic *Psammomys* and on factors involved in the regulation of insulin secretion, as outlined above, are needed in order to clarify the role of the pancreas in the aetiology of diabetes in this nutrition-dependent animal model of NIDDM.

ACKNOWLEDGMENTS

This work was supported by grants from The Israel Science Foundation, The Israel Ministry of Health, The Wolfson Foundation and The Hebrew University-Hadassah Diabetes Research Center.

REFERENCES

1. Duckworth, W. C., Solomon, S. S., and Kitabchi, A. E., 1972, Effect of chronic sulfonylurea therapy on plasma insulin and proinsulin levels, *J. Clin. Endocrinol. Metab.* 35:585–591.
2. Gorden, P., Hendricks, C. M., and Roth, J., 1974, Circulating proinsulin-like component in man: increased proportion in hypoinsulinaemic states., *Diabetologia* 10:469–474.
3. Mako, S. E., Starr, J. I., and Rubenstein, A. H., 1977, Circulating proinsulin in patients with maturity onset diabetes, *Am. J. Med.* 63:865–869.
4. Ward, W. K., LaCava, E. C., Paquette, T. L., Beard, J. C., Wallum, B. J., and Porte, D. Jr., 1987, Disproportionate elevation of immunoreactive proinsulin in type 2 (non-insulin-dependent) diabetes mellitus and in experimental insulin resistance, *Diabetologia* 30:698–702.
5. Yoshioka, N., Kuzuya, T., Matsuda, A., Taniguchi, M., and Iwamoto, Y., 1988, Serum proinsulin levels at fasting and after oral glucose load in patients with type 2 (non-insulin-dependent) diabetes mellitus, *Diabetologia* 31:355–360.
6. Deacon, C. F., Schleser, M. S., Ballmann, M., Willms, B., Conlon, J. M., and Creutzfeldt, W., 1988, Preferential release of proinsulin relative to insulin in non-insulin-dependent diabetes mellitus, *Acta Endocrinol (Copenh)* 119:549–554.
7. Temple, R. C., Carrington, C. A., Luzio, S. D., Owens, D. R., Schneider, A. E., Sobey, W. J., and Hales, C. N., 1989, Insulin deficiency in non-insulin-dependent diabetes, *Lancet* 1:293–295.
8. Clark, P. M., Levy, J. C., Cox, L., Burnett, M., Turner, R. C., and Hales, C. N., 1992, Immunoradiometric assay of insulin, intact proinsulin and 32–33 split proinsulin and radioimmunoassay of insulin in diet-treated type 2 (non-insulin-dependent) diabetic subjects, *Diabetologia* 35:469–474.
9. Levy, J. C., Clark, P. M., Hales, C. N., and Turner, R. C., 1993, Normal proinsulin responses to glucose in mild type II subjects with subnormal insulin response, *Diabetes* 42:162–169.
10. Glauber, H. S., Henry, R. R., Wallace, P., Frank, B. H., Galloway, J. A., Cohen, R. M., and Olefsky, J. M., 1987, The effects of biosynthetic human proinsulin on carbohydrate metabolism in non-insulin-dependent diabetes mellitus, *N. Engl. J. Med.* 316:443–449.
11. Kosaka, K., Kuzuya, T., Akanuma, Y., and Hagura, R., 1980, Increase in insulin response after treatment of overt maturity-onset diabetes is independent of the mode of treatment, *Diabetologia* 18:23–28.
12. Hidaka, H., Nagulesparan, M., Klimes, I., Clark, R., Sasaki, H., Aronoff, S.L., Vasquez, B., Rubenstein, A.H., and Unger, R.H., 1982, Improvement of insulin secretion but not insulin resistance after short term control of plasma glucose in obese type II diabetics, *J. Clin. Endocrinol. Metab.* 54:217–222.
13. Vague, P., and Moulin, J. P., 1982, The defective glucose sensitivity of B-cell in non-insulin dependent diabetes: improvement after twenty hours normoglycemia, *Metabolism* 31:139–142.
14. Glaser, B., Leibovich, G., Nesher, R., Hartling, S., Binder, C., and Cerasi, E., 1988, Improved beta-cell function after intensive insulin treatment in severe non-insulin-dependent diabetes, *Acta Endocrinol (Copenh)* 118:365–373.
15. Yoshioka, N., Kuzuya, T., Matsuda, A., and Iwamoto, Y., 1989, Effect of dietary treatment on serum insulin and proinsulin response in newly diagnosed NIDDM, *Diabetes* 38:262–266.
16. Bonner-Weir, S., Trent, D. F., and Weir, G. C., 1983, Partial pancreatectomy in the rat and subsequent defect in glucose induced insulin release, *J. Clin. Invest.* 71:1544–1553.
17. Grill, V., and Rundfeldt, M., 1986, Abnormalities of insulin responses after ambient and previous exposure to glucose in streptozotocin-diabetes and dexamethasone-treated rats. Role of hyperglycemia and increased B-cell demands, *Diabetes* 35:44–51.
18. Leahy, J. L., Cooper, H. E., Deary, D. A., and Weir, G. C., 1986, Chronic hyperglycemia is associated with impaired glucose influence on insulin secretion. A study in normal rats using chronic in vivo glucose infusions, *J. Clin. Invest.* 77:908–915.
19. Kergoat, M., Bailbe, D., and Portha, B., 1987, Insulin treatment improves glucose-induced insulin release in rats with NIDDM induced by streptozocin, *Diabetes* 36:971–977.

20. Rossetti, L., Shulman, G. I., Zawalich, W., and DeFronzo, R. A., 1987, Effect of chronic hyperglycemia on in vivo insulin secretion in partially pancreatectomized rats, *J. Clin. Invest.* 80:1037–1044.
21. Leahy, J. L., Halban, P. A., and Weir, G. C., 1991, Relative hypersecretion of proinsulin in rat model of NIDDM, *Diabetes* 40:985–989.
22. Leahy, J. L., and Weir, G. C., 1991, Beta-cell dysfunction in hyperglycaemic rat models: recovery of glucose-induced insulin secretion with lowering of the ambient glucose level, *Diabetologia* 34:640–647.
23. Leahy, J. L., 1993, Increased proinsulin/insulin ratio in pancreas extracts of hyperglycemic rats, *Diabetes* 42:22–27.
24. Unger, R. H., and Grundy, S., 1985, Hyperglycaemia as an inducer as well as a consequence of impaired islet cell function and insulin resistance: implications for management of diabetes, *Diabetologia* 28:119–121.
25. Adler, J. H., Kalman, R., Lazarovici, G., Bar-On, H., and Ziv, E., Achieving predictable model of type 2 diabetes in the sand rat, in *Lessons from Animal Diabetes III*, E. Shafrir, Editor. 1991, Smith-Gordon: London. p. 212–214.
26. Shafrir, E., and Gutman, A., 1993, Psammomys obesus of the Jerusalem colony: A model for nutritionally induced non-insulin-dependent diabetes, *J. Basic Clin. Physiol. Pharmacol.* 4:83–99.
27. Kalderon, B., Gutman, A., Levy, E., Shafrir, E., and Adler, J. H., 1986, Characterization of stages in development of obesity-diabetes syndrome in the sand rat *(Psammomys obesus)*, *Diabetes* 35:717–723.
28. Marquie, G., Duhault, J., and Jacotot, B., 1984, Diabetes mellitus in sand rats *(Psammomys obesus)*. Metabolic pattern during development of the diabetic syndrome, *Diabetes* 33:438–443.
29. Kanety, H., Moshe, S., Shafrir, E., Lunenfeld, B., and Karasik, A., 1994, Hyperinsulinemia induces a reversible impairment in insulin receptor function leading to diabetes in the sand rat model of NIDDM, *Proc. Natl. Acad. Sci. USA* 91:1853–1857.
30. Kalman, R., Ziv, E., Adler, J. H., Lazarovici, G., and Bar-On, H., 1993, The efficiency of the sand rat metabolism is responsible for the development of obesity and diabetes, *J. Basic Clin. Physiol. Pharmacol.* 4:57–68.
31. Kahn, S. E., McCulloch, D. K., Schwartz, M. W., Palmer, J. P., and Porte, D. J., 1992, Effect of insulin resistance and hyperglycemia on proinsulin release in a primate model of diabetes mellitus, *J. Clin. Endocrinol. Metab.* 74:192–197.
32. Lacy, P. E., and Kostianovsky, M., 1967, Method for the isolation of intact islets of Langerhans from rat pancreas, *Diabetes* 16:35–39.
33. Kaiser, N., Corcos, A. P., Tur-Sinai, A., Ariav, Y., and Cerasi, E., 1988, Monolayer culture of adult pancreatic islets on extracellular matrix: Long term maintenance of differentiated B-cell function, *Endocrinology* 123:834–840.
34. Gadot, M., Leibowitz, G., Shafrir, E., Cerasi, E., Gross, D. J., and Kaiser, N., 1994, Hyperproinsulinemia and insulin deficiency in the diabetic Psammomys obesus, *Endocrinology* 135:610–616.
35. Seino, S., Fu, Z. Z., Marks, W., Seino, Y., Imura, H., and Vinik, A., 1986, Characterization of circulating insulin in insulin autoimmune syndrome, *J. Clin. Endocrinol. Metab.* 62:64–69.
36. Cohen, R. M., *et al.*, 1986, Proinsulin radioimmunoassay in the evaluation of insulinomas and familial hyperproinsulinemia, *Metabolism* 35:1137–1146.
37. DeFronzo, R. A., 1988, The triumvirate: β-cell, muscle, liver. A collusion responsible for NIDDM, *Diabetes* 37:667–687.
38. DeFronzo, R. A., Bonadonna, R. C., and Ferrannini, E., 1992, Pathogenesis of NIDDM: A balanced overview, *Diabetes Care* 15:318–368.
39. Bennett, P. H., Rushforth, N. B., Miller, M., and LeCompte, P. M., 1976, Epidemiologic studies of diabetes in the Pima Indians, *Recent Progr. Horm. Res.* 32:333–376.
40. Cook, D. L., and Taborsky, J. G. J., B-cell function and insulin secretion, in *Diabetes Mellitus. Theory and Practice*, H. Rifkin and J.D. Porte, Editor. 1990, Elsevier Science Publ. Co., Inc.: New York. p. 86–103.
41. Like, A. A., and Miki, E., 1967, Diabetic syndrome in sand rats IV. Morphologic changes in islet tissue, *Diabetologia* 3:146–166.
42. Porte, D., Jr., 1991, Banting lecture 1990: β-cells in type II diabetes mellitus, *Diabetes* 40:166–180.
43. Leahy, J. L., Bumbalo, L. M., and Chen, C., 1993, Beta-cell hypersensitivity for glucose precedes loss of glucose-induced insulin secretion in 90% pancreatectomized rats, *Diabetologia* 36:1238–1244.

50

ALTERED SECRETORY RESPONSIVENESS OF BRIN-BD11 CELLS CULTURED UNDER HYPERGLYCAEMIC CONDITIONS IS NOT READILY REVERSED BY SUBSEQUENT CULTURE IN LOWER GLUCOSE CONCENTRATIONS

Alison M. Wilson, Christopher R. Barnett, and Peter R. Flatt

Diabetes Research Group
School of Biomedical Sciences
University of Ulster
Coleraine, Co Londonderry, N. Ireland, United Kingdom BT52 1SA

INTRODUCTION

The complex interaction of nutrient stimuli on the pancreatic B-cell results in the appropriate amount of insulin being secreted to maintain glucose homeostasis. In non-insulin-dependent diabetes mellitus (NIDDM), defects in the regulatory mechanisms of in sulin secretion make a major contribution to the metabolic disorders associated with the disease (Kahn and Porte, 1990). Possible molecular mechanisms underlying pancreatic B-cell dysfunction in NIDDM include site-specific defects in the stimulus-secretion pathway and alterations of B-cell function consequent to changes in external influences on the B-cell (Flatt *et al.*, 1994). Studies in man and experimental animals both *in vivo* and *in vitro* have indicated that long-term exposure to a hyperglycaemic environment results in a gradual impairment of insulin secretion (Leahy *et al.*, 1992; McClenaghan *et al.*, 1996; Barnett *et al.*, 1993, 1994). Such observations support the concept of glucose toxicity and the view of hyperglycaemia as an inducer, as well as a consequence of B-cell dysfunction (Unger and Grundy, 1985). Recent studies indicate that there may be species variation in the susceptibility to the detrimental effects of a hyperglycaemic environment (Eizirik and Sandler, 1992; Eizirik *et al.*, 1989). These observations raise two important considerations. Firstly, species differences may reflect differences in endogenous mechanisms which protect against the effects of glucose toxicity. Secondly, the deleterious effects of hyperglycaemia may be manifest in genetically susceptible B-cells where increased functional strain is imposed on existing weakspots in the insulin secretory pathway. In this study we investi-

Physiology and Pathophysiology of the Islets of Langerhans, edited by Soria.
Plenum Press, New York, 1997.

gated the effects of hyperglycaemia on insulin secretory responsiveness of the novel clonal B-cell line, BRIN-BD11 (Flatt *et al.*, 1993). Possible reversal of the glucose toxic effects by subsequent culture at lower glucose concentrations were also examined.

MATERIALS AND METHODS

Insulin secreting BRIN-BD11 cells, derived from the electrofusion of New England Deaconess Hospital (NEDH) rat islet cells and RINm5F cells (Barnett *et al.*, 1993), were routinely cultured in RPMI 1640 medium containing 11.1 mmol/l D-glucose (Gibco Life Technologies, UK), supplemented with 10% (v/v) foetal calf serum (Gibco Life Technologies, UK) and 1% (v/v) gentamicin (Sigma Chemical Co. Ltd). BRIN-BD11 cells were harvested and seeded into 75 cm^2 tissue culture flasks (Corning Ltd, UK) and cultured in RPMI 1640 medium containing 11.1 mmol/l or 66.6 mmol/l D-glucose for 72 hours. After each 24 hour period the culture medium was replaced with fresh medium to maintain the media glucose concentration. Following the 72 hours culture period, the cells were harvested and seeded (200,000 cells/well) into 24 well tissue culture plates (Nunc Ltd, UK). The cells cultured at 11.1 mmol/l D-glucose were maintained in medium with this concentration. However, the cells initially cultured at 66.6 mmol/l D-glucose were seeded into two 24 well tissue culture plates. One 24 well plate of cells was cultured with medium containing 11.1 mmol/l D-glucose and the other with medium containing 66.6 mmol/l D-glucose. All cells were cultured for a further 24 hours in the new medium. After this culture period the media were removed, the cells washed and pre-incubated (40 minutes) with Krebs Ringer Bicarbonate Buffer (KRB), pH 7.4, containing 1.1mmol/l D-glucose. Investigation of insulin secretion during 20 minute incubations with KRB containing 1.1mmol/l–16.7mmol/l D-glucose was performed using the cells cultured at 11.1 mmol/l and 66.6 mmol/l D-glucose. Acute 20 minute incubations were also performed with KRB, pH 7.4 containing; either 1.1 mmol/l D-glucose or 16.7 mmol/l D-glucose; 1.1 mmol/l D-glucose plus 10 mmol/l L-alanine; 1.1 mmol/l D-glucose plus 25 mmol/l potassium chloride. The amount of insulin secreted during these incubations and the total intracellular insulin content were determined by radioimmunoassay using rat insulin as standard (Flatt and Bailey, 1981).

RESULTS

The BRIN-BD11 cells cultured in RPMI-1640 medium containing 66.6 mmol/l D-glucose did not display altered cell growth or morphological characteristics compared with cells cultured at 11.1 mmol/l D-glucose. BRIN-BD11 cells cultured at 11.1 mmol/l D-glucose displayed a progressive concentration-dependent insulin secretory response to increasing glucose concentration (Figure 1). In contrast, those cellules cultured in RPMI-1640 media containing 66.6 mmol/l D-glucose displayed a defective response to increasing D-glucose concentration (Figure 1).

Evaluation of the insulin response to both alanine (10 mmol/l) and a depolarising concentration (25 mmol/l) of potassium chloride revealed a highly significant ($P < 0.001$) depression in responsiveness of the cells cultured at 66.6 mmol/l D-glucose compared to cells cultured at 11.1 mmol/l (Figure 2). This was not completely ameliorated by subsequent culture of the cells for 24 hours in RPM I-1640 containing 11.1 mmol/l D-glucose (Figure 2).

Measurement of the cellular insulin content under the three culture conditions revealed a highly significant depression ($P < 0.001$) in the cells cultured at 66.6 mmol/l

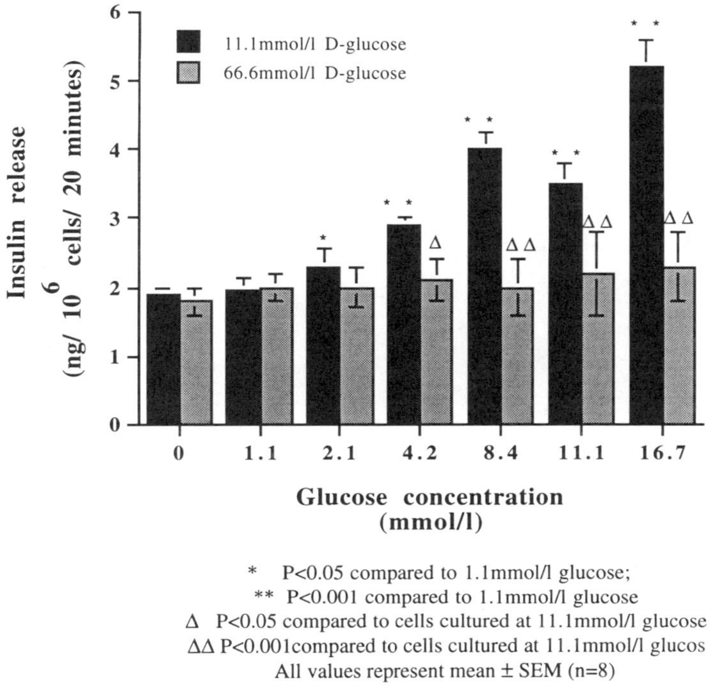

Figure 1. Acute effects of glucose on insulin release from BRIN-BD11 cells cultured at 11.1 mmol/l or 66.6 mmol/l D-glucose for 96 hours. *P < 0.05 compared to 1.1 mmol/l glucose; **P < 0.001 compared to 1.1 mmol/l glucose; $^{\Delta}$P < 0.05 compared to cells cultured at 11.1 mmol/l glucose; $^{\Delta\Delta}$P < 0.001 compared to cells cultured at 11.1 mmol/l glucose. All values represent mean ± SEM (n = 8).

D-glucose compared to those cultured at 11.1 mmol/l D-glucose (Figure 3). Culture of cells for 24 hours at 11.1mmol/l D-glucose following 72 hrs culture at 66.6 mmol/l D-glucose resulted in a small but insignificant increase in insulin content. Comparison of the amount insulin secreted during 20 minutes to the total cellular insulin content indicated that the cells were secreting less than 10% of their total cellular insulin during the test incubations.

DISCUSSION

The concept of glucose toxicity has received much attention during recent years (Unger and Grundy, 1985; Rossetti *et al.*, 1990; Yki-Järvinen, 1992). The current evidence indicates that culture of human islets in hyperglycaemic conditions has detrimental effects on normal secretory responsiveness (Ezirik *et al.*, 1992). However, these effects appear to display marked species variation (Ezirik *et al.*, 1989, 1992). Investigation of glucose toxicity using clonal insulin secreting cell lines may overcome many of the problems associated with differences between human islets and hose derived from various other species. However, most clonal insulin secreting cell lines display defective insulin secretion responsiveness, particularly to glucose.

Selection of an appropriate cell line for *in vitro* investigation of glucose toxic effects must take these factors into consideration. The BRIN-BD11 cell line, used in the present

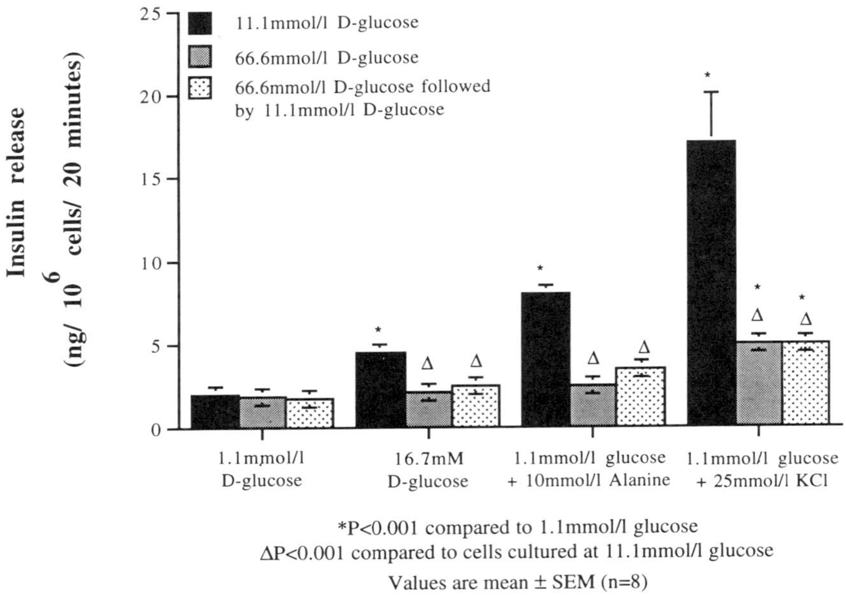

Figure 2. Acute effects of glucose, alanine, and a depolarising concentration of KCl on insulin release from BRIN-BD11 cells cultured at 11.1 mmol/l or 66.6 mmol/l D-glucose for 72 hours followed by an additional 24 hours at 11.1 mmol/l or 66.6 mmol/l D-glucose. $^*P < 0.001$ compared to 1.1 mmol/l glucose; $^{\Delta}P < 0.001$ compared to cells cultured at 11.1 mmol/l glucose. Values represent mean ± SEM (n = 8).

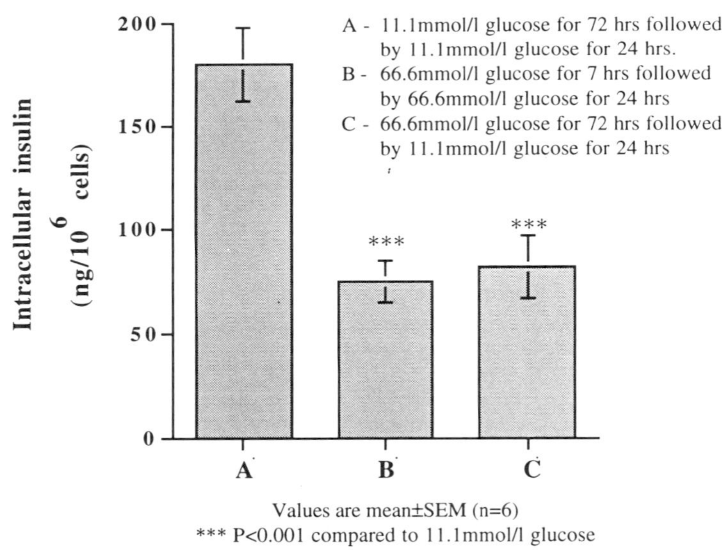

Figure 3. Intracellular insulin content of BRIN-BD11 cells following culture in RPMI-1640 media containing 11.1 mmol/l glucose for 96 hours, 66.6 mmol/l glucose for 96 hrs, or 66.6 mmol/l glucose for 72 hrs followed by 11.1 mmol/l glucose for 24 hrs. Values are mean ± SEM (n = 6). $^{***}P < 0.001$ compared to 11.1 mmol/l glucose.

study, is derived from the rat, a species susceptible to glucose toxicity. These cells display a pronounced step-wise insulin secretory responsiveness to increasing glucose concentration (Figure 1; Barnett *et al.*, 1993). The results of this investigation clearly indicate that the culture of BRIN-BD11 cells at high glucose concentration has marked detrimental effects on responsiveness to a range of secretagogues. The decreased responsiveness of the cells cultured at 66.6 mmol/l glucose is not a result of decreased cellular insulin content as all cells are secreting less than 10% of their total cellular insulin. Furthermore these effects were not readily reversed by subsequent culture at 11.1 mmol/l D-glucose indicating induction of a possible lasting defect in the stimulus-secretion coupling pathway. Additional studies are currently being performed to evaluate this possibility by attempting to counter the glucose toxic effects by subsequent culture at lower glucose concentrations for a more protracted period of time. The glucose concentration used in this study to induce glucose toxicity is several fold higher than encountered in poorly controlled diabetes mellitus. However, recent studies indicate that the glucose toxic effects on BRIN-BD11 cells can be manifest in culture conditions of 22 mmol/l D-glucose (Flatt *et al.*, 1994).

CONCLUSION

Culture of BRIN-BD11 insulin secreting cells in a hyperglycaemic environment produces marked alterations in insulin responsiveness. The molecular basis for the pronounced

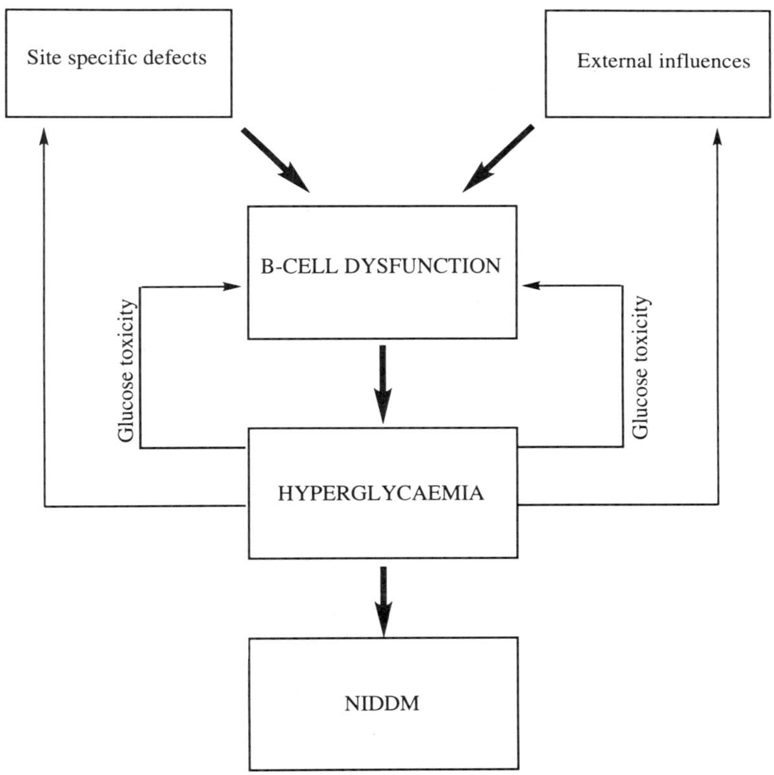

Figure 4. Model for the interactions between site-specific defects, external influences and glucose toxicity in B-cell dysfunction.

interruption of the normal pathway for insulin secretion is currently under investigation. Whether this represents a general, non-specific effect, or a site specific interaction of the glucose molecule has yet to be determined. Glucose toxicity appears to be species-dependent indicating that the deleterious effects may be manifest in genetically susceptible B-cells where increased functional strain is imposed on existing weakspots in the insulin secretory pathway. A possible model for the interactions between site-specific defects, external influences and glucose toxicity in B-cell dysfunction and NIDDM is outlined in Figure 4.

REFERENCES

Flatt, P. R. and Bailey, C. J. (1981) Development of glucose intolerance and impaired plasma insulin repsonse to glucose in obese and hyperglycaemic (ob/ob) mice. Horm. Metab. Res. 13:556

Barnett, C. R., Wilson, A. M., McClenaghan, N. H., Yoon, T. W., Swanston-Flatt, S. K., Ah-Sing, E. and Flatt, P. R. (1993). Effects of chronic hyperglycaemia on the function of insulin-secreting cells maintained in tissue culture. Diabetic Medicine Suppl 3, 10: S24

Barnett, C. R., Wilson, A. M., McClenaghan, N. H., Yoon, T. W., Swanston-Flatt, S. K. and Ah-Sing, E. (1994) Impaired insulin secretory responsiveness of BRIN-D11 cells cultured at high glucose concentrations. Diabetic Medicine. 20:164

Eizirik, D. L., Korbutt, G. S. and Hellerstrõm, C. (1992) Prolonged exposure of human pancreatic islets to high glucose concent rations *in vitro* impairs B-cell function. J. Clin. Invest. 90:1263

Eizirik, D. L. and Sandler, S. (1989) Sustained exposure to toxically damaged mouse pancreatic islets to high glucose does not increase B-cell dysfunction. J. Endocrinology 123:47

Flatt, P. R., Abdelwahab, Y. H. A., Wilson, A. M., Barnett, C. R., O'Harte, F. P M. and Swanston-Flatt, S. K. (1994) Site-specific defects and glucose toxicity in pancreatic B-cell dysfunction of non-insulin-dependent diabetes mellitus. in: "Frontiers of Insulin Secretion and Pancreatic B-cell Research". Eds. P. R. Flatt, S. Lenzen, Smith-Gordon & Co. Ltd, London, pp. 481–489

Kahn, S. E. and Porte, D., Jr, (1990) The pathophysiology of type II (non-insulin-dependent) diabetes mellitus: Implications for treatment. In: Ellenberg and Rifkin's Diabetes Mellitus: Theory and Practice Rifkin, H. and Port, D. Jr, eds., 4th edn., Elsevier, New York

Leahy, J. L., Bonner-Weir, S. and Weir, G. C. (1992) B-cell dysfunction induced by chronic hyperglycaemia; current ideas on mechanism of impaired glucose-induced insulin secretion. Diabetes Care 15:442

McClenaghan, N. H., Barnett, C. R., Ah-Sing, E., Abdel-Wahab, Y. H. A., O'Harte, F. P. M., Yoon, T.-W., Swanston-Flatt, S. K., and Flatt, P. R. (1996) Characterization of a novel glucose-responsive insulin-secreting pancreatic B-cell line, BRIN-BDII, produced by electrofusion. Diabetes 45:1132–1140

Rossetti, L., Giaccari, A. and DeFonzo, R. A. (1990) Glucose toxicity. Diabetes Care 13:610

Unger, R. H. and Grundy, S. (1985) Hyperglycaemia as an inducer as well as a consequence of impaired islet cell function and in sulin resistance: implications for the management of diabetes. Diabetologia 28:119

Yki-Järvinen, H. (1992) Glucose toxicity. Endocrine Reviews 13:415

51

B-CELL HYPERRESPONSIVENESS TO GLUCOSE IN NIDDM DURING PREDIABETES

Yoshihiko Sato, Fujiki Ishihara, Kiyoshi Hashizume, and Toru Aizawa

Department of Geriatrics Endocrinology and Metabolism
Shinshu University School of Medicine
Matsumoto, Japan

INTRODUCTION

It is not clear what is the initial metabolic abnormality in obese non-insulin-dependent diabetes mellitus (NIDDM). Recently established rat strain with naturally occurring obese NIDDM, Otsuka Long-Evans Tokushima Fatty (OLETF) rats,[1] possesses remarkable resemblance to obese NIDDM in humans. Namely, the rats initially develop obesity, hyper-insulinemia, and glucose intolerance, and later, becomes hypoinsulinemic with diabetic renal pathology similar to end-stage renal lesion found in humans.[1] Furthermore, development of glucose intolerance is virtually 100% in male OLETF,[1] indicating the rats are useful for the delineation of initial metabolic abnormality in obese NIDDM. We examined 3 w-old (non-obese, euglycemic and normoinsulinemic) male OLETF rats in the present study, and found marked hyperresponsiveness of the B-cell to glucose *in vitro*.

MATERIALS AND METHODS

Male OLETF and its control strain Long-Evans Tokushima Otsuka (LETO) rats were obtained from Otsuka Pharmaceutical Co. (Tokushima, Japan) through Dr. Kawano.[1] Pancreatic islets were isolated and used in the incubation experiments as described.[2] In brief, 5 islets/tube were incubated in Krebs-Ringer bicarbonate buffer (KRBB) for 75 min at 37°C with various concentration of glucose. The ATP-sensitive K^+ (K^+ATP) channel-independent glucose action was evaluated by stimulating diazoxide (150 mM) -pretreated islets with 25 mM K^+ plus high concentration of glucose as reported.[2] Glucose oxidation was determined at 37°C by incubating 20 islets/tube with 0.8 mCi D-[^{14}C(U)] glucose for 60 min with ambient glucose concentration of 27.8 mM as reported previously.[3] Insulin was determined by radioimmunoassay. Data are expressed as mean ± SD.

Physiology and Pathophysiology of the Islets of Langerhans, edited by Soria.
Plenum Press, New York, 1997.

Table 1. Insulin content of pancreatic islets and glucose oxidation by the islet cells

Animal	Insulin content ng/islet	Glucose converted to CO_2 pmoles/20 islets/60 min
OLETF	34.7 ± 10.3	457.4 ± 55.4
LETO	33.6 ± 3.9	498.1 ± 143.8

Data are not significantly different between the 2 groups of islets.

RESULTS AND DISCUSSION

Three week-old OLETF rats are non-obese, and euglycemic and normoinsulinemic at oral glucose tolerance test; at the age of 27 w, they are obese and hyperglycemic without exception as reported (data not shown).[1] Thus, 3 w-old OLETF rats are at prediabetic phase and, at the same time, destined to develop obese NIDDM.

Islet insulin content and glucose oxidation by the islet cells are not significantly different between OLETF and LETO (Table 1). Basal insulin release (with 3 mM glucose) is comparable between the 2 groups of islets (Table 2), whereas insulin release in response to 27.8 mM and 40 mM glucose are markedly greater in the islets of OLETF than in those of LETO (Table 2). Such hyperresponsiveness to glucose is not found when the islets are stimulated by glucose in a K^+ATP channel-independent manner (Table 2).

This is the first study of B-cell function in population destined to develop obese NIDDM during non-obese, euglycemic and normoinsulinemic phase. Our data strongly suggest that exaggerated B-cell responsiveness to glucose is the initial abnormality in such population. Because not only plasma glucose but also plasma insulin are normal in OLETF, *in vivo* insulin sensitivity is considered normal. Furthermore, insulin content and glucose metabolism of the islets is not increased. Thus, we hypothesize that exaggerated B-cell response to glucose is an intrinsic abnormality of exocytosis in the B-cell of OLETF, leading to obesity, insulin resistance and glucose intolerance. The K^+ATP channel-independent branch of glucose-induced signaling is not exaggerated, at least during the prediabetic phase, in the B-cell of obese NIDDM.

Such hypothesis is distinct from a generally held view on the etiology of obese NIDDM in human,[4] in which insulin resistance is believed to be the initial abnormality and hyperinsulinemia is considered to be the secondary abnormality. Our data obtained in a rat model of obese NIDDM indicate that the sequence of events is in fact opposite: hyperresponsiveness of the B-cell develops first and insulin resistance may ensue. Exaggerated B-cell response to glucose is unequivocally present during non-obese, euglycemic,

Table 2. Glucose-induced insulin release by pancreatic islets *in vitro*

	Insulin release (pg/islet/75 min) — untreated islets glucose (mM)			Diazoxide (150 mM) — pretreated islets[a] glucose (mM)
Animal	3.0	27.8	40	27.8
OLETF	194 ± 61	3263 ± 807[b]	5084 ± 1646[c]	4700 ± 1761
LETO	278 ± 73	2027 ± 877	1919 ± 769	4517 ± 2412

[a]Diazoxide was present during the preincubation (30 min) and throughout the experimental incubation period. K^+ concentration during glucose stimulation was 25 mM in case of diazoxide-pretreated islets and insulin release in response to [3 mM glucose plus 25 mM K^+] was subtracted from that in response to [27.8 mM glucose plus 25 mM K^+].

[b] and [c], $P < 0.05$ and 0.01, respectively, compared to the corresponding values of the islets of LETO rats.

and normoinsulinemic phase. Because OLETF rats are phenotypically identical to patients with obese NIDDM, we hypothesize that hyperresponsiveness to glucose is the initial metabolic abnormality in such patients as well.

CONCLUSIONS

In a newly established rat model of NIDDM, OLETF rat,[1] pancreatic B-cell is hyperresponsive to glucose *in vitro* before the development of obesity, glucose intolerance and hyperinsulinemia. We hypothesize that this is the *intrinsic* abnormality of insulin release mechanism in the B-cell.

ACKNOWLEDGMENTS

This work was supported by a Grant-in-Aid for Scientific Research from the Ministry of Education, Science and Culture, Japan. We wish to thank Otsuka Pharmaceutical Co. and Dr. Kawano for generous gift of OLETF and LETO rats.

REFERENCES

1. K. Kawano, T. Hirashima, S. Mori, Y. Saitoh, M. Kurosumi, and T. Natori, Spontaneous long-term hyperglycemic rat with diabetic complications. Otsuka Long-Evans Tokushima Fatty (OLETF) stain. *Diabetes* 41:1422 (1992).
2. Y. Sato, T. Aizawa, M. Komatsu, N. Okada, and T. Yamada, Dual functional role of membrane depolarization/Ca^{2+} influx in rat pancreatic B-cell. Diabetes 41:438 (1992).
3. M.L. McDaniel, S. King, S. Anderson, J. Fink, and P.E. Lacy, Effect of cytochalasin B on hexose transport and glucose metabolism in pancreatic islets. *Diabetologia* 10:303 (1974).
4. R.A. DeFronzo, R.C. Bonadonna, and E. Ferrannini, Pathogenesis of NIDDM. A balanced overview. *Diabetes Care* 15:318 (1992).

INSULIN TREATMENT PREVENTS ADAPTATION OF THE ENDOCRINE PANCREAS TO PREGNANCY

T. R. Koiter, S. Wijkstra, H. Moes, and G. C. J. van der Schaaf-Verdonk

Division of Reproductive Biology
Department of Obstetrics and Gynaecology
Groningen University Hospital
PO Box 30.001
9700 RB Groningen, The Netherlands

INTRODUCTION

During pregnancy in the rat the insulin sensitivity of the maternal tissues decreases, thereby increasing the demand for insulin (Leturque et al. 1989). At the same time the insulin production and release increases (Koiter et al. 1989). These phenomena are associated with a transient increase in islet-cell proliferation (Dunger et al. 1989). It has been suggested that placental lactogens directly stimulate β-cell function and the proliferation of islet cells (Nielsen et al. 1986; Parsons et al. 1992). Alternatively, placental lactogens, by increasing the demand for insulin (Freinkel 1985), indirectly cause the increase in insulin production and cell-proliferation in the islets. This hypothesis of increased insulin demand was tested by investigating how insulin production and cell-proliferation change when exogenous insulin was infused in pregnant rats at such a rate that the demand for insulin was fully met.

MATERIALS AND METHODS

Wistar rats were subcutaneously (Alzet osmotic minipumps; model 2001) infused with 4.8 IU human insulin (NOVO)/day from day 8 to day 14 of pregnancy. In the freely moving rats with indwelling atrial catheters insulin and glucose plasma concentrations were monitored before during and after administration of an iv glucose load (0.5 g/kg) both before and after the insulin treatment. Insulin was measured by double antibody radioimmunoassay using a rat standard (R 171; 20.7 IU/mg; NOVO). Glucose was measured by the glucose-oxidase/peroxidase method (Boehringer Mannheim).

In another series of experiments 5-bromo-2-deoxyuridine (BrdU; 30 mg) was iv infused over 24 h on various days of pregnancy before and after the insulin treatment.

Physiology and Pathophysiology of the Islets of Langerhans, edited by Soria.
Plenum Press, New York, 1997.

Immediately after the BrdU-infusion the animals were sacrificed and the pancreata were excised, cut in three and rapidly frozen. Cryostat sections (4 µm) were immunostained for BrdU-positive cells, as previously described (Harms et al. 1986). The sections were counterstained with Celestine's blue and Mayer's haematoxylin. Islet sizes were measured by a television-based computerized image-analysing technique in 1 head, 1 tail and 1 body section of each animal (5 animals/group) for determination of the proportion of endocrine/exocrine tissue. More than 1000 islet-cells were counted in randomly chosen islets for determination of the proportion of BrdU-positive cells. In separate cryostat sections beta cells were immunostained using a polyclonal antibody against bovine insulin and the proportion of insulin-positive/-negative tissue was determined in the same way.

Also cryostat sections (10 µm) were attached to SuperFrost/Plus slides (Menzel-Gläser, Germany). After proteinase-K digestion the slides were hybridized at 30°C in 40% formamide, using a complementary oligoprobe for rat-proinsulin-mRNA (Chen et al. 1989). The probe was labeled with digoxigenin and made visible by immunostaining (Boehringer Mannheim). For each animal in about 10 medium- to large-sized islets the absorption was measured using an automatic scanner (Wolters et al. 1980). The total area of mRNA-positive cells was measured in the same way as in the BrdU-sections.

RESULTS AND DISCUSSION

The insulin treatment caused death by resorption of about 60% of the foetusses. The surviving foetusses were slightly growth-retarded. These effects were probably caused by the low plasma glucose levels induced by the insulin treatment.

During pregnancy basal insulin levels (after a 2-h fast) did not change. The insulin treatment induced hyperinsulinaemia (187 ± 24 mIU/l in insulin-treated day-14 pregnant rats vs 69 ± 9 mIU/l plasma in control pregnant rats). After cessation of the insulin treatment at day 14, basal insulin levels were temporarily decreased for one day, but then regained the pre-treatment values.

Basal glucose levels were decreased during the second half of pregnancy. Insulin treatment induced severe hypoglycaemia (1.8 ± 0.2 mM in insulin-treated day-14 pregnant rats vs 4.9 ± 0.3 mM in control pregnant rats). After cessation of the treatment basal glucose levels of the insulin-treated rats were lower than in non-pregnant control rats, but remained until the end of pregnancy slightly higher than those in control rats at the same days of pregnancy.

Glucose tolerance was not affected by pregnancy. It was decreased in the insulin-treated rats after cessation of the treatment for the duration of the experiment (day 20), the area under the curve of the glucose response being about twice as much as in the control rats at the same days of pregnancy.

Plasma insulin responses, as determined at 5 min after injection of the glucose load, increased in the second half of pregnancy. After cessation of the insulin treatment the insulin responses of insulin-treated rats were strongly suppressed. They only partially recovered in the following days (see Fig. 1). The low insulin-responsiveness of the insulin-treated animals was probably the cause of the reduced glucose tolerance observed in these animals.

The proportion endocrine tissue/exocrine tissue was increased to 1.5 ± 0.2% (non-pregnant control rats: 1.0 ± 0.1%) during the second half of pregnancy. During insulin treatment it was decreased to 0.6 ± 0.05%. After cessation of the treatment it was increased to 2.5 ± 0.5 and 1.9 ± 0.4% on days 18 and 20 (pregnant control rats: 1.4 ± 0.2% and 1.1 ± 0.1%).

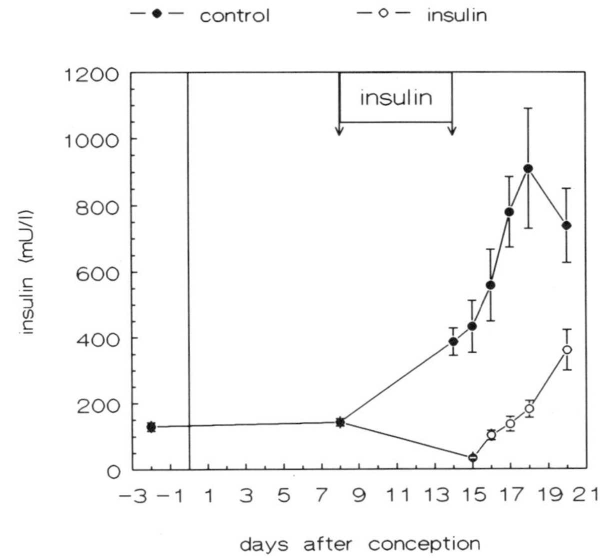

Figure 1. Effect of gestation and insulin treatment of the increment of the insulin plasma concentration, 5 min after intravenous injection of glucose (0.5 g/kg; n = 4–16).

Proinsulin-mRNA concentrations in the islets, as measured by percentage extinction, did not change during pregnancy, but the amount of mRNA-positive pancreatic tissue was increased from 0.8% to 1.4% during the second half of pregnancy. During the insulin treatment virtually no proinsulin-mRNA could be detected. After cessation of the treatment the mRNA concentrations were slightly decreased, but the amount of mRNA-positive cells was increased over the values of the pregnant control rats on day 20 (see Fig. 2).

Similar observations were made in sections immunostained for insulin. Only in insulin-treated rats about 0.7 ± 0.05% of the pancreatic tissue still stained positive for insulin vs 1.7 ± 0.2% in the day-14 pregnant control rats and 1.1 ± 0.2% in non-pregnant control

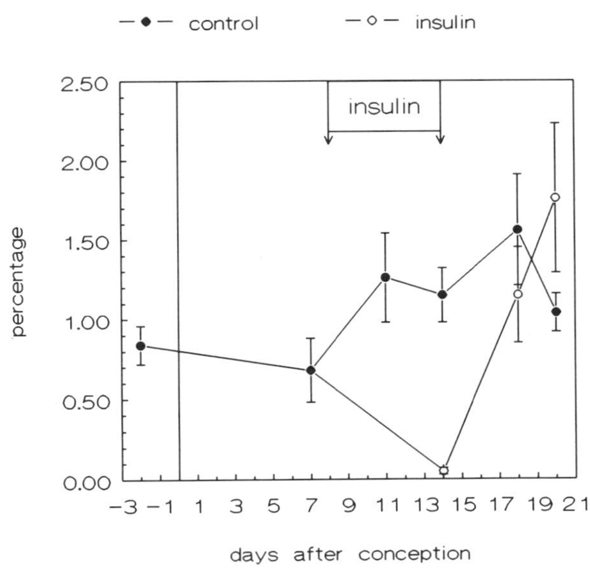

Figure 2. Effect of gestation and insulin treatment on percentage of proinsulin-mRNA-positive tissue in the pancreas (n = 4–6).

rats. After cessation of the insulin treatment insulin-positive tissue increased again and amounted to 1.6 ± 0.4% and 1.7 ± 0.3% on days 18 and 20 vs 1.6 ± 0.2% and 1.3 ± 0.2% in control pregnant rats.

These results show that the changes in the proportion endocrine/exocrine tissue can be explained by changes in beta cell mass. Furthermore, complete recovery of insulin synthetic capacity is apparently not sufficient for full recovery of the insulin secretory response after insulin treatment. This suggests that the treatment also somehow affected the insulin secretory mechanism, which may take longer to recover.

The suggestion of a defect in the insulin-secretory mechanism induced by the insulin treatment is supported by measurements of total pancreatic insulin content. In non-pregnant rats, as well as in day-14 pregnant rats the pancreas contains about 1.4 ± 0.2 IU of insulin. On day 20 insulin content had risen to 2.2 ± 0.2 IU. During insulin treatment insulin content declined to 0.2 ± 0.1 IU on day 14 and recovered to 2.4 ± 0.2 IU on day 20 after cessation of the treatment. Apparently, also full recovery of pancreatic insulin stores after insulin treatment is not sufficient to ensure a normal high insulin response to an intravenous glucose load on day 20 of pregnancy.

Islet-cell proliferation was increased during the second half of pregnancy with a peak at day 14. During insulin treatment proliferation was suppressed by about 60%. After cessation of the treatment proliferation increased as yet, with a peak at day 18 (see Fig. 3). It is likely that most of the proliferating islet-cells are beta cells (Bonner-Weir et al. 1989).

These observations, that supply of exogenous insulin prevents the adaptations of the endocrine pancreas to pregnancy and that these adaptations occur as yet after cessation of the insulin treatment, appear to support the hypothesis that the increased demand for insulin causes the changes in beta cell function and proliferation during pregnancy. Yet, it cannot wholly be excluded that the observed suppression of insulin synthesis and release and of cell proliferation by exogenous insulin is simply due to lack of energy. It is possible that at the low glucose concentrations present during insulin treatment, glucokinase cannot generate sufficient amounts of phosphorylated glucose for cell metabolism (Malaisse 1983; Matschinsky 1990).

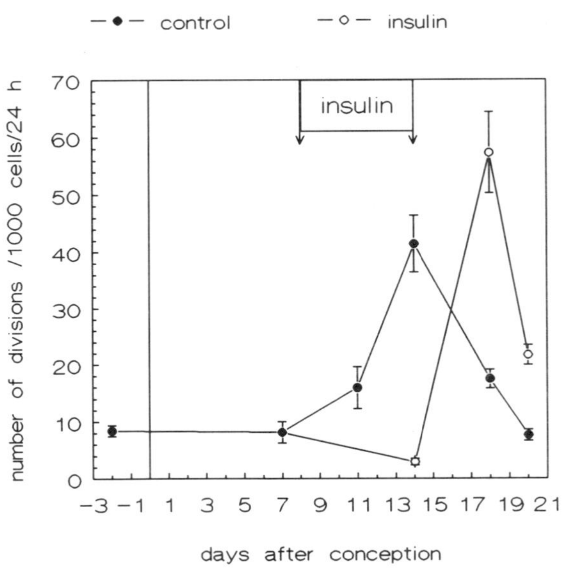

Figure 3. Effect of gestation and insulin treatment on the proliferation of pancreatic islet-cells (n = 4–6).

CONCLUSIONS

In pregnant rats exogenous insulin prevents the various adaptations of the endocrine pancreas to the condition of pregnancy, such as increased insulin production and release and increased islet-cell proliferation. It also induces desensitization of the β-cells (Grodsky 1989). However, the adaptations occur as yet after cessation of insulin treatment. Yet, due to lack of recovery of the β-cells from insulin-induced desensitization, normalization of insulin release is prevented. It is suggested that the studied adaptations of maternal glucose metabolism to pregnancy are largely explained by an increased demand for insulin rather than by any direct effects of placental factors on the endocrine pancreas.

REFERENCES

Bonner-Weir, S., Deery, D., Leahy, J. L., and Weir, G. C., 1989, Compensatory growth of pancreatic β-cells in adult rats after short-term glucose infusion, *Diabetes* 38:49–53.

Chen, L., Komiya, I., Inman, L., McCorkle, K., Alam, T., and Unger, R. H., 1989, Molecular and cellular responses of islets during perturbations of glucose homeostasis determined by in situ hybridization histochemistry, *Proc. Nat. Acad. Sci. USA* 86:1367–1371.

Dunger, A., Lucke, S., Besch, W., and Hahn, H. J., 1989, The rat pancreatic B-cell during pregnancy and after delivery, *Int. J. Feto-Mat. Med.* 2:55–61.

Freinkel, N., 1985, Metabolic Changes in pregnancy, In: Wilson, J. D., and Foster, D. W. (Eds), Williams Textbook of Endocrinology, 7th Ed., W. B. Saunders Company, Philadelphia, p. 438–451.

Grodsky, G.M., 1989, A new phase of insulin secretion. How will it contribute to our understanding of β-cell function, *Diabetes* 38:673–678.

Harms, G., van Goor, H., Koudstaal, J., de Ley, L., and Hardonk, M. J., 1986, Immunohistochemical demonstration of DNA-incorporated 5-bromodeoxyuridine in frozen and plastic embedded sections, *Histochemistry* 85:139–143.

Koiter, T. R., Poelstra, K., Scheringa, M., van der Schaaf-Verdonk, G. C. J., Steffens, A. B., and Schuiling, G. A., 1989, Glucose and insulin responses during mixed meals or infusion of glucose in pregnant and lactating rats, *Physiol. Behav.* 46:881–887.

Leturque, A.P., Ferré, P., Satabin, P., Kervran, A., and Girard, J., 1980, In vivo insulin resistance during pregnancy in the rat, *Diabetologia* 19:521–528.

Malaisse, W. J., 1983, Insulin release: The fuel concept, *Diab. Metabol.* 9:313–320.

Matschinsky, F. M., 1990, Glucokinase as glucose sensor and metabolic signal generator in pancreatic β-cells and hepatocytes, *Diabetes* 39:647–652.

Nielsen, J. H., Nielsen, V., Pedersen, L. M., and Deckert, T., 1986, Effects of pregnancy hormones on pancreatic islets in organ culture, *Acta Endocrinol. (Kbh.)* 11:336–341.

Parsons, J. A., Brelje, T. C., and Sorenson, R. L., 1992, Adaptation of islets of Langerhans to pregnancy: increased islet cell proliferation and insulin secretion correlates with the onset of placental lactogen secretion, *Endocrinology* 130: 1459–1466.

Wolters, G. H. J., Pasma, A., Konijnendijk, W., and Bouman, P. R., 1980, Effects of calcium manipulation and glucose stimulation on a histochemically detectable mobile calcium fraction in isolated rat pancreatic islets, *Histochemistry* 66:125–135.

Part VIII. ISLET GROWTH, REGENERATION, AND TRANSPLANTATION

53

ISLET TRANSPLANTATION

Gregory S. Korbutt,[1] Garth L. Warlock,[1] and Ray V. Rajotte[1,2]

[1]Department of Surgery
Surgical-Medical Research Institute
[2]Department of Medicine
University of Alberta
1074 Dentistry/Pharmacy Building
Edmonton, Alberta TOG 2N8

INTRODUCTION

Insulin-dependent (type 1) diabetes mellitus (IDDM) is caused by a progressive destruction of insulin-producing β cells in the pancreatic islets of Langerhans.[1] Destruction of β cells appears to be mediated by a cell selective autoimmune reactivity which can be triggered by environmental factors in genetically predisposed individuals,[2] *leading to a life-long dependence on insulin therapy*. Despite current modes of treatment, IDDM patients experience episodes of abnormally high blood glucose levels.[3] These recurrent hyperglycemia episodes have been suggested to cause the development of chronic lesions which can result in renal failure, blindness, heart disease, neuropathy, and atherosclerosis.[4] In recent years a predominant focus of diabetes research has been to attempt and develop new forms of treatment which prevent the disabling neurovascular complications of the disease. Recently, through tight control of blood glucose levels, the Diabetes Control and Complications Trial demonstrated that long-term intensive insulin treatment was associated with a reduction in the risk of developing diabetes-related complications.[5] However, this therapy can result in harmful side effects due to hypoglycemia and may be difficult to achieve in all IDDM patients.[5] Furthermore, the intensive involvement required for monitoring and providing therapy for these patients may exceed the capabilities of many individuals and their health care providers. An attractive alternative is to transplant insulin-producing tissue, which can offer a more physiological approach for precise restoration of glucose homeostasis, thereby reversing the metabolic and neurovascular complications of diabetes.

PANCREAS TRANSPLANTATION

A brief overview of what has been achieved with pancreas transplantation is in order, since it provides a standard to compare islet transplantation and it defines the efficacy that

Physiology and Pathophysiology of the Islets of Langerhans, edited by Soria.
Plenum Press, New York, 1997.

clinical transplantation has on correcting basal hyperglycemia and reversing the serious complications of IDDM. Transplantation of the vascularized pancreas was first reported in 1966[6] and by June of 1993 a total of 4,799 cases were reported to the International Pancreas Transplant Registry.[7] Transplantation of the pancreas can restore normoglycemia[8] and result in normal levels of glycosylated hemoglobin.[9] Functioning grafts have been shown to decrease the progression of diabetic glomerulopathy[10] and autonomic nerve dysfunction[11,12] as well as to improve quality of life.[13–15] This form of treatment has been ineffective in preventing retinopathy[16] and almost 50% of the successfully transplanted patients exhibit impaired glucose tolerance curves.[17–19] Pancreas transplantation also requires a complex surgical procedure and life-long immunosuppression. Because of this, pancreas transplantation has been restricted to cases with advanced chronic lesions,[20] since the risks associated with the procedure can exceed those of diabetes itself. Furthermore, allograft rejection has been reported in 40% of the patients within the first 3 years,[20] and HLA-identical grafts were shown to elicit recurrence of autoimmune reactivity in IDDM recipients.[21] Therefore, even though considerable progress has been made with whole organ pancreas transplantation, a simpler and safer method is needed to restore metabolically adequate insulin-producing tissue which can function long-term.

EXPERIMENTAL ISLET TRANSPLANTATION

Why Islet Transplantation?

Compared with vascularized pancreatic grafts, transplantation of isolated islet cells offers a number of advantages in that donor tissue can be tested and pretreated before implantation, thus permitting the possibility of preparing grafts which have specific metabolic and immunological characteristics. The risks and morbidity associated with islet cell transplantation is also significantly lower than that of implanting pancreatic grafts, since the transplant procedure involves an injection of the insulin-producing tissue into a well vascularized circulatory bed.

Preparation and Transplantation of Islet Grafts

In 1911,[22] Bensley stained islets within the guinea pig pancreas with a number of dyes so that they could be picked free of surrounding acinar tissue. Hellerström in 1964[73] first described a method to microdissect viable islets from the rat pancreas. A significant contribution to the advancement of islet isolation was made by Moskalewski,[24] who used theenzyme collagenase to digest and subsequently isolate islets from freshly-chopped guinea pig pancreas. Lacy and Kostianovsky[25] then introduced intraductal distension of the pancreas as a refinement in the collagenase digestion of pancreatic tissue. Rodent islets were originally purified by hand-picking from the dispersed digest,[24] then density gradient centrifugation was found to be more effective for islet purification.[25] Sucrose gradients were initially used,[25] however, Ficoll has now become the gradient of choice because it provides a more suitable osmotic environment.[26,27] This basic approach has now been used for the past two decades by a wide number of research groups for preparing purified rat islet suspensions. In recent years, delivery of collagenase into the pancreatic duct followed by a stationary digestion has yielded a high number of viable islets from both mouse[28] and rat[29,30] pancreata.

The first successful attempt at experimental islet transplantation was reported by Ballinger and Lacy.[31] Transplantation of 400 to 600 isogeneic islets into the peritoneal cavity or the thigh muscle of streptozotocin-induced diabetic rats produced a significant reduction in hyperglycemia and glycosuria.[31] These findings were later confirmed by Reckard and Barker,[32] who were able to completely normalize blood glucose levels in rats following intraperitoneal injection of 800 to 1200 islets. Kemp and co-workers,[33] however, showed there was a physiological advantage to transplant islets into the liver. They found that 800 islets only partially ameliorate diabetes when placed intraperitoneally, but when embolized into the liver via the portal vein, plasma insulin levels and glucose homeostasis were completely normalized. Since then basal glycemia has also been normalized in rodents with chemically-induced diabetes by implantation of islets into the pancreas,[34] as well as in a variety of ectopic sites such as the spleen, testicles, brain, thymus, and renal subcapsular space.[35–38] Transplantation of isolated islets into a highly vascular bed with portal venous drainage, however, has resulted in a more rapid return to normoglycemia as compared to the peritoneum, muscle, or subcutaneous areas.[33,39] In 1976, Pipeleers-Marichal et al.[40] demonstrated that the time required to achieve normal blood glucose levels varied with the number of islets transplanted. Others have also documented that in diabetic rats the size of the islet cell implant affects the rapidity and extent of metabolic normalization.[41,42] The results of the above series of investigations established that complete and permanent reversal of diabetes in rodents was feasible by transplantation of isolated islets of Langerhans.

The success that was achieved in rodent islet isolation was not obtainable when attempted in larger animals, as these techniques proved to be ineffective for the more dense fibrous pancreas found in larger species, including man. It was soon realized that in order to promote effective clinical trials, techniques for islet isolation must be evaluated in a large animal model which simulates the compactness of the human pancreas. Several laboratories therefore began exhaustive efforts utilizing the canine pancreas as a preclinical model for developing methods for human islet isolation.

Mirkovitch and Campiche[43] were the first to report that autotransplants of partially digested canine pancreatic fragments into the spleen could achieve normoglycemia in pancreatectomized recipients. Using similar procedures, autografts of dispersed pancreatic fragments prepared by enzymatic digestion and mechanical dispersion were shown by other investigators to reverse the diabetic state in dogs,[44–47] however, when these impure preparations were injected into the liver via the portal vein complications occurred, including: portal hypertension, elevated liver enzymes, systemic hypotension and disseminated intravascular coagulation.[48,49] More efficient means of digesting the large mammalian pancreas were subsequently developed when collagenase was introduced into the duct by direct injection[50–52] or through continuous perfusion.[53–57] This effective delivery of the collagenase to the connective tissue stroma of the islet-acinar interface, resulted in a greater separation of islets from the surrounding exocrine tissue. Using these methods for pancreas digestion, successful intraportal autotransplantation of purified canine islets became a reality.[53,55,57] These technical advancements have also been used for human pancreas which has allowed for the isolation of large numbers of viable human islets.[51,52,56] These procedures consist of three distinct steps, including: 1) delivery of collagenase via the pancreatic duct; 2) gentle mechanical dissociation; and 3) density gradient centrifugation. A more automated procedure of human islet isolation has also been described,[58] which was shown to simplify the isolation process and enhance islet recovery. Both the automated digestion protocol and the manual procedure have now been used successfully for preparing viable human islet grafts for transplantation.

Numerous techniques have been tested for human islet purification, including filtration,[51] elutriation, density gradient centrifugation[51,52,56,58,59] fluorescence-activated sorting,[60] and the use of lectins that bind magnetic microspheres to exocrine tissue.[61] Since all of these procedures are associated with varying degrees of islet purification and recovery, most laboratories have selected density gradient centrifugation as the preferred method for islet purification.

Islet Allografts

Compared with whole organ transplantation, grafting of isolated islets offers more alternatives for developing strategies to prevent allograft rejection. Donor tissue can be pretreated to reduce its immunogenicity and it can be placed in immunoisolation devices or transplanted into immunopriviledged sites. Isolated islets have been pretreated to reduce their immunogenicity by eliminating or inactivating MHC class II bearing cells, which are known to exert potent immunostimulatory effects.[62–64] A number of ways of pretreating islets have been demonstrated in rodent models. Selective destruction of Ia expressing or dendritic cells in isolated mouse islets was reported by Faustman et al.,[65,66] by using a cell specific antibody-mediated cytotoxicity reaction. When transplanted, these islets remained functional in allogeneic recipients[65,66] however, untreated control islets also reversed the diabetic state in 20% of recipients,[65] suggesting that the selected recipients were low responders to donor islet alloantigens. Furthermore, this approach was not successful when attempted by other laboratories[67] and was shown to require temporary cyclosporine treatment to prevent islet allorejection in rats.[68] The use of ultraviolet light to inactivate allostimulatory cells was used by Lau et al.[67,70] who was able to prolong survival of islet allografts,[69] although in rats with much stronger allogeneic response, temporary immunosuppression was required for survival of donor tissue.[70]

Tissue culture has also been used to reduce islet immunogenicity, either at 24°C[71] or at 37°C in the presence of a gaseous phase containing 95% oxygen.[72] Lacy demonstrated that culture at 24°C for 7 days prolonged survival of allogeneic rat islets, provided the recipients received a single injection of antilymphocyte serum.[71] Interestingly, Markmann et al. has shown that the reduced immunogenicity of rat islets cultured at 24°C is correlated to a reduction in endocrine cell class I MHC antigen expression rather than to the depletion of class II positive cells.[73] Warnock et al.[74] reported that low temperature culture of canine islet allografts in combination with low doses of cyclosporine improved survival, however, grafts promptly failed after cessation of cyclosporine treatment. Furthermore, human islet allografts were also rejected despite the use of immunosuppression and low temperature culture for 7 days.[75] These studies therefore indicate that although pretreatment can prevent islet allograft rejection in mice and rats, its efficacy in other species is highly dependent upon immunosuppressive treatment.

The main rationale for pretreating donor islets is to eliminate the need for continuous immunosuppression, since current immunosuppressive protocols are associated with impaired β cell function,[76–78] reduced islet graft revascularization[79,80] and long-term side effects such as nephrotoxicity and malignancy.[81,82] In contrast, prolonged rat islet cell allograft function has been observed in the absence of immunosuppression when donor islets were pretreated by the purification of endocrine islet cell grafts.[83] Using autofluoresence-activated cell sorting, Pipeleers et al. reported that highly enriched islet endocrine cell aggregates survived as allografts without immunosuppression in 11 of 13 streptozotocin-treated rats over a 20 week follow-up.[83] Even though this approach represents a means of reducing islet allograft rejection, its relevance and application to larger animal models or man, where larger quantities of donor islet cells are required, still needs to be evaluated.

Prevention of islet allorejection has also been accomplished by placing tissue in immunoisolation devices constructed of semipermeable membranes separating donor islets from the recipients immune system. These devices consist of synthetic semi-permeable membranes which allow diffusion of low molecular weight substances (i.e. glucose, insulin) yet exclude cellular contacts between donor and host cells as well as passage of large molecular weight molecules (i.e. immunoglobulins). Islets have been immunoisolated by placing them in: biohybrid chambers anastomosed to the vascular system[84]; diffusion chambers,[85,86] and microcapsules.[87,88] Recently, the progress with these devices has been published in a review by Lanza et al.[89] Although progress has been made at preventing both islet allo- or xenorejection, many technical problems still need to be overcome before this approach can be used successfully in a clinical setting.

In an effort to prevent islet allorejection, many sites have been explored for their potential of offering some privilege against immune attack of islet allografts. Dispersed pancreatic islet cells cultured for 1 day at 26°C were shown to restore normoglycemia following intracerebral allotransplantation in diabetic rats[90,91] When implanted into the testes, islet allograft survival was extended as compared to tissue placed intraportally.[92] Another site which permitted prolonged islet allograft survival is the thymus.[93] Posselt et al.[93] showed that freshly-isolated islets survived as allografts when they were placed intrathymically in combination with a single injection of antilymphocyte serum. Furthermore, this procedure resulted in a state of donor-specific unresponsiveness, since subsequent islet grafts from the same donor strain were not rejected when grafted in sites other than the thymus.[93] The authors hypothesized[93] that the maturation of T cell precursors in a thymic environment containing foreign alloantigens may produce a selective unresponsiveness or tolerance towards the donor antigen. They as well as others have provided support for this view, by demonstrating that intrathymic inoculation of either allogeneic bone marrow[94] or splenic cell membrane antigens[95] with a single dose of antilymphocyte serum, induces an unresponsive state that permits survival of a subsequent pancreatic islet allograft to an extrathymic site. These studies on the prevention of islet allograft rejection have provided novel strategies for permitting long-term allograft survival without the need for chronic immunosuppression, which has now stimulated attempts for their application in man.

Recurrence of Diabetes

Animal models of IDDM have proven useful for testing the effect of islet transplantation in a spontaneous form of the disease. In the BB rat, either culture at 24°C for 14 days[96] or the preparation of purified islet endocrine cells[97] has allowed for prolonged survival of MHC-incompatible grafts when recipients received temporary immunosuppression. Using similar methods, MHC-compatible islet grafts did not survive,[96,97] suggesting that in the BB rat disease recurrence is MHC restricted. However, other studies have shown that the disease recurrence is not MHC restricted in BB rats.[98,99] In addition, reversal of diabetes in BB rats has also been accomplished by transplanting encapsulated allogeneic Wistar islets without the use of immunosuppression.[100] Similarly, intrathymic transplantation of either MHC-compatible or -incompatible donor islets was shown to consistently reverse hyperglycemia in BB rats.[101] It was also shown that intrathymic islet transplantation in neonatal or young diabetic prone BB rats prevents the development of spontaneous diabetes.[102,103] In the NOD mouse, a single injection of either complete Freund's adjuvant or bacillus Calmette-Guerin (an attenuated strain of Mycobacterium bovis) can prevent recurrence of diabetes in syngeneic islet grafts.[104,105] The transfusion of autoreactive T cell clones has also been shown to prevent the recurrence of insulitis and development of diabetes in pancreatic islet-grafted NOD mice.[106] Taken together, these data suggest that the immune mechanisms that cause β cell-specific disease recurrence can be suppressed effectively without the use of chronic immunosuppression, which is important as strategies are developed for the treatment of young juvenile diabetics.

CLINICAL ISLET TRANSPLANTATION

Since 1974, 206 adult human islet allografts have been performed in both European and North American centers.[107] However, in the past 5 years there has been a surge of interest in clinical islet transplantation, so that the total number of transplants performed worldwide by year has progressively increased. For example, in the period of 1974 to 1988 77 islet allografts were conducted, whereas from 1989 to December 31, 1993, 129 transplants were undertaken.[107] Due to the increase in number of islet transplants, the need for maintaining an international registry was soon realized, and the Islet Transplantation Registry (ITR) was therefore established in 1989 at the University of Giessen, Germany.

Until 1989, virtually all attempts to correct basal hyperglycemia in man failed.[108–110] The poor outcome with the initial attempts at human islet transplantation was attributable to implantation of an insufficient β cell mass, since reliable techniques were lacking for the preparation of large quantities of viable human islets. However, during the past 4 to 5 years, several cases have been reported where human islet transplantation has corrected basal hyperglycemia, rendering recipients insulin-independent for varying periods of time (Table 1).[75,110-121] This recent success is largely due to the availability of more reproducible methods for isolating and purifying islets from the human pancreas.[51,56,58] In addition, progress in preserving donor islet tissue before transplantation, either at 24°C[75] or by cryopreservation,[122] has also contributed to the success of clinical islet transplantation.

Recipients of human islet allografts have been type 1 diabetics with a kidney graft, nonuremic IDDM patients, or pancreatectomized patients receiving a liver graft due to upper abdominal exenteration (Table 1). Insulin-independence for more than 2 weeks was obtained in 5 of 10 pancreatectomized recipients and in 8 of 35 cases of type 1 diabetes (Table 1). Islet function in type 1 diabetes was not influenced when the implantation occurred after (IAK) or simultaneous (SIK) to a kidney graft, but those who received islet

Table 1. Effect of islet transplantation in human subjects with type 1 or pancreatectomy induced diabetes

Recipient	Type of transplant	Success rate[a]	Period (months)[b]	Reference
Type 1 diabetes	Allograft			
	SIK	3/19	4–24	111–117
	IAK	5/13	0.5–5	75,116–118
	NRF	0/3	—	118
Pancreatectomized	Allograft[c]	5/10	9–16	111,121
	Autograft	9/22	8–90	119,120

[a]Number of recipients with insulin-independence for more than 2 weeks over total number of published cases.
[b]latest reported time-point with insulin independency.
[c]In combination with a liver graft.
IAK = islet transplant after kidney graft; SIK = simultaneous islet and kidney transplant; NRF = non-renal failure (islet implant alone).

grafts only, exhibited the lowest success rate. The small number of transplants performed in these groups does not allow for a concise conclusion at this time. Successful results were usually observed when islets were provided from multiple donors.[112,113,116,118] Furthermore, when cryopreserved islets were combined with freshly-isolated tissue, an increase in the incidence of recipients obtaining insulin-independence was seen.[113,118] Overall, these results suggest that the improved success of islet transplantation in type 1 diabetics is mainly due to the provision of a sufficient β cell mass.

Gores et al. recently documented two successful cases of prolonged insulin-independence in type 1 diabetics who received unpurified islet tissue obtained from a single donor.[115] Similarly, unpurified pancreatic fragments have also been used as autografts for patients who underwent a partial or complete pancreatectomy due to chronic pancreatitis (Table 1).[119,120] Insulin-independence was achieved in 9 of 22 of these autografted recipients for a period extending from 8 to 90 months posttransplantation (Table 1). It remains uncertain whether insulin is being secreted by the remaining pancreatic remnant and if the impurity of the grafts will be deleterious to long-term function, as few of these recipients have remained insulin independent for over a year.[119] Furthermore, this subset of patients is quite different than those with long-term IDDM since they exhibit metabolic and immunological characteristics clearly distinct from type 1 diabetes. When islets are transplanted into IDDM patients the grafts are exposed to a more hostile environment due to the poor potential for revascularization, the presence of peripheral insulin resistance, and the possibility for recurrence of autoimmune destruction. These differences may therefore explain the higher success rate observed in islet transplantation after pancreatectomy versus allotransplants in patients with advanced IDDM. Whilst the data on pancreatectomized islet recipients does demonstrate that islet transplantation has the ability to induce euglycemia in man, an increased islet mass or improved methods to engraft the islets will likely be required to successfully treat the majority of type 1 diabetics.

Irrespective of the relatively low success of human islet transplantation, the results demonstrate that this form of therapy is capable of correcting hyperglycemia in man following either auto- or allotransplantation. It has also been shown by our group[113] and by others[118] that insulin independence can be achieved long-term and that islet allograft function can normalize glycosylated hemoglobin, which supports the concept that it can potentially achieve the fundamental aim of restoring carbohydrate metabolism. The transplantation and successful engraftment of a sufficient islet cell mass may, however, become a limiting factor, since multiple donors are presently being used to treat one recipient. For this reason, unique methods and approaches are required in order to meet the future for widespread clinical application.

Supply of Islet Tissue

In order to prepare sufficient number of islet grafts, clinical transplant centers will need to rely upon methods of successfully transporting pancreata from one center to another. The preparation of viable human islet cell grafts will thus depend on the ability to preserve β cell survival between the removal of donor pancreata and their processing in the laboratory. The University of Wisconsin (UW) solution is presently the preferred media for whole organ pancreas preservation, however, whether it is optimal for cold storage prior to islet cell isolation is still uncertain. In order to examine if the cold storage solution can influence the yield of insulin-producing tissue, Korbutt and Pipeleers[123] determined the number of viable β cells that could be isolated from freshly-harvested and 24 hour cold-preserved rat pancreata. Organs stored in UW yielded 40% less β cells than organs processed without prior storage.[123] On the other hand, recovery of β cells was not reduced when pancreata were preserved in Collins solution containing bovine serum albumin and benzamidine (CAB solution).[123] These isolated β cells preparations were structurally intact and exhibited the same functional properties as freshly-isolated cells.[123] Although these results can not be extrapolated to human organs, they suggest that CAB solution offers a testable condition which may potentially improve the recovery of human islet cells.

Based upon calculations of the total islet mass within a human pancreas,[1] many islet isolation procedures rarely recovery more than 50% of the islet mass. A limiting step in the whole process has been the lack of effective lots of collagenase. In an effort to overcome this problem, the practice in many laboratories has been to conduct a series of trial and error digestions until a batch of collagenase is found which provides satisfactory results. Because it is unclear as to which enzymes in collagenase are useful for isolating islets, this approach usually involves testing many lots, which is extremely expensive and labor intensive. Recently, a report by Wolters et al.[124] demonstrated that proteases play a critical role in the activity of collagenase during the digestion of rat pancreatic tissue. This study concluded that the presence of both collagenase and proteases are required for successful islet isolation, but it remains uncertain as to what the optimal composition of the various enzymatic preparations should be for a consistent reproducible digestion. Therefore, further research is needed to identify and characterize the active components present within collagenase and possibly develop more standardized products for future clinical use.

Once successfully isolated, some form of tissue bank will be needed which will permit one to store supplemental islets in order to augment marginally adequate grafts for transplantation into an individual recipient. Presently, the only method for successful long-term storage of pancreatic islet cell grafts is through cryopreservation. Initially developed in our laboratory for rodent and canine islets,[122] we have subsequently modified these protocols for preserving human islets.[122] The procedure of cryopreservation consists of three distinct steps, including: 1) addition of a cryoprotectant; 2) freezing and thawing of tissue; and 3) return of tissue to physiological medium. The best outcome has been obtained by using dimethyl sulfoxide as the cryoprotectant in combination with slow cooling and rapid thawing,[122] These techniques have now added flexibility to clinical islet transplantation by allowing for the collection and storage of viable human islets, so that tissue can be pooled from multiple donors for treating individual recipients.

If islet transplantation becomes a widespread treatment for diabetes, the supply of cadaveric human pancreata will become a major limiting step. In an attempt to overcome this supply problem, animal islet tissue is being considered for xenotransplantation across concordant or widely discordant species barriers.[37,38] A clinical trial on transplantation of cultured fetal pig islet cells into immunosuppressed diabetic patients was initiated by Anderson and associates[125] in Sweden. Although there was no evidence to indicate engraftment of the fetal cells, all patients tolerated the procedure well and no adverse side effects were recorded.[125] Nevertheless, more effective means of immunosuppression and/or immunoisolation are required before xenotransplantation of islet tissue becomes a clinical reality. Lastly, an additional source of insulin-producing tissue can possibly be obtained through the design of cellular engineering experiments. Recently, Newgard et al.[126] have successfully transferred the Glut-2 gene into an insulinoma cell line. These experiments provide evidence that different types of somatic cells can possibly serve as vehicles that mimic the production and secretion of insulin with characteristics similar to normal human β cells. Ultimately, the availability of genetically engineered insulin-producing cells could solve the problem of donor supply for the treatment of IDDM.

CONCLUSION

The present state of islet cell transplantation illustrates that over the past two decades this field has had many advancements. Twenty years ago, hyperglycemia was corrected in rats with chemically-induced diabetes by intraportal transplantation of isogeneic islets. Today, islet transplantation has moved into the clinical arena, resulting in insulin-independence long-term in many type 1 diabetics. Technical progress has been achieved in the isolation and cryopreservation of human islets, which has enabled many centers to establish islet transplantation programs.

The clinical potential of islet transplantation will only be fully realized by its capacity to correct glucose homeostasis and to prevent the development of chronic complications associated with diabetes. Ideally, islet transplantation should occur at an early stage of the disease, since these patients could benefit the most. However, the selected treatment should not introduce new hazardous risks to the patient. The avoidance of chronic immunosuppression is definitely the ideal scenario for islet transplantation and studies in animal models suggest that this can be accomplished by various approaches. Clinical trials should now determine whether such methods can prolong islet allograft survival in man without the need for chronic immunosuppression. Even though the transfer of these approaches to a clinical setting is far from being perfect, the establishment of concise, well controlled step-by-step protocols in both basic and clinical research can potentially facilitate their application in man.

ACKNOWLEDGMENTS

Support was provided by the Alberta Foundation of Diabetes Research, the Alberta Heritage Foundation for Medical Research, the Juvenile Diabetes Foundation International, the Medical Research Council of Canada, and the Muttart Diabetes Research and Training Centre. G.S. Korbutt is a recipient of a Canadian Diabetes Association Postdoctoral Fellowship Award. The authors are grateful to Colleen Gardner for invaluable secretarial assistance.

REFERENCES

1. W. Gepts, Pathological anatomy of the pancreas in juvenile diabetes mellitus, *Diabetes* 14:619–633 (1965).
2. G.S. Eisenbarth, Type 1 diabetes mellitus. A chronic autoimmune disease, *N. Engl. J. Med.* 314:1360–1368 (1986).
3. D.M. Nathan, The rationale for glucose control in diabetes mellitus, *Endocrinol. Metab. Clin. North Am.* 21:221–235 (1992).
4. D.M. Nathan, Long-term complications of diabetes mellitus, *N. Engl. J. Med.* 23:1676–1685 (1993).
5. American Diabetes Association, Position Statement, Implications of the diabetes control and complications trial, *Diabetes* 42:1555–1558 (1993).
6. W.D. Kelly, R.C. Lillehei, F.K. Merkel, Y. Idezuki, F.C. Goetz, Allotransplantation of thé pancreas and duodenum along with the kidney in diabetic nephropathy, *Surgery* 61:827–837 (1967).
7. D. Sutherland, A. Gruessner, K. Moudry-Munns, International Pancreas Transplant Registry Report, *Transplant. Proc.* 26:407–411 (1994).
8. H. Katz, M. Homan, J. Velosa, R. Robertson, R. Rizza, Effects of pancreas transplantation on postprandial glucose metabolism, *N. Engl. J. Med.* 327:1278–1283 (1991).
9. R.P. Robertson, Perspectives in diabetes: pancreas transplantation in humans with diabetes mellitus, *Diabetes* 40:1085–1089 (1991).

10. R.W. Bilous, S.M. Mauer, D.E.R. Sutherland, J.S. Najarian, F.C. Goetz, M.W. Steffes, The effects of pancreas transplantation on the glomerular structure of renal allografts in patients with insulin-dependent diabetes, *N. Engl. J. Med.* 321:80–85 (1989).
11. X. Navarro, W.R. Kennedy, R.G. Loewenson, D.E.R. Sutherland, Influence of pancreas transplantation on cardiorespiratory reflexes, nerve conduction, and mortality in diabetes mellitus, *Diabetes* 39:802–806 (1990).
12. W.R. Kennedy, X. Navarro, F.C. Goetz, D.E.R. Sutherland, J. S. Najarian, Effects of pancreatic transplantation on diabetic neuropathy, *N. Engl. J. Med.* 322:1031–1037 (1990).
13. C.L. Zehrer, C.R. Gross, Quality of life of pancreas transplant recipients, *Diabetologia* 34(Suppl.l):S145–S149 (1991).
14. W. Piehimeier, M. Bullinger, J. Nusser, A. Konig, W.D. Illner, D. Abendroth, et al., Quality of life in type 1 (insulin-dependent) diabetic patients prior to and after pancreas and kidney transplantation in relation to organ function, *Diabetologia* 34(Suppl.l):S150–S157 (1991).
15. D.M. Nathan, H. Fogel, D. Norman, P.S. Russell, N. Tokoff-Rubin, F.L. Delmonico, et al., Long-term metabolic and quality of life results with pancreatic/renal transplantation in insulin-dependent diabetes mellitus, *Transplantation* 52:85–89 (1991).
16. R.C. Ramsay, F.C. Goetz, D.E.R. Sutherland, S.M. Mauer, L.L. Robison, H.L. Cantrill, et al., Progression of diabetic retinopathy after pancreas transplantation for insulin-dependent diabetes mellitus, *N. Engl. J. Med.* 318:208–214 (1988).
17. F.H. Wright, J.L. Smith, S.A. Ames, B. Schanbacher, R.J. Corry, Function of pancreas allografts more than 1 year following transplantation, *Arch. Surg.* 124:796–800 (1989).
18. R. Landgraf, J. Nusser, R.L. Riepl, F. Fiedler, W.D. Illner, D. Abendroth, W. Land, Metabolic and hormonal studies of type 1 (insulin-dependent) diabetic patients after successful pancreas and kidney transplantation, *Diabetologia* 34(Suppl.l):S61–S67 (1991).
19. P. Morel, K.L. Brayman, F.C. Goetz, D.M. Kendall, K. Moudry-Munns, C. Chau, et al., Long-term metabolic function of pancreas transplant and influence of rejection episodes, *Transplantation* 51:990–1000 (1991).
20. R.P. Robertson, Pancreatic and islet transplantation for diabetes — cures or curiosities?, N. *Engl. J. Med.* 327:1861–1868 (1993).
21. R.K. Sibley, D.E.R. Sutherland, F. Goetz, A.F. Michael, Recurrent diabetes mellitus in the pancreas iso- and allograft. A light and electron microscope and immunohistochemical analysis of four cases, *Laboratory Invest.* 53:132–144 (1985).
22. R.R. Bensley, Studies on the pancreas of the guinea pig, *Am. J. Anat.* 12:297–388 (1911).
23. C. Hellerström A method for the microdissection of intact pancreatic islets of mammals, *Acta Endocrinol.* 45: 122–132 (1964).
24. S. Moskalewski, Isolation and culture of the islets of Langerhans of the guinea pig, *Gen. Comp. Endocrinol.* 5:342–353 (1965).
25. P.E. Lacy, M. Kostianovsky, Method for the isolation of intact islets of Langerhans from the rat pancreas, *Diabetes* 16:35–39 (1967).
26. A. Lindall, M. Steffes, R. Sorenson, Immuno-assayable insulin content of subcellular fractions of rat islets, *Endocrinology* 85:218–223 (1969).
27. D.W. Scharp, C.B. Kemp, M.J. Knight, W.F. Ballinger, P.E. Lacy, The use of Ficoll in the preparation of viable islets of Langerhans from the rat pancreas, *Transplantation* 16:686–689 (1973).
28. M. Gotoh, T. Maki, T. Kiyoizumi, S. Satomi, A.P. Monaco, An improved method for isolation of mouse pancreatic islets, *Transplantation* 40:437–438 (1985).
29. R. Sutton, M. Peters, P. McShane, D.W.R. Gray, P.J. Morris, Isolation of rat pancreatic islets by ductal injection of collagenase, *Transplantation* 42:689–691 (1986).
30. M. Gotoh, T. Maki, S. Satomi, J. Porter, S. Bonner-Weir, C.J. O'Hara, A.P. Monaco, Reproducible high yield of rat islets by stationary in vitro digestion following pancreatic ductal or portal venous collagenase injection, *Transplantahon* 43:725–730 (1987).
31. W.F. Ballinger, P.E. Lacy, Transplantation of intact pancreatic islets in rats, *Surgery* 72:175–186 (1972).
32. C. Reckard, C. Barker, Transplantation of isolated pancreatic islets across strong and weak histocompatibility barriers, *Transplant. Proc.* 5:761–763 (1973).
33. C.B. Kemp, M.J. Knight, D.W. Scharp, W.F. Ballinger, P.E. Lacy, Effect of transplantation site on the results of pancreatic islet isografts in diabetic rats, *Diabetologia* 9:486–491 (1973).
34. A. Hayek, G.M. Beattie, Intrapancreatic islet transplantation in experimental diabetes in the rat, *Metabolism* 41:1367–1369 (1992).
35. D.W.R. Gray, P.J. Morris, Developments in isolated pancreatic islet transplantation, *Transplantion* 43:321–331 (1987).
36. R. W. Nason, R.V. Rajotte, G .L. Warnock, Pancreatic islet cell transplantation: past, present and future, *Diabetes Res.* 7:1–11 (1988).

37. P.E. Lacy, Status of islet cell transplantation, *Diabetes Rev.* 1:76–92 (1993).
38. D.G. Pipeleers, B. Keymeulen, G.S. Korbutt, Islet transplantation, *in:* "The Diabetes Annual/8," S. Marshall, P. Home, eds., Elsevier Science Publishers, Amsterdam, pp. 299–330 (1994).
39. B.N. Gray, E. Watkins, Isolated islet transplantation in experimental diabetes, *Austr. J. Exp. Biol. Med. Sci.* 54:57–70 (1976).
40. M.A. Pipeleers-Marichal, D.G. Pipeleers, J. Cutler, P.E. Lacy, D.M. Kipnis, Metabolic and morphologic studies in intraportal-islet-transplanted rats, *Diabetes* 25: 1041–1051 (1976).
41. B. Keymeulen, H. Teng, M. Vetri, F. Gores, P. In't Veld, D.G. Pipeleers, Effect of donor islet mass on metabolic normalization in streptozotocin-diabetic rats, *Diabetologia* 35:719–724 (1992).
42. D.T. Finegood, B.W. Tobin, J.T. Lewis, Dynamics of glycemic normalization following transplantation of incremental islet masses in streptozotocin-diabetic rats, *Transplantation* 53:1033–1037 (1992).
43. V. Mirkovitch, M. Campiche, Successful intrasplenic autotransplantation of pancreatic tissue in totally pancreatectomized dogs, *Transplantation* 21:265–269 (1976).
44. A.J. Matas, D.E.R. Sutherland, M.W. Steffes, J. S. Najarian, Short-term culture of adult pancreatic fragments for purification and transplantation of islets of Langerhans, *Surgery* 80: 183–191 (1976).
45. E. Kolb, R. Ruckert, L. Largiader, Intraportal and intrasplenic autotransplantation of pancreatic islets in the dog, *Eur. Surg. Res.* 9:419–420 (1977).
46. G.J. Kretschmer, D.E.R. Sutherland, A.J. Matas, M.W. Steffes, J.S. Najarian, The dispersed pancreas: Transplantation without islet purification in totally pancreatectomized dogs, *Diabetologia* 13:495–502 (1977).
47. G.J. Kretschmer, D.E.R. Sutherland, A.J. Matas, T.L. Cain, J.S. Najarian, Autotransplantation of pancreatic islets without separation of exocrine and endocrine tissue in totally pancreatectomized dogs, *Surgery* 82:74–81 (1977).
48. G.J. Kretschmer, D.E.R. Sutherland, A.J. Matas, W.D. Payne, J.S. Najarian, Autotransplantation of pancreatic fragments to the portal vein and spleen of totally pancreatectomized dogs: A comparative evaluation, *Ann. Surg.* 187:79–86 (1978).
49. D.G. Mehigan, W.R. Bell, G.D. Zuidema, J.C. Eggleston, J.L. Cameron, Disseminated intravascular coagulation and portal hypertension following pancreatic islet autotransplantation, *Ann. Surg.* 191:287–293 (1980).
50. J. Noel, A. Rabinovitch, L. Olson, G. Kyriakides, J. Miller, D.H. Mintz, A method for large scale, high yield isolation of canine pancreatic islets of Langerhans, *Metabolism* 31:184–187 (1982).
51. D.W.R. Gray, P. McShane, A. Grant, P.J. Morris, A method for isolation of islets of Langerhans from the human pancreas, *Diabetes* 33:1055–1061 (1984).
52. D.W. Scharp, P.E. Lacy, E. Finke, B. Olack, Low-temperature culture of human islets isolated by the distension method and purified with Ficoll or Percoll gradients, *Surgery* 102:869–879 (1987).
53. A. Horaguchi, R.C. Merrel, Preparation of viable islet cells from dogs by a new method, *Diabetes* 30:455–458 (1981).
54. G.L. Warnock, R.V. Rajotte, A.W. Procyshyn, Normoglycemia after reflux of islet-containing pancreatic fragments into the splenic vascular bed in dogs, *Diabetes* 32:452–459 (1983).
55. G.L. Warnock, R.V. Rajotte, Critical mass of purified islets that induce normoglycemia after implantation into dogs, *Diabetes* 37:467–470 (1988).
56. G.L. Warnock, D.K. Ellis, R.V. Rajotte, I. Dawidson, S. Baekkeskov, J. Egebjerg, Studies of the isolation and viability of human islets of Langerhans, *Transplantation* 45:957–963 (1988).
57. D.B. Kaufman, P. Morel, M.J. Field, S.R. Munn, D.E.R. Sutherland, Purified canine islet autografts. Functional outcome as influenced by islet number and implantation site, *Transplantahon* 50:385–391 (1990).
58. C. Ricordi, P.E. Lacy, E.H. Finke, B.J. Olack, D.W. Scharp, Automated method for isolation of human pancreatic islets, *Diabetes* 37:413–420 (1988).
59. S.P. Lake, D. Bassett, A. Larkins, J. Revell, K. Walczak, J. Chamberlain, G.M. Rumford, N.J.M. London, P.S. Veitch, P.R.F. Bell, R.F.L. James, Large-scale purification of human islets utilizing discontinuous albumin gradient on IBM 2991 cell separator, *Diabetes* 38(Suppl.1):143–145 (1989).
60. D.W. Gray, W. Gohde, N. Carter, T. Heiden, P.J. Morris, Separation of pancreatic islets by fluorescence-activated sorting, *Diabetes* 38(Suppl.1):133–135 (1989).
61. S. Winto-Morbach, K. Ulrichs, G. Leghausen, W. Muller-Rucholtz, New principle for large-scale preparation of purified human pancreas islets, *Diabetes* 38(Suppl.1):146–149 (1989).
62. W.E.F. Klinikert, J.H. LaBadie, J.P. O'Brien, C.F. Beyer, W.E. Bowers, Rat dendritic cells function as accessory cells and control the production of a soluble factor required for mitogenic responses of T lymphocytes, *Proc. Natl. Acad. Sci. USA* 77:5414–4518 (1980).
63. R.I. Lechler, J.R. Batchelor, Restoration of immunogenicity to passenger cell-depleted kidney allografts by the addition of donor strain dendritic cells, J. *Exp. Med.* 155:31–41 (1982).
64. S.C. Knight, J. Mertin, A. Stackpoole, J. Clark, Induction of immune responses in vivo with small numbers of veiled (dendritic) cells, *Proc. Natl. Acad. Sci. USA* 80:6032–6035 (1983).

65. D. Faustman, V. Hauptfield, P. Lacy, J. Davie, Prolongation of murine islet allograft survival by pretreatment of islets with antibody directed to Ia determinants, *Proc. Natl. Acad. Sci.* USA 78:5156–5159 (1981).
66. D.L. Faustman, R.M. Steinman, H.M. Gebel, V. Hauptfield, J.M. Davie, P.E. Lacy, Prevention of rejection of murine islet allografts by pretreatment with anti-dendritic cell antibody, *Proc. Natl. Acad. Sci. USA* 81: 3864–3868 (1984).
67. P.F. Gores, D.E.R. Sutherland, J.L. Platt, F.H. Bach, Depletion of donor IA+ cells before transplantation does not prolong islet allograft survival, J. *Immunol.* 137:1482–1485 (1986).
68. R. Terasaka, P.E. Lacy, V. Hauptfeld, R.P. Bucy, J.M. Davie, The effect of cyclosporin A, low-temperature culture, and anti-Ia antibodies on prevention of rejection of rat islet allografts, *Diabetes* 35:83–88 (1986).
69. H. Lau, K. Reemtsma, M.A. Hardy, Prolongation of rat islet allograft survival by direct ultraviolet irradiation of the graft, *Science* 223:607–608 (1984).
70. H. Lau, K. Reemtsma, M.A. Hardy, The use of direct ultraviolet irradiation and cyclosporin in facilitating indefinite pancreatic islet allograft acceptance, *Transplantation* 38:566–569 (1984).
71. P.E. Lacy, J.M. Davie, E.H. Finke, Prolongation of islet allograft survival following in vitro culture (24°C) and a single injection of ALS, *Science* 204:312–313 (1979).
72. K.M. Bowen, S.J. Prowse, K.J. Lafferty, Successful allotransplantation of mouse pancreatic islets to nonimmunosuppressed recipients, *Diabetes* 29(Suppl.1):98–104 (1980).
73. J.F. Markmann, J. Tomaszewski, A.M. Posselt, M.M. Levy, M. Woehrle, C.F. Barker, A. Naji, The effect of islet cell culture in vitro at 24°C on graft survival and MHC antigen expression, *Transplantation* 49:272–277 (1990).
74. G.L. Warnock, K.D. Dabbs, M.S. Cattral, R.V. Rajotte, Improved survival of in vitro cultured canine islet allografts, *Transplantion* 57:17–22 (1994).
75. D.W. Scharp, P.E. Lacy, J.V. Santiago, C. S. McCullough, L. G. Weide, L. Falqui, et al., Insulin independence after islet transplantation into type 1 diabetic patient, *Diabetes* 39:515–518 (1990).
76. R.P. Robertson, Cyclosporin-induced inhibition of insulin secretion in isolated rat islets and HIT cells, *Diabetes* 35:1016–1019 (1986).
77. S.L. Gillison, S.T. Bartlet, D.L. Curry, Inhibition by cyclosporin of insulin secretion — A beta cell specific alteration of islet tissue function, *Transplantion* 52:890–895 (1991).
78. G.L. Viviani, M.G. Borgoglio, I. Fontana, A. Borgoglio, Azathioprine decreases insulin secretion in human islets, *Transplant. Proc.* 21:2714–2716 (1989).
79. R.C. Merrel, M.E. Mahoney, G. Basadonna, L.F. Cobb, M. Maeda, Failure of canine islet allografts and autografts with cyclosporine, *Surgery* 98:324–329 (1985).
80. P. Rooth, I. Dawidson, K. Lafferty, K. Diller, J. Armstrong, et al., Prevention of detrimental effect of cyclosporin A on vascular growth of transplanted pancreatic islets with verapamil, *Diabetes* 38(Suppl.1): 202–205 (1989).
81. I. Penn, Cancers following cyclosporin therapy, *Transplantahon* 43:32–35 (1987).
82. G. Feutren, M.J. Mihatch, I.K. Bread, Risk factors for cyclosporin-induced nephropathy in patients with autoimmune diseases, N. *Engl. J. Med.* 326:1654–1660 (1992).
83. D.G. Pipeleers, M. Pipeleers-Marichal, B. Vandbrabandt, S. Duys, Transplantation of purified islet cells in diabetic rats. II. Immunogenicity of allografted islet β-cells, *Diabetes* 40:920–930 (1991).
84. A.P. Monaco. T. Maki, H. Ozato, M. Carreta, S.J. Sullivan, K.M. Borland, et al., Transplantation of islet allografts and xenografts in totally pancreatectomized diabetic dogs using the hybrid artificial pancreas, *Ann. Surg.* 214:339–362 (1991).
85. J.J. Altman, P. McMillan, P. Callard, P.M. Galletti, A bioartificial pancreas prevents chronic complications of diabetes in rats, *Am. Soc. Artif. Intern. Organs* 32:145–147 (1986).
86. R.P. Lanza, K.M. Borland, P. Lodge, M. Carretta, S.J. Sullivan, T.E. Muller, et al., Treatment of severely diabetic pancreatectomized dogs using a diffusion-based hybrid pancreas, *Diabetes* 41:886–889 (1992).
87. W. M . Fritschy, J. H . Stubbe, G .H. J. Wolters , R. Van Schilfgaarde, Glucose tolerance and plasma insulin response to intravenous glucose infusion and test meal in rats with microencapsulated islet allografts, *Diabetologia* 34:542–547 (1991).
88. P. Soon-Shiong, E. Feldman, R. Nelson, J. Komtebedde, O. Smidsrod, G. Skjak-Braek, et al., Successful reversal of spontaneous diabetes in dogs by intraperitoneal microencapsulated islets, *Transplantation* 54:769–774 (1992).
89. R.P. Lanza, S.J. Sullivan, W.L. Chick, Islet transplantation with immunoisolation, *Diabetes* 41:1503–1510 (1992).
90. W.J. Tze, J. Tai, Successful intracerebral allotransplantation of purified pancreatic endocrine cells in diabetic rat, *Diabetes* 32:1185–1187 (1983).
91. W.J. Tze, J. Tai, Intrathecal allotransplantation of pancreatic endocrine cells in diabetic rats, *Transplantation* 41:531–534 (1986).

92. H.P. Selawry, K. Whittington, Extended allograft survival of islets grafted into intra-abdominally placed testis, *Diabetes* 33:405–406 (1984).
93. A.M. Posselt, C.F. Barker, J.E. Tomaszewski, J.F. Markmann, MA Choti, A. Naji, Induction of donor unresponsiveness by intrathymic islet transplantation, *Science* 249:1293–1295 (1990).
94. A.M. Posselt, J.S. Odorico, C.F. Barker, A. Naji, Promotion of pancreatic islet allograft survival by intrathymic transplantation of bone marrow, *Diabetes* 41:771–775 (1992).
95. T. Qian, R. Schachner, M. Brendel, S. Shen Kong, R. Alejandro, Induction of donor-specific tolerance to rat islet allografts by intrathymic inoculation of solubilized spleen cell membrane antigens, *Diabetes* 42:1544–1546 (1993).
96. M. Woehrle, J. F. Markmann, W.K . Silvers , C .F. Barker, N. Naji, Transplantation of cultured pancreatic islets to BB rats, *Surgery* 100:334–341 (1986).
97. D. Pipeleers, M. Pipeleers-Marichal, H. Markholst, A. Hoorens, G. Kloppel, Transplantation of purified islet cells in diabetic BB rats, *Diabetologia* 34:390–396 (1991).
98. S.J. Prowse, D. Bellgau, K.J. Lafferty, Islet allografts are destroyed by disease occurrence in the spontaneous diabetic BB rat, *Diabetes* 35: 110–114 (1986).
99. E.J. Weringer, A.A. Like, Immune attack on pancreatic islet transplants in the spontaneous diabetic biobreeding/Worchester (BB/W) rat is not MHC restricted, J. *Immunol.* 134:2383–2386 (1985).
100. M. Fan, Z.P. Lum, X.W. Fu, L. Levesque, I.T. Tai, A.M. Sun, Reversal of diabetes in BB rats by transplantation of encapsulated pancreatic islets, *Diabetes* 39:519–522 (1990).
101. A.M. Posselt, A. Naji, J.H. Roark, J.F. Markmann, C.F. Barker, Intrathymic islet transplantation in the spontaneously diabetic BB rat, *Ann. Surg.* 214:363–373 (1991).
102. A.M. Posselt, C.F. Barker, A.L. Friedman, A. Naji, Prevention of autoimmune diabetes in the BB rat by intrathymic islet transplantation at birth, *Science* 256:1321–1324 (1992).
103. S.T. Koevary, M. Blomberg, Prevention of diabetes in BB/Wor rats by intrathymic islet injection, *J. Clin. Invest.* 89:512–516 (1992).
104. T. Wang, B. Singh, G.L. Warnock, R.V. Rajotte, Prevention of recurrence of IDDM in islet-transplanted diabetic NOD mice by adjuvant immunotherapy, *Diabetes* 41:114–117 (1992).
105. J.R.T. Lakey, B. Singh, G.L. Warnock, R.V. Rajotte, BCG immunotherapy prevents recurrence of diabetes in islet grafts transplanted into spontaneously diabetic NOD mice, *Transplantation* 57:1213–1217 (1994).
106. T. Utsugi, M. Nagata, T. Kawamura, J. Yoon, Prevention of recurrent diabetes in syngenic islet-transplanted NOD mice by transfusion of autoreactive T lymphocytes, *Transplantation* 57:1799–1804 (1994).
107. International Islet Transplant Registry, Newsletter No. 5, B.J. Hering, C. Geier, A.O. Schultz, R.G. Bretzel, K. Federlin, eds. vol. 4: March (1994).
108. B.J. Hering, C.C. Browatzki, A. Schultz, R.G. Bretzel, K.F. Federlin, Clinical islet transplantation — registry report, accomplishments in the past and future research needs, *Cell Transplantation* 2:269–282 (1993).
109. B.J. Hering, R.G. Bretzel, K. Federlin, Current status of clinical islet transplantation, *Horm. Metab. Res.* 20:537–545 (1988).
110. G.L. Warnock, R.V. Rajotte, Human pancreatic islet transplantation, *Transplantation Rev.* 6:1–8 (1992).
111. C. Ricordi, A.G. Tzakis, P.B. Carroll, Y. Zeng, H.L. Rodriguez Rilo, R. Alejandro, et al., Human islet isolation and allotransplantation in 22 consecutive cases, *Transplantation* 53:407–414 (1992).
112. G.L. Warnock, N.M. Kneteman, E. Ryan, R.E.A. Seelis, A. Rabinovitch, R.V. Rajotte, Normoglycemia after transplantation of freshly isolated and cryopreserved pancreatic islets in type 1 (insulin-dependent) diabetes mellitus, *Diabetologia* 34:55–58 (1991).
113. G.L. Warnock, N.M. Kneteman, E. Ryan, A. Rabinovitch, R.V. Rajotte, Long-term follow-up after transplantation of insulin-producing pancreatic islets into patients with type 1 (insulin-dependent) diabetes mellitus, *Diabetologia* 35:89–95 (1992).
114. P.F. Gores, J.S. Najarian, E. Stephanian, J.J. Lioveras, S.L. Kelley, D.E.R. Sutherland, Insulin independence in type 1 diabetes after transplantation of unpurified islets from single donor with 15-deoxyspergualin, *Lancet* 341:19–21 (1993).
115. P.F. Gores, J.S. Najarian, E. Stephanian, J.J. Lioveras, S.L. Kelley, D.E.R. Sutherland, Transplantation of unpurified islets from single donors with 15-deoxyspergualin, *Transplant. Proc.* 26:574–575 (1994).
116. R. Alejandro, S. Strasser, V. Esquenazi, G. Burke, J. Nery, J. Miller, E.T. Shapiro, C. Ricordi, D. Mintz, Long-term survival of intraportal islet allografts in type 1 diabetes mellitus. In: Pancreatic Islet Cell Transplantation (C. Ricordi, ed.). R.G. Landes Co., Austin, pp. 410–413 (1994).
117. C. Socci, C. Ricordi, V. Di Carlo, L. Falqui, P. Maffi, G. Pozza, A.M. Davalli, A. Secchi, Substitution of the endocrine pancreatic function in IDDM patients by allotransplantation of fresh islets: the Milan experience. In: Pancreatic Islet Cell Transplantation (C. Ricordi, ed.). R.G. Landes Co, Austin, pp. 414–422 (1994).
118. D.W. Scharp, P.E. Lacy, J.V. Santiago, C.S. McCullough, L.G. Weide, P.J. Boyle, et al., Results of our first nine intraportal islet allograft in type 1, insulin-dependent diabetic patients, *Transplantation* 51:76–85 (1991).

119. A.C. Farney, J.S. Najarian, R.E. Nakhleh, G. Lloveras, M.J. Field, P.F. Gores, et al., Autotransplantation of dispersed pancreatic islet tissue combined with total or near-total pancreatectomy for treatment of chronic pancreatitis, *Surgery* 110:427–439 (1992).
120. K.L. Pyzdrowski, D.M. Kendall, J.B. Halter, R.E. Nakhleh, D.E.R. Sutherland, R.P. Robertson, Preserved insulin secretion and insulin independence in recipients of islet autografts, N. *Engl. J. Med.* 327:220–226 (1992).
121. A.G. Tzakis, C. Ricordi, R. Alejandro, Y. Zeng, J.J. Fung, S. Todo, Pancreatic islet transplantation after upper abdominal exenteration and liver replacement, *Lancet* 336:402–405 (1990).
122. R.V. Rajotte, G.L. Warnock, M.G. Coulombe, Islet cryopreservation methods and experimental results in rodents, large animals, and humans, *in:* "Transplantation of the Endocrine Pancreas in Diabetes Mellitus," R. van Schilfgaarde, M.A. Hardy, eds., Elsevier, Amsterdam, pp. 125–135 (1988).
123. G.S. Korbutt, D.G. Pipeleers, Cold storage of rat pancreas before purification of islet β-cells, *Diabetes* 41: 299–307 (1992).
124. G.H.J. Wolters, G.H. Vos Scheperkeuter, J.H.M. Van Deijmen, R. Van Schilfgaarde, An analysis of the role of collagenase and protease in the enzymatic dissociation of the rat pancreas for islet isolation, *Diabetologia* 35:735–742 (1992).
125. A. Andersson, S. Sandler, Fetal pancreatic transplantation, *Transplant. Rev.* 6:20–38 (1992).
126. S. Ferber, H. Beltrandeltio, J.H. Johnson, R.J. Noel, L.E. Cassidy, S. Clark, T.C. Becker, S.D. Hughes, C.B. Newgard, Glut-2 gene transfer into insulinoma cells confers both low and high affinity glucose-stimulated insulin release, *J. Biol. Chem.* 269:11523–11529 (1994).

54

THE SYNGENEIC ISLET TRANSPLANTATION TO STUDY PHYSIOLOGY AND PATHOPHYSIOLOGY OF PANCREATIC β-CELLS

Hans J. Hahn and Beate Kuttler

Department of Medical Cell Biology
Institute of Diabetes "G. Katsch"
Medical School
University of Greifswald
17495 Karlsburg, Germany

INTRODUCTION

Several years ago, techniques have been developed for isolation of pancreatic islets from rodent pancreas[1,2] in order to permit in vitro studies on the mechanism and events involved in the formation, storage, and release of insulin by pancreatic B-cells and other hormones produced by the islet cells[3]. A natural outgrowth of this development was to determine whether transplants of isolated islets into inbred strains of rodents (syngeneic transplantation), with experimentally induced diabetes, would achieve and maintain normoglycaemia in the recipients. Since the pioneering work of Lacy[4], who demonstrated the successful reversal of diabetes with syngeneic islet grafts, studies were performed to determine the effect on diabetic complications, as they occur in rodents. The islet transplants prevented or reversed many of the complications caused by hyperglycaemia, thus the possibility was raised to utilize pancreatic islets for transplantation in diabetic patients[4–6]. In consequence, primary experimental, and later clinical research was concentrated on the development of methods for mass isolation of islets, for immunological procedures, which allowed allogeneic or xenogeneic transplantation without continuous immunosuppression, and for clinical application in diabetic patients. Even, if the ultimate goal of islet transplantation is to cure diabetic patients, the syngeneic islet transplantation can be used to improve our understanding of pancreatic B-cells in normal and abnormal conditions. This review will summarize some results obtained when fetal, neonatal or adult pancreatic islets were grafted into inbred animals.

Physiology and Pathophysiology of the Islets of Langerhans, edited by Soria.
Plenum Press, New York, 1997.

PHYSIOLOGY OF GRAFTED PANCREATIC ISLETS

If enough pancreatic B-cells were transplanted into hyperglycaemic inbred animals and into a site (intraportally, beneath the kidney capsules, into spleen, intraperitoneally), which permits engraftment, normoglycaemia is achieved within 3–5 days. The normoglycaemia is normally maintained life-long and accompanied by a normal glucose tolerance. Morphological investigations of the graft, which have been performed in rodents up to 2 years after transplantation, reveal pancreatic B-cells fullfilled with secretory granules containing insulin (Fig.1). The long-term survival of islet grafts, which is responsible for long-term compensation of glycaemia supports the assumption of a long-term function of the heterotopically grafted tissue, which presumes a sufficient supply with nutrients and oxygen, a sufficient transport of secreted hormones, and a sufficient renewal rate of the cells. Indeed, when livers with grafted islets are perfused 3 months after transplantation insulin is biphasically released in response to glucose[7], and glucagon is biphasically released in response to arginine[8]. Detailed investigations reveal a "physiological hormone response" already 2 weeks after transplantation, as depicted for insulin in Fig. 2, which is maintained up to 12 months after transplantation in response to glucose and other stimuli (Fig. 2)[9,10]. Such an early biphasic insulin secretion can only be realized, when the capillarization has been finished. Indeed, experimental investigations clearly demonstrate that heterotopically grafted islets are not only capillarizised within 7 days[11], but also the intra-islet portal system perfusing the pancreatic islets sequentially from B- to A/D-cells can be reestablished[12]. Furthermore, morphological investigations reveal the reinnervation of islet

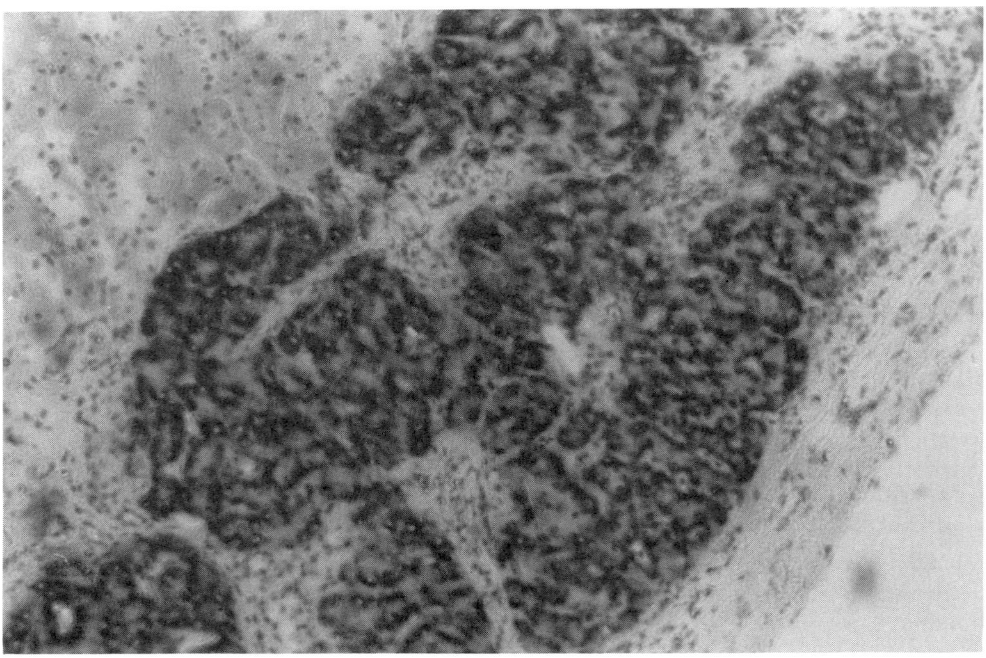

Figure 1. Syngeneic islet graft 120 d after transplantation stained with a monoclonal insulin antiboby, which is visualized by APAAP-technique. The darkly stained cells are insulin-containing pancreatic B-cells (magnification × 160).

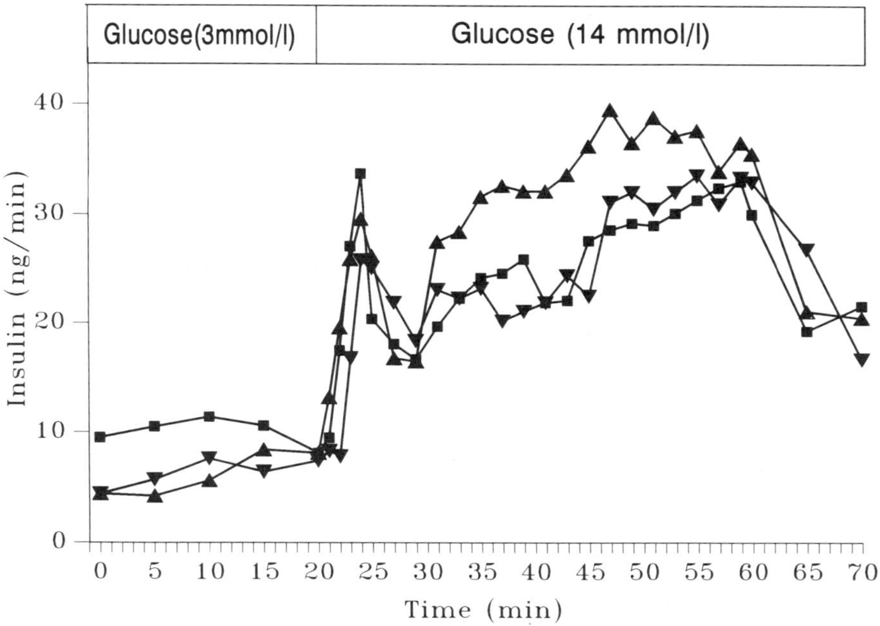

Figure 2. Pancreatic islets (LEW.1W) are intraportally grafted into streptozotocin-diabetic LEW.1W rats. 0,5 mo (■—■), 6 mo (▲—▲) or 12 mo (▼—▼) after the transplantation the livers are perfused with 3 mmol/l or 14 mmol/l glucose to investigate insulin secretion (n = 5–6 experiments) (taken from 9, with permission).

grafts[13,15], which regulates insulin secretion e.g. by sympathetic nerves[15] (Fig. 3). Consequently, the grafted islets are characterized by an oscillatory hormone secretion[9,16], as also observed in perfused pancreas or in vivo. Taken together, there is a vast amount of evidence that syngeneic grafted pancreatic islets respond like the endocrine pancreas despite of a heterotopical location. This makes it possible to create a B-cell enriched suborgan, which can be investigated for years, and which responds to metabolic or hormonal alterations of the recipients, e.g. pregnancy or hyperglycaemia[10].

IMMUNOLOGICAL OR TOXICOLOGICAL INVESTIGATIONS ON SYNGENEIC PANCREATIC ISLET GRAFTS

Following the hypothesis that not the pancreatic B-cells, but endogenous lymphoid cells (passenger leucocytes, dendritic cells, macrophages) are the cells inducing an allogeneic or xenogeneic immune response, which inaugurates the islet destruction, vast amounts of experiments were performed to kill selectively the immune cells within the islet with the hope that such islets with a reduced immunogenecity may be outwit the immune system. The selectivity of procedures is based on a different sensitivity of immune and endocrine cells against an exogenous attack, and side effects on pancreatic B-cells are excluded by investigations of e.g. hormone secretion, synthesis and/or content in vitro. When, for example, pancreatic islets are irradiated or treated with antibodies directed to MHC epitopes, neither the islet metabolism, nor the hormone secretion are altered in vitro[17,18]. However, the syngeneic transplantation of such pretreated islets reveal a shortened

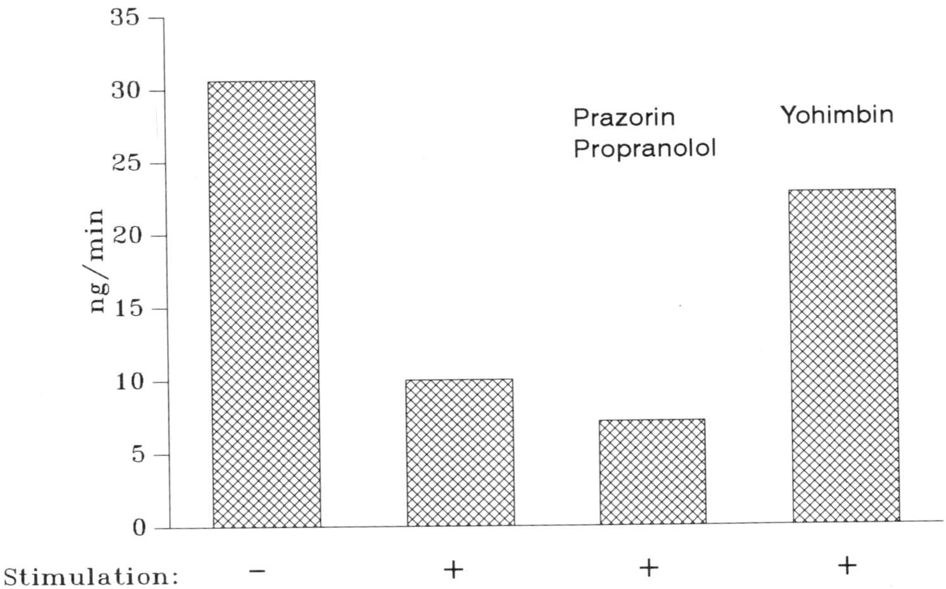

Figure 3. 3 months after intraportal islet transplantation the livers are perfused in situ with 14 mmol/l glucose to measure insulin secretion. Electrical stimulation of sympathetic hepatic nerves starts after 25 min for 2 ms. The insulin secretion is given as integrated area between 25th and 29th min. In 2 series of experiments the perfusate contains either the α_1 antagonist prazosin and the β-blocker propranolol or the α_2-adrenergic blocker yohimbin, which prevents the nerve stimulation-dependent inhibition of glucose-stimulated insulin secretion (taken from 15, with permission).

graft survival[17–19] (Fig. 4), indicating delayed cell defects, which are not seen in the normally applied methods to characterize the pancreatic B-cell function. Furthermore, when e.g. such control experiments, as the syngeneic islet transplantation, are not performed, the results of allogeneic islet grafting could be misinterpreted.

The grafted islets are as sensitive as pancreatic B-cells to toxins as for example streptozotocin and alloxan. When drugs exert toxic effects on pancreatic B-cells, such deterioration can be observed both in the native endocrine pancreas and the syngeneic graft, as depicted in Tab. 1 for Cyclosporin A, which exerts toxic side effects on pancreatic B-cells leading to an increase of plasma glucose[20]. An accumulated amount of altered pancreatic B-cells, which can be simply prepared eg from the kidney capsules, originates an exellent material for further investigations. Thus, the syngeneic islet transplantation can be used for toxicological investigations to confirm or exclude direct or indirect effects on the endocrine cells of pancreatic islets.

THE SYNGENEIC ISLET TRANSPLANTATION TO STUDY AND TO PREVENT PANCREATIC B-CELL DESTRUCTION IN AUTOIMMUNE DIABETES

The observation of pancreatic B-cell destruction after pancreas transplantation into diabetic nonimmunosuppressed monozygotic twins, which was accompanied by an insulitis in the graft, is a strong evidence for an autoimmune origin of diabetes mellitus[21].

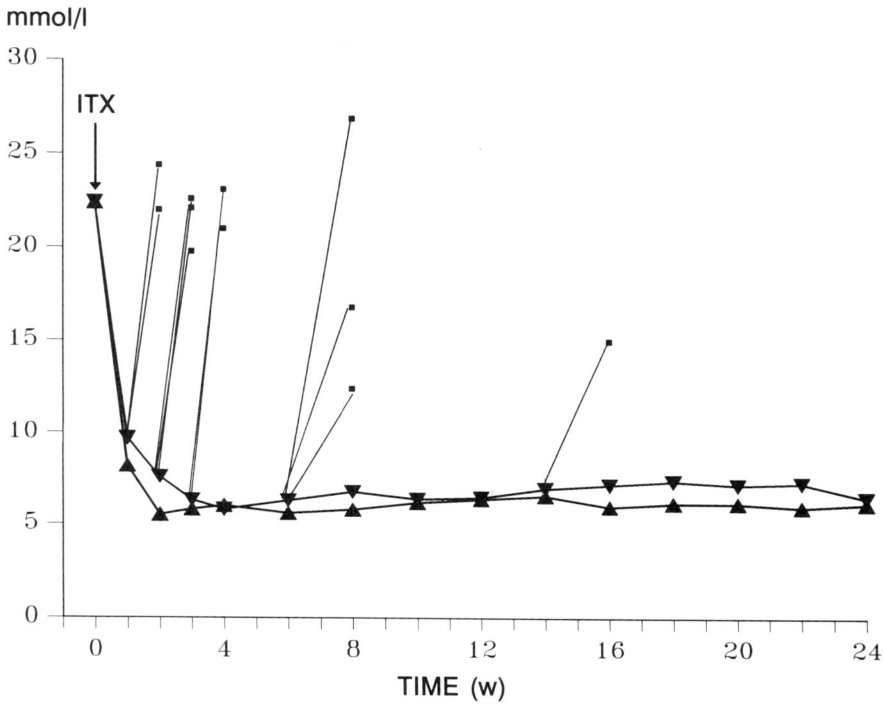

Figure 4. Pancreatic islets are irradiated (▼—▼, n =12) in vitro (25 Gy) or stayed untreated (▲—▲, n = 10). The islets are syngeneicly grafted into STZ-diabetic recipients. Whereas the nonirradiated islets maintain normoglycaemia up to 24 weeks, the recipients with the irradiated islets relapse into hyperglycaemia (●, 11/12 animals). (taken from 17, with permission).

Table 1. Normal Wistar rats or STZ-diabetic Wistar rats with a syngeneic islet graft (3 weeks after transplantation) were treated for 3 weeks with 50 mg/kg b.w. Cyclosporin A. The treatment decreases plasma, pancreas, and graft insulin content and increases postprandial glycaemia. (**P < 0.01 in comparison to vehicle-treated animals)

		Wistar rats		Islet-grafted Wistar rats	
Treatment		Vehicle	CS-A	Vehicle	CS-A
N		10	9	6	6
Time	d	21	21	21	21
Dosis	mg/kg	0	50	0	50
Plasma glucose	mmol/l	7.9 ± 0.2	10.5 ± 0.8**	7.4 ± 0.4	11.2 ± 0.4*
Plasma insulin	pmol/l	233 ± 29	50 ± 18**	264 ± 41	39 ± 11*
Pancreatic insulin	pmol/mg	18.5 ± 2.0	6.2 ± 0.6**		
Graft insulin	pmol			18352 ± 1245	5430 ± 751**

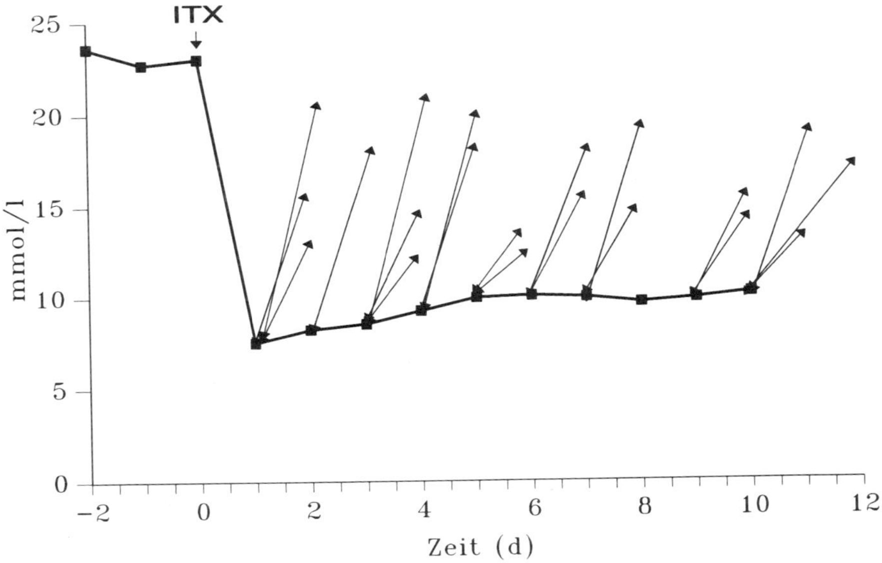

Figure 5. Spontaneously diabetic NOD-mice (2–4 weeks diabetes) are grafted beneath the kidney capsules with 1000 NOD-mice islets. The recipients (n = 20) relapse into hyperglycaemia within 2 weeks.

Animal experiments in BB rats[22] or NOD-mice (Fig. 5) confirme the destruction of syngeneic pancreatic B-cells after islet transplantation by relapse into hyperglycaemia within 3 weeks (Fig. 5). The destruction of the B-cells grafted into spontaneously diabetic animals cannot be the result of an allogeneic cell-mediated mechanism, as the rejection process, but is the result of the restimulated autoaggressive immune system after reapplication of the antigen (pancreatic B-cells). The restimulation may simulate the natural process leading to insulin-dependent diabetes, which is characterized by phases of B-cell destruction due to repeated restimulation of the autoaggression interrupted by phases of tolerance redevelopment[23]. The discontinuity of the process is also supported by the confirmation of insulitis accompanied by a reduced B-cell volume density and pancreatic insulin content in prediabetic BB-rats[24] as well as in animals, which escaped diabetes onset[23]. Consequently, such animals which cured pancreatic B-cell destruction spontaneously[25], do also accept a syngeneic islet graft[22,26].

Among the cells, which could be observed within pancreatic islets (insulitis) and which may be involved in pancreatic B-cell destruction, macrophages, CD4 T-cells, CD8 T-cells and NK-cells can be identified in both newly diagnosed diabetic and prediabetic animals[24,27]. Detailed immunocytochemical characterizations reveal an activated state in the majority of the invading cells (e.g., the expression of IL-2 receptor on T-lymphocytes). When a syngeneic islet graft is investigated at relapse into hyperglycaemia, the graft is characterized by a reduced number of pancreatic B-cells (Fig. 6A), a decrease of graft insulin content[22], and a marked insulitis (Fig. 6A). The immunocytochemistry of such grafts reveal macrophages, which are located at the graft periphery, T-cells, which do invade the graft and no NK-cells. Among the T-cells, only CD4 T-cells invade the graft (Fig. 6B), whereas CD8 T-cells are only occassionally observed (Fig. 6C). We conclude from these experiments that CD4 T-cells are directly cytotoxic and involved in pancreatic B-cell destruction. Indeed, when splenocytes obtained from newly-diagnosed

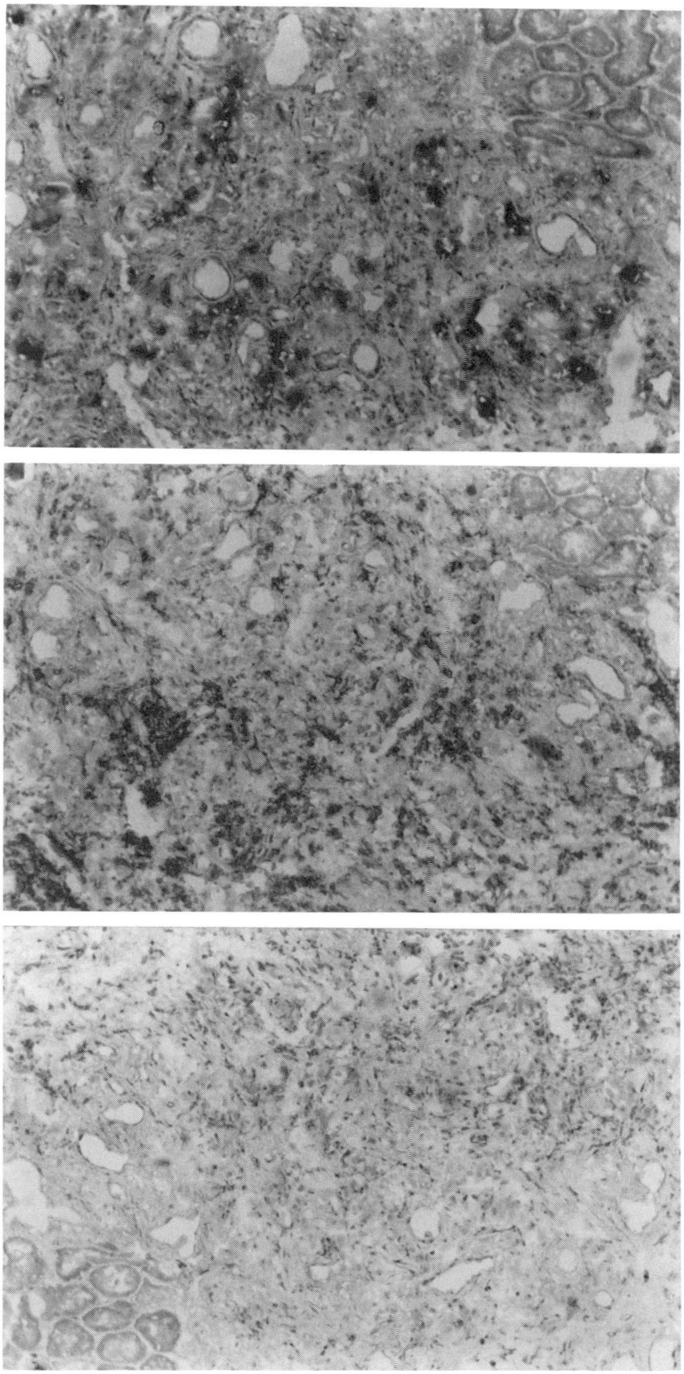

Figure 6. Morphology of a BB/OK rat islet graft (magnification × 160) at relapse into hyperglycaemis of the BB/OK recipient. **(A)** The number of darkly stained pancreatic B-cells is markedly reduced, whereas the number of mononuclear cells (MNC) is enhanced. **(B)** The majority of MNC are CD4 T-cells, whereas **(C)** CD8 T-cells cannot be observed.

diabetic animals are incubated with ^{51}Cr-prelabeled pancreatic islets, the lymphocytes caused a MHC-dependent increase of specific chromium release in the majority of investigated animals.

Concequently, the treatment of prediabetic animals with antibodies directed to the CD4 epitope prevents diabetes development[29]. Also, when newly-diagnosed diabetic patients are treated with anti CD4 antibodies the remaining C-peptide can be maintained[29].

The syngeneic islet transplantation into spontaneously diabetic animals, which is an excellent model of experimental prediabetes, can also be successfully used to investigate new strategies of immunomodulation to prevent and/or to treat autoagressive destruction of pancreatic B-cells. Thus, by means of a temporary anti IL-2 receptor therapy in combination with low Cyclosporin A doses, we could demonstrate not only the interruption of pancreatic B-cell destruction, but also the redevelopement of tolerance directed to the endogenous pancreatic B-cells[30].

Summarizing the review, we want to stress that the syngeneic islet transplantation is a suitable model to study long-term effects on pancreatic B-cells in vivo and to investigate the natural process of autoimmune pancreatic B-cell destruction and its immunomodulatory prevention.

ACKNOWLEGMENT

The authors want to thank Dr. S. Lucke (IfD, Karlsburg) for preparation of microphotographs, Prof. Dr. W. Blech and Dr. W. Hildebrandt (Department of Biochemistry, University of Halle, Germany) for the investigations of insulin secretion on islet grafted livers, Dr. A. Gardemann (now Department of Clinical Chemistry, University of Gießen, Germany) and Prof. Dr. L. Cossel and Prof. Dr. F. Wohlrab (Department of Pathology, University of Leipzig, Germany) for the work on reinervation of grafted islets. The original work quoted in the review was supported by the Ministry of Health of former GDR and by WIP/KAI e.V. (018297/M).

REFERENCES

1. S. Moskalewski: Isolation and culture of the islets of Langerhans of the guinea pig. Gen&Comp.Endocrinol. 5: 342–348 (1965).
2. P.E. Lacy, and M. Kostianovsky: A method for the isolation of intact islets of Langerhans from the rat pancreas. Diabetes 16: 35–39 (1967).
3. H.J. Hahn: Die isolierte Langerhanssche Insel, ein Modell zur Untersuchung der Insulinsekretion in vitro. Endokrinol. 71: 308–329 (1978).
4. W.F. Ballinger and P.E. Lacy. Transplantation of intact pancreatic islets in rats. Surgery 72: 175–186 (1972).
5. D.W.R. Gray and P.J. Morris: Developments in isolated pancreatic islet transplantation. Transplantation 43: 321–329 (1987).
6. P.E. Lacy: Studies of islet cell transplantation. Diab. Rev. 1: 75–92 (1993).
7. H.J. Brömme, H.J. Hahn and W. Blech: Biphasic release of insulin from islets of Langerhans after their transplan-tation into the liver of rats, Horm. Metab. Res. 20: 138–140 (1988).
8. H.J. Brömme, H.J. Hahn, S. Lucke, W. Hildebrandt and W. Blech: Arginine stimulated insulin and glucagon release from islets transplanted into the liver of diabetic rats. Horm. Metab. Res. 21: 587–589 (1989).
9. W. Hildebrandt: Thesis, Medical Faculty University Halle (1994).
10. A. Dunger, C. Kauert, H.J. Brömme, W. Hildebrandt, W.Blech and H.J. Hahn: Functional response of a limited β-cell mass to long-term hypgerglycemia. Pancreas 9: 186–192 (1994).
11. M.D.Menger, P. Vajkoczy, R. Leiderer, S. Jäger and K. Messmer: Influence of experimental hyperglycemia on microvascular blood perfusion of pancreatic islet isografts. J. Clin. Invest. 90: 1361–1369 (1992).

12. M.D. Menger, P. Vajkoczy, C. Beger, and K. Messmer: Orientation of microvascular blood flow in pancreatic islet isografts. J. Clin. Invest. 93: 2280–2285 (1994).
13. N. Noda, K. Ina, Y. Yasunami, S. Ryu, J. Ono and R. Takaki:Reinnervation of intraportal islet allografts in rats. Transplantation 55: 664–665 (1993).
14. O. Korsgren, A. Andersson, L. Jansson, and F. Sundler Reinnervation of syngeneic mouse pancreatic islets transplanted into renal subcapsular space. Diabetes 41: 130–135 (1992).
15. A. Gardemann, K. Jungermann, V. Große, L. Cossel, F.Wohlrab, H.J. Hahn, W. Blech and W. Hildebrandt: Intraportal transplantation of pancreatic islets into livers of diabetic rats: Reinnervation of islets and regulation of insulin secretion by the hepatic sympathetic nerves. Diabetes 43: 1345–1352 (1994).
16. E.T. Shapiro, S. Strasser, and K.S. Polonsky: Persistence of oscillatory insulin secretion in denervated islet cell autografts. Transplantation 52: 574–575 (1991).
17. D. Heinzmann: Die Wirkung einer einzeitigen Bestrahlung mit ^{60}Co auf Parameter des Glukosestoff-wechsels in vivo und auf Funktionen der isolierten Langerhansschen Insel in vitro. Thesis, Med. Acad. Magdeburg (1987).
18. B. Kuttler, S. Schmidt, I. Klöting and O. Stark: In vitro and in vivo behaviour of rat islets of Langerhans treated with MHC antisera and complement. Exp. Clin. Endocrinol. 89: 83–88 (1987).
19. M. Gotoh, T. Kanai, K. Dono, J. Porter, T. Maki and A.P. Monaco: Gamma-irradiation as a tool to reduce immunogenicity of islet allo- and xenografts. Horm.Metab.Res. Suppl. Ser. 25: 89–92 (1990).
20. J. Mason: Pharmocology of cyclosporine (Sandimmune)-VII. Pathophysiology and toxicology of cyclosporine in humans and animals. Pharmacol. Rev. 42: 423–434 (1989).
21. R.K. Sibley, D.E.R. Sutherland, F. Goetz, and A.F. Michael: Recurrent diabetes mellitus in the pancreas iso- and allograft. A light and electron microscopic and immunohistochemical analysis of four cases. Lab. Invest. 53: 132–144 (1985).
22. H.J. Hahn, C. Kauert, A. Dunger, B. Kuttler, and T. Diamantstein: Interleukin 2 receptor targeted immunotherapy in the prevention of autoimmune beta-cell destruction as observed in diabetic BB/OK rats grafted with BB/OK rat islets. Autoimmunity 5: 139–142 (1989).
23. H.J. Hahn, S. Lucke, B. Kuttler, A. Dunger, H.D. Volk, and T. Diamantstein: Investigations of diabetes-prone normoglycaemic BB rats. Lessons from animal diabetes 3: 30–33 (1990).
24. S. Lucke, W. Besch, C. Kauert, and H.J. Hahn: The endocrine pancreas of BB/OK-rats before and at diagnosis of hyperglycaemia. Exp. Clin. Endocrinol. 91: 161–170 (1988).
25. B. Kuttler, A. Dunger, H.D. Volk, T. Diamantstein and H.J. Hahn: Prevention and suppression of autoimmune pancreatic beta-cell destruction in BB rats by syngeneic lymphocytes obtained from long-term normoglycaemic donors. Diabetologia 34: 74–78 (1991).
26. B. Kuttler, C. Mathieu, M. Waer, H.J. Hahn, and R. Bouillon: Lack of disease recurrence in diabetic BB/PFD rats after syngeneic islet transplantation. Autoimmunity 15: 107–112 (1993).
27. H.J. Hahn, J. Gerdes, S. Lucke, L. Liepe, C. Kauert, H.D.Volk, H.H. Wacker, S. Brocke, H. Stein, and T. Diamantstein: Phenotypical characterization of the cells invading pancreatic islets of diabetic BB/OK rats: effect of interleukin 2 receptor-targeted immunotherapy. Eur. J. Immunol.18: 2037–2042 (1988).
28. H. Wanka, B. Kuttler, and H.J. Hahn: Is the in vitro destruction of pancreatic islets MHC-dependent? Diabetologia 36: Suppl. 19, A9 (1993).
29. H.J. Hahn, B. Kuttler, F. Laube, and F. Emmrich: Anti-CD4 therapy in recent-onset IDDM. Diab. Metab. Rev. 9: 323–328 (1993).
30. T. Diamantstein, and H.J. Hahn: Interleukin-2 receptor- targeted immune therapy. In: Monoclonal antibodies and peptide therapy in autoimmune diseases.(ed. J.F. Bach) Marcel Dekker, Inc. N.Y., Basel, Hong Kong, pp. 295–318 (1993).

55

BETA CELL REPLICATION AND MASS IN ISLET TRANSPLANTATION

Eduard Montaña,[1] Susan Bonner-Weir,[2] and Gordon C. Weir[2]

[1]Endocrine Unit, CSUB-Hospital Bellvitge
08907 L'Hospitalet de Llobregat, Barcelona, Spain
[2]Research Division, Joslin Diabetes Center
and The Department of Medicine, New England Deaconess Hospital and Brigham and Women's Hospital, Harvard Medical School
Boston, Massachusetts 02215

INTRODUCTION

The first successful transplants of islet cells in diabetic patients have been reported recently[1–4]. However, restoration of normoglycemia is often not achieved or has limited duration. Failure of islets autotransplanted in large animals[5] suggests that nonimmunological factors, such as limited growth capacity could play a role in the limited survival of islet transplants in diabetic patients. One of the major problems in human islet transplantation is that a greater quantity of islet tissue is required than had been predicted on the basis of beta cell measurements in diabetes[6]. The reasons for the need of such a large amount of islet tissue are not known. In addition, a critical islet mass must be transplanted to achieve normoglycemia with continued success being dependent upon the number of initially transplanted islets[7–9]. An unknown factor in these considerations is the growth capacity of transplanted islets. A limitation in the growth capacity of transplanted islets compared to endogenous pancreatic islets could lead to continuous loss of beta cell mass and failure of the graft. We studied the beta cell replication and mass in short term successful islet tranplants and the capacity of transplanted beta cells to modify their replication and mass in response to changes in metabolic demand.

METHODS

Two groups of experiments were performed. In the first group, streptozocin diabetic C57BL/6 mice were transplanted with 150 or 300 syngenic islets under the kidney capsule. The expectation was that transplantation of 300 islets would achieve normoglycemia while 150 islets would be an inadequate number to restore normoglycemia in the diabetic

Physiology and Pathophysiology of the Islets of Langerhans, edited by Soria.
Plenum Press, New York, 1997.

recipients. Grafts were harvested 10, 18 or 30 days after transplantation. In the second group of experiments male Lewis rats were transplanted with 500 syngeneic islets under the kidney capsule, and/or underwent a 95% pancreatectomy. Pancreatectomy was performed to increase the metabolic demand placed on already transplanted islets. Rats were used in these experiments to avoid the technical problems of extensive pancreatectomies in mice. The following groups of rats were studied: (1) Tx-Px group: rats were transplanted and 14 days later underwent a 95% pancreatectomy; grafts and pancreatic remnants were harvested 28 days after transplantation; (2) Tx group: rats were transplanted and grafts and pancreas were harvested 14 or 28 days later; (3) Px group: rats underwent 95% pancreatectomy and pancreatic remnants were harvested 14 days later.

Islets were isolated by collagenase digestion, separated by a density gradient and hand picked under a stereomicroscope. Only islets more than 75 and less than 250 μm in diameter were collected. The islets were transplanted under the left kidney capsule on the day of the isolation. A 95% partial pancreatectomy was performed by gentle abrasion with cotton applicators being careful to leave major blood vessels intact[10]. On the day of graft removal animals were injected with 5-bromo-2′deoxyuridine (BrdU) (Sigma), 100 mg/kg body weight IP, and 6 hour later the graft was removed. The kidney capsule surrounding the graft was incised and removed with the graft. In rat experiments, animals were killed after graft removal and the pancreas or the pancreatic remnants were excised. Grafts and pancreases were weighed and processed for immunocytochemistry.

Sections of graft and pancreas were double stained by immunoperoxidase with a monoclonal antibody anti-BrdU and a cocktail of antibodies (anti-glucagon, -somatostatin and -pancreatic polypeptide). On the stained sections, beta cell replication was measured by counting beta cells and BrdU positive beta cells. Results were expressed as the percentage of BrdU positive beta cells. At least 1200 cells were counted per graft or pancreas. Individual beta cell area, a measure of beta cell size, was determined by planimetry on immunoperoxidase stained sections of grafts and isolated islets. Beta cell mass was measured by point counting morphometry on immunoperoxidase stained sections of graft and endogenous pancreas.

Results were expressed as mean and standard error of the mean ($\bar{x}$ ± SEM). For comparisons between two groups the unpaired Student's t test (two tailed) was used and for multiple comparisons the one-way analysis of variance (ANOVA) was used. A p value of less than 0.05 was considered significant.

RESULTS

Beta Cell Replication, Area and Mass When a Sufficient or an Insufficient Beta Cell Mass Is Transplanted

As expected, 300 islets restored normoglycemia in STZ-diabetic mice while the mice receiving only 150 islets remained severely hyperglycemic. In normoglycemic mice beta cell replication in transplanted islets was similar to replication in normal pancreas, beta cell area increased significantly 30 days after transplantation (305 ± 13 μm^2 vs 271 ± 14 μm^2, $p < 0.01$) and beta cell mass in the graft remained constant throughout the follow-up. In contrast, beta cell replication was increased 10 days after transplantation in the group receiving 150 islets (1.39 ± 0.11%); however, beta cell replication decreased to basal levels at 18 (0.68 ± 0.06%) and 30 days (0.72 ± 0.11%) despite similar severe hyperglycemia at all the point times (over 20 mmol/l). Individual beta cell area did not change

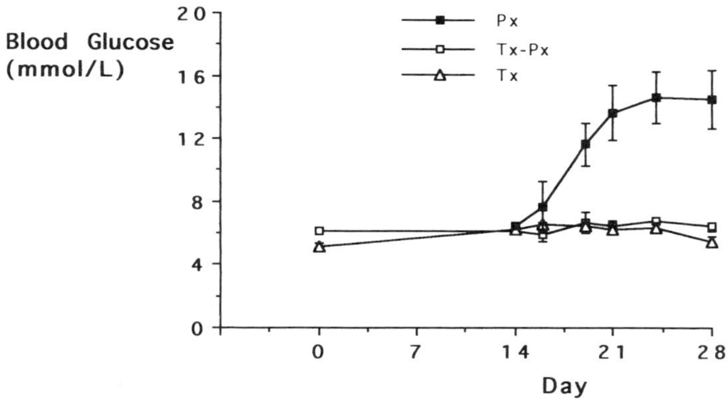

Figure 1. Evolution of fed glucose in rat experimental groups. Day 0: transplantation of 500 islets (Tx-Px and Tx groups). Day 14: 95% pancreatectomy (Tx-Px and Pxgroups) Values are mean ± SEM (adapted with permission from J Clin Invest 1994;93:1577).

in these groups, but total beta cell mass was reduced by day 10 (0.31 ± 0.07 mg) and day 30 (0.17 ± 0.03 mg) compared to the initially transplanted beta cell mass (0.46 ± 0.06 mg) ($p < 0.001$).

Beta Cell Replication, Area, and Mass after Increased Metabolic Demand

Pancreatectomy induced severe hyperglycemia in Px group. In contrast, hyperglycemia was prevented in Tx-Px group by the previous transplantation of 500 islets. Blood glucose in this group was not different from glucose in normal rats nor Tx group during the follow up (Figure 1).

Beta cell replication was increased in transplanted islets from Tx-Px group (1.15 ± 0.12%) compared to pancreatic islets from normal non-transplanted rats (0.38 ± 0.05%) and to transplanted beta cells from Tx group (0.64 ± 0.07%) ($p < 0.001$) (Figure 2). Beta cell replication in the pancreatic remnant of this Tx-Px group was increased (1.01 ± 0.25%) compared to Px group (0.65 ± 0.18%) and to the pancreas of Tx (0.40 ± 0.11%) and normal (0.38 ± 0.05%) groups ($p < 0.05$) (Figure 3). When experimental animals were analyzed individually, it was apparent that replication in transplanted beta cells and in pancreatic beta cells was similar and the presence of a positive correlation between repli-

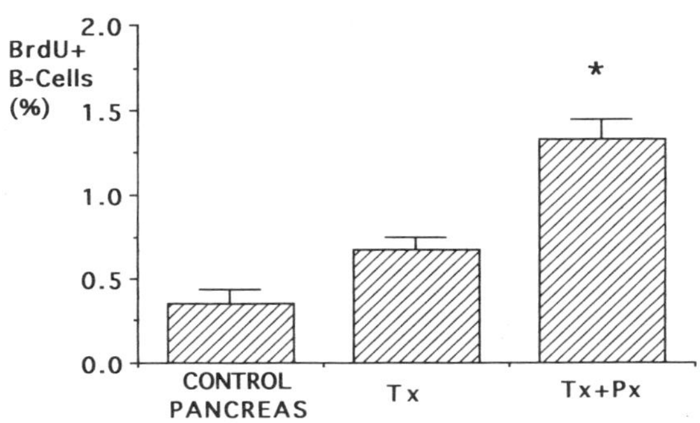

Figure 2. Beta cell replication in normal pancreas and in transplanted islets in Lewis rats. Values are mean ± SEM. *p < 0.001 between Tx-Px group and the other groups (adapted with permission from J Clin Invest 1994; 93: 1577).

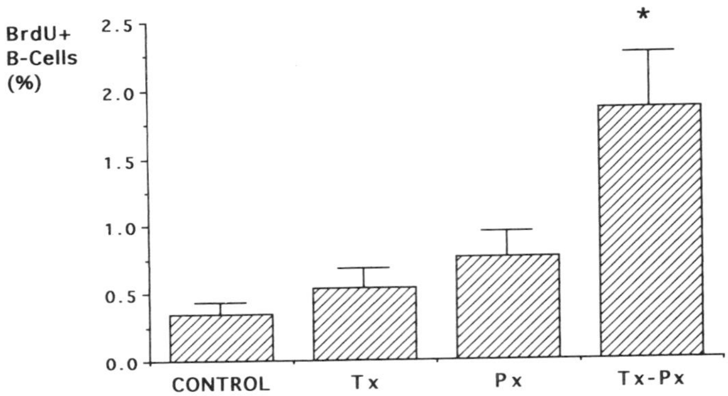

Figure 3. Beta cell replication in endogenous pancreatic beta cells. Values are mean ± SEM. *p < 0.001 between Tx-Px group and the other groups (adapted with permission from J Clin Invest 1994; 93: 1577).

cation in both locations was established ($r = 0.55$, $p = 0.003$). Individual beta cell size was increased in transplanted islets from Tx-Px group (311 ± 14 μm^2) compared to Tx group: 252 ± 12 μm^2 or to beta cell area in isolated islets (239 ± 10 μm^2) ($p = 0.001$). Transplanted beta cell mass increased in Tx-Px (1.81 ± 0.51 mg) rats compared to Tx group: 0.78 ± 0.17 mg) ($p < 0.05$). Beta cell mass in Tx-group grafts was reduced to 74% of the initially transplanted beta cell mass (1.05 ± 0.07 mg, p = NS) (Figure 4).

DISCUSSION

We studied the replicative capacity of transplanted beta cells in normoglycemia and hyperglycemia and the evolution of beta cell mass over the first weeks after transplantation. In addition, we analyzed the capacity of transplanted beta cells to respond to increased metabolic demand. When normoglycemia was restored after transplantation the replication of transplanted beta cells was similar to that of pancreatic beta cells of normal animals and the graft beta cell mass remained stable. In contrast, persistance of hypergly-

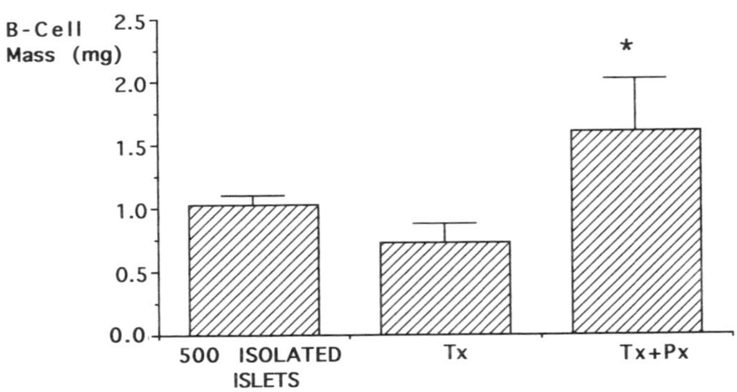

Figure 4. Beta cell mass in rat transplanted islets. 500 Isolated Islets: show the initially transplanted beta cell mass. Values are mean + SEM. $p < 0.05$ between Tx-Px and Tx groups (adapted with permission from J Clin Invest 1994; 93: 1577).

cemia after transplantation resulted in a limitation of beta cell replication and a progressive reduction of the grafted beta cell mass. When already engrafted beta cells were challenged with an increased metabolic demand after 95% pancreatectomy they were able to maintain normoglycemia by increasing their replication and size and the total beta cell mass in the graft. Beta cell response in transplanted islets was similar to that of islets in the endogenous pancreas, indicating that normal growth capacity was preserved in beta cells after short term transplantation.

In the mouse experiments we used a model that reproduces two different situations in islet transplantation: (1) transplantation of a minimum amount of beta cells to achieve normoglycemia, and (2) transplantation of an insufficient beta cell mass to restore normoglycemia. When normoglycemia was achieved after transplantation, beta cell replication was similar to that of the pancreas of normal animals. It is interesting to note that replication of transplanted beta cells in normoglycemic conditions was rather similar at different time points after transplantation. The values were also similar to those of beta cells transplanted into normoglycemic non-pancreatectomized rats. Beta cell mass was maintained when normoglycemia was restored after transplantation into diabetic mice. By day 30 after transplantation individual beta cell size was increased in this group indicating that hypertrophy of transplanted beta cells was also contributing to preservation of beta cell mass.

When a insufficient beta cell mass was transplanted into diabetic mice we found an increased replication after 10 days of hyperglycemia. This increase was probably being driven by hyperglycemia[11–13] but could not be maintained at later time points despite the persistence of hyperglycemia, indicating that a limitation of growth capacity can occur in transplanted beta cells when hyperglycemia is maintained. Transplanted beta cell mass was progressively reduced in this group, despite the initially increased beta cell replication and the maintained beta cell size, suggesting that an increased beta cell destruction was taking place. Therefore, our results suggest that chronic hyperglycemia led to an increase beta cell death in transplanted islets.

We used the partial pancreatectomy model to create a situation of increased metabolic demand on transplanted islets. Beta cells transplanted into normal rats increased their replication and size when a 95% pancreatectomy was performed and total beta cell mass almost tripled. Beta cell response to pancreatectomy in the grafted islets was similar to that of islets in the endogenous pancreas, indicating that normal growth capacity was preserved in beta cells after transplantation.

The increase in replication and size of transplanted beta cells after pancreatectomy in Tx-Px rats resulted in increased beta cell mass. The severe hyperglycemia that followed pancreatectomy in Px group was prevented in Tx-Px rats by the prior transplantation of 500 islets. Thus, transplanted beta cells were able to compensate for the increased metabolic demand placed upon them by the surgical reduction of endogenous beta cell mass. It is not clear, however, how beta cells sensed this increased metabolic demand. The concept of adaptive beta cell proliferation has been used to suggest that functional demand is a mechanism of control of beta cell replication[14]. Glucose is a well known stimulus for beta cell replication both in vitro[12,13] and in vivo[11], and hyperglycemia is present in most of the conditions in which adaptive beta cell proliferation occurs. However, hyperglycemia was not detected in Tx-Px group. The results resemble the islet growth described in other situations of increased metabolic demand where hyperglycemia is not detected, such as 40% and 60% pancreatectomies[15,16] or pregnancy[17]. Subtle elevations in blood glucose could have been responsible for increased beta cell replication in Tx-Px rats. Moreover, in addition to glucose, other mediators may also have contributed to increase beta cell proliferation. The identification of these mediators could open the possibility for interventions to modulate the growth of transplanted beta cells.

The capacity of transplanted beta cells to respond to changes in metabolic demand and the similarity between their replicative response and that of endogenous non-transplanted beta cells has important implications for islet transplantation. In clinical transplantation, different factors may modify the metabolic demand placed on transplanted beta cells. For instance, episodes of acute rejection decrease the transplanted beta cell mass and higher doses of immunosuppressive drugs can increase insulin resistance and impair beta cell function or islet cell DNA replication[18,19]. It is therefore encouraging to find that transplanted beta cells are able to respond effectively to severe reductions in beta cell mass. Moreover, if the transplantation method could be optimized it may be possible to obtain a successful result with a smaller number of islets, thus alleviating the islet shortage that currently limits transplantation efforts.

CONCLUSIONS

When normoglycemia is achieved after transplantation, the replication of transplanted beta cells is similar to that of endogenous pancreatic beta cells and beta cell mass remains constant in the first weeks after transplantation. Persistance of hyperglycemia after transplantation results in a limitation of grafted beta cells replication and progressive reduction of the mass of transplanted beta cells, suggesting increased beta cell death.

Transplanted beta cells are able to respond to changes in metabolic demand. Transplanted beta cells responded effectively to severe reductions in beta cell mass preventing the development of hyperglycemia after pancreatectomy. Increased metabolic demand resulted in increased replication and size of transplanted beta cells and was associated with an increased beta cell mass in the graft. The response of transplanted islets was similar to that of endogenous pancreatic beta cells suggesting that normal growth capacity is preserved in transplanted beta cells.

ACKNOWLEDGMENTS

This work was supported by grants DK-35449 and DK-36836 from the National Institutes of Health, a grant from the Juvenile Diabetes Foundation and grant FIS 93/0329 from the Ministry of Health of Spain.

REFERENCES

1. Scharp D.W., Lacy P.E., Santiago J.V., McCullough C.S., Weida L.G., Boyle P.J., Falui L., Marchetti P., Ricordi C., Gingerich R.L, Jaffe A.S., Cryer P.E., Hanto D.W., Anderson C., and Flye M.W., 1991, Results of our first nine intraportal islet allografts in type 1, insulin-dependent diabetic patients, *Transplantation* 51:76–86.
2. Warnock G.L., Kneteman N.M., Ryan E., Seelis R.E.A., Rabinovitch A., and Rajotte R.V., 1991, Normoglycemia after transplantation of freshly isolated and cryopreserved pancreatic islets in type 1 (insulin-dependent) diabetes mellitus, *Diabetologia* 34:54–58.
3. Socci C., Falqui L., Davalli A.M., Ricordi C., Braghi S., Bertuzzi E., Maffi P., Secchi A., Gavazzi F., Freschi M., Magistretti P., Socci S., Vignali A., Di Carlo V., and Pozza G., 1991, Fresh human islet ransplantation to replace pancreatic endocrine function in type I, insulin-dependent diabetic patients, *Acta Diabetol* 28:151–157.

4. Gores P.F., Najarian J.S., Stephanian E., Lloveras J.J., Kelley S., and Sutherland D.E.R., 1993, Insulin independence in type I diabetes after transplantation of unpurified islets from a single donor with 15-deoxyspergualin, *Lancet* 341:19–21.
5 Alejandro R., Cutfield R.G., Shienvold F.L., Polonsky K.S., Olson L., Dillberg J., Miller J., and Mintz D.H., 1986, Natural history of intrahepatic canine islet cells autografts, *J Clin Invest* 78:1339–1348.
6 Weir G.C., Bonner-Weir S., and Leahy J.L., 1990, Islet mass and function in diabetes and transplantation, *Diabetes* 39:401–405.
7 Warnock G.L., and Rajotte R.V., 1988, Critical mass of purified islets that induce normoglycemia after implantation into dogs, *Diabetes* 37;467–470.
8 Warnock G.L., Dabbs K.D., Evans M.G., Gattral M.S., Kneteman N.M., and Rajotte R.V., 1990, Critical mass of islets that function after implantation in a large mammalian, *Horm Metab Res* (Suppl 25):156–161.
9 Kaufman D.B., Morel P., Field M.J., Munn S.R., and Sutherland D.E.R., 1990, Importance of implantation site and number of islets transplanted on functional outcome following autotransplantation in a canine model, *Horm Metab Res* (Suppl 25):162.
10 Bonner-Weir S., Trent D.F., and Weir G.C., 1983, Partial pancreatectomy in the rat and subsequent defect in glucose-induced insulin secretion, *J Clin Invest* 71:1544–1553.
11 Bonner-Weir S., Deery D., Leahy J.L., and Weir G.W., 1989, Compensatory growth of pancreatic B-cells in adult rats after short term glucose infusion, *Diabetes* 38:49–53.
12 Swenne I., 1983, Effects of aging on the regenerative capacity of pancreatic beta cells of the rat, *Diabetes* 32:14–19.
13 Swenne I., 1982, The role of glucose in the in vitro regulation of cell cycle kinetics and proliferation of fetal pancreatic B-cells, *Diabetes* 31:754–760.
14 Hellerstrom C., Swenne I., and Andersson A., 1987, Islet cell replication and diabetes, *in:* "The pathology of the endocrine pancreas in diabetes," P.J. Lefebvre and D.G. Pipeleers, ed., Springer-Verlag, Heidelberg.
15 Leahy J.L., Bonner-Weir S., and Weir G.W., 1988, Minimal chronic hyperglycemia is a critical determinant of impaired insulin secretion after an incomplete pancreatectomy, *J Clin Invest* 81:1407–1414.
16 Lee H.C., Bonner-Weir S., Weir G.C., and Leahy J.L., 1989, Compensatory adaptation of partial pancreatectomy in the rat, *Endocrinology* 124:1511–1515.
17 Parsons J.A., Brelje T.A., and Sorenson R.L., 1992, Adaptation of islets of Langerhans to pregnancy: increased islet cell proliferation and insulin secretion correlates with the onset of placental lactogen secretion, *Endocrinology* 130:1459.
18 Andersson A., Borg A., Hallberg A., Hellerstrom C., Sandler S., and Schnell A., 1984, Long-term effects of cyclosporin A on cultured mouse pancreatic islets, *Diabetologia* 27:66–69.
19 Kojima Y., Sandler S., and Andersson A., 1986, Cyclosporine inhibits mouse islet cell replication, *Transpl Proc* 18:37–39.

56

ISLET GROWTH AFTER PANCREATIC FRAGMENTS AUTOTRANSPLANTATION INTO THE DOG'S SPLEEN

How Can the Engrafted Islet Mass Satisfy the Demand for Its Specific Products?

Mário L. C. Madureira*

Departments of Surgery, Experimental Surgery and Pathology
University of Oporto School of Medicine
Oporto, Portugal

INTRODUCTION

The prospective mechanisms by which the transplanted islet mass may satisfy an increased demand for its specific products must be, as in the pancreas *in situ* the hypertrophy or the increase of the synthetic and secretion mechanisms of the islet cells, their replication or their eventual regeneration from ductal precursors[1–4]. The endocrine cells, particularly the engrafted B-cells, when stressed evolve to exhaustion specially in the case of a critical islet mass engrafted[5–8]. A wave of islet cell replication may go on[9,10] and we know that the engrafted islet cell mass can duplicate in two weeks[11], but the potential of that mechanism is obviously limited[1], so its efficacy for the stabilization of the metabolic state is largely dependent on the islet mass engrafted[7,8]. A nesidioblastic process from "precursor" ductal cells is a common finding with the cultured and engrafted fetal and neonatal pancreases[12,13] and the neogenesis of B-cells from adult ductal cells has been recently reported[14] Culture experiments, histochemical and ultrastructural studies conjugated with the molecular biology[15] may be the best methods for the study of the global characteristics of the morphogenetic mechanisms of the pancreatic regenerative process, of its promoters, for identifying the nature of the "precursor cells" and for the characterization of transition cells of the acinar and islet differentiation. The purpose of this work is to present preliminar evidence that the neogenesis of islet cells is a complementary mechanism for the growth of the engrafted adult islet tissue.

* Correspondence should be addressed to Mário L. C. Madureira, M.D., Apartado 2282, 4204, Porto, Codex, Portugal.

Physiology and Pathophysiology of the Islets of Langerhans, edited by Soria.
Plenum Press, New York, 1997.

MATERIALS AND METHODS

Enzymatic digested adult pancreatic fragments autotransplanted into the spleen of totally and near-totally (90%) pancreatectomized dogs[16,17].

Plan of the Morphological Study

We have studied the spleen of height dogs until the five day, of fourteen hyperglycemic dogs that were sacrificed or died spontaneously between the 1st and 8th weeks, and of 23 normoglycemic dogs exclusively grafted with collagenase digested pancreatic fragments that were subjected to test-splenectomy at the 4th (5 dogs), 8th (12 dogs), 24th (4 dogs), 36th (1 dog) and 48th (1 dog) weeks, these ones fundamentally basing the ultrastructural study, being in mind to discard the glucotoxic effects on ductal and endocrine cells.

Light Microscopy

The splenic tissue was fixed in Bouin's solution and set in paraffin; the sections were stained with hematoxylin-eosine (H.E.), periodic acid-Schiffs (P.A.S.), aldehyde-fuchsin (A.F.), A.F./Green-Light, and A.F./Orange-G.

Electron Microscopy

The splenic fragments, almost exclusively derived from splenectomized normoglycemic dogs, were fixed in glutaraldehyde 3% with a Millonig phosphate buffer, and enbedded in epon. Semithin sections were stained with toluidine blue and ultrafine sections were stained with Reynold's lead citrate.

RESULTS

The global characteristics of the fate of the inoculated pancreatic tissue studied by light and electron microscopy have demonstrated a pancreatic regeneration whose morphogenetic process was very similar to that of the fetal pancreas *in situ*[18–21], with acinar and a polyendocrine differentiation. We have identified ductal-acinar, ductal-islet, islet (B, A_2, D and F-cells), mixed-islet, acinar-islet and G-cells in the regenerated exocrine structures.

The acinar-islet phenotype was characterized in all islet cell-types identified in ductules, G-cells included [B-ac, A_2-ac, D-ac, F-ac (PLATE) and G-ac cells]. Simultaneous with this remarkable cellular pleomorphism, an extensive intracytoplasmic "dissolution" of the zymogen granules in acinar, ductal-acinar, ductal-acinar-islet and acinar-islet cells has been characterized, that did not seem to affect their fine ultrastructural characteristics.A progressive rarefaction of the exuberant regenerated exocrine structures coincident with cystic degenerative signs, apoptosis of acinar and ductal cells were also characterized, with the selective survival and growing predominance of ductal-acinar-islet buds with B, A_2 and D differentiation, distinct islets, aggregates of islet-cells or solitary islet-cells dispersed in the splenic pulp.

In this extraductal islet tissue, besides the B, A_2 and D cell-types of the normal adult dog's islet, we have also recognized differentiating B-cells in maturing islet structures, very rare insular cell-types or never reported in the adult dog's islet were also putatively

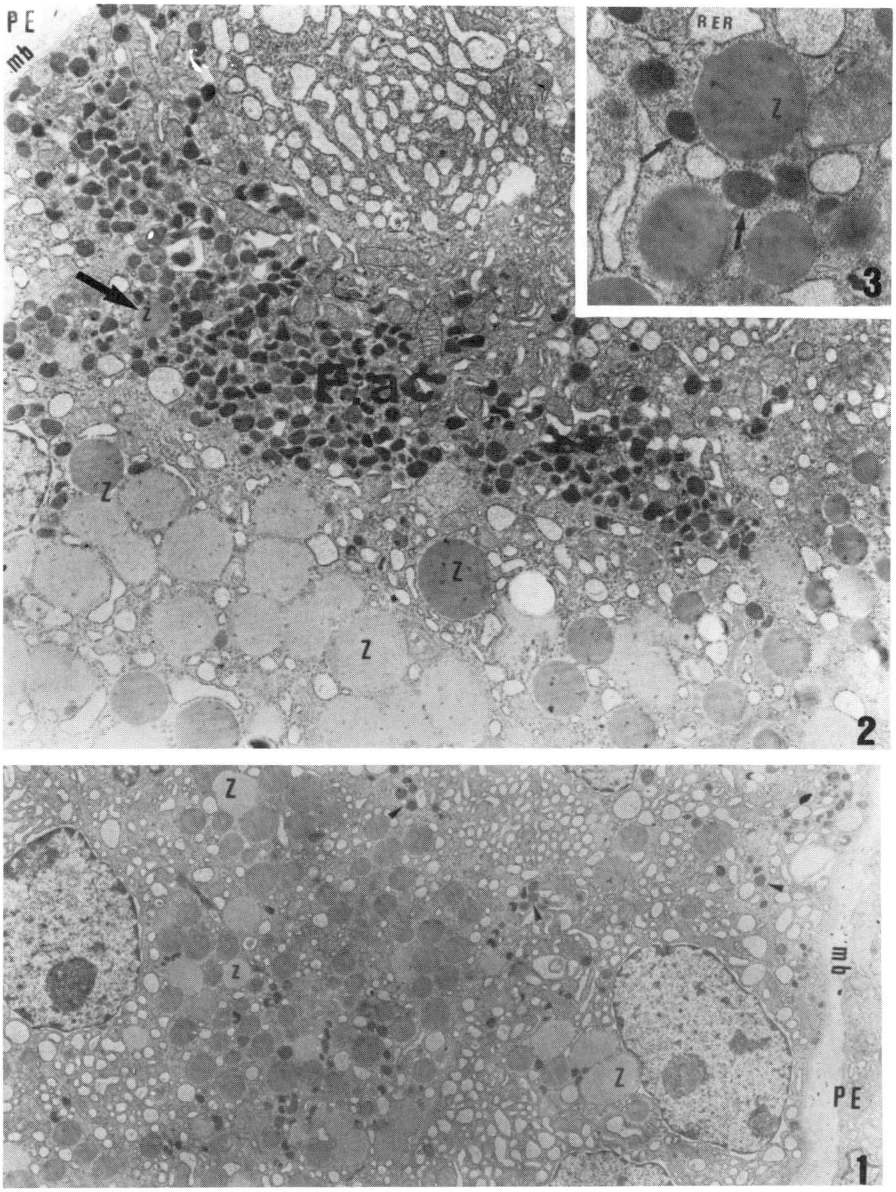

PLATE (Figures 1, 2, 3): Ductal structure in the spleen of a normoglycemic dog at four weeks.

Figure 1. Large view with only erraticaly dispersed F-type endocrine granules (arrowheads) intermingled with zymogen granules dissolving in the cytoplasm (Z); ductal basement membrane (mb); splenic pulp (P.E.). Electron microscopy [1 cm = 1.6 μm].

Figure 2. In another cut of the same structure, the growing number of polimorphous endocrine granules shapes true cells: F-cell (F-ac) with a solitary zymogen granule (thick-arrow/z) yet denoucing it's acinar-islet nature. In the neighbour ductal-acinar-cells, endocrine granules of the same type (arrowheads) and an extensive intracytoplasmic dissolution and fusion of the zymogen granules (Z); surrouding ductal basement membrane (mb); splenic pulp (PE). Electron microscopy [1 cm = 1 μm].

Figure 3. Detail with zymogen granules (Z) admixed with F-type granules (arrows), these ones with a granular texture, a medium to high electron density and a tight-fitting membrane; vesiculous R.E.R. (RER). Electron microscopy [1 cm = 0.6 μm].

identified, like mixed endocrine cells of the A_2-B, A_2-D and B-D types, G-cells and mixed acinar-islet cells of the D-acinar type.

DISCUSSION

The first question is the criticism and evaluation of these results. At the technical level, more specific and precise methods are necessary to identify all cell-types and the first steps of the islet and acinar differentiation, but mixed acinar-islet cells do exist in the engrafted pancreatic tissue. At the theoretical level the discussion about the ontogeny of these cells remains and is well known[22,23]. Our study of the fate of the autotransplanted pancreatic tissue in the spleen of the adult pancreatectomized dog demonstrated an exuberant acinar regeneration and a nesidioblastic process, both modulated by the restrictive conditions imposed by the splenic location[24] and possibly also regulated by the recipient diabetic model, in particularly by the pancreatectomies and the gastrointestinal hormones[11,24–27].The described cellular pleomorphism was also suggesting the concept of an occasional and transitory acinar-islet phenotype for all islet cell-types, G-cells included[28–30] and that the regenerated acinar phenotype[31] could not persist in the specific environment offered by our experimental model.

CONCLUSIONS

The relative importance of the islet cell regeneration needs to be considered and evaluated, but as the islet cell replication, seems also an intrinsically limited mechanism[1,3,32], so the first goal of the islet transplantation, a maximum of islet mass engrafted, remains a basic concept.

ACKNOWLEDGMENTS

This work is part of a Research Program on Transplantation of The Endocrine Pancreas supported by the Gulbenkian Foundation and the Instituto de Investigação Científica (I.N.I.C.)

REFERENCES

1. J. Logothetopoulos, Islet cell regeneration and neogenesis, in: "Handbook of Physiology, Sec. 7, Endocrinology, Vol. 1, Endocrine Pancreas, pp.67", O. R. Greep, E. B. Astwood, D. F. Steinner, N. Freinkel, S. R. Geiger, Am. Phys. Soc., Washington, D.C. (1972)
2. L. Rosenberg, D. Dafoe, J. Turcote, Enhancing hamster pancreatic isolation by induction of nesidioblastosis, Transplant. Proc., 19: 907 (1987)
3. M. Marx, W. Schmidt, M. Herrmann, R. Goberna, Electron microscopic studies on the existence of the so-called "acinar-islet cells" in the regenerating pancreas of the rat, Horm. Met. Res., 2: 204 (1970)
4. S. Oya, L. Diaz-Flores, M. J. Gayoso, Transformation ducto-insular en pancreas en regeneration, Morfologia Normal y Patologica, Sec. A: 141 (1977)
5. S. M. Griffin, D. Alderson, J. R. Farndon, Long-term metabolic follow-up with different preparations of islet autografts, Diabetes 38 [Suppl 1]: 305 (1989)
6. R. Alejandro, R. G. Cutfield, F. L. Shienvold, K. S. Polonsky, J. Noel, L. Olson, J. Dillberger, J. Miller, D. H. Mintz, Natural history of intrahepatic canine islet cell autografts, J. Clin. Invest. 78: 1339 (1986)

7. D. B. Kaufman, P. Murel, M. J. Field, S. R. Munn, D. E. R. Sutherland, Purified canine islet autografts: functional outcome as influenced by islet number and implantation site, Transplantation 50: 385 (1990)
9. R. C. Griffith, D. W. Scharp, B. K. Hartman, W. B. Ballinger, P. E. Lacy, A morphologic study of intrahepatic portal-vein islet isografts, Diabetes 26: 201 (1977)
10. A. Mellgren, A. H. S. Landström, B. Petersson, A. Andersson, The renal subcapsular site offers better growth conditions for transplanted mouse pancreatic islet cells than the liver or spleen, Diabetologia 29: 670 (1986)
11. E. Montana, S. Bonner-Weir, G. C. Weir, Transplanted beta-cell replication and mass increase after 95% pancreatectomy, "Fourth International Congress on Pancreas and Islet Transplantation", Amsterdam, The Netherlands, Abstracts, 15.1 (1993)
12. R. W. Dudek, N. Freinkel, N. Lewis, C. Hellerström, R. Johnson, Morphologic study of cultered pancreatic fetal islets during maturation of the insulin stimulus-secretion mechanism, Diabetes [Suppl 1] 29: 15 (1980)
13. A. Lazarow, L. J. Wells, A-M. Carpenter, O. D. Hegre, R. J. Leonard, R. C. McEvoy, Islet differentiation, organ culture and transplantation, Diabetes 22: 877 (1973)
14. R. W. Dudek, I. E. Lawrence Jr., R. S. Hill, R. C. Johnson, Induction of islet cytodifferentiation by fetal mesenchime in adult pancreatic epithelium, Diabetes 40: 1041 (1991)
15. D. F. Steiner, D. E. James, Cellular and molecular biology of the beta cell, Diabetologia 35 [Suppl 2]: S41 (1992)
16. G. J. Kretschmer, D. E. R. Sutherland, A. J. Matas, M. W. Steffes, J. S. Najarian: The dispersed pancreas: transplantation without islet purification in totally pancreatectomized dogs, Diabetologia 13: 495 (1977)
17. D. G. Mehigan, G. D. Zuidema, J. L. Cameron, Pancreatic islet transplantation in dogs: Critical factors in technique, Am. J. Surg. 141: 208 (1981)
18. A. A. Like, L. Orci, Embriogenesis of the human pancreatic islets: light and electron microscopic study, Diabetes 21 [Suppl 2]: 511 (1972)
19. R. L. Pictet, W. J. Rutter, Development of the embryonic endocrine pancreas, in :"Handbook of Physiology, Sec. 7, Endocrinology, Vol. 1, Endocrine Pancreas, pp. 25", O. R. Greep, E. B. Astwood, D. F. Steinner, N. Freinkel, S. R. Geiger, Am. Phys. Soc., Washington, D.C. (1972)
20. N. S. Track, C. Creutzfeldt, M. Bokermann, Enzymatic functional and ultrastructural development of the exocrine pancreas. 2- The human pancreas, Comp. Biochem. Physiol. 51 (A): 95 (1975)
21. L-I. Larsson, J. F. Rehfeld, F. Sundler, R. Hakânson, Pancreatic gastrin in foetal and neonatal rats, Nature 262: 609 (1976)
22. N. M. Le Douarin, On the origin of pancreatic endocrine cells (Minirewiew), Cell 53: 169 (1988)
23. S. Alpert, D. Hanahan, G. Teitelman, Hybrid insulin genes reveal a developmental lineage for pancreatic endocrine cells and imply a relationship with neurons, Cell 53: 295 (1988)
24. K. Motojima, N. Kohara, J. Maeda, M. Yamaguchi, T. Kanematsu, A comparison of exocrine and endocrine function after pancreatic fragments autotransplantation into splenic pulp, portal vein, and hepatic parenchima, Transplantation 53: 527 (1992)
25. R. N. Melmed, R. C. Turner, S. J. Holt, Intermediate cells of the pancreas. 2- The effects of dietary soybean trypsin inhibitor on acinar-B cell structure and function in the rat, J. Cell Sci. 13: 279 (1973)
26. R. E. Brown, W. J. S. Still, Acinar-islet cells in the exocrine pancreas of the adult cat, Am. J. Digest. Diseases 15: 327 (1970)
27. Y. Yanatory, T. Fujita, Hyperthrophy and hyperplasia in the endocrine and exocrine pancreas of rats fed soybean trypsin inhibitor or repeatedly injected with pancreozymin, Arch. Histol. Jap. 39: 67 (1976)
28. von L. Cossel, Intermediate cells in the adult human pancreas. Contribution to the transformation of differentiated cells in vertebrates, Wirchows Arch. (Cell Path.) 47: 313 (1984)
29. R. N. Melmed, Intermediate cells of the pancreas. An appraisal. Gastroenterology 76: 196 (1979)
30. E. H. Leduc, E. E. Jones, Acinar-islet transformation in mouse pancreas, J. Ultrastructure Res. 24: 165 (1968)
31. R. Müller, R. Laucke, B. Trimper, von L. Cossel, Pancreatic cell proliferation in normal rats studied by in vivo autoradiography with H^3-thymidine.Wirchows Arch. B. Cell Pathol. 59: 133 (1990)
32. S. Bonner-Weir, D. F. Trent, G. C. Weir, Partial pancreatectomy in the rat and subsequent defect in glucose-induced insulin release, J. Clin. Invest. 71: 1544 (1983)

THE USE OF IMMUNOMAGNETIC SEPARATION FOR SECONDARY PURIFICATION OF PANCREATIC ISLETS

A Comparison of Different Magnetic Fields in the Rat

Joanna E. Davies,* Julie C. Chamberlain, Sue Swift, Roger F. L. James, Nicholas J. M. London, and Gavin S. M. Robertson

Department of Surgery
University of Leicester
Clinical Sciences Building, Leicester Royal Infirmary
Leicester LE2 7LX, United Kingdom

INTRODUCTION

Current human islet purification methods utilise differences in buoyant-density to purify islets from non-endocrine tissue. Using continuous density gradients, yields of approximately 250,000 islets per pancreas can be routinely obtained. However, with accepted protocols for human pancreatic islet transplantation requiring the intraportal infusion of 8–10,000 islets per recipient kg, such yields are clearly inadequate to allow successful transplantation on a one donor to one recipient basis, a central goal for researchers if islet transplantation is to become clinical reality.

In order to address this problem we elected to adapt current immunomagnetic cell separation techniques to the isolation of rat islets with a view to developing a secondary purification technique that could be applied to human islet isolation in conjunction with density gradients.

METHODS

M-450 Dynabeads® were coated with LDS10, an IgM monoclonal antibody raised against rat acinar tissue, at a concentration of 8mg/mg at pH9.6. Rat pancreatic digest was

* Address for correspondence: Joanna E. Davies, Department of Surgery, University of Leicester, Clinical Sciences Building, Leicester Royal Infirmary, Leicester LE2 7LX, United Kingdom.

prepared by intraductal distension with collagenase enzyme[1], and in order to allow the preparation of standard aliquots of digest for the comparative experiments the islets were purified by density gradient purification[2]. Standard aliquots of digest were then prepared by handpicking 300 islets from the purified sample and adding an estimated 10,000 exocrine fragments.

Dynabeads were incubated for 20 minutes with the aliquots of digest in 0.5 ml RPMI-1640 culture medium (Northumbria Biologicals, Cramlington, UK) on a Spiromix 5® (Denley, Billingshurst, U.K.) at a ratio of 500 beads per exocrine particle. At the end of this incubation a control sample was examined microscopically to check the labelling of tissue with beads.

During each comparative experiment, 0.5 ml aliquots of immunomagnetically labelled digest suspension were released from a pasteur pipette into the top of a 10 ml conical tube containing 9 ml of RPMI. The aliquot was allowed to drift under gravity through a magnetic field generated by varying numbers and configurations of permanent iron boron neodymium magnets arrayed outside the tube (Figure 1). The magnetically labelled tissue was visibly removed as it entered the magnetic field. After 10 minutes to allow the islets to settle to the bottom of the tube a fine pasteur pipette was used to aspirate the islets in the bottom 2 ml of medium as the first non-magnetic fraction (NMF1). The remaining 7.5 ml RPMI was then aspirated in the same way as NMF2, before removing the 10 ml tube from the magnetic field and resuspending the tissue held in the magnetic field as the magnetic fraction (MF).

The tissue in the three fractions (NMF1, NMF2 and MF) was then assessed for its islet and exocrine content by sonicating the tissue and assaying the insulin content by radioimmunoassay based on the method of Hales and Randle[3] and the amylase content by the Phadebas® amylase test (Pharmacia Diagnostics AB, Uppsala, Sweden.).

In the first comparison the effect of increasing the density of the RPMI using BSA together with vibrating the pipette containing the digest during the release process (in an effort to reduce tissue clumping prior to release) was then investigated using both the bipolar and quadripolar magnetic fields. Six experiments were performed in each group to allow statistical analysis of the results.

In the second comparison, the effect on the islet purification process of altering the configuration of the quadripolar field was examined and the effect of fields in which two, three or four magnets repelled each other were compared (see legend for Figure 3).

In examining each method, 6 release experiments were performed to allow comparison of the percentage of islets and exocrine tissue trapped in the magnetic fraction by the various release and magnetic field parameters. The medians were calculated for each group of 6, and the Mann-Whitney U test used to compare the percentages of exocrine tissue removed and islets trapped.

RESULTS

Releasing the digest into a bipolar magnetic field using a hand-held pasteur pipette removed a median of 94% of the exocrine tissue but trapped 43% of the islets (Figure 2). However, when a bipolar magnetic field with vibration and BSA was used, there was a significant decrease in the removal of exocrine tissue ($p=0.005$) as a result. The effective removal of exocrine tissue could be restored (88%) by using a quadripolar magnetic field (NNNN). In a series of 12 release experiments using this combination, a median of 88% of the exocrine tissue was removed with only 23% of the islets being trapped.

The effect of releasing the digest with vibration and BSA and altering the configuration of the quadripolar magnetic field is shown in Figure 3 The use of four repelling magnets (NNNN) produced less islet trapping in the magnetic fraction than any of the following

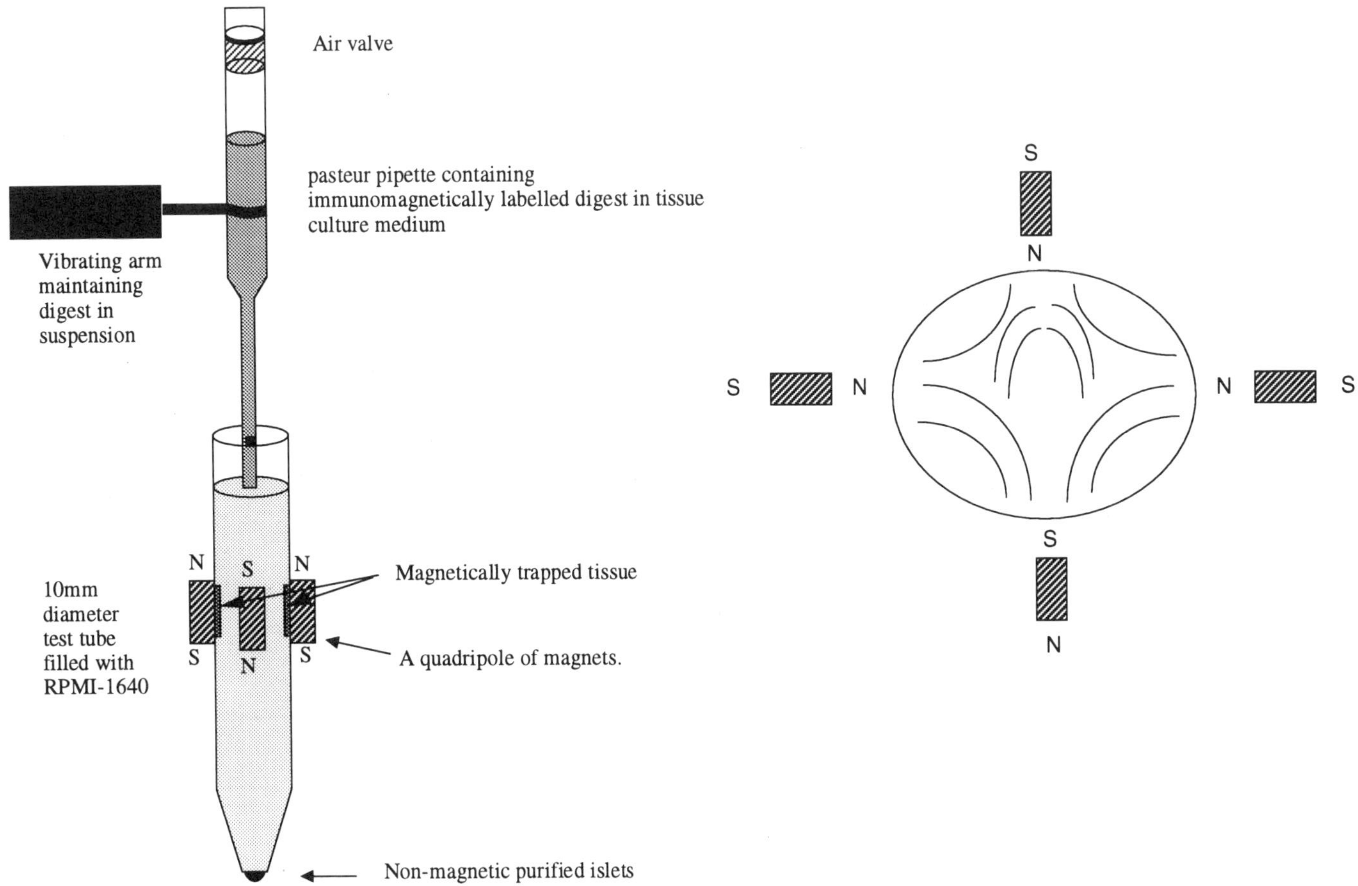

Figure 1. Shows a diagrammatic representation of the separation system used. The digest is released from the Pasteur pipette into a 10 ml conical test-tube and allowed to drift through the magnetic field. The islets settle to the bottom of the test-tube, as the "non-magnetic fraction." The quadripolar magnetic field created by 1 pair of magnets attracting and the other pair repelling (NNNS) is also shown.

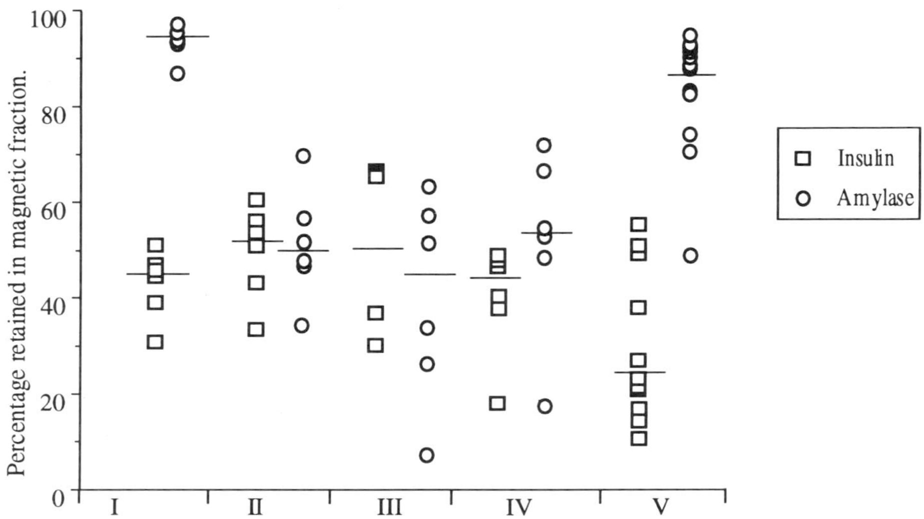

Figure 2. Comparison of methods of digest release into **(I)** two repelling magnets with no vibration or BSA, **(II)** a bipolar magnetic field using vibration alone, **(III)** a bipolar magnetic field using BSA alone, **(IV)** a bipolar filed using vibration and BSA, and **(V)** a quadripolar filed using vibration and BSA. The percentages of amylase and insulin containing tissue trapped by the magnet are plotted, with the median shown as a line.

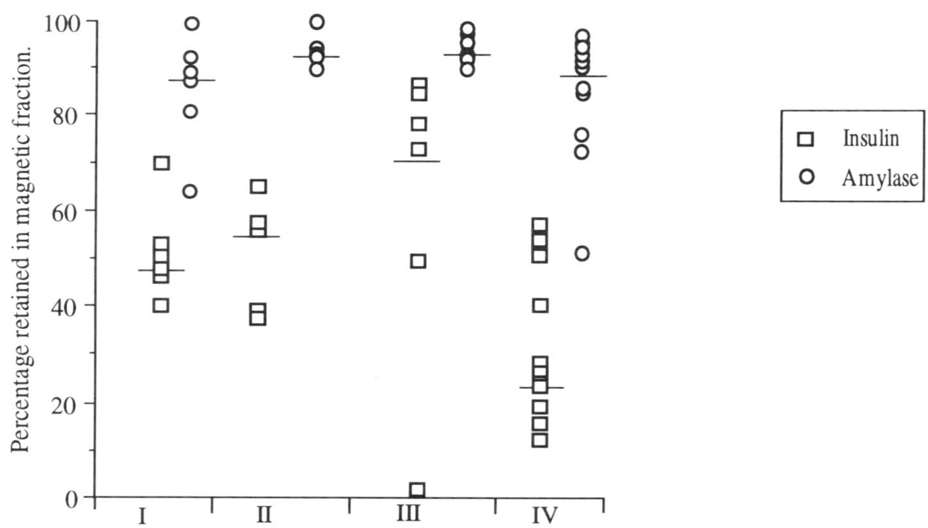

Figure 3. Shows the results obtained using a quadripole of magnets in various configurations **(I)** NNSS opposite magnets attracting, **(II)** NNNS one pair of opposing magnets attracting, one pair repelling, **(III)** NSNS opposing magnets repelling but neighbouring magnets attracting, **(IV)** NNNN all magnets repelling each other. The percentages of amylase and insulin containing tissue trapped by the magnet are plotted, with the median shown as a line.

configurations; NNSS where opposite magnets attracted each other (p=0.04), NNNS (as shown in Figure 2) with one opposing pair of magnets attracting and one repelling (p=0.13) or NSNS in which opposite magnets repelled but neighbouring magnets attracted each other (p=0.05).

DISCUSSION

In summary, the use of vibration and BSA when releasing the digest significantly reduced the percentage of islets trapped in the magnetic fraction, but a quadripolar magnetic field was necessary to maintain adequate immunomagnetic exocrine tissue removal under these conditions.

Immunomagnetic cell separation procedures are rapid, gentle and highly reproducible, providing an alternative and much more specific method of separating the components of the pancreatic digest based on specific differences in cell surface antigens.

Using monoclonal antibodies produced in our Department we have been able to produce reliable binding of M450-Dynabeads to exocrine tissue, allowing immunomagnetic labelling of the exocrine component of the digest. The results of this work show subsequent passage of this digest through a magnetic field can be reliably used to remove almost 90% of the exocrine tissue with yields of up to 80% of the islets. This is considerably better than the results so far achieved using any other method.

The use of immunomagnetic islet purification as a secondary purification procedure in conjunction with initial density dependent 'debulking' of the pancreatic digest, could significantly increase the yield of purified islets from each human pancreas. The recent description of large scale continuous density gradients for density dependent islet purification[4], produces a series of gradient fractions of increasing density some of which contain pure islets followed by some which contain large numbers of islets but are heavily contaminated with exocrine tissue making them unsuitable for transplantation. These could be further purified by using immunomagnetic separation techniques to increase the yield of islets produced from a single donor pancreas.

In conclusion therefore the adaptation of immunomagnetic cell separation techniques for islet purification provides a highly reliable and specific method of increasing islet yields which could be expected to improve the results of human islet transplantation.

ABBREVIATIONS

The following abbreviations have been used:

BSA	Bovine serum albumin
MF	Magnetic fraction
N	North magnetic pole
NMF	Non-magnetic fraction
RPMI-1640	Roswell Park Memorial Institute
S	South magnetic pole

ACKNOWLEDGMENTS

We would like to thank the Juvenile Diabetic Foundation and the British Diabetic Association for supporting our work.

REFERENCES

1. Sutton R, Peters M, McShane P, Gray DWR, Morris PJ. Isolation of rat pancreatic islets by ductal injection of collagenase. Transplantation 1986; 42: 689.
2. Lake SP, Anderson J, Chamberlain J, Gardner SJ, Bell PRF, James RFL. Bovine serum albumin density gradient isolation of rat pancreatic islets. Transplantation 1987; 43: 805.
3. Hales CN, Randle PJ. Immunoassay of insulin with insulin antibody precipitate. Biochemistry 1963; 88: 137.
4. Robertson GSM, Chadwick DR, Contractor H, Rose S, Chamberlain R, London NJM. Optimisation of the Cobe 2991 cell processor for islet isolation using linear continuous density gradients. Acta Diabetol 1993; 30: 175.

TRANSPLANTATION OF SYNGENIC PANCREATIC ISLETS INTO RATS WITH STREPTOZOTOCIN INDUCED NON INSULIN DEPENDENT DIABETES MELLITUS

Maria Angeles Tormo,[1] Danielle Bailbé,[2] Patricia Serradas,[2] Catherine Saulnier,[2] Bernard Portha,[2] and Jose Enrique Campillo[1]

[1]Department of Physiology
University of Extremadura
Apartado 108
06071 Badajoz, Spain
[2]Laboratory of Physiology of Nutrition
CNRS URA 307
University Paris 7
France

INTRODUCTION

An important concept in understanding the pathogenesis of Non Insulin Dependent Diabetes Mellitus (NIDDM) has recently emerged: the concept that hyperglycemia is not only the principal metabolic derangement of diabetes but also a pathogenetic factor in its own right. Once it develops, either from insulin deficiency or from insulin resistance, hyperglycemia will exacerbate both defects, thereby closing a pathologic feedback loop[1]. Recognition of the important pathogenetic role of hyperglycemia per se in the evolution of NIDDM has important therapeutic implication. First normalization of the plasma glucose profile, should lead to an impairment in insulin secretion in NIDDM subjects. In fact significant improvements in insulin secretion and insulin action have been demonstrated after weight loss, sulfonylurea administration or insulin therapy, each of these therapeutic interventions leading to an improvement of glycemic control[2].

It has not yet been shown, however, that the defects can be completely reversed and it is unclear at the moment whether recovery of insulin secretion and action are maintained after cessation of the treatment. Accordingly, the present study aimed at investigating first if islet graft is an apropriate tool to normalize blood glucose and insulin levels in a model of non insulin dependent diabetes and second if there is any benefit for the functioning of the residual pancreas.

Physiology and Pathophysiology of the Islets of Langerhans, edited by Soria.
Plenum Press, New York, 1997.

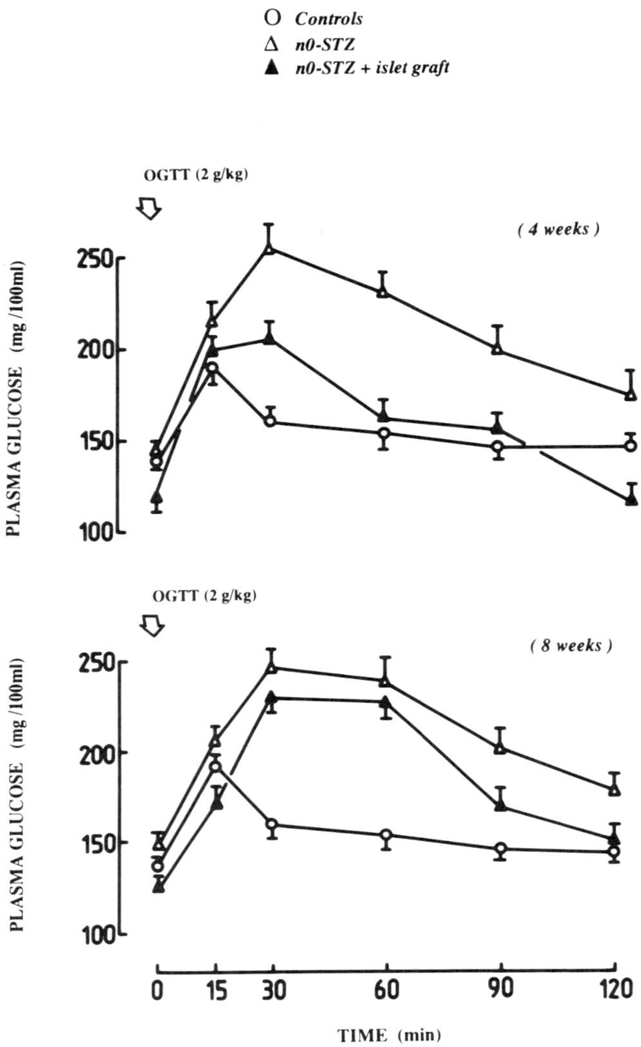

Figure 1. Plasma glucose levels measured after oral glucose administration to control (n = 6), diabetic (n = 8) and diabetic grafted (n = 8) rats at the 4th and 8th week of study.

MATERIALS AND METHODS

Male from highly inbred rats of Lewis strain were used in this study. A very mild form of NIDDM, was generated by injecting (i.p.) rats on the day of their birth with 100 mg/kg of streptozotocin (n0-STZ). By 8 weeks of age and thereafter, n0-STZ rats showed mild basal hyperglycemia, marked abnormal response to intraperitoneal or intravenous glucose tolerance tests and a 50% decrease in pancreatic insulin stores without changes in pancreatic glucagon stores[1].

Pancreatic islets were isolated from normal rats by collagenase digestion method (collagenase P, 3 mg/pancreas, Boehringer Mannheim). Groups of 100 islets were cultured at 37°C in a humidified atmosphere free floating for 2 days in 1640 RPMI medium supplemented with 10% calf serum, 2 mmol/l glutamine and antibiotics. After 48 h of culture, 1000 islets were implanted beneath the kidney capsule of sodium pentobarbital anesthetized diabetic and non diabetic rats[3].

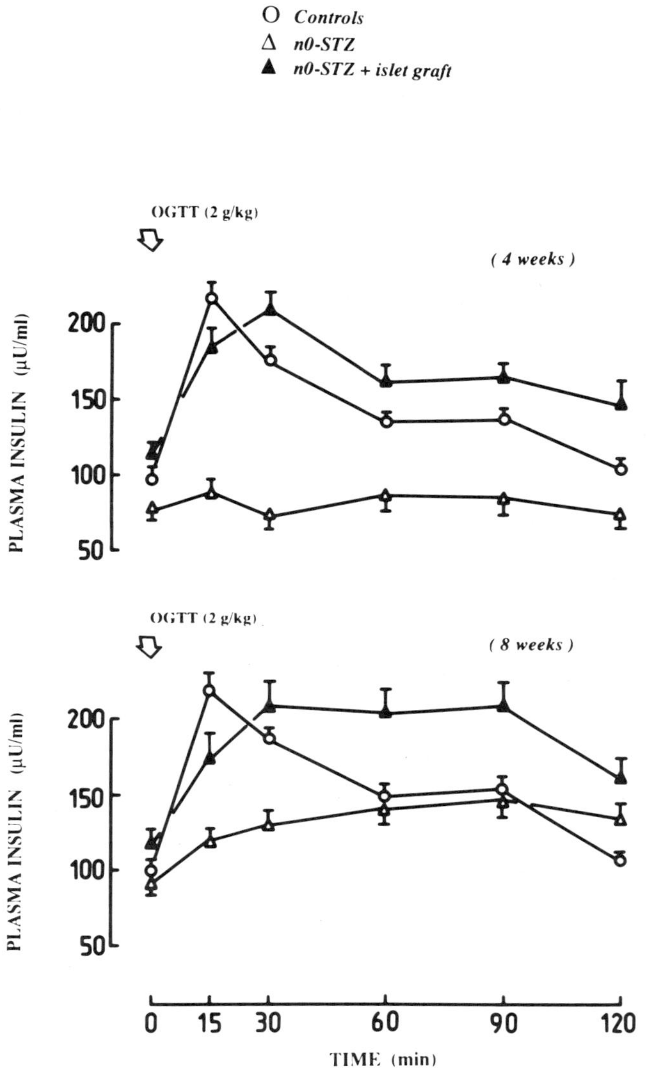

Figure 2. Plasma insulin levels measured after oral glucose administration to control (n = 6), diabetic (n = 8) and diabetic grafted (n = 8) rats at the 4th and 8th week of study.

Endocrine graft function was monitored by weekly determination of plasma glucose (Glucose oxidase method) and body weight. After 4 and 8 weeks, an oral glucose tolerance test (OGTT) was performed. Insulin values were determined by radioimmunoassay using rat insulin as standard (Novo).

At the end of study, the in vitro insulin release by the recipient pancreas was evaluated by using the isolated and perfused pancreas method[4].

RESULTS

In control rats, fasting blood glucose remained low and constant during the 8 weeks period. Diabetic rats showed high blood glucose levels around 10 to 12 mmol/l. After pancreatic islets transplantation, blood glucose levels were significantly reduced and remained low during the whole period of study. As shown in Figures 1 and 2, after oral glucose

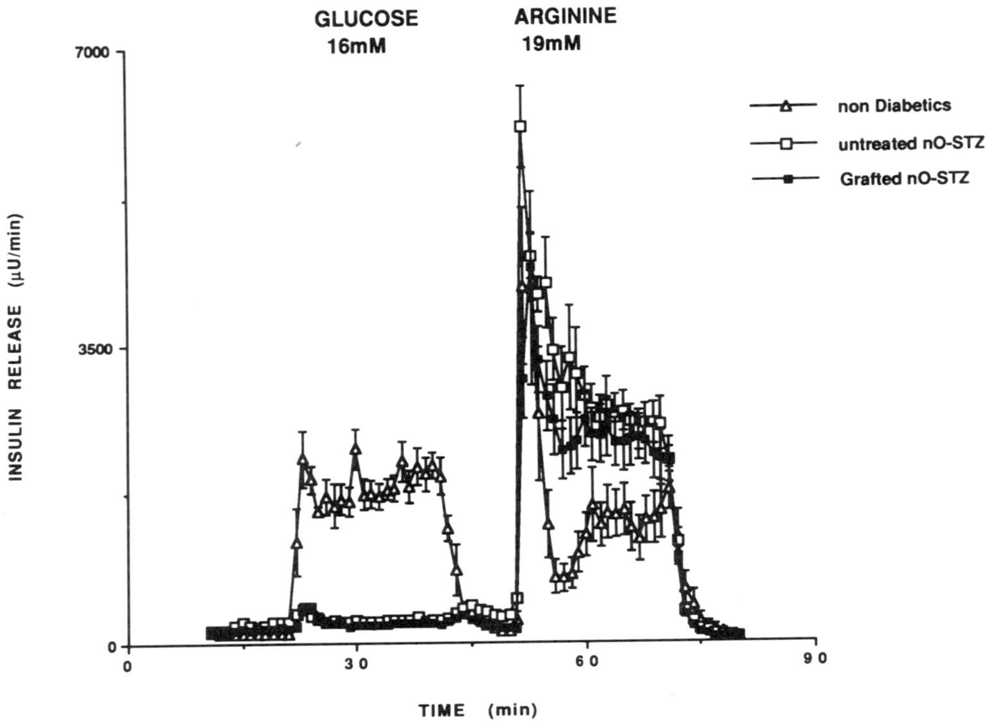

Figure 3. Insulin released by in vitro perfused pancreas isolated from control (n = 6), diabetic (n = 8) and diabetic grafted (n = 8) rats after 8th weeks of study.

administration, a clear glucose intolerance was observed in non transplanted diabetic rats and an absence of a clear insulin secretory response. At the 4th and 8th weeks of study, glucose tolerance was normal in diabetic transplanted rats and insulin secretory response was similar to that observed in control rats.

Figure 3 shows the insulin released by perfused pancreas in response to stimulation with glucose and arginine from rats under the various experimental conditions at 8th weeks of study. The insulin secretion (μU/min) in response to 16.7 mmol/l glucose was 1646 ± 145 in control rats, 32 ± 5 in non grafted diabetic and 111 ± 20 in grafted diabetic rats. The insulin secretion in response to arginine 19 mmol/l was 1477 ± 280 in control, 2771 ± 227 in non grafted diabetic and 2309 ± 265 in grafted diabetic rats.

CONCLUSIONS

By 10 weeks of age and thereafter, the rats that received 100 mg/kg of STZ on the day of birth (n0-STZ) showed mild basal hyperglycemia, marked glucose intolerance in response to oral glucose, and a lack of insulin response to glucose both in vivo and by the isolated perfused pancreas. By contrast, the n0-STZ diabetic rats revealed to be hypersensitive to arginine induced insulin secretion in vitro.

The transplantation of 1000 cultured pancreatic islets beneath the kidney capsule resulted in a normalization of basal plasma glucose values and a clear impairment of glucose tolerance after oral glucose load was observed. In the grafted diabetic rats, the in vivo insulin secretion in response to oral glucose was similar to that recorded in control non diabetic rats, but the in vitro insulin secretion in response to 16.7 mmol/l glucose was severely reduced.

Insulin secretion in response to 16.7 mmol/l glucose was significantly higher ($p<0.02$) in grafted versus non grafted diabetic rats suggesting that the pancreatic islets transplantation used to normalize plasma glucose levels could lead to some degree of improvement in glucose induced insulin release.

In vitro insulin release in response to 19 mmol/l arginine was significantly increased in the n0-STZ diabetic rats versus that measured in control rats.

REFERENCES

1. B. Portha, O. Blondel, P. Serradas, R. McEvoy, M.H. Giroix, M. Kergoat, D. Bailbé, The rat model of non insulin dependent diabetes induced by neonatal streptozotocin. *Diabète & Metabolisme* 15: 61–75 (1989).
2. R.A. Fronzo, The triumvirate: B-cell, muscle and liver. A collusion responsible for NIDDM, *Diabetes* 37: 610–687 (1989).
3. O. Korsgreen, L. Janson, A. Andersson, Effects of hyperglycemia on function of isolated mouse pancreatic islets transplanted under kidney capsule, *Diabetes* 38: 510–515 (1989).
4. E.K. Sussman, G.D. Vaughan, R.F. Timmer, An in vitro method for studying insulin secretion in the perfused isolated rat pancreas, *Diabetes* 15: 466–472 (1966).

59

EFFECTS OF CAFFEINE ON GLUCOSE-STIMULATED INSULIN RELEASE FROM ISLET TRANSPLANTS

Chun-Liang Shi

Department of Histology and Cell Biology
University of Umea
S-901 87 Umea
Sweden

INTRODUCTION

Islet transplantation has long been regarded as a promising approach for ameliorating type-1 diabetes. Despite progress in developing procedures for isolating donor islets[1–3], immunosuppressive agents[4–6], and techniques for immuno-isolation[7–9], the overall success has not yet been overwhelming. The possibility that dislocation and denervation alters the properties of donor islets has received little attention. The extent to which islets behave normally at an ectopic site remains a basic question.

We have observed that transplantation of islets from pancreas to kidney induces several alterations of B-cell function[10;Shi,unpublished work]. A relatively decreased first phase of glucose-stimulated insulin release, a transient drop of secretion in response to glucose, and a stimulatory "off-response" to glucose withdrawal were frequently recorded. Islets transplanted under the kidney capsule also exhibited decreased responses to acetylcholine[11].

Since acetylcholine is a potentiatior of normal insulin secretion, the question arose as to whether transplanted islets show an attenuated responsiveness to potentiators in general. In the present study, this question was addressed by examining the effect of caffeine on glucose-stimulated insulin release from islets transplanted under the kidney capsule.

MATERIALS AND METHODS

Adult male NMRI mice (ALAB, Sollentuna, Sweden) and inbred female BALB/c mice (Bomhåltgård, Denmark) were used. The NMRI mice are not strictly inbred but sufficiently homogenous to tolerate intra-strain transplantation without immunosuppression. Groups of 150 (BALB/c) or 300 (NMRI) collagenase-isolated islets were cultured

Physiology and Pathophysiology of the Islets of Langerhans, edited by Soria.
Plenum Press, New York, 1997.

overnight and implanted beneath the left kidney capsule in syngeneic (BALB/c) and subsyngeneic (NMRI) transplantation experiments. Batches of 50 fresh islets were also studied for comparative purposes.

Three or twelve weeks after transplantation, grafts were removed under general anaesthesia, placed in a perifusion device[12], and perifused at a rate of 1 ml/min with Krebs-Ringer bicarbonate buffer (pH 7.4, 37°C) gassed with oxygen-carbon dioxide (95:5). In one set of experiments, fresh islets or grafts were stimulated with 16.7 mmol/l D-glucose alone or in combination of 1 or 5 mmol/l caffeine for 60 min. In another set, a self-control experimental protocol was used. After 40 min of basal secretion at 2 mmol/l D-glucose, fresh islets or grafts were sequentially perifused with 11 mmol/l D-glucose for 20 min, 2 mmol/l D-glucose for 20 min, and 11 mmol/l D-glucose plus 1 mmol/l caffeine for 20 min.

A similar self-control protocol was also used to determine the interaction between caffeine and acetylcholine. Fresh islets or grafts were stimulated with 11 mmol/l D-glucose, first in the absence and then in the presence of 10 μmol/l acetylcholine plus 10 μmol/l eserine. In test groups, 1 mmol/l caffeine was present throughout, while control experiments were performed without caffeine.

Samples of effluent were collected to determine secretory rates. Grafts were extracted in acid ethanol to measure their insulin content. Insulin was assayed radio-immunologically. Results are given as mean values together with the corresponding range (n = 2) or SEM (n > 2).

RESULTS

After perifusion, untransplanted fresh islets contained 148 ± 10 (NMRI, 6 expts.) and 121 ± 15 (BALB/c mice, 10 expts.) ng of insulin per islet. For grafts the corresponding values were 16 ± 3 (NMRI 3 weeks, 6 expts.), 45 ± 4 (BALB/c 3 weeks, 8 expts.), and 37–51 (BALB/c 12 weeks, 2 expts.) ng of insulin per transplanted islet.

In fresh NMRI mouse islets, 16.7 mmol/l glucose induced a biphasic insulin release that was potentiated by 1 or 5 mmol/l caffeine in a dose-dependent manner, notably during the second, prolonged phase (Fig. 1, Table 1). Secretion from NMRI-mouse islet grafts was also clearly potentiated by caffeine. In fact, both during the first and second phases, the grafts appeared hyper-reponsive to the potentiator.

When untransplanted islets from BALB/c-mice were exposed to only 11 mmol/l D-glucose and 1 mmol/l caffeine according to a self-control experimental protocol, the effect of

Table 1. Effect of caffeine on basal and stimulated insulin secretion[a]

Group	Caffeine mmol/l	Basal ng/10 min per islet	First phase ng/10 min per islet	Second phase ng/50 min per islet
Grafts				
	0	0.01 ± 0.00	0.02 ± 0.00	0.28 ± 0.08
	1	0.02 ± 0.01	0.18 ± 0.03	1.78 ± 0.39
	5	0.05 ± 0.01	0.33 ± 0.15	3.65 ± 1.04
Fresh islets				
	0	0.12 ± 0.10	1.39 ± 0.78	4.85 ± 0.44
	1	0.14 ± 0.00	0.62 ± 0.06	8.76 ± 0.23
	5	0.39 ± 0.08	1.41 ± 0.05	16.61 ± 1.70

[a]Insulin secretion was calculated by integration of perifusion profiles in Fig. 1. Mean ± half range for 2 experiments in all groups.

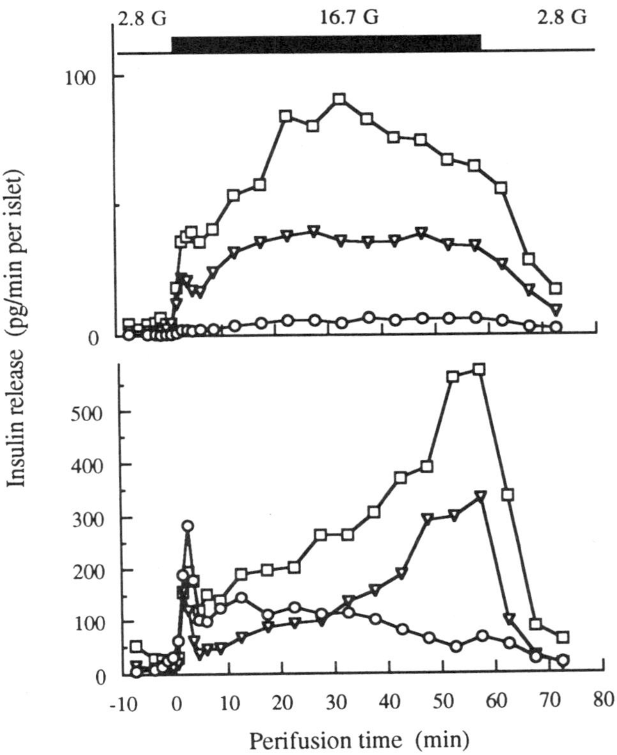

Figure 1. Effects of caffeine on glucose-induced insulin release. Fresh islets (lower panel) or 3-week-old grafts (upper panel) from NMRI mice were perifused as described in Materials and Methods. The change of glucose (G) concentration is indicated by top horizontal bars. The perifusion medium contained 0 (circles), 1 (triangles) or 5 mmol/l (squares) caffeine throughout. Mean values of 2 experiments.

caffeine was barely discernible (Figs. 2 and 3). However, under the same conditions, 12-week (Fig. 2) and 3-week (Fig. 3) old BALB/c grafts exhibited potentiatory responses to caffeine.

In the absence of caffeine, 3-week old BALB/c grafts reacted less strongly to acetylcholine than did untransplanted islets (Fig. 3 and Table 2). The addition of 1 mmol/l caffeine did not enhance the potentiating effect of acetylcholine, whether in untransplanted or transplanted islets (Fig. 3). Rather, the interaction between caffeine and acetylcholine appeared negative.

Table 2. Effect of glucose (G), alone or in combination with caffeine (C) and acetylcholine (ACh) on glucose-induced insulin secretion[a]

Group	G	G + ACh	G + C	G + ACh + C
Fresh islets	31.6 ± 2.9 (6)	429.6 ± 79.6 (6)	69.0 ± 10.9 (2)	222.5 ± 72.5 (2)
Grafts	56.5 ± 11.9 (4)	120.0 ± 18.2 (4)	108.0 ± 5.9 (2)	101.1 ± 12.7 (2)

[a] Insulin secretion rates (pg/min per islet) were calculated by integrating the perifusion profiles in Fig. 3 and averageing over time. Mean value ± SEM or half range for the numbers of experiments in parentheses.

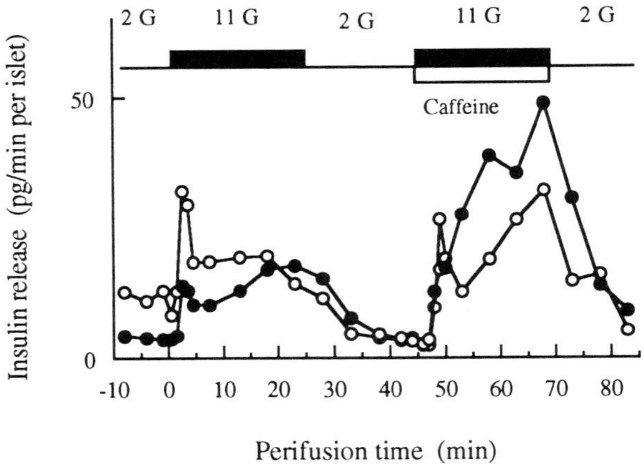

Figure 2. Effect of caffeine on glucose-induced insulin release. Fresh islets (open circles) or 12-week old grafts (solid circles) from BALB/c mice were exposed to two pulses of 11 mmol/l glucose, first in the absence then in the precence of 1 mmol/l caffeine. During the two pulses of glucose stimulation, the integrated output of insulin was 0.46 (islets, no caffeine), 0.51 (islets, caffeine), 0.33 (grafts, no caffeine), and 0.81 (grafts, caffeine) ng/20 min. Mean values of 2 experiments.

DISCUSSION

More than a hundred years ago, Hédon[13] reported the successful transplantation of a vascularized pancreas autograft in the dog. Normoglycemia was maintained after the remaining part of the pancreas had been removed. Islets transplanted as free grafts have since proven effective in ameliorating experimental diabetic conditions, at least in rodents[14,15]. Many such experiments in vivo, as well as numerous observations on isolated islets in vitro, suggest that the glucostat function of the B-cell is largely independent of the cell's normal innervation and anatomical surrounding. Nevertheless, studies on islet grafts removed from the transplantation site have revealed a decreased in vitro potentiatory responsiveness to acetylcholine[10,11]. It seems therefore possible that severing the islets from their normal vagal input induces changes in the secretory mechanisms in the B-cells. However, it is not known whether the relative refractariness to acetylcholine is due to receptor-linked alterations or reflects perturburations of more distal events in the secretory signal chains.

Calcium ion, cyclic AMP, and diacylglycerol are generally envisaged as the major messengers controlling the distal events of insulin secretion. Whereas cholinergic agents are likely to act via diacylglycerol and calcium, caffeine most probably affects cyclic AMP and calcium. Under normal conditions, the interplay between B-cell messenger systems is believed to be positive. Thus calcium, cyclic AMP and diacylglycerol have been postulated to interact synergistically in the process of stimulus-secretion coupling[16]. Yet, inhibitory effects of caffeine on cytoplasmic calcium oscillations induced by cholinergic agonists have been reported[17,18]. Such interference could perhaps explain why caffeine did not enhance, but rather seemed to decrease, the potentiating action of acetylcholine in the present study.

Most importantly, however, the present results show that the glucose-induced insulin release from transplanted islets was quite sensitive to the potentiating action of caffeine in the absence of acetylcholine, suggesting that the grafted B-cells maintained a well func-

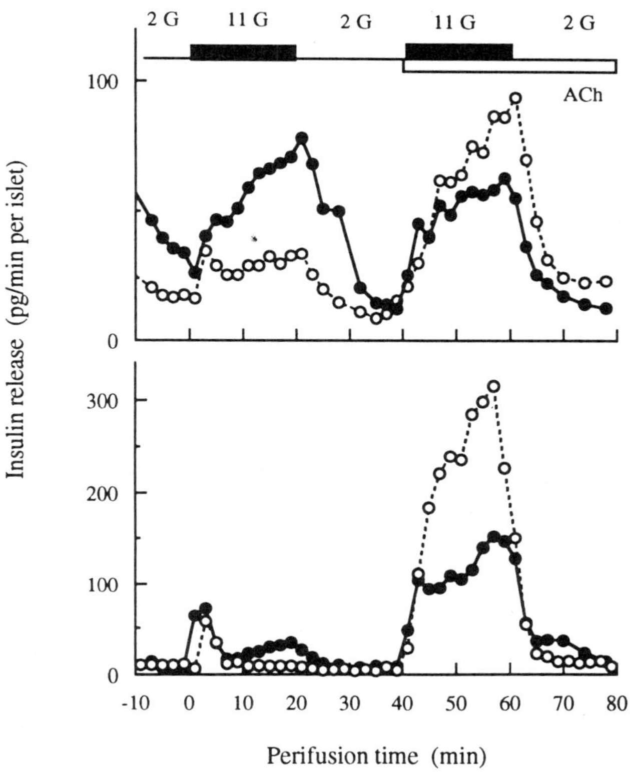

Figure 3. Effects of caffeine and acetylcholine (ACh) on glucose-induced insulin release. Fresh islets (lower panel) and 3-week old grafts (upper panel) from BALB/c mice were exposed to two pulses of 11 mmol/l glucose, first in the absence and then in the precence of 10 μmol/l ACh plus 10 μmol/l eserine. Solid circles indicate that 1 mmol/l caffeine was included throughout, and open circles represent perifusion without caffeine. Mean values of 2–6 experiments.

tioning machinery for insulin discharge. Therefore, it seems logical to assume that the decreased responsiveness to acetylcholine is either due to a downregulation or dysfunction of receptors, or reflects some disturbance of the cholinergic signal pathway influencing the intracellular calcium.

CONCLUSION

In mouse islets transplanted to the kidney, the glucose-induced insulin secretion exhibits a diminished potentiatory responsiveness to acetylcholine but not to caffeine. The displacement and denervation of transplanted islets is likely to affect either the cholinergic receptors or their mediated influence on intracellular calcium.

ACKNOWLEDGMENTS

This work was supported by the Swedish Medical Research Council (12x-2288), the Swedish Diabetes Association, and the Sahlberg Foundation.

REFERENCES

1. Gray, D. W., Warnock, G., Sutton, R., Peters, M., McShane, P., and Morris, P. J., 1986, Successful autotransplantation of isolated islets of Langerhans in the cynomolgus monkey, *Br. J. Surg.* 73:850–853.
2. Warnock, G. L., and Rajotte, R. V., 1988, Critical mass of purified islets that induce normoglycemia after transplantation into dogs, *Diabetes* 37:467–470.
3. Ricordi, C., Lacy, P. E., and Scharp, D. W., 1989, Automated islet isolation from human pancreas, *Diabetes* 38 (suppl 1):140–142.
4. Ishizuka, J., Gugliuzza, K. K., Wassmuth, Z., Hsieh, J., Sato, K., Tsuchiya, T., Townsend Jr., C. M., Fish, J. C., and Thompson, J. C., 1993, Effects of FK506 and cyclosporine on dynamic insulin secretion from isolated dog pancreatic islets, *Transplantation* 56:1486–1490.
5. Xenos, E. S., Casanova, D., Sutherland, D. E., Farney, A. C., Lloveras, J. J., and Cores, P. F., 1993, The in vivo and in vitro effect of 15-deoxyspergualin on pancreatic islet function, *Transplantation* 56:144–147.
6. Sandberg, J. O., Eizirik, D. L., Tracy, D. E., and Andersson, A., 1993, Treatment with interleukin-1 receptor antagonist protein prolongs mouse islet allograft survival, *Diabetes* 42:1845–1851.
7. Scharp, D., Mason, N., and Sparks, R., 1984, Islet immuno-isolation. The use of hybrid artificial organ to prevent islet tissue rejection, *World J. Surg.* 8:221–229.
8. Monaco, A.P., Maki, T., Ozato, H., Carretta, M., Sullivan, S.J., Borland, K.M., Mahoney, M.D., Chick, W.L., Muller, T.E., Wolfrum, J., and Solomon, B., 1991, Transplantation of islet allografts and xenografts in totally pancreatectomized diabetic dogs using the hybrid artificial pancreas, *Ann. Surg.* 214:339–362.
9. Lanza, R. P., Butler, D. H., Borland, K. M., Staruk, J. E., Faustman, D. L., Solomon, B. A., Muller, T. E., Rupp, R. G., Maki, T., Monaco, A. P., and Chick, W. L., 1991, Xenotransplantation of canine, bovine, and porcine islets in diabetic rats without immunosuppression, *Proc. Natl. Acad. Sci. U.S.A.* 88:11100–11104.
10. Taljedal, I.-B., Shi, C.-L., and Rooth, P., 1994, Functional aspects of mouse islets transplanted to the kidney, *Diabetologia* 37 (Suppl. 2):S112–S116.
11. Shi, C.-L., Rooth, P., and Taljedal, I.-B., 1993, Desensitization to acetylcholine in mouse islet grafts: an in vitro perifusion study, *Acta Endocrinol. (Copenh.)* 128 (Suppl. 1):18.
12. Shi, C.-L., Rooth, P., and Taljedal, I.-B., 1993, Protective effects of verapamil on mouse islets transplanted under the kidney capsule, *Transplantation* 56:1491–1495.
13. Hédon, E., 1892, Greffe sous-cutanée du pancréas; ses résultats au point de vue de la théorie du diabète pancréatique, *Compt. rend. Soc. Biol.* 678–680.
14. Ballinger, W. F., and Lacy, P. E., 1972, Transplantation of intact pancreatic islets in rats, *Surgery* 72:175–186.
15. Kemp, C. B., Knight, M. J., Scharp, D. W., Ballinger, W. F., and Lacy, P. E., 1973, Transplantation of isolated islets into the portal vein of diabetic rats, *Nature* 244:447.
16. Prentki, M., and Matschinsky, F. M., 1987, Ca2+, cAMP, and phospholipid-derived messengers in coupling mechanisms of insulin secretion. *Physiol. Rev.* 67:1185–1248.
17. Toescu, E. C., O'Neill, S. C., Petersen, O. H., and Eisner, D. A., 1992, Caffeine inhibits the agonist-evoked cytosolic Ca2+ signal in mouse pancreatic acinar cells by blocking inositol trisphosphate production, *J. Biol. Chem.* 267:23467–23470.
18. Lund, P.-E., and Gylfe, E., 1994, Caffeine inhibits cytoplasmic Ca2+ oscillations induced by carbachol and guanosine 5′-O-(3-thiotriphosphate) in hyperpolarized pancreatic β-cells, *Naunyn-Schmiedeberg's Arch. Pharmacol.* 349:503–509.

INDEX